Mind and Brain

Books by William R. Uttal

Real Time Computers: Techniques and Applications in the Psychological Sciences

Generative Computer Assisted Instruction (with Miriam Rogers, Ramelle Hieronymus, and Timothy Pasich)

Sensory Coding: Selected Readings

The Psychobiology of Sensory Coding

Cellular Neurophysiology and Integration: An Interpretive Introduction

An Autocorrelation Theory of Form Detection

The Psychobiology of Mind

A Taxonomy of Visual Processes

Visual Form Detection in 3-Dimensional Space

Foundations of Psychobiology (with Daniel N. Robinson)

The Detection of Nonplanar Surfaces in Visual Space

The Perception of Dotted Forms

On Seeing Forms

The Swimmer: An Integrated Computational Model of a Perceptual-Motor System (with Gary Bradshaw, Sriram Dayanand, Robb Lovell, Thomas Shepherd, Ramakrishna Kakarala, Kurt Skifsted, and Greg Tupper)

Toward A New Behaviorism: The Case against Perceptual Reductionism

Computational Modeling of Vision: The Role of Combination (with Ramakrishna Kakarala, Sriram Dayanand, Thomas Shepherd, Jaggi Kalki, Charles Lunskis Jr., and Ning Liu)

The War between Mentalism and Behaviorism: On the Accessibility of Mental Processes

The New Phrenology: On the Localization of Cognitive Processes in the Brain

A Behaviorist Looks at Form Recognition

Psychomyths: Sources of Artifacts and Misrepresentations in Scientific Cognitive Neuroscience

Dualism: The Original Sin of Cognitivism

Neural Theories of Mind: Why the Mind-Brain Problem May Never Be Solved

Human Factors in the Courtroom: Mythology versus Science

The Immeasurable Mind: The Real Science of Psychology

Time, Space, and Number in Physics and Psychology

Distributed Neural Systems: Beyond the New Phrenology

Neuroscience in the Courtroom: What Every Lawyer Should Know about the Mind and the Brain

Mind and Brain: A Critical Reappraisal of Cognitive Neuroscience

Mind and Brain

A Critical Appraisal of Cognitive Neuroscience

William R. Uttal

The MIT Press
Cambridge, Massachusetts
London, England

For information about special quantity discounts, please email special_sales@mitpress.mit.edu

This book was set in Stone Sans and Stone Serif by Toppan Best-set Premedia Limited. Printed and bound in the United States of America.

Library of Congress Cataloging-in-Publication Data

Uttal, William R.
Mind and brain : a critical appraisal of cognitive neuroscience / William R. Uttal.
    p. ; cm.
Includes bibliographical references and indexes.
ISBN 978-0-262-01596-7 (hardcover : alk. paper)
1. Cognitive neuroscience. 2. Learning—Physiological aspects. I. Title.
[DNLM: 1. Mental Processes—physiology. 2. Brain—physiology. 3. Brain Mapping.
4. Neurosciences—history. 5. Neurosciences—trends.   BF 441]
QP360.5.U86   2011
612.8′233—dc22

                                                          2010053615

The views, opinions, and/or findings contained in this book are those of the author and should not be construed as an official U.S. Army Research Institute position, policy, or decision unless so designated by other official documentation.

10   9   8   7   6   5   4   3   2

For Mitchan

"Were our minds and senses so expanded, strengthened, and illuminated, as to enable us to see and feel the very molecules of the brain; were we capable of following all their motions, all their groupings, all their electric discharges, if such there be; and were we intimately acquainted with the corresponding states of thought and feeling, we should be as far as ever from the solution of the problem, 'How are these physical processes connected with the facts of consciousness?' The chasm between the two classes of phenomena would still remain intellectually impassable. Let the consciousness of love, for example, be associated with a right-handed spiral motion of the molecules of the brain, and the consciousness of hate with a left-handed spiral motion. We should then know, when we love, that the motion is in one direction, and, when we hate, that the motion is in the other; but the 'Why ?' would remain as unanswerable as before."
—John Tyndall, 1871, p. 87[1]

"That the mental processes may be due to cerebral activities we may believe, but with what anatomical elements the individual mental processes may be connected we do not know. Notwithstanding our ignorance, it would appear best and most scientific that we should not adhere to any of the phreno-logical systems, however scientific they may appear to be on the surface. We should be willing to stand with Brodmann, believing that mind is a function or an attribute of the brain as a whole, or is a con-comitant of cerebral operations, but I at least am unwilling to stand with the histological localizationists on the ground of a special mental process for special cerebral areas or for special cerebral cell groups."
—Shepard Ivory Franz, 1912

"There is no greater impediment to a unified cognitive neuroscience than our inveterate Aristotelian tendency to consider cognitive functions as separate entities. For more than a century, experimental psychologists have been successfully dissecting them. It should be obvious, however, that the success in defining, classifying, and experimentally manipulating any given cognitive function does not imply a separate neural structure for it. Common sense, psychophysics, and experimental psychology provide ample evidence that all cognitive functions are interdependent. Perception depends on memory and attention, memory depends on perception, language depends on all three, and intelligence is served by all of the above plus reasoning, and so on. Also interdependent must be, of course, their neural foundations."
—Joaquin M. Fuster, 2000, p. 52

"There is an explanatory gap between our knowledge of the brain and what we know first-hand of ourselves, and it is difficult to imagine what kind of finding would bridge that gap. That there should be a neurological basis for our mental life is not controversial. But that beginning insight also seems to exhaust the contribution of brain scans to our self-understanding."
—Matthew B. Crawford, 2007, p. 78

1. I am grateful to Stanley Klein of the University of California-Santa Barbara for calling this prescient quotation to my attention.

Contents

Foreword

Everyone knows that the brain is in the head and that the mind is the product of the brain—no brain, no mind; malfunctioning brain, defective mind. But reflection on this unique organ—this "enchanted loom," or "great raveled knot," to use Sherrington's (1942) colorful metaphors—prompts many questions. Why, for example, is the brain all "scrunched up" in one spot within the skull? Might there not be some advantages to having it distributed throughout the body, as the nervous system, as a whole, is? Distributed systems work perfectly well in the world of computers, even without any centralized control element. Might it not be advantageous to have pockets of computing power located close to the extremities where much of the action is, rather than having all that power located in one small area at one end of the body. (It was once held that Diplodocus, a dinosaur about 80 to 90 feet in length, had one brain in its head and another at the base of its spine because, given the relatively leisurely rate at with which neural impulses travel, the head was too far away from the tail to control it in a timely fashion. Whether the bulge at the end of the end of the spine actually housed a second brain is now disputed.) Another of the mysteries of the brain is why its surface has such a convoluted shape, with more of the cerebral cortex—the two-millimeter thick layer of gray matter that covers the entire cerebrum—within the fissures than on the surface.

Presumably, the brain is in the head, and the cortex is folded in on itself, as it is, because there is some biological advantage of it being in this location and shaped this way. One advantage of having the cortex in the smallest possible space is that of minimizing the time required for the transmission of neural impulses between its most widely separated parts. Laid out flat, the cortex would cover an area of about two square feet; scrunched up in the skull, the greatest distance between any two points is roughly 6 inches, and the average distance between random points is, of course, much less than that. A possible cause of the convolutions is that the cortex has experienced an explosive growth relative to the brain's inner portions, and there is some reason for it to remain relatively thin. The only way this could happen within the confines of the skull would be for the outer layer to fold in on itself. This idea gains plausibility from the fact that the human brain differs from those of other mammals more with respect to its gray matter than with respect to other parts.

Whatever the reasons for the brain's location and shape, the question that trumps all others is: just how does the brain make the mind? Many inquisitive minds have pondered this question over the ages—minds pondering the basis of the existence of minds. I said that everyone knows that the mind is the product of the brain, but perhaps in that I misspoke. The nature of the relation between brain and mind is an old and abiding enigma. Some would say that the brain *is* the mind. Others would deny the existence of the mind, dismissing its apparent existence as an epiphenomenon. I take it as the prevailing view among modern neuroscientists, however, that the brain does, indeed, make the mind. Few, if any, would dispute the assumption that the brain, somehow, gives rise to sensation, perception, cognition, volition, and other psychological experiences or states. The persisting challenge is to determine precisely how the brain does this.

Exactly when people began to suspect that the brain had something to do with sensory experience and thinking is unknown, but it probably predates recorded history. Did neolithic humans have enough of an idea of the role of the brain—or whatever they thought inhabited the head—in determining mental states to motivate them to develop the practice of boring a hole in the skull for therapeutic or other purposes? No one knows. One guess is that they adopted the practice in the belief that it relieved severe head pain or lessened the occurrence of mysterious behavior, such as might be caused by epilepsy.

The ancient Greeks entertained a variety of notions regarding the function of the brain. Among the first to identify it as the organ essential to sensation, intelligence, and thought was Alcmaeon, who lived during the fifth century BC. Plato endorsed this idea in *The Republic*, locating reason (one part of the tripartite soul, the other two parts being spirit and desire) in the head. Aristotle described the function of the brain—which he believed to be the coolest organ of the body—as that of cooling body moisture, which had been turned into vapor by the sun's heat. He, like the fifth-century BC Sicilian philosopher-scientist Empedocles before him, considered the seat of intelligence to be the heart.

During the second century AD, renowned Roman physician Galen took exception to Aristotle's description of the brain as a cooling system and proclaimed it to be the source of mental activity. Not surprisingly, this did not settle the matter, and the Alcmaeonic-Platonic-Galenic view did not become universal, or nearly so, until relatively modern times. In common parlance the heart is still cited as the organ that houses our innermost beliefs, knowledge, and passions; and it is not always clear to what extent such references are intended to be metaphorical. In the seventeenth century René Descartes famously proclaimed the pineal gland to be the abode of the soul and the mediator between mind and body. His basis for this view was belief that this gland is the only structure within the brain that does not exist in duplicate and his mistaken assumption that animals do not have pineal glands.

Dissections of the brains of cadavers (some claim also of those of live prisoners) were performed as early as the third or fourth century BC by the Greek philosopher-physicians Herophilus and Erasistratus (the latter is credited with distinguishing between sensory and motor nerves). Although outlawed at times in certain places (e.g., ancient Rome), autopsies and dissections provided increasing knowledge of human anatomy and physiological functions throughout the Middle Ages and until the present day.

The idea that different regions of the brain might serve different purposes dates back at least to the Middle Ages (Kemp, 1996). Interest in the possibility of associating specific functions with different brain areas began in the nineteenth century, when localizing was done primarily by studying the effects on various psychological functions of injuries to different parts of the brain and sometimes by creative speculation. Thomas Willis, a seventeenth-century English physician and author of *Cerebri Anatome* (1664), believed memory to be located in the cortical gyri of the cerebrum (rather than the cerebellum), because, he observed, it is the temples and fore part of the head, not the back, that we rub when we wish to remember something. German physician Franz Joseph Gall (1758–1828) developed the idea of inferring psychological properties from the detailed shape of a person's skull into a pseudoscience, remnants of which persist.

Perhaps the first serious attempts to localize functions in the brain by empirical means should be considered to be those of the French physician, Paul Broca (1824–1889), who performed postmortem examinations of the brains of people suffering from paralysis and aphasia. Broca's pioneering contribution has been acknowledged by the designation of a region of the left (or dominant) temporal lobe of the brain just posterior to the inferior frontal gyrus, critical to speech, as Broca's area. Carl Wernicke (1848–1905) pointed to an area posterior to Broca's as essential to language understanding; again the basis of the localization was study of the effects of localized injury.

Undoubtedly the most widely publicized incident involving the study of localized brain function as a consequence of an accident was the horrific injury suffered by Phineas Gage in 1848. Gage, about 25 at the time, was using a straight iron bar to tamp blasting powder in a hole in preparation for blasting rock from a roadbed at a railroad construction site. The powder exploded prematurely, launching the bar, which passed through Gage's head destroying much of his frontal cortex. Gage remained conscious through the ordeal and lived as a physically able person for an additional 12 years. Much has been written about the effects of the trauma on Gage's personality and mental capability. According to a recent account (Macmillan, 2000), reports of its effects include many claims for which there is little factual evidence, and the actual effects were not as devastating as the more sensational reports portrayed them to be.

As medical knowledge increased and surgical procedures became more sophisticated, it became feasible to study brain functions in less opportunistic and passive ways. Pioneering work was done by Canadian neurosurgeon Wilder Penfield (1891–1976), who made a practice of stimulating the exposed cortex of persons undergoing brain surgery under local anesthesia and recording their responses. In this way he was able to pinpoint areas that were to be excised to control epileptic seizures. Over time he compiled detailed maps of primary sensory and motor areas of the cortex.

The emerging belief that the frontal, or prefrontal, cortex was unessential to normal mental functioning, but at the same time was somehow responsible for various types of psychotic behavior or states, led in the 1930s and 1940s to a rash of frontal lobotomies, a procedure for the development of which in 1936 Egas Moniz received the Nobel Prize in 1949. A stunningly dark chapter in the annals of twentieth-century medicine is the story of Walter Freeman's infamous "ice-pick lobotomies," of which he is said to have performed between 3,000 and 4,000, often in showman style, over a period of less than 20 years. Lobotomies typically had the desired effect of quelling psychotic episodes—replacing violent behavior with docility—but at the cost of destroying people's personalities. They fell out of fashion with the appearance of antipsychotic drugs in the mid-1950s.

Development of the ability to deliver a mild electrical impulse to precise areas of the brains of animals via implanted electrodes led to much experimental exploration of the brain in efforts to associate specific areas with specific functions. Among the better-known results of these efforts was the serendipitous discovery by James Olds and Peter Milner (1954; Olds, 1956, 1958) that rats would relentlessly press a bar in order to experience whatever they were experiencing when a mild current was delivered to the septal area of their brains. This discovery yielded the notion of a pleasure center within the brain and launched a to-date unsuccessful search for a reliable method of stimulating it chemically in humans for therapeutic or hedonistic purposes (Stix, 2009).

Among the more interesting discoveries in brain science to have been made in the twentieth century was the effect on brain function of the separation of the two cerebral hemispheres by transection of the corpus callosum, as a means of controlling otherwise uncontrollable epileptic seizures. Roger Sperry (1913–1994) and colleagues explored the effects of this operation on the subsequent functioning of the "split brain," many of which gave a picture of two brains working independently. This work, for which Sperry received the Nobel Prize in 1932, and research following directly from it have been documented extensively by Sperry's student and collaborator, Michael Gazzaniga (e.g., 1970, 1998).

Despite the crude techniques available, the study of brain function over the centuries produced considerable knowledge about, and immense fascination with, the brain. Wouldn't it be wonderful and illuminating to be able to observe what is going on in one's brain *while* one is sensing a touch on one's arm, perceiving the red of a strawberry, recalling yesterday's baseball game or an event in one's childhood, searching one's memory for a temporarily forgotten name, or feeling euphoric or sad or guilty or proud. Thanks to the breathtaking strides that have been made in neural imaging, a technology that barely existed a few years ago, this idea has morphed from the realm of fantasy to that of working science. But what does it mean to observe the activity of the brain? At what precisely should one want to look? The firing of individual neurons? The activity at neural synapses? The patterns of signal transmissions among neuron clusters? Changes in the gross level of activity of specific regions of the cortex or of identifiable "organs" within the brain?

What does one look for in the hope of finding the biological resting place of a specific memory? A reverberating neural circuit? Changes in the diameters of axons or dendrites with resulting changes in propagation characteristics such as resistance or conductance? Evidence of proliferation of synaptic terminals? Establishment of new intercellular connections? Changes in the properties of the conducting surfaces of neurons? Changes in the rate of production of different types of neurotransmitter substances? Changes in the arrangement of nucleotides on RNA or DNA molecules? Effects of the "second messenger" nucleotide cyclic adenosine monophosphate (AMP)? Patterns of activity of hormones such as adrenocorticotropic hormone (ACTH) and the melanocyte-stimulating hormone (MSH)? The chemical activity of glial cells? The operation of isolatable subsets of neurons—"neural cliques?" Something else?

The questions seem endless, but one is inclined to assume that whatever one chooses to observe, one is sure to learn much that is both intrinsically interesting and useful. Little wonder that the development of sophisticated noninvasive techniques for observing ongoing brain activity has everyone wanting to take a look. The opportunities presented by these techniques have been seized enthusiastically by researchers, and a great deal of work is exploiting them for the purpose of identifying areas and structures within the brain that are involved in the production of specific psychological states and experiences. But the apparent richness of the possibilities prompts other questions. Are there limits—practical and/or theoretical—to what one can discover about the mind by observing the behavior of the brain? What can one reasonably hope to learn about psychological processes and experiences through the use of brain imaging techniques?

In *Mind and Brain: A Critical Appraisal of Cognitive Neuroscience*, William Uttal addresses questions of these sorts and casts a sharp critical eye on what appears to be a trend toward more and more work on brain mapping, spurred by technological developments, at the expense of less and less utilization of conventional experimental studies of psychological phenomena per se. He does not argue that brain imaging devices and techniques are worthless. To the contrary, he characterizes their development as among the more important diagnostic and scientific developments ever and acknowledges their unique and revolutionary role in alleviating human suffering. But he raises many questions regarding their use in the study of psychological—especially cognitive—processes. What, he asks, is the likelihood that brain imaging techniques will add value to existing behavioral science research? Is this type of research worth the amount of attention it is receiving relative to that being received by other types of research aimed at understanding cognition? Are realistic assumptions being made about the knowledge and understanding of cognitive processes and experiences that these techniques are likely to produce? Are the results of the research that is being done being interpreted objectively and the practical implications of those results being assessed and reported responsibly?

Mind and Brain is an ambitious and gutsy effort to confront these and closely related questions. In Uttal's words, his aim is "to critically evaluate to what extent brain imaging and other recording techniques have informed scientific psychology"—to consider, in particular, whether "these new technologies offer us an expedited pathway to the great question of how the brain makes the mind."

One learns early in the book—in the Preface—that Uttal's answer to the last question is unequivocally negative; in the remainder of the book he makes a case to convince the reader that that conclusion is warranted. Readers of *The New Phrenology*, Uttal's earlier book on the same topic, will not find this surprising. *Mind and Brain: A Critical Appraisal of Cognitive Neuroscience* is an update of *The New Phrenology* in that it covers a great deal of work involving the use of brain imaging techniques that has been done since the latter was published, but it is more than an update by virtue of addressing a broader range of relevant topics.

The case that Uttal makes is many faceted. It deals with technical and methodological issues that are relevant to the application of brain imaging to the study of cognitive processes, including the costs and cumbersomeness of imaging equipment, difficulty in controlling independent variables, questionable reliability of data processing (the subtraction technique) and interpretation, difficulty of measuring the intensity or amplitude (as distinct from location) of brain activity, uncertainty regarding precisely what type of neural activity brain images represent, temporal differences between experienced cognitive states and presumably associated brain image patterns, inter- and intrasubject variability in recorded brain activity ostensibly representing the same cognitive states or activities, and the complexity of techniques that are used to analyze brain imaging data.

He argues that the brain's neural network is too complex and the observational instruments at our disposal too blunt to permit study at a level of specificity that would warrant hope of discovering how the brain makes the mind. Moreover, the limitation, he contends, may be more than a temporary one; the complexity of brain networks may be beyond analysis:

> It may represent an intractable problem that neither new measuring devices nor computational engines could ever begin to unravel. There are too many uncertainties, too many neurons, too many idiosyncratic connections (e.g., the brain is not neatly organized as is a simple crystalline structure) for us to ever be able to understand its detailed organization and how, specifically, this complex information pattern produces the reality we call mind.

Uttal considers most cognitive constructs (attention, memory, emotion) to be insufficiently precisely defined to admit of matching them up with specific brain locations or processes. He is skeptical of the numerous taxonomies of learning and memory that have been proposed, questioning whether the various "types" that have been identified are truly distinctive. He contends that the functions that researchers of brain imaging generally are trying to locate have been identified by specific psychological models, and if the models were to change, it would make for considerable confusion.

Among several important distinctions that Uttal makes, none is more central to his position than the distinction between the questions of *where* and *how*. Much of his critique deals with the prospects of answering the *where* question—the localization of brain regions responsible for specified mental states or experiences—and his conclusion is that the prospects of answering it satisfactorily are not good. He argues that it is theoretically impossible to associate any particular brain activation site or pattern of activation uniquely with any particular cognitive state because even the simplest of thoughts typically activates many areas of the brain, and any given area is likely to be activated by many different psychological processes. "In fact, as some scholars have pointed out, brain images tell us little more than that there is some brain activity when our minds are active. . . . However, as far as specifying the specific neural processes that are the coded equivalents of mind, virtually all such cumulative measures of brain activity are bankrupt."

But suppose we *could*, or sometime in the future *will*, answer the *where* question. Would this bring us any closer to an answer of the question of *how*? As Uttal puts it, "What does knowing what part of the brain is activated by some stimulus or task tell us about how that part encodes mental activity?" What if we had (or sometime in the future acquire) the techniques to observe the activity of neurons and their interactions at whatever level of detail desired? Is it reasonable to suppose that at some point we would see that the activity that is observed must give rise to mental states we all experience?

What would it mean to *explain* consciousness and subjective experience in terms of neural activity? That learning does not require consciousness has been known for some time. In *Design for a Brain*, W. Ross Ashby (1952/1960) attributes his failure to use "consciousness and its related subjective elements" in his book, despite his intention to deal with how the brain learns, to the fact that "at no point have I found their introduction necessary" (p. 11). Norbert Wiener (1964) addressed the possibility of the existence of machines that learn and reproduce themselves in his book, *God and Golem, Inc.* Many instances of machine learning have been documented in the meantime, and the self-replicating capability is an active area of research. The possibility of machines becoming self-aware, once the purview of science fiction, has been getting increasing attention from scientists with a futuristic bent. The June 2010 issue of *Scientific American* includes the development of machine self-awareness in its list of "12 events that will change everything" (Greenemeier, 2010). If machines become self-aware, some argue, they will surely discover and act upon the possibility of reproducing themselves in ever better (more intelligent, more powerful) forms, and what this would portend for human beings, who can say?

For present purposes the question of interest is this: how could one ever know for sure whether a machine was aware of itself or conscious in the sense in which people are aware of themselves and conscious? Its ability to claim to be conscious and to behave *as though* it were conscious is hardly compelling evidence. Imagine not knowing what a brain is but having the opportunity to observe one (natural or artificial) in action at any level of detail one desires. What might one expect to see in the activity of the molecules that make up the neurons, and those that carry the electrochemical signals down the axons and across the synapses—individually or collectively—or in the detailed behavior of complex neural circuits, that would convince one that consciousness is the necessary result? I find it difficult to imagine what it could be. It seems to me not unlikely that we will never solve the mystery of consciousness. To some, acceptance of this possibility undoubtedly would be a cause for disappointment or despair. I am not among them.

Uttal objects to what he sees as overstatements of what has been learned about human cognition through brain imaging studies, and in doing so he does not mince words. "[A]ll putative extrapolations from behavioral to neuroscientific mechanism are vastly underdetermined inferences from data that do not provide the logical or empirical constraints necessary to draw robust conclusions." Further, he contends "Cognitive neuroscience, despite considerable ballyhoo, does not yet have the tools with which to deal with a complex system such as the brain. . . . Of particular concern are the unjustifiably strong conclusions drawn from noisy data, a characteristic of much of the research currently being carried out in this field."

We psychologists (including neuroscientists among us), Uttal says in a variety of ways, are good at fooling ourselves into believing that we have made progress in understanding details of the neural substrate of behavior and cognition when we really haven't. He speaks of the seductiveness of brain images and their tendency to add persuasive weight to a report. (It seems a safe bet that *neuroscience* sounds more scientific than *psychology* or even *cognitive science*, at least to the general public and probably to many scientists as well.)

It is arguably a major failing of human reasoning that in judging the benefit that has been derived from any effort to achieve some goal, or good, we too often fail to consider nonobvious negative effects the effort may have had, or what might have been accomplished if the same energy had been expended on alternative goals. Uttal argues that to the extent that work on brain mapping is motivated by the assumption that this is an effective avenue to a better understanding of cognition, much of it is not worth the opportunity costs (represented by alternative paths not taken) it incurs.

Is Uttal right in this assessment? I don't know. What I do know is that *Mind and Brain: A Critical Appraisal of Cognitive Neuroscience* is a scholarly, incisive, thought-provoking book. This will surprise no one who has read any of the many other substantive provocative books Uttal has written. In this book, Uttal raises hard questions about the nature of science, about how one should decide what is worth doing, about prioritizing among the possibilities, about how to determine whether progress is being made—especially about whether progress is being made in understanding cognition. Whatever the future of brain mapping, I believe that in *Mind and Brain: A Critical Appraisal of Cognitive Neuroscience* Uttal has done an extraordinarily valuable service in articulating a host of issues that deserve attention from anyone with a more-than-passing interest in the age-old and ever-new question of how the brain makes the mind.

Raymond S. Nickerson
Tufts University

References

Ashby, W. R. [1952] (1960). *Design for a brain* (2nd ed.). New York: Wiley.

Gazzaniga, M. S. (1970). *The bisected brain*. New York: Appleton-Century-Crofts.

Gazzaniga, M. S. (1998). Split brain revisited. *Scientific American, 279*(1), 35–39.

Greenemeier, L. (2010). Machine self-awareness: What happens when robots start calling the shots? *Scientific American, 302*(6), 44–45.

Kemp, S. (1996). *Cognitive psychology in the Middle Ages*. Westport, CT: Greenwood Press.

Macmillan, M. (2000). *An odd kind of fame: Stories of Phineas Gage*. Cambridge, MA: MIT Press.

Olds, J. (1956). Pleasure center in the brain. *Scientific American, 195*(4), 105–116.

Olds, J. (1958). Self-stimulation of the brain. *Science, 127*, 315–324.

Olds, J., & Milner, P. (1954). Positive reinforcement produced by electrical stimulation of the septal area and other regions of rat brain. *Journal of Comparative and Physiological Psychology, 47*, 419–427.

Sherrington, C. S. (1942). *Man on his nature*. Cambridge, UK: Cambridge University Press.

Stix, G. (2009). Turn it up, dear. *Scientific American, 300*(5), 22–23.

Wiener, N. (1964). *God & Golem, Inc.: A comment on certain points where cybernetics impinges on religion*. Cambridge, MA: MIT Press.

Preface

There is no greater fascination on the part of humanity than with the brain mechanisms that might explain our minds. What, we all ask, could possibly account for our personal awareness of the world of which we are a part? There are so many examples of this fascination in both popular culture and the scientific literature that it would be impossible to catalog them. Whether our personal answers to the great question of what we are mentally are to be found in religion, spirituality, philosophy, physiology, or psychology, the question is undoubtedly asked by virtually all of us at one time or another.

One of the most important developments in scientific history is that increasing numbers of people are attempting to answer this age-old question in terms of the biology of the nervous system and, in particular, of the nature of that magnificent organ—the human brain. The brain is probably the most complex system that has ever been discovered. Its complexity possibly rivals that of the universe and probably exceeds it in terms of the potential range and diversity of interconnections and interactions.

Cognitive neuroscience is the current manifestation of the theologies, philosophies, and sciences that have long been concerned with the relation between our minds and our brain. It asks (or should ask) questions such as:

1. How does the brain make the mind and control behavior?
2. What is the level of analysis of the brain that is the most likely basis of our cognitive processes?
3. How do traumatic brain injuries inform us about the relation of the mind and the brain?
4. How do surgically induced lesions inform us about the relation of the mind and the brain?
5. How do EEGs and brain imaging techniques inform us about the relation of the mind and the brain?
6. What is the significance of different patterns of activity on the brain when a person is stimulated or tasked?
7. Can brain imaging provide an alternative approach (to behavioral techniques) with which to measure, control, and predict behavior? Does it add value to the behavioral measures?

8. Given that the dominant current theory is that the mind can be parsed into relatively independent "modules" whose mechanisms can be localized in circumscribed regions of the brain, what is the current state of this theory?

9. What implications do new findings on the distribution of neural responses, brain "holism," and cognitive inaccessibility have on the dominant theories of cognitive psychology and their efforts to discover the underlying neural mechanisms of our cognitive activities?

10. What is the current state of the empirical findings from brain imaging–cognitive comparisons? Does their lack of reliability and modest correlations justify their use as predictors of performance and abilities? Do they provide a coherent pathway to understanding the mind-brain problem?

11. Are we drawing appropriate interpretations and inferences from the empirical findings that have been forthcoming over the last two centuries in particular?

12. What does the future hold for cognitive neuroscience? Is it reasonable to think of a non-neuroreductive scientific psychology? In other words, can psychological science exist and prosper without neuroscience?

13. What is the likelihood that cognitive neuroscience as we conceptualize it today will be applicable to the many social and medical problems facing humanity?

The goal of this book is to consider some of the many alternative answers that have been provided to some of these questions. The strategy used here is framed in the form of a critical review of both cognitive neuroscience's past history and its modern developments. A particular interest is considering the possible role of the newest technological development—brain imaging—in studying the relationship between the mind and the body. Unfortunately, the explosive growth of this new mode of research has not been accompanied by a comprehensive and synoptic evaluation of the huge number of studies that have been published in the past two decades. To do so coherently, however, requires that we also consider the history of cognitive neuroscience prior to the invention of modern brain imaging devices, especially functional magnetic resonance imaging (fMRI). This includes consideration of the psychological and more conventional approaches to what used to be called physiological psychology.

My purpose, therefore, is to take a cut at a synoptic synthesis of this substantial body of scientific literature. This is not going to be an easy task; results are varied and numerous, and, as I point out in the body of this book, not only is there a substantial amount of inconsistency in the research findings, but there is also great conceptual confusion about the significance of virtually every one of the multitude of reported experiments.

At the outset I must accept the fact that it is impossible to cover all of the relevant literature. However, by selecting appropriate exemplars, I hope that it will be possible to come to a reasonable conclusion about the current status of what clearly is a time of major developments in cognitive neuroscience. Having no vested interest on my own part with regard to particular findings or specific theories, I hope what I can offer is an objective evaluation of the state of the field a decade or so into the twenty-first century.

Nevertheless, I also have to acknowledge that I come to this project with a somewhat negative bias. It appears to me that there has been far too much hyperbole and far too little critical analysis of what our experimental outcomes really mean. This has been a major problem throughout the history of cognitive neuroscience and promises to continue to be one well into the current period. I am not now convinced of the validity (defined in its most formal sense) of much of these data and even less so of the interpretations that are often attached to them.

Despite this skepticism, there has been enough empirical progress to support a major transformation in thinking about the role of brain imaging in cognitive neuroscience. That change has been from an almost phrenological orientation in which separate cognitive modules were thought to be localized in narrowly circumscribed locales in and on the brain. Recent research studies, especially those in which the results of many different experiments were combined (meta-studies), have shown that the response to even the most carefully controlled stimulus is much more widely distributed on and in the brain than hitherto thought.

In an older work (Uttal, 2001), I argued against localization on technical and conceptual grounds. In a more recent work (Uttal, 2009), I showed how recent research made this point even more emphatically and led to the conclusion that the modular-localization hypothesis had to be replaced by one that emphasized both widespread distribution of brain representations and a more unified view of psychological mechanisms.

If there is an overarching assumption driving the ideas expressed in this book, it is my focus on the failures of reductionism—both to cognitive modules and to neural mechanisms. I am now convinced that finding support for both cognitive modularism and neuroreductionism is a much more difficult task than hitherto assumed and that we actually know far less in both domains than many think we do.

In my earlier books I tried to identify the pitfalls associated with efforts to proclaim the nature of hypothetical cognitive processes on the basis of behavioral observations. In this present work I emphasize the search for some explanation of the increasing variability of empirical findings with regard to their reduction to neural mechanisms. There is still too much uncertainty about some of the most basic findings from studies that attempt to assign specific functions to specific brain regions (or to systems made up of localized functions) to uncritically accept much of the present literature. This book is a modest effort to resolve some of the present problems generated by mental inaccessibility and neural complexity.

This present work has a somewhat different orientation than the two earlier ones. After introducing my philosophy of mind-brain relations and discussing some of the general problems faced by cognitive neuroscience, I carry out a review of specific brain-behavioral studies to see how well they have informed us in our search for mind-brain relations. Although a major effort will be directed at recent imaging studies, the present situation becomes understandable only in the context of the history, both psychological and neuroscientific, that has led us to the present situation.

There are a few general points that I should like to make in these introductory comments. First, as a psychologist, I must express the opinion that scientific psychology is at risk in the current context of brain imaging—the newest fad in its long history.[1] An important question is—do neuroscientific findings inform psychology, or does psychological knowledge inform neuroscience? As I progress through the discussions in this book, I have become increasingly convinced that neuroscience is much more dependent on psychology than psychology is dependent on neuroscience and that with the uncertainties of precise cognitive process definitions and the innate problems we have controlling cognitive states, there is substantial reason for caution. Indeed, beyond the sensory and motor systems, neuroscience has done little, in the opinion of many of us, to resolve any of the great questions of psychology. On the other hand, it is virtually impossible to carry out a meaningful experiment in cognitive neuroscience without guidance from psychological findings and theories.

Am I biased? Of course, I am. I am coming at the problems of cognitive neuroscience from a perspective that may be unusual among my colleagues. Where they seek affirmation of their findings and theories, I seek negation; I challenge the empirical outcomes and interpretative theories. Where their work is based on a set of usually implicit assumptions, I seek to make the assumptions explicit and in doing so often find contradictions at the most basic level of understanding.

Despite some who would read this criticism of cognitive neuroscience as a generalized attack on both experimental psychology and neuroscience, I hope I can make it clear to my readers that I am a strong and positive proponent of the kinds of empirical research that I discuss in this book. Much of the data, the findings, and the results obtained over the last century are relatively solid scientific facts that provide us with a picture of human nature that was not possible in the speculative periods that preceded it. As I show throughout this book, however, there is somewhat less assurance that PET or fMRI images are reliable and valid indicators of psychologically meaningful patterns of brain activity. The difficulty is in large part with the theories that have proliferated over this same time period—theories that have been proposed to explain psychological processes with neural mechanisms. I argue that most of these theories cannot be discriminated from each other for a number of reasons. First, the anatomic structures to which they refer are rarely adequately demarcated, and their activities are, to a degree not yet fully realized, unreliable and unreplicated.

Second, the data are complex, and the systems involved not adequately simplified by assumptions such as "pure insertion"—the idea that the removal of one portion of a complex process leaves all of the other components in their original state.

Third, none of the neuroscientific theories so far proposed is sufficiently quantitative or precise to account for the vagaries of the data. Indeed, most psychological theories do not have identifiable neural postulates that can be tested. Therefore, at the same time, they all permit too much leeway in accommodating contradictory information and do not constrain our theories when opposing discoveries occur. Furthermore, without specific neural postulates, it is rare, indeed, when psychological controversies can be resolved by neurophysiological techniques. The major exceptions to this generalization occur in the sensory and motor domains where the research issues are of neural transmission codes rather than of the neural equivalents of our cognitive processes. In general unless a psychological theory has specific neurophysiological postulates, it is neutral with regard to underlying mechanisms. By "neutral" I mean that it is underdetermined; that is, it does not contain sufficient information to discriminate between plausible neural mechanisms. Underdetermination also plagues any reductionist approaches using behavior and mathematical models as well.

Fourth, there is a lot of cherry picking exhibited in the field; references are selected to provide support for arguments that on close inspection are only a small part of the relevant literature. I must admit that I cannot avoid this problem; my strategy is also to select a few particularly salient reports and deal in depth with each of them for each of the topics considered here. My bibliography will happily be shortened to the hundreds from the tens of thousands by this selective approach; however, more important is the fact that a detailed dissection of a few studies will often uncover hidden design flaws, internally inconsistent findings, and illogic that might have otherwise been overlooked.

This then brings me to a highly personal admission. Whenever one attempts to survey such a broad and complex field of science as cognitive neuroscience, it is very difficult to be sure that one has interpreted all of the reports within the frame of reference intended by the authors. I am sure that there may be discrepancies between their stated conclusions and my own evaluations of their findings. In some cases, I am probably to blame, but in others I am convinced that some investigators have read far too much into what are variable and inconsistent results. In some cases I am sure that differences in initial assumptions may also account for differing interpretations. I also apologize in advance to all of those authors whose publications are overlooked because of the sheer volume of the literature, as well as to those who may feel I have not expressed their point of views correctly.

Obviously, when one samples from such a broad literature, the selection may be unbalanced. I am aware of that problem and admit that I have often sought out articles and reports (the number of which is growing every week it seems) that were critical or that illustrated the variability or uncertainty of the empirical findings. However, the huge variety of stimuli, analytical methods, and experimental conditions makes the results far more variable and complex than anticipated. Indeed, if one examines the literature very carefully, there is a remarkable absence of real replication. This problem is exacerbated by the fact that very small changes in experimental protocol can produce very large changes in results. This problem is even further compounded by the complexity of the brain itself. An emerging generalization is that even the most peripheral parts of the brain are so heavily interconnected with higher levels that it is often difficult to tease out their separate roles.

Finally, another personal note: I am fully aware that the strongly critical approach I take in this book will not be well received by many of my fellow cognitive neuroscientists. However, I am becoming increasingly aware that the field in which we labor is heavily contaminated with both our hopes and our implicit, a priori assumptions. This does not mean that the study of behavior or brain anatomy, chemistry, and physiology will not continue to lead to understanding about their respective fields. It is the current failure to establish robust links between the cognitive and neural domains that is the problem.

If the analysis I present here provides the basis for a more realistic, constructive, and conservative evaluation of what we have accomplished in cognitive neuroscience, or even stimulates some discussion about the possible flaws in traditional and modern research, I will feel that the effort has been worthwhile. With these caveats in place, I now turn to the task at hand—a critical appraisal of the field of cognitive neuroscience in the twenty-first century.

Acknowledgments

The initial stimulus for this book came from a conversation I had with two of my University of Hawaii colleagues, M. E. (Jeff) Bitterman and Peter Balsam (also of Columbia University). Jeff, Peter, and I had gotten into the habit of discussing outlandish ideas about psychology and neuroscience. Despite the enormous activity in the field of cognitive neuroscience, it quickly became apparent that there was a lacuna to be filled—it seemed that there was a need for a critical evaluation of the field from an objective point of view. I owe much to those original conversations. Indeed, my last eight summers have been spent as a visiting colleague at the Bekesy Laboratory of Neurophysiology at the University of Hawaii. These visits were made possible through the efforts of my friend and colleague, Patricia Couvillon. I am deeply grateful to Pat for her intellectual and administrative support during this period. Nor can I ignore the warm aloha hospitality of the many members of the laboratory staff who made this such a rich personal experience.

This book was written with contract support from the U.S. Army Research Institute for the Behavioral and Social Sciences, a document known as W91WAW-09-C-0091. I especially acknowledge the support of Paul A. Gade, chief of the Basic Research Unit of the U.S. Army Research Institute for the Behavioral and Social Sciences for his intellectual support as this book developed over the last year. Paul also took on the onerous task of reading many manuscript chapters adding to the precision of my language and the crispness of my logic.

I also want to express my appreciation to a number of my academic colleagues. Duncan Luce of UC Irvine provided guidance and wisdom for several chapters. David S. Leland of Pitzer College made many useful comments on an early draft of chapter 1. Gary Greenberg of The University of Wichita has been a constant supporter of my work, however much he disagreed with some of my views. Gary provided advice and references to some extremely useful material that helped me challenge some modern ideas about the mind-brain relation. Individual chapters were read and commented on by John Reich. Raymond Nickerson read the whole manuscript and made many useful suggestions with a degree of diligence that was probably greater than anyone else prior to publication; I am eternally indebted to him for cleaning up some of my ideas and grammar. Needless to say, none of these friends and colleagues bears any responsibility for some of the conceptual flaws that still will be found scattered throughout this book.

Many others have influenced me over the years sometimes by their writing and sometimes by means of a brief comment expressed in much less formal settings. It is amazing how a few words can stimulate a decade-long research project.

For the last 11 years, since my retirement from Arizona State University, I have enjoyed the continued support of my home department—Industrial Engineering. I am deeply grateful to a succession of department chairs and college deans for their willingness to provide a home for my work. It could not have continued without their confidence that what I was doing was worthwhile, however distant it may have been from their organizational charter.

My appreciation for my colleagues and our interactions in our little "metaphysical society" continues unabated. My discussions with Peter Killeen, David Hestenes, Mike McBeath, Art Glenberg, Federico Sanabria, and Warren Van Egmond, played an important role in the development of my ideas. John Reich's invitation to join a comparable social-science–oriented discussion group also helped me to develop some of the strategies of critical thinking that were useful in writing this book.

Finally, my dear wife continues to provide a home environment and what seems to be an unending amount of patience with me. Without her, nothing would have happened. And so, once again, I lovingly dedicate this book to her.

1 Introduction

1.1 Some Background

In the past decade and a half important new developments in instrumentation capable of studying the functioning brain have appeared. These devices, most notably positron emission tomography (PET) and functional magnetic resonance imaging (fMRI) but also now including such exotic tools as magnetoencephalography, now unquestionably make it possible to study the anatomy and physiology of the brain (among other organ systems) better than ever before. There is no question that brain imaging devices represent one of the most important diagnostic and scientific developments of all time. Human suffering has been alleviated to a degree because of these devices in a way that is comparable only to the introduction of anesthesia or the purification of public water supplies. MRI machines are capable of tracking brain transmitter distribution, spotting potential weaknesses in circulation, defining the tracts connecting distant regions, and, to an as yet unknown degree, determining regions of heightened metabolic activity that may be associated with cognitive activity.

Despite this abundant progress, it must be clearly understood that anatomic and physiological images are not direct measurements or indicators of cognitive processes. Indeed, their meaning as correlations of our mental life is open to a wide variety of disputes, empirical inconsistencies, and internal uncertainties.

Nevertheless many researchers in the field of cognitive neuroscience argue that brain images can be used to study the neural foundations of our mental activities in a way that had hitherto been beyond the hopes of even the most imaginative researchers. Supplanting the older techniques of the electroencephalograph (EEG) and the event-related potential (ERP), these new techniques promised to provide a means of studying the function of the brain as it carries out its adaptive cognitive processes. However, many of us are beginning to believe that it is a promise yet to be fulfilled. In this book I critically examine just what has happened and what we have learned from the astonishingly large corpus of published experiments in which brain images are compared to cognitive processes.

The argument that brain imaging techniques will revolutionize cognitive science is based on the idea that they are direct measurements of salient brain activity during controlled cognitive activities. Many applications of brain imaging have been proposed, some of which are thought to offer alternative, if not better, means of measuring cognitive states and processes than those provided by the traditional psychological methods. Many of these suggestions thus promise what are considered to be objective measures of what had traditionally been limited to subjective measures of mental states.

However, there are others who believe that there are substantial unresolved problems with and limitations of this approach that suggest that some of the initial expectations may be unachievable not only in the short run but also in the distant future. The problems arise in many guises and include some that are conceptual, some that are technical, and some that are empirical. This gradually emerging awareness has led to a somewhat belated critical examination of the plausibility of the assumption that brain imaging techniques will permit us to "read the mind" of a human being or even to find adequately correlated biological markers for particular cognitive states.

The current book considers the role that brain imaging has made or might make to cognitive neuroscience. It is a new embodiment of what had hitherto been known as physiological psychology. The complexity and variability of human behavior have made progress in this field difficult to evaluate and even to conceptualize. Clearly, any novel method of evaluating, predicting, and controlling behavior would be of extreme interest—if it could be shown that these methods work or are likely to work in the future. This is the crux of the problem faced by modern cognitive neuroscience—what is the likelihood that brain imaging techniques will be able to bring added value to the existing behavioral science research? How deep should be our science's commitment to techniques that many researchers believe are deeply flawed and, despite their popularity, are neither theoretically nor empirically seminal nor even, in some cases, possible?

An important goal of this book, therefore, is critically to evaluate the extent to which brain imaging and other recording techniques have informed scientific psychology. This is not just an empirical problem; there is a profound theoretical question lurking in the background—what is the likelihood that we will be able to add to the fundamental theory of the mind-brain question using these powerful methods? In other words, do these new technologies offer us an expedited pathway to the great question of how the brain makes the mind?

Although the ultimate answer to the possibility of supplementing, if not substituting, brain research for behavioral research is going to be primarily empirical (will it work?), it must also be appreciated that there are major philosophical and logical issues raised whenever one has the audacity to compare mental and neural activities. There is no denying that this is a task of universal interest and monumental implications, but at least a few scholars agree that at present there has been limited conceptual progress despite the great diversity and number of empirical studies. We can no more ignore some of the imponderable foundation philosophical concepts that are involved than we can the limits of the technology. Given the current state of our knowledge, it may indeed be that our choice of the "correct" level of analysis, whether it is behavioral or neural, may be instrumental in interpreting the meaning as well as the applicability of what are complex and indirect experiments. Clearly, this is a problem of extreme complexity, and resolving it will be instrumental in the future development of scientific psychology as well as neuroscience.

The primary question—how does the brain make the mind?—cannot be studied in isolation. Cognitive neuroscience may have a short history, but it evolved not only from a century or so of physiological psychology but also from a longterm concern with the basic question. Therefore, other tasks in this book will be to review and evaluate the history of the cognitive neurosciences that preceded the invention of the imaging devices. The observation that much of this earlier work is also deeply flawed adds some depth of understanding to why modern imaging techniques have so far failed to achieve some of their most extravagant claims.

1.2 The Great Question—The World Knot

The greatest scientific question of all time, the one to which most human attention has been directed over the millennia, is—how are our minds and our brains related? The profundity of the question has led to its being referred to by Arthur Schopenhauer (1788–1860) as the "world knot."

Although there is considerable debate about the reality of the mind (see for example the article by Schlinger, 2005), to deny its reality or to declare it merely epiphenomenal would be to make human existence meaningless. Furthermore, there is at least one piece of solid evidence that the mental processes are real. That singular piece of evidence is that each of us is endowed with a personal awareness, a process that has come under many names. Whatever the term used—mind, mentality, soul, ego, self, intellect, consciousness, awareness, sentience, psyche, or cognition—we all have first-hand knowledge of what it is that we are talking about when we use any one of these words. There is no way that we could deny the reality of the mind because proof positive exists within each of us—our own sentience. We could not do so without destroying the meaningfulness of our ability to converse and interact at many different social levels.

However, as much as I am convinced that my mind exists, I have long ago resigned myself to the fact that defining the mind is an unachievable goal. These days I look upon it as a process of the brain analogous to rotations being a feature of material devices called wheels—albeit infinitely more complicated. In other words mind is neither nothing more nor nothing less than a function of the material brain.

Despite this near universal appreciation of the reality of mental activities, the description of the mind and the explanation of its neural origins have proven to be extremely difficult challenges for the science that has grown over the centuries to study them. That science is psychology, not the psychology of the therapeutic couch or inferred, but inaccessible, cognitive entities but the hard science of observable behaviors. If the interests of psychological science are combined with neurophysiological science, we refer to this science as physiological psychology, psychobiology, or, most recently, cognitive neuroscience. A major question that is implicit in this discussion is—can (or should) psychology exist without its neural co-studies? More precisely, what do psychology and neuroscience offer each other?

Psychology, confronted as it is by enormous obstructions and difficulties in constructing explanations of mental phenomena, has fractionated into a number of subsciences that have taken many different and often idiosyncratic directions over the years. Schools of thought have proliferated, and over time, strategic collaborations with other sciences have repeatedly formed.

At the root of cognitive psychology, however, has been the assumption that the nature of the mind (or its effects) can be studied experimentally. A further special assumption of modern cognitive neuroscience is that we will also be able to determine the neural conditions that lead to the mind. On the basis of this premise it is argued that, in principle, we should be able to understand the neural mechanisms that account for mental and behavioral activities. It is not yet clear whether or not this goal can or will be achieved; only time will tell. What we can discern now are the intellectual and philosophical roots that underlie the neuroreductionist goal of explaining mind in terms of the brain and the many obstacles that prevent us from achieving that goal.

The most fundamental root of all of these questions lies not in the laboratory but in speculative ontology—a major division of metaphysical philosophy. Ontology is that branch of metaphysics that deals with the philosophy of reality, of the nature of existence itself. The ontology of cognitive neuroscience is especially complex for two reasons: first, we have no direct access to or empirical evidence of the mind (Uttal, 2007); we have only indirect evidence from which we must infer its nature and construct hypotheses concerning its function. Second, mental activity is not sufficiently constrained by behavioral observations so that a robust analysis can be made of it into modular elements: in other words, all of our cognitivist-reductionist theories of mind are underdetermined.

Many questions for which we have no current answers, therefore, lay solely within the confines of the speculative philosophy that we call ontology. In the place of specific empirical answers to some of these most profound questions, philosophers have over the centuries tried to establish certain beliefs about the nature of reality that are based on whatever relevant knowledge is available and rational and logical arguments and derivations that may make these beliefs plausible, even if pure speculation cannot confirm them.

In cognitive neuroscience there is a major ontological assumption that, however controversial, guides the day-by-day activities of laboratory researchers as well as those who conjure up new theories of the relation between the mind and the brain. That basic assumption is that, however inexplicable it may be at the moment, the brain makes the mind. Although we do not know how, it is widely accepted that a complete neural explanation is, in principle, possible. Those who labor in the laboratory rarely make this monistic assumption explicit, and yet few cognitive neuroscientists would challenge this fundamental idea.[1]

Nevertheless, the assumption of mind-brain equivalence is without any compelling empirical foundation; none of the required tests of necessity and sufficiency have ever been carried out to confirm it generally or specifically. However likely it may seem, there is no evidence other than plausibility and reason to support this foundation assumption.

This profound foundation assumption comes in two parts (box 1.1). The first part is a general hypothesis, implicitly honored by all cognitive neuroscientists. It asserts that any mental or cognitive activities and processes as well as all of those that control behavior are the functions, the outcomes, or the results of the activities of the nervous system. Herein is the foundation assumption of what ontologists would refer to as monism or physicalism or mind-brain neuroreductionism.

Only those who believe in some kind of dualism would deny this part of the basic ontological postulate. (See Uttal, 2004, for a more complete discussion of the impact of dualistic thinking throughout history on theology, philosophy, and psychology.) This assumption links the worlds of the mind and the nervous system into a single inseparable reality; one part is structure, and the other is function. We can no more conceptually separate the two than we can separate the circular motion of a wheel from the wheel itself. This does not mean, however, that the two sciences—psychology and neuroscience—are inseparable empirically. Despite the ontological, in principle, inseparability, practical considerations (e.g., complexity) may keep these two scientific paths separate. Examining this issue is also a part of the challenge faced in this book.

The essential point of the first part of the basic ontological postulate is that the function cannot exist without some kind of equivalent physical structure. Our minds are products of our nervous system, and any idea of the consciousness or mind existing after the deterioration of the brain is without merit. Indeed, without this kind of mind-brain[3] monism the whole cognitive neuroscience enterprise would be meaningless and pointless; we could never be sure that our studies were not contaminated by other forces that were totally out of our control and totally unaccounted for in our experimental protocols.

Beyond the general mind-brain, monistic postulate just described lies the second part— one that is much more specific. It is the hypothesis that our minds are not just functions

Box 1.1
The Two Parts of the Basic Ontological Postulate

> 1. All mental processes are the outcome of neural activity.
> 2. All mental processes are the outcome of the microscopic interactions and actions of the great neuronal networks of the brain.[2] This is the proper level of analysis of the mind-brain problem.

of our material nervous system (the first part) but that they are the specific result of the cumulative integration and interaction of complex and innumerable <u>neuronal</u> activities that go on in the brain as opposed to other levels of <u>neural</u> activity.

It is this complex and intricate pattern of neuronal activity and interactions that cognitive neuroscientists assert becomes or *is* mind; it is in the complex network of neurons that memories are stored, that decisions are made, that personalities are forged, and that behavior is controlled. It is there that the physiological actions are transmuted in some mysterious way into all of the many kinds of mental states, processes, feelings, and faculties that grace human existence. The mind, according to this postulate, arises out of the complex interactions of billions of component parts in ways that we do not now know and possibly may never to be able to know.[4] The relation between the brain and the mind, cognitive neuroscientists agree, is something akin to the Sherrington's (1940/1963) "enchanted loom":

The brain is waking and with it the mind is returning. It is as if the Milky Way entered upon some cosmic dance. Swiftly the head-mass becomes an enchanted loom where millions of flashing shuttles weave a dissolving pattern, always a meaningful pattern, though never an abiding one; a shifting harmony of sub-patterns. (p. 178)

This is beautiful poetry but hardly a rigorous scientific finding; it is simply a vague metaphor for the point being made by the second part of the basic ontological postulate.

This piece of poetry by Sherrington aside for the moment, the general principle expressed in the second postulate is widely held by contemporary psychologists and neuroscientists. The modern version of the idea was probably first expressed by McCulloch and Pitts (1943) and Pitts and McCulloch (1947) in their pioneering work on the logic of networks and then in a follow-up on form recognition by such networks. However, the first specifically neuroscientific expression of the second postulate was published by Hebb (1949). In it he suggested specific patterns of neural interaction as the basis of cognitive activities. His theoretical neurophysiology was based on his elaboration of what had originally been a psychological principle—Thorndike's (1931) "Law of Effect."[5] This purely psychological observation was that repeated practice led to enhanced behavioral strength. Hebb argued that this law must also have a neural equivalent and in 1949 presciently formulated the following neural equivalent of it:

When an axon of cell A is near enough to excite a cell B and repeatedly or persistently takes part in firing it, some growth process or metabolic changes takes [*sic*] place in one or both cells such that A's efficiency, as one of the cells firing B, is increased. (Hebb, 1949, p. 62)

Hebb then went on to suggest that the "growth process" was the increased growth of synapses as they were exercised. This idea—that it is the change in synaptic conductivity that accounts for the changes in the neural network—is the basis of most physiological theories of learning and memory. Synaptic conductivity changes can account for short-term memory by invoking reverberating circuits that fade as the temporary synaptic changes lose the transient "potentiation." Long-term memories are accounted for by permanent changes in conductivity so that the information in the synaptic patterns becomes locked in. Martin, Grimwood, and Morris (2000) present a compelling argument that such synaptic changes are necessary but that "little data currently support the notion of sufficiency" (p. 649).

Hebb, nevertheless, made some remarkable speculative leaps from this foundation idea of neural networks. He postulated the existence of "cell assemblies"—a "diffuse structure" of neurons in the brain that was created as a result of use and one that could encode complex responses. To this construct he added the notion of the "phase sequence"—a series of cell assemblies that actually was the level at which "thoughts" became extant. It is important to reiterate that the empirical evidence for these hypothetical neuronal net structures is as nonexistent now as it was then.

Many contemporary scholars also followed in Hebb's footprints. In a recent debate in a popular magazine Koch and Greenfield (2007)[6] argued from two opposed speculative points of view in attempting to answer the question—"How does consciousness happen?" Their answers were almost the same but differ in one main way; Koch argues that consciousness occurs when a specific set of neurons in a specific part of the brain fires in a specific manner. Greenfield argues that the brain produces consciousness when neurons in all parts of "the brain are synchronized into coordinated assemblies, and then disband."

Both hypotheses share a common principle, what I have referred to as the second part of the basic ontological postulate—the plausible, but unsubstantiated, idea that it is the arrangement of the great neuronal networks in the brain that accounts for consciousness, their term for the mind.

The distinctive anatomical attribute that distinguishes between their two theories, on the other hand, is the degree to which the neural network of the brain producing consciousness is localized or distributed. However, they do not differ with regard to the level of analysis; both assume that it is based on the detailed state and interactions of the neuronal network of the brain.

Despite the disclaimer in Koch and Greenfield's joint paper that neither one is "is attempting to explain how consciousness arises" (p. 83), in fact both are actually operating at pretty much the same level at which Hebb was at the beginning of the neural network days. Both are proposing ingenious, but nonspecific and untestable, hypotheses that closely conform to the ontological postulates presented earlier. Both make the same foundation assumptions, and both suggest ways that such assumptions might be implemented. However, neither makes any specific statements about the details of how the neural networks produce the mind. Their speculative contributions are plausible and reasonable; however, they are without any empirical support. Koch is very explicit about this in their joint article when he says:

Neuroscience does not yet understand enough about the brain's inner workings to spell out exactly how consciousness arises from the electrical and chemical activity of neurons. Thus, the first big step is to determine the best neural correlates of consciousness (NCC)—the brain activity that matches up with specific conscious experiences. (pp. 76–77)

In this manner he retreats back to confront the traditional problems faced by all cognitive scientists. First, all of the problems faced by correlation methods are once again brought to our attention; second, the brain measures—the NCCs—to which he alludes are generally drawn from irrelevant levels of analysis such as brain images, EEGs, and other cumulative methods; and,third there is no direct access to the conscious experiences that permits us to directly compare mental and neural events. The details of the neural networks, however gracefully and eloquently expressed, are totally finessed. Indeed, with considerable justification, we may conclude that Koch and Greenfield's ideas are, perhaps, less specific than were those of Hebb!

It is in this context that the greatest misunderstanding of the current brain imaging approach becomes crystal clear. In a recent paper (Posner & Rothbart, 2007) extolling the importance of the Hebbian tradition dealing with neuronal networks, it was suggested that brain imaging "also probes neural networks that underlie all aspects of human thought, feeling and behavior" (p. 5). Unfortunately, there is a disconnect here between the Hebb *neuronal* network model and the *neural* network of brain regions at which brain imaging techniques operate: the Hebbian network is a network of *microscopic* neurons. The networks that are studied with, for example, an fMRI system, are combinations of *macroscopic* brain regions that actually tell us very little about how the brain makes the mind. Nor do brain images tell us anything about the details of the network of neurons. In fact all of the salient details of their function are lost by the processes of accumulation and summation that characterize such techniques as fMRIs and EEGs. It is entirely possible for two totally different neuronal network states to produce the same fMRI response. Thus, there is no functional relation between an fMRI image and the activity of the critical and essential network of neurons that Hebb so presciently pointed out must be the psychoneural equivalent of a cognitive process. In short, the macroscopic neural networks studied with fMRI systems are not the same as the microscopic neuronal networks that cannot (because of their complexity) be studied at all. To link them together is nothing other than a neuroscientific pun.

It should be clear now that the second part of the ontology postulate is widely, but not universally, held among cognitive neuroscientists. For reasons that have more to do with available technology than with either philosophy, logic, or empirical findings, many other theorists place the essential transformation process between brain and mind at other levels of activity such as single neurons, wavelike fields of activity, or activated chunks of the brain. These alternative hypotheses must be appreciated to be temporary surrogates for the impenetrable neuronal net hypothesis. It is the information processing by highly complex microscopic neural networks, rather than any of these alternative measures cum theories, that is the core of the foundation premise of modern cognitive neuroscience.

The main difficulty that makes the neuronal network hypothesis into a postulate (as opposed to a robust empirically observed fact) is that the combinatorial complexity of the brain's neuronal network is so extreme that it cannot be studied directly. The true psychoneural identity level of activity—the idiosyncratic and exceedingly complex interaction of so many neurons—at which brain becomes mind is computationally intractable. As a result, alternative theoretical approaches such as single-cell or field measurements are called into play simply because they are measurable with available measuring instruments. Ethologists refer to this kind of behavior as displacement activity—one does what one can when one cannot do what one should do!

Complexity being what it is, this is not necessarily a criticism of the state of our science. It is no more a problem than the relativistic limit on the speed of light or the second law of thermodynamics' prohibition of perpetual motion machines. Complexity is becoming better understood and increasingly appreciated as being supremely frustrating to the kind of scientific analysis to which cognitive neuroscientists aspire. However, it is important that we realize the implications of the inaccessibility and noncomputability of the neuronal network. These constraints have profound implications for theory and practice in cognitive neuroscience, the way it has developed, and how it will continue to do so in the future.

However widespread is the acceptance among cognitive neuroscientists of this second part of the ontological postulate—the mind is an emergent factor from the interactions among the vast number of neurons[7] that make up the brain—it must also be reiterated that there is no proof of it, and it has to be considered as an unprovable assumption rather than a provable fact. There is no empirical proof in which necessity and sufficiency of the network have been proven; nor is there any computer simulation that exhibits any of the properties of consciousness.[8] Although we cannot prove the second part of the ontological postulate, there is no plausible alternative explanation available at the present time, only details of how neurons might interact at local levels or speculations about the overall nature of the network in the style proposed by Koch and Greenfield (2007). This is why it is presented here as an ontological postulate or presumption, plausible and reasonable, but not proven and probably not provable.

This second part of the basic ontological postulate is critical (along with the practical limits of what we can do) in determining not only the nature of our theories but our day-to-day activities in the laboratory. The elusiveness of empirical answers to the question of the essential level of analysis is the basic reason that the mind-brain problem (how does the brain make the mind?) remains unanswered and why there is such an abundance of questionable theoretical speculation and flawed empirical research in this field.

Unfortunately, the presumed level of brain activity (the interactions among a vast number of neurons) at which we believe the salient information processes are carried out that become sentience, consciousness, and mental activities of all kinds is exactly the level at which our research techniques are least adequate; the most fundamental reason, as noted, being the extraordinary complexity and numerousness of the involved neurons and the idiosyncratic nature of every neuron-to-neuron interaction.

As a result, neuroscientists have turned to other techniques to provide grist for their theoretical mill. All of the most frequently used methods epitomized by the fMRI or the

EEG, however, share a common difficulty—they pool the responses from the many neurons that make up the brain into cumulative, global measures. In doing so, they lose all of the critical information about the neuron-to-neuron interactions that make up the crucial activities of the brain. All, therefore, are not operating at the level of analysis at which the predominant current opinion suggests is the one at which mind and brain activity are most closely associated—the details of the interactions between myriad individual neurons of the brain. It is a practical problem—there are just too many of them—that restricts this approach.

Another main technological alternative is the use of microelectrodes to study the action of individual neurons. This method has been a powerful tool in helping us understand the nature of the components of the neural networks of the brain (the individual neurons) but from the very narrow perspective of the one-micron-wide point of a microelectrode. However microelectrodes offer little information about the interactive organization of the great numbers of neurons that are involved in even the simplest thought. Indeed, the ability to record from a single electrode has driven a major theoretical tradition based on the idea that single neurons can encode complex cognitive processes. This theoretical hypothesis seems also to be based on a flimsy empirical foundation.

In summary, these two ideas—the general first part of the ontological postulate stating that the mind is a function of the brain and the second more specific part that it is the detailed pattern of neuronal interactions that represents or encodes mental activities and processes—with all of their uncertainties seem to be our best current answers to the mind-brain problem.

It should not be inferred that these two postulates are merely topics for philosophers to mull: they exert an enormous influence on the development of theory and the choice of experimental protocols. By so specifying the relevant level of analysis, we can see that two corollaries immediately emerge. First, assigning mind to very complex neural interactions suggests that almost all of the work that has been done and can be done in the future using brain images is aimed at the wrong level of analysis. Because the old phrenological idea of localized cognitive process encoding modular cognitive processes also seems to be on its last legs, it can be expected that attempts to correlate cognition[9] with brain images will also diminish just as the enthusiasm for the EEG as an entrée into the mind has moderated over the years. Rather than these cumulative, pooled, and integrated signals, we should be attending, if we could, to the detailed patterns of activity of a myriad of neuronal interactions.[10]

Second, the computational and combinatorial aspects of the neuronal net hypothesis suggest that the problem as posed by the ontological postulates is intractable. The best that can be hoped for is that there will be some neural correlates of cognitive processes observed with these integrated global measures that may serve as useful biological markers in certain restricted situations (box 1.2).

To summarize, the main point made here is that a priori no macroscopic brain imaging or electrical recording activity, no matter how direct it may seem to be in recording the activity of the brain, can *in principle* provide solutions to the mind-brain problem. The basic

Box 1.2

Two Corollaries of the Basic Ontological Postulate

> 1. Brain imaging techniques are formulated at the wrong level of analysis and thus cannot provide answers to the mind-brain problem.
> 2. The neuronal network approach is computationally intractable and thus cannot provide answers to the mind-brain problem.

reason for this conceptual barrier is that the current technology used by these methods is operating at the wrong level of analysis. Whereas brain imaging produces cumulative signals, the essence of the mind is more likely to be found in the microdetails of idiosyncratic neuronal interactions. This clash is between the innumerable states of a discrete network and a single cumulative state in which all of these microscopic activities have been pooled at the cost of great information loss.

In the section that follows, I show how these basic postulates can have a far-reaching effect on our thinking about the relation between the mind and the brain.

1.3 Implications of the Ontological Postulate

This section is concerned with the implications of the two parts of the ontological postulate; first the brain is the organ of mind, and, second, the level of analysis at which that equivalence is manifested is to be found in the details of the great network of interacting neurons. Of the first part, little more need be said. One is either a monistic physical materialist or one is a nonmaterialist dualist.[11] If one denies the idea expressed in this part of the postulate, then the whole enterprise of cognitive psychology is a meaningless and uncontrollable mess. For purely theoretical reasons, the second part of the ontological postulate should be the focus of the entire cognitive neuroscience enterprise. That it is not is due to the practical problems dealing with its great complexity.

1.3.1 Implication for Philosophy

Dualism comes in many guises: one can resort to theology or such traditional philosophical concepts as Descartes's substance dualism, Geulincx's and Malebranche's occasionalism, or Leibniz's parallelism, on the one hand, or turn to more modern ideas such as Eccles's tripartite reality, Chalmers's naturalistic, or Kripke's versions of dualism, as well as certain interpretations of Davidson's supervenience.[12]

The adoption of any of these dualistic stances by some philosophers, although this point is likely to be disputed, is inconsistent with the whole motivation behind cognitive neuroscience. It seems completely illogical to expect that one could carry out experiments attempting to study the mind-brain relation guided by the presumption that they represented two different kinds of reality. To suggest that mind and brain, in fact, are not causally or otherwise intimately related to the degree of identity or equivalence would invalidate the very essence of cognitive neuroscience.

This then brings us to the second part of the ontological postulates. Having accepted the proposition that the mind and the brain are two parts of the same basic reality, what more can be said about the specific nature of that relation? The answer to this query, the second part of the ontological postulate asserts, is that they are related in the way that a mechanism and its function are related. In this particular case the ontological assertion is that the salient mechanism is the intricate interconnection pattern of the myriad of neurons that make up the great networks of the brain. This level of analysis is complex and is probably beyond analysis and specific explanation for the reasons I have already mentioned. Indeed, it may represent an intractable problem that neither new measuring devices nor computational engines can ever begin to unravel. There are too many uncertainties, too many neurons, too many idiosyncratic interconnections (e.g., the brain is not neatly organized as is a simple crystalline structure) for us to ever be able to understand its detailed organization and how, specifically, this complex information pattern produces the reality we call mind.

This approach has profound implications for understanding what cognitive neuroscience has achieved and what still remains mysterious and unknown. If we are to accept the second part of the ontological postulate, then almost all of the other approaches to studying the relation between the mind and the brain are being carried out at the wrong level of analysis.

For compelling practical and historical reasons neuroscientists have turned to other more global measures such as the EEG, the ERP, and most recently the brain imaging procedures such as fMRI and PET. All of these methods, however, share a common difficulty—they pool the responses from the many neurons that make up the brain into cumulative, global measures. In doing so, they lose all of the critical information that makes up the salient activities of the brain. All, therefore, are not operating at the level of analysis at which the predominant current opinion suggests is the one at which mind and brain activity are most closely associated.

If this analysis is correct, then all of the work using the molar, integrated, cumulative measures of brain activity is misdirected, and the resulting findings must be considered to be irrelevant in the search for solutions to the mind-brain problem. This is as serious an impediment to scientific understanding as acceptance of dualism would be.

There is implicit in these comments another important and essential point—the fact that it is the pattern of information transactions, not the biochemistry of individual neurons, that accounts for the emergence of consciousness or mind. For example, although we know a lot about the biochemistry of the neuron and of the synapse and can explain the details of the transfer of information along an axon or from cell to cell, these are properties of the microscopic components of the nervous system; the particular technology is not essential to an information-processing system's function. By themselves, therefore, these properties tell us little about the mind-brain problem—only about the details of the particular bio-chemical mechanisms of the components of which the brain is made. Just as a material from which a transistor is made tells us nothing about the program that is being run on a computer, even the most detailed knowledge of the biochemistry of a neuron tells us nothing about how the overall system is representing mental processes. In some unlikely ideal world, should we be able to build a brain-like structure capable of mimicking all of the complex informational processes and interactions, albeit with a completely different technology than the sodium-potassium-chloride chemistry our brains use, such a system would presumably be able to "think" or "perceive" as well as we do and may even be "con-scious." The point is that it does not matter what component technological units are being used; only the arrangement and interactions of those elements are of consequence in rep-resenting "mind."

This, then brings us to the next step in this preliminary philosophical study of the nature of mind-brain reality—that of the epistemology of cognitive neuroscience. That is, how can we know (i.e., what strategies can we use to learn about) the critical mind-brain interactions. Epistemologists have different goals and consider different topics then do ontologists. Rather than contemplating what is, they are concerned with the limits on our ability to know what is; that is, given postulates such as those proposed by the ontologists, what does this mean to our ability to study the mind-brain problem (among many others) and to understand, to learn, to describe, or to explain the properties of the mind and the brain. In other words, what is it logically possible for psychologists to do given the ontological pos-tulates as starting points?

Few practicing experimental psychologists or cognitive neuroscientists struggle with such questions. They go about their various projects questioning only how data can be gathered or explained. Their epistemology is an empirical one; decisions are made on the basis of what works or what appears to work—their epistemology is an unredeemably practical one. Nevertheless, they, too, are bound by the epistemological constraints. More or less implicitly, without overt awareness, all cognitive neuroscientists and psychologists constantly make certain practical assumptions within this context of unspoken and implicit epistemological conundrums about what they can learn from their experiments.

In the following pages I distinguish between those epistemological issues that guide psychology and those that guide the neuroreductionist efforts of cognitive neuroscientists.

1.3.2 Implications for Psychology

To understand how the two ontological postulates affect the course of scientific psychology, it is important to express a major epistemological principle (box 1.3). Before dealing with the impact of this postulate on psychology, I must consider a very special idea—accessibility and its antithesis, inaccessibility. The issue being dealt with here is how much access do we have to mental processes? Can we gain access to (i.e., measure) the nature of mental

Box 1.3

The First Epistemological Postulate for Psychology

> Mental processes are private and are not accessible to any form of measurement, either experimental or introspective.

processes, or are we forever constrained from any direct measurement of the mind? Let me now spell out in detail some of the arguments for both of the two interpretations.

Arguments for Inaccessibility

The argument for the inaccessibility of the mind revolves around the fact that the mind, by definition, is a private personal experience. Since there is no detailed explanation (beyond the second part of the ontological postulate) of the relation between the physical structure and processes of the brain and our individual and private experience of being, sentience, or awareness, there is no instrument that we can attach to or scan the head that will directly measure mental processes. As many psychologists have written previously, mind is an *intrapersonal* and not an *interpersonal* phenomenon. The only possible way that we can begin to get any, however defective, insight into the mind of another person is by means of that individual's introspective reports or by observing that person's behavior.

However, both introspection and drawing inferences from behavioral observation are well known to be deeply flawed methodologies. Researchers such as Nisbett and Wilson (1977) had shown four decades ago that people are not aware of their own logical processes and mental strategies. The reasons for this introspective blindness are manifold but include false memory construction (Loftus, 1996) and the automatic (i.e., unconscious or preconscious) nature of many behavioral processes (Bargh, 1997). Whatever the reasons, and there are many others, it is clear that people cannot always accurately report the logic or reasons they used to arrive at a decision. For some phenomena, for example those associated with the basic qualitative state of such experiences as color or pitch, it is not possible to reconstruct with words what it is that a person is experiencing. Introspection, therefore, must be ruled out as an effective means of accessing mental states.

The main alternative means of accessing mental states is to draw indirect inferences from publically observable behavior. However this strategy, too, is deeply flawed. The reasons behind this assertion are equally numerous and include these:

• There is a well-known engineering principle (that holds for human behavior as well as pieces of electronic equipment) that the inner workings of an unopened "black box" cannot be determined by comparing the box's input to its output. The relation between input and output cannot in principle tell us anything definitive about the functional changes that may be occurring in the box. This is well known to engineers and should be to psychologists.

• The reason for this generalization is that the mechanism inside either a piece of hardware or the human mind is underdetermined by the behavioral observation. That is, there is not enough information in behavior to precisely and uniquely determine inner mechanisms. There are many possible (and far too many plausible) explanations for each behavioral observation. No convergence of observations can lead to an answer to the problem of internal structure. Indeed, additional observation often leads to even more plausible and possible explanations than had been contemplated originally.

• Human behavior is characterized by enormous variability when compared to other sciences. Individual results are not sufficiently repeatable. Therefore, there remains a serious question concerning the reliability as well as the validity of many psychological measurements.

• Human behavior is not bound by robust, stable, universal laws of time, space, and number in the way physical phenomena are. There is, therefore, no way that an entirely external observation can be associated with an inaccessible experience. Physics can generally do this, but its success depends on the assumption that the laws of physics are the same everywhere—in the internal microscopic world as well as distant macroscopic universes.[13]

• Behavior, as expressed in the literature of experimental psychology is not adequately linked to the associated mental activities. People can intentionally or unintentionally display behavior that is quite contrary to what they are really thinking. Questionnaires, stage plays, and the courtroom all present examples that illustrate how separated one's thoughts can be from one's utterances. Even the best experimental protocols do not provide robust constraints or necessarily even plausible links between behavior and the underlying thoughts.

• Mental faculties and components are "hypothetical constructs" (MacCorquodale & Meehl, 1948) created by psychologists to describe behavior and, therefore, may not exist in some physical or psychobiological sense.

• Finally, the complexities of both behavior and the neuronal mechanism are so great that there is no computational way in which they can be linked. There is no one-to-one correspondence among measurable behavior, mental activity, and brain responses.

Arguments for Accessibility

The honorable epistemological opposition argues that these arguments are too stringent and demanding and that much is lost when we limit ourselves by assuming mental inaccessibility. Although the words may differ in the many arguments, the ubiquitous core argument for accessibility is that consciousness exists, and without assuming accessibility we would be denied any hope of measuring and explaining it. By denying accessibility, they argue, we lose one of the main raisons d'être of psychological science as well as basic matters of our own humanity. In any event proponents of accessibility argue that the links between mind and behavior are solid enough for us to draw good inferences.

Herein lies the core of the greatest debate in psychology—the one between behaviorism and cognitive mentalism. It is here that the empirical and theoretical strategies of these two great schools of psychological thought diverge. My argument in the present context is that they so diverge primarily because of their differing stances on the epistemological question—are the process and activities of the mind accessible?

The issue has been debated for many years, and the opposing answers to it are based on beliefs and assumptions more comparable to ontological and epistemological speculation than on any empirical evidence. On one side of the debate are those who traditionally have been called mentalists and more recently cognitive mentalists. Mentalism is based on an initial epistemological assumption asserting that mind is sufficiently directly accessible to be studied by introspective or experimental assay techniques. Behaviorists, in opposition, accept that the mind is not directly accessible and, therefore, that we can only observe and measure the final outcome of mental activity—behavior. From that point the respective strategies of the two approaches to the study of the problems of interest to psychology are set in a conceptual concrete.

The arguments for and against behaviorism and mentalism, respectively, can be summed up in the following brief lists abstracted from my earlier work (Uttal, 2000).

The Essential Arguments against Mentalism
1. There is a lack of public availability, objectivity, and repeatability for metaphysical or mental processes.
2. Mentalism leads to homunculus or infinite regression arguments.
3. Mentalism produces unprovable hypothetical constructs.
4. The empirical data argue against the accessibility of mental processes.
5. Mentalism requires complex experimental designs and unprovable assumptions that produce fragile data.
6. Mentalism arises because of the vested interests of its humanist, theological, and personal protagonists or from the professional needs of psychotherapists.

The Essential Arguments against Behaviorism
1. There is only a limited range of behaviorist psychology.
2. Behaviorism dehumanizes humans.
3. Behaviorism is too "mechanical" or is "not sufficiently mechanical."
4. Behaviorism is not a step forward.
5. Behaviorism overemphasizes the environment and underemphasizes heredity as a source of behavior.
6. Behaviorism is nothing more than common sense.
7. Behaviorism is antidemocratic.
8. Behaviorism is antireligious.

Clearly, none of these arguments is compelling by itself. They all depend in large part on an original decision to accept or reject accessibility. Having said that, it is important not to try to finesse this issue, but, instead, to take the bull by the horns and make a value judgment. In my opinion most of the arguments against behaviorism and its attendant inaccessibility are wishes and hopes rather than scientific arguments. They dote on humanistic judgments about the desirability of understanding the human condition.

The arguments against mentalism, on the other hand, have a greater degree of scientific robustness and support (or are supported by) the idea of inaccessibility. Without any question, however, it is the acceptance or denial of the epistemological postulate of accessibility that directs and guides one to either behaviorism or mentalism. My opinion is that psychology would be better off scientifically being behaviorist rather then mentalist. I go so far as to make it an epistemological postulate asserting my preference for behaviorism (box 1.4).

There is another way in which these two postulates impact on thinking in psychology. Because, according to the second part of the ontological postulate and the first epistemological postulate, the brain level at which mind is embodied is that of the great and unanalyzable neural network and that mental processes are not directly accessible, there are few constraints on how we might assume the mind-brain to be structured. Coupled with the great complexity of the system, this means that we are relatively unfettered in making certain further assumptions concerning the nature of the organization of the mind-brain. Two of these assumptions stand out in the history of psychology—separability and analyzability. Because we cannot deal with the whole complex system with all of its interacting parts and variables at once, we fall back on Descartes's admonition to break the system into parts. This leads to two extremely potent, but highly questionable, governing assumptions. The first is that the mind is modular; that it is made up of quasi-independent units—the faculties and processes that are explored in conventional psychological experiments. The second is that the neural equivalents of these mental modules are located in particular parts of the brain.

Throughout the history of cognitive psychology and its predecessors, up to and including the early days of the brain imaging movement, experiments have been based on these two assumptions. The search was on—find the areas of the brain that were activated by such cognitive processes as "solve a problem," "decide which candidate you prefer," "think about a loved one," or "think about a cow." As the discussion in this book progresses it will become clear that modularization and localization are no longer tenable interpretations. In their place two alternative statements must be substituted. First, mental components cannot be

Box 1.4

The Second Epistemological Postulate for Psychology

> Psychology is better served by a behaviorist approach that dotes on the observable parameters of human activity rather than the inferences of a reductionist mentalism.

analyzed into independent and separable cognitive modules; to do so in a Cartesian sense belies the interactive complexity of our thoughts. It is likely that we will begin to realize the mental modules represent a convenient organizing principle but do not necessarily reflect the actual nature of our mental activities. Because compelling evidence for neither modularization nor holism is yet available, I also characterize this idea as an epistemological postulate (box 1.5).[14]

1.3.3 Implications for Neuroscience

Just as the choice of one's theoretical psychological stance depends on certain assumptions about the accessibility and modularity of the mind, the choice of one's neuroreductionist stance depends on the second part of the ontological postulate—that the instantiation of the mind is to be found in the actions and interactions of the many neurons of the great networks in the brain.

There is rapidly accumulating empirical evidence that the range of brain regions involved in even the simplest thought is widely distributed throughout the brain as summarized as The First Epistemological Postulate for Neuroscience (box 1.6). This assertion, however, is much less speculative and represents the first of the postulates driving neuroscientific research.

As these holist ideas (the mind must be treated more as a whole than as a system of separable modules, and the brain activities associated with a thought are widely distributed) have increasingly begun to percolate into experiment and theory, the epistemological situation has gotten much worse. A diffusely distributed system is not conceptually simpler than a system of discrete nodes. Furthermore, distribution complicates the search for an objective neural correlate of any behavioral activity. Since multiple regions are involved, distribution has led to the use of complex pattern recognition analysis methods that were far more challenging and the results of which were far less certain than those based on the

Box 1.5

The Third Epistemological Postulate for Psychology

> Although convenient as a means of experimental protocol simplification, mental processes are not modular and cannot be divided up into quasi-independent entities.

Box 1.6

The First Epistemological Postulate for Neuroscience

> Brain activity associated with mental activity is broadly distributed on and in the brain. The idea of phrenological localization must be rejected and replaced with a theory of broadly distributed neural systems accounting for our mental activity.[15]

simple modular and localizationist ideas of the past. Some investigators (e.g., Hilgetag, O'Neil, & Young, 1996) have suggested that the situation is actually much worse than just being "more complicated." They argued that the analysis of a heavily interconnected system of cooperating and interacting regions in the manner cognitive neuroscience may require might not be possible in fundamental principle. Instead, they argue that the situation would get increasingly complicated (not less so) as more and more experiments are carried out.

Brain images, it must be clearly understood, still provide us only with the capability to search for highly variable locales of activation that may be associated with vaguely defined cognitive processes. It is important to remember that no matter how complex the analysis, brain images essentially search only for answers to the "where" question. The essence of the mind-brain problem, however, is still the "how" question, and it is not yet clear just what the "where" question tells us about the mind-brain problem.

Just as it is necessary to invoke an additional epistemological postulate in order to understand the roots of psychology, it is also necessary to invoke another basic assumption to define one's approach to neuroscience. In the case of psychology, as I noted earlier, the additional epistemological assumption concerns the inaccessibility of the intrapersonal events we designate as mental. Depending on one's choice, it was a more or less logical progression from the respective assumptions of accessibility or inaccessibility to the kind of empirical and theoretical research to be pursued. If one accepted the intrinsic arguments for inaccessibility, the challenges to cognitive psychology were not just practical but of deep principle; inaccessibility denied even the hope of a remote future in which we might find some way to even indirectly measure the attributes of the mind.

The comparable supplemental epistemological assumption underlying modern cognitive neuroscience, however, is a practical one rather than one of deep principle. It is the respective answer to the query—is it possible to measure or examine the details of the neural network that is the basic psychoneural equivalent of mental activity? This supplementary epistemological postulate for neuroscience can be formalized as shown in box 1.7. Although this postulate may well run counter to the current Zeitgeist, a strong argument supporting this postulate can be made based on combinatoric arguments.

Inherent in any such postulate, of course, is the possibility that, at some unforeseeable future time, unexpected developments may make possible what is currently impossible in

Box 1.7
The Second Epistemological Postulate for Neuroscience

> Because of their great complexity and number, it is not possible for us to analyze the great neuronal networks of the brain in a way that would permit us to identify the neural equivalent of any kind of mental activity at this microscopic level of analysis.

practice. Nevertheless, the reality today is that there is no practical way to analyze such a complex and irregular network, and some mathematical arguments concerning combinatorics and computability strongly suggest that this is a reasonable working rule for the near and perhaps even for the far-distant future.

What are these arguments supporting the second epistemological postulate for neuroscience? Some of them are these:

• The kinds of network problems that are observed in the brain are known to be computationally intractable *in practice*. They are not infinitely complex (which would introduce an *in principle* constraint) but merely so consuming of any conceivable computational power that they could never be solved. This is equivalent to what complexity theorists call an NP complete problem, a problem that cannot be solved in any determined amount of time.
• Few of our neural network simulations scale up. That is, the simple models we are able to program onto a computer typically fall apart or saturate in one way or another when we try to increase the number of interacting simulated neurons beyond a few hundred.
• Efforts to simplify the difficulties inherent in these problems (e.g., by assuming regularity, adding additional nonbiological constraints, or by breaking it up into smaller parts) do not work.[16]

There are really no good counterarguments to these practical constraints on understanding the neuronal basis of the mind. What actually happens is that investigators implicitly accept the limitations and then turn to alternative experimental and theoretical strategies. They implicitly accept the monumental barriers to the direct evaluations of these complex neuronal networks and utilize whatever measuring devices are available (e.g., the EEG or the fMRI), whether or not these devices are operating at the appropriate level of analysis. In so doing, often without realizing it, they are accepting the unanalyzability of the neuronal network—the second epistemological postulate for neuroscience—and opt for some alternate, but questionable, strategy that does not even promise to answer the essential mind-brain problem. It is important to point out again that this does not imply an "in principle" rejection of the second ontological assumption; instead it is simply a practical and necessary response to the fact that studying the microdetails of the neuronal network is not an effective strategy.

1.4   Some Relevant Conceptual Issues

1.4.1   The Seductive Attractiveness of Brain Images

A major issue in cognitive neuroscience concerning the use of brain images such as the fMRI is that their impact on our science may be far more than they deserve. That is, we are seduced by the pretty pictures and the seeming "face validity" that these images seem to offer. For example it is now established (McCabe & Castel, 2008) that people are more likely to accept the credibility of a published report when a brain image rather than an informationally equivalent graph or table is used. Roskies (2008) referred to brain images as perpetuating an "illusion of inferential proximity" that makes us feel we know something about something that, in fact, actually remains inscrutable.[17]

Weisberg, Keil, Goodstein, Rawsdon, and Gray (2008), arguing in a similar vein, suggested that neuroscientific information itself, even if it is not relevant, made a theory more acceptable than when that kind of information was withheld. This effect was maximum when the judging subjects were not expert in the field beings discussed. These authors warned especially against the problems posed for nonexperts in evaluating neuroscience information added as decorations to scientific story.

The point is that the attractiveness and the seeming, but illusory, directness of these images give them a conceptual and scientific impact that they may not entirely deserve. Their charm, their novelty, and their pictorial splendor tend to overwhelm critical consideration of the serious epistemological issues revolving around the limits of what these images can actually tell us. It is only in recent years that the empirical facts have begun to raise further questions about some of the facile misinterpretations of their meaning.

It can be argued that the widespread and uncritical acceptance of the brain image as a measuring tool of cognitive processes is based on a widespread misunderstanding of the actual progress that has been made in linking results from the two fields. Although cognitive neuroscience journals have been flooded with publication of what are often very preliminary reports, the neural basis of cognition and the neural activity depicted by brain images operate at vastly different conceptual levels. We do not yet understand what either of these differences means or how we might link them together.

In short, there is no theory or putative explanation that yet explains how mental processes emerge from neural ones. There is, instead, an emerging corpus of scientific opinion that the mind-brain problem is intractable due to the complexity of the neural interconnections that actually lie at its core. The misunderstanding that we have made more progress on this fundamental issue than we have is also exacerbated by the hyperbolic and exaggerated popularization of very preliminary or unsubstantiated scientific findings by the press and the lay community.

1.4.2   The Problem of Defining Mental Processes

One of the most serious impediments to unraveling the mind-brain problem is that mental states are very difficult to precisely define. In fact many of the cognitive processes that we wish to correlate with either surgical interventions or brain images are merely neologisms for experimental results or hypothetical constructs used to flesh out some speculative psychological theory. To compare the objective neurological data with such poorly defined, and often arbitrary, mental entities stretches logical analysis to its limits. The actual connection is so loose that it is all too easy to carry out what are, in retrospect, misleading comparisons. It is also possible in systems as complex as this to find empirical support for almost any theory.

The problem is that the history of psychology is filled with a huge vocabulary for a large number of different psychological faculties, traits, or modules. Yet there has been no clear development of a coherent taxonomy or classification system for psychology comparable to the Linnaean one in biology or Mendeleev's in chemistry. Instead, idiosyncratic and obscure terms come and go as psychologists suggest new hypothetical entities, study them until they are no longer of interest, and then move on to some other topic. Words like "acquisitiveness" or "ego" have now been replaced by such equally vague concepts as "consciousness" or "attention." Only operationally defined terms such as "reaction time" or "percent correct" tell us anything and then only about the behavior of the organism.

The issue of definition becomes extremely vexing when a comparison is made between a mental activity and a brain response, especially if it is uncertain just what mental processes are being invoked and how such obscure processes as "attention" and "perception" actually are different or independent of each other (if they are). The point is that it becomes difficult to locate in the material brain what are little more than hypothetical constructs or tags attached to experimental protocols.

This issue raises serious practical problems of interpretation in any mental process–brain response comparison. For example, a study purportedly of people's preferences for a cola or a political candidate may end up measuring a brain response that has nothing directly to do with our preferences per se but may be measuring some subtle aspect of a general emotional response or of some previous experience. This misdirection to an irrelevant aspect of the cognitive state plays havoc with any attempt to use a brain image as an indicator of mental activity as well as any effort to develop a coherent theory of mind-brain relations.

In a more general sense, it raises questions about the validity of any purported neural measure of any cognitive process. If there is always the possibility (because of poor definitions) that we are measuring something other than what we thought we were, no matter how reliable the findings, those findings may be theoretically meaningless. In short, poor definition of mental entities degrades the validity of any neural correlations with those nebulous cognitive processes. To note that it also makes independent stimulus control more difficult is simply to restate the obvious.

1.4.3   The One-to-Many Issue

It is becoming increasingly clear that many different cognitive processes can activate the same area or system of areas of the brain. (For example, see the work of Culham & Kanwisher, 2001.) Thus, if the available findings are limited to answers to questions about "where" a response is occurring, it is theoretically impossible to exclusively associate any particular brain activation site or pattern of activation with any particular cognitive state. In the words of Poldrack (2006), it is extremely difficult because the putative location of a cognitive module is not unique, to use "reverse inference" to assign specific mental meanings to even the most discrete and reliable brain activations. Any attempt to do so, according to Poldrack, is "deductively invalid." He goes on to say that it "still can provide some information," but this depends on the empirical "selectivity of activation" (p. 59).

This is a very important, but largely overlooked, point. It raises severe limitations for any attempt to "read a person's mind" by measuring brain responses. First, multiple functionality of single brain regions disassociates specific brain responses from particular cognitive processes as a matter of principle. That is, activation in any particular brain region cannot be solely assigned to any particular cognitive process when that brain area is involved in representing many different cognitive processes.

Second, the one-to-many problem adds to the practical difficulty of assigning either qualitative or quantitative significance to what are often only modest correlations in brain image-cognitive process comparisons. No matter how carefully an experimenter controls the salient experimental variables,[18] there must necessarily always be other forces operating to modulate the response of a given brain region. Efforts to use brain imaging in legal proceedings as a "lie detector" to mitigate culpability are invalidated from the outset by this principle.

1.4.4   The Many-to-One Issue

Just as the fact that many psychological tasks and stimuli can simultaneously activate a single brain region (and, therefore, we cannot in principle say that any particular neural activity or place is a unique indicator of any particular kind of mental activity), it must also be remembered that it is likely that many behaviors or cognitive processes may be instantiated by a number of different and redundant brain mechanisms. We have little knowledge about the full range of brain regions that may be equivalent or substitutable for each other. However, we do have plenty of evidence that many different regions of the brain are activated during any kind of cognitive task. Furthermore, we also know that under extreme conditions (such as damage due to ischemic stroke) some regions of the brain are capable of taking over functions of damaged regions. Whether or not this redundancy under the extreme conditions of a stroke is also implicitly or explicitly present under normal conditions remains an important question for cognitive neuroscience.

The potential for redundant representation strongly suggests that cognitive processes need not be encoded by the same neural mechanisms in different people. Just as there are different cognitive strategies to solve a particular problem, it is probably the case that many different brain regions or clusters of brain regions may account for a particular behavioral outcome. This is what we refer to as the many-to-one principle. This is also what is meant by the general underdeterminative nature of behavioral responses—behavior cannot tell us what brain mechanism is active just as activations of brain regions do not tell us which mental process is active. Behavior by itself is neutral with regard to underlying mechanisms.

This limitation on our understanding is also known, as I have discussed earlier, as the "black box problem." To know precisely what mechanism is inside the black box, one must open the box. Unfortunately, for mind-brain theorists, even after imaging the brain, the complexity of the system and the variability of the responses are so great that our path to understanding is blocked by another kind of virtual "closeness"—complexity.

1.4.5 The Sign-Code Distinction

Over the years (starting with Uttal, 1967) I have repeatedly pointed out that there are two possible meanings—signs and codes—of the correlated neurophysiological responses that are obtained when one compares brain activity to cognitive processes. A "sign" is a correlate of brain activity that indicates that something is happening neurophysiologically, but it is only a candidate to be the "psychoneural equivalent" of the associated mental activity. That is, a sign may be correlated neural activity in response to stimulus or mental task. However, it has not been established that it is *the* neural activity that specifically results in or *is* the cognitive experience itself. It does not encode, represent, or in any way is it the equivalent of the mental experience. All that a sign does is to tell us that there is a recordable brain response to some stimulus or cognitive state.

A sign may be used in powerful ways to measure some property of brain activity and possibly even someday serve as a biomarker of some dysfunctional cognitive activity. However, it does not necessarily explain or represent the mechanism by means of which brain activity is transmuted into mental activity. In short, the concept of a sign reminds us that not all neural responses recorded from the brain are psychobiologically relevant.

On the other hand I have designated a correlated neurological response that *is* the psychoneural equivalent of some mental activity as a "code." A code is a measure of neural activity that is the actual mechanism of whatever cognitive process is being manipulated. It is the necessary and sufficient mechanism, not merely a concomitant or correlated sign, of some mental activity. In short, it is the neural activity whose activity *is* the mental activity.

Distinguishing between a sign and a code is not an easy task given that either may correlate highly with brain activity. To determine that something is a code requires that we prove both its necessity and its sufficiency, an empirical task of considerable difficulty. Clearly, because the requirements for a code are so high, there are very few that have been robustly identified in the cognitive neuroscience literature beyond the transmission codes of the sensory and motor systems. The study of higher-level cognitive processes remains virtually untouched by such progress.

It now seems clear that most of the molar,correlated brain responses, whether they are EEGs or fMRIs, are signs. In fact, as some scholars have pointed out, brain images tell us little more than that there is some brain activity when our minds are active, an idea that is hardly surprising given the ontological postulates discussed earlier. However, as far as specifying the specific neural processes that are the coded equivalents of mind, virtually all such cumulative measures of brain activity are bankrupt. The persisting question is—what does knowing what part of the brain is activated by some stimulus or task tell us about how that part might encode mental activity?

1.5   Some Relevant Technical Issues

The conceptual, occasionally philosophical, issues discussed in the previous sections raise serious questions about the applicability of brain imaging devices to the measurement of cognitive processes. There are, in addition, a number of purely technical issues that complicate the matter further. These issues and challenges arise not because of any subtle logical or epistemological uncertainties but because of well-documented and tangible issues with the day-to-day details of using brain imaging devices to conduct research on cognitive processes. The technical issues collectively also provide serious challenges to any optimism to the use of brain imaging as a means of evaluating such poorly defined psychological faculties as learning, attention, perception, personality, thinking, intelligence, level of learning, decision making, or other complex, high-level cognitive states. The following paragraphs discuss some of the technical issues that still bedevil research efforts to correlate brain images and cognitive states.

1.5.1   Cumbersome Procedures

However beautiful a colorful brain image may eventually turn out to be, it is the final result of a massive investment in time and money. The PET system, for example, not only requires the detector system itself, but also a radioisotope- generating capability to produce the injectable radioactive materials and a computer facility to process the raw data from that detector. (The medical and ethical issues of using such an invasive procedure, furthermore, should not be minimized.)

The complexity and expense of MRI systems are also well appreciated, but the major issue of invasiveness associated with the PET procedure is largely overcome by MRI systems. Functional MRIs are totally noninvasive; no one has ever shown any deleterious physical effects from the large magnetic fields used to orient the protons of the body's atoms other than being hit by an errant piece of metal attracted by the powerful magnetic fields surrounding the device. Nevertheless, there are a number of practical issues in their use that also make the process cumbersome, complicated, and expensive.

It takes an extended period of time to produce a single fMRI image with most current techniques. Furthermore, subjects must cooperate to an extreme degree including remaining motionless and attending to a single cognitive theme for the duration of the measurement in what can be an acoustically noisy and highly constricted environment. Even the slightest head or respiratory movements can distort the final image (Raz et al., 2005). Furthermore, because of the extended time required to collect the data in an fMRI-based experiment, the number of subjects is usually relatively low compared to behavioral evaluations.

Perhaps most significant, however, is the remarkable lack of control over the cognitive tasks that serve as the independent variables in experiments comparing cognitive states and brain images—a lack of control that is also the bane of many psychology researchers. It is not always possible to know that the instructions to carry out a specific cognitive activity are being followed. Both effortful (is the subject trying to play some other game than that designed by the experimenter?) and inadvertent (did the subject not understand the instructions?) actions can lead to a lack of control of both the experimental and control conditions.

1.5.2 The Subtraction Issue

Although there have been recent improvements in quantification of the responses obtained with brain imaging devices, the basic research paradigm remains: determine how the brain response differs when a subject is thinking about "nothing" (the control condition) and when the subject is carrying out a specified mental task (the experimental condition). Examples of the latter are making a decision, carrying out mental arithmetic, or thinking about a specific object such as a "cow." The general procedure is to subtract the control condition ("don't think about a cow") from the experimental condition ("think about a cow"). The idea is that only the salient aspects of the response will show up in the difference image; all irrelevant and unchanging portions will disappear because they remain the same and sum to nothing. Despite the array of modern statistical approaches and analytic methods for producing a brain image, in the final analysis it is the subtractive difference between the control and experimental conditions that is the methodological kernel of this or, for that matter, any other cognitive neuroscience experiment using imaging techniques. The frailties of this kind of subtractive logic have been more or less obvious to many investigators in the field since Van Orden and Paap's (1997) cogent criticism, but many still ignore its basic limitation. Most important of all is the fact that the resulting brain images are themselves the cumulative activity of uncountable numbers of neuronal responses. Thus, the observation that an area may null out and leave no trace in the difference image does not mean that its detailed activity was the same in both the experimental and control conditions. The nature of the underlying neuronal network state may change considerably and still produce zero difference scores. Furthermore, the logic of the subtraction process can be subverted because it is highly likely that the detailed activity in two sequential (i.e., the control and experimental) conditions would be different simply because time had elapsed between the two measurements.

However, there is something even more basic and fundamental at work here that should perplex anyone using the subtraction method. The assumption that the baseline conditions during the "control" condition remain stable is highly questionable. In an article that deserves much wider attention, Stark and Squire (2001) pointed out that one possible control condition—what was supposed to be the inactive rest period between experimental conditions—was highly unstable in learning experiments. That is, what were assumed to be repeatable baseline conditions that one could subtract from the experimental condition were, in fact, very variable. Stark and Squire pointed out that in some experimental protocols (those involving the medial temporal lobe among others) it was possible for the baseline rest condition to be so variable that it could actually change the sign of the difference between the control and the experimental activations.

Closely related to this problem with the subtraction process is the prevailing but erroneous idea that the brain is inactive when not involved in mental activity. The whole thrust of the subtraction process is that no change in the activation pattern indicates no difference in the salient neural activity. In a recent article Raichle (2010) summarized the earlier discovery (Binder et al., 1999; Fransson, 2006) of the "default" mode—extensive amounts of brain activity during rest. Raichle pointed out that "60 to 80% of all energy used by the brain—occurs in circuits unrelated to any external event" (p. 47). If this is so, it raises questions about what the absence of an activation measured with an fMRI machine actually means in terms of the blood oxygen level dependent (BOLD) level itself and the fundamental idea that blood oxygenation varies with neural activity in the way we thought it did. What the concept of resting or default activity further raises is that this ongoing activity is being confounded with the evoked activations! If the subtraction method is thus flawed and BOLD measurements are associated not only with stimulus-evoked neural activity but also with background activity, the whole edifice of this kind of brain imaging could be called into question.

It must also be appreciated that whatever advanced data-processing techniques (for example, multidimensional scaling or general linear models) are used to analyze the effects of a number of different variables are only methods that help to organize the data; they are not reductive analyses of the anatomy or structure of the involved brain mechanisms. (This insightful comment has been attributed to Professor Anne Anastasi.)

If one adds to this situation the problems of the loss of information when one pools data and the fact that different regions of the brain may interact by reinforcing, inhibiting, or disinhibiting another region's response, it is clear that we are confronting a tangle that at least a few of us now believe to be bordering on the inscrutable and unanalyzable. The bottom line is that the basic subtraction method is so deeply flawed that it makes much of the research using this method highly questionable.

1.5.3 The Paucity of Quantification

Another major issue faced by any investigator who wishes to use brain image responses as indicators of changes in behavior (for example, degree of learning) is that the magnitude of most brain images and measures has not yet been adequately related quantitatively to the cognitive responses these images are supposed to measure. Indeed, it may not be possible to do so. There are many discontinuities, thresholds, multiple influences, and nonlinearities that make it extremely difficult to use variations in brain image contrast as a quantitative scale of cognitive activity. Because of the many factors that can distort the amplitude of the fMRI signal, there is a paucity in the literature of results in which the magnitude of the brain image response has been used as a scale of different levels of either activation or cognitive activity. In most cases the brain image is used as an indication of where something is occurring rather than how much of that activity is occurring.

Specific calibrated values for the extent and magnitude of the brain response are regularly confounded by the arbitrary choice of thresholds at which focal responses are accepted as being biologically significant. So far, because the brain image device is primarily used to determine the location of activations, and because the brain responses are magnified or suppressed in a highly nonlinear manner, it will be extremely difficult to directly relate the amplitude of a brain response to the subjective magnitude of a perception or the degree of learning a subject has achieved.[19] The best we can do is to say that this or that brain area may be involved in some way.

A typical approach at the present time is to scale (and artificially color) a brain image based on statistical tests such as the z-score or the number of voxels that are at or above some criterion level. (The images may be presented as contour maps in which the color or height corresponds to intensity differences.) However, should the relation be grossly non-linear, such a measure would lose much of its integrity as an indicator of the amplitude of a response. Such a distortion should be expected in a complex and presumably nonlinear system such as the brain. Other problems arise when one attempts to use tests of statistical significance because of their sensitivity to deviations from normality and because normality is unlikely in the processes mapped by brain imaging or EEG systems. Behavioral measures, on the other hand, are far more direct and scalable than brain responses.

A related problem concerning the use of a brain image as a measurement of cognitive function is that the degree of contrast is determined by a substantial number of different factors, some known and some unknown, that prohibit simple interpretations of the quantitative relation between the cognitive state and the neural response. The strength of the magnet, the material being scanned, and the choice of the time constant measured all can and do introduce nonlinearities that preclude simple scaling. The implication is that brain images are actually most often qualitative and rarely quantitative. In short an irregular scale devoid of a specific metric defining the interval size does not provide the necessary basis for quantification of the magnitude of a brain response, regardless of method.

It is also important to appreciate that the mere fact that numbers can be assigned to some variable does not mean that a quantitative relation exists between the numbers and that variable. An irregular interval or the absence of a nonarbitrary zero can lead to gross distortions of the meaning of a series of data points. This lack of robust quantitative scaling should affect any decision to supplement neural responses for behavioral ones in any serious way. Ignoring these limits on measurement can lead to mistaking an illusion of measurement for a quantified scale simply because numbers can be "assigned." Such a mistake would be especially significant in the context of learning; it could lead us to ignore a precise behavioral measure (for example, "percent correct") for an imprecise, seductive, and ill-quantified, variation in a brain image. Although the brain image promises to add objectivity to the behavioral measure with its panoply of high-tech equipment, it is, in fact, far more removed from that which is to be measured (the cognitive process) than is the behavioral measure.

The situation is much more complex and challenging than usually appreciated. To prove that there is a causal relation between two variables requires tests of sufficiency and necessity that are elusive. To prove that a measure is valid (actually measuring what you think is being measured) is also a demanding and difficult task. Philosophers and logicians have tangled with the problem of validity for centuries without complete success. It is all too easy to succumb to the siren call of "face validity" and to assume that *what is being measured* is *what is intended to be measured* simply because *it can be measured*.

In the context of this background the task of relating neural responses and cognitive processes for psychology is far more complex than generally appreciated. Dingman and Sporn (1964), for example, in a specific effort to consider how we might confirm that a particular molecule, neuron, or locus in the brain was the locus of the memory engram presciently proposed the following tests:

We suggest that the following criteria must be satisfied in order to demonstrate that a given molecule, set of molecules, structure, or set of structures is indeed [the site of] a permanent memory trace: (i) It must undergo a change of state in responses to the experience being remembered. (ii) The altered state must persist as long as the memory can be demonstrated. (iii) Specific destruction of the altered state must result in permanent loss of the memory. (p. 26)

Such rigorous tests for cognitive neuroscientific relations of any kind are rarely, if ever, satisfied. Therefore Dingman and Sporn concluded that all such suggestions that there is a specific memory storage region or mechanism must be "highly circumstantial" (p. 26). Considering the way data are collected today in many comparable kinds of experiments, we must also agree that many of the reported relations using imaging techniques also remain "circumstantial."

Other authors (e.g., Martin, Grimwood, & Morris, 2000) have also described a set of criteria that they feel must be met to establish a particular neural mechanism as the site of a memory. Their criteria are paraphrased in table 1.1.

Martin, Grimwood, and Morris's criteria are even more stringent than Dingman and Sporn's. Indeed they appear to be based on the assumption that it is possible to manipulate the synaptic connectivity of a complex neuronal system in a detailed way—an assumption that is clearly untenable at present. This impossibility is especially evident in the mimicry criterion. Therefore both sets of criteria are actually inappropriate to the problem at hand. Each represents the protocol of an unexecutable Gedanken experiment, rather than a scientific plausibility.

A more subtle problem concerns the misidentification of neural activity that seems superficially to have the same shape and dimensionality as a behavioral response.

Table 1.1
Stringent criteria for establishing neural-cognitive correspondences

---

Detectability   Some change in synaptic efficiency must be detected somewhere in the nervous system.

Mimicry   If we could imitate the synaptic pattern, the memory would be the same as the real pattern.

Anterograde alteration   Anything that prevents the synaptic pattern from forming should prevent the formation of a memory.

Retrograde alteration   Anything that alters the synaptic pattern should change the memory.

Paraphrased from Martin, Grimwood, & Morris (2000).

Isomorphism has been used by cognitive neuroscientists for years as an acceptance criterion of a putative relation between neural and mental variables. If there is a similarity in the shape or time course of two functions, then this similarity is taken as evidence that one represents the other. Nevertheless, if there is any single principle we have learned from the study of sensory processes, it is that there is no need to assume that the dimensions used by the stimulus are the same as those used by the neural responses; similarity of functional shape or even of dimensionality is not good evidence of a causal relation. Thus, for example, although a stimulus may be continuously varying in magnitude, it is not only possible but well established that the actual neural representation of the associated cognitive response may be encoded by some other neural dimension such as recruitment, spatial location, or even temporal sequence.

The bottom line of this lack of robust quantification is that it is unlikely that we will find a means of manipulating brain images so that they can be used as a scaled quantitative measure of a cognitive activity such as the degree of training, intelligence, aptitude, or personality. Although some coarse and indirect measures may be observed to correlate (typically with rather low coefficients) with cognitive capabilities, the search for a brain image displaying a quantifiable scale that meets all of the conditions for good measurement of such subtle psychological properties as "leadership" is unlikely to succeed.

1.5.4   Indirectness of Measurement

A related technical issue concerns the degree to which brain images are direct or indirect measures of the neural codes for cognitive processes. As with the earlier methods such as EEG, there has always been a presumption on the part of researchers that the brain images are especially potent tools because they are "direct" measures of the brain's activities. Unlike many of the earlier methods that used autonomic indicators (e.g., the polygraph), which were obviously secondary and indirect measures of brain and cognitive activity, the fMRI, for example, seems at first glance to be a direct measure of the activity of the brain. Thus modern brain images have assumed a kind of face validity that belies what we now know to be their actual indirectness as measures of brain activity.

There remains considerable controversy in the field concerning the exact relation of the brain image both to the brain's metabolism and to the information processing carried out by neuronal networks. The chain of logical and functional connections between a thought and an fMRI brain image is much longer than generally appreciated. In retrospect we now appreciate that the fMRI is as distant as the galvanic skin response or pulse rate from cognitive processes. Although there is little question that the brain images are measures of some aspect of the brain's neurobiological activity, how direct or indirect they may be remains open to question. The issue of directness becomes even more controversial when we make the leap to cognition.

An argument can be made that the responses captured by fMRI systems are logically quite distant from the essential information processes that are assumed to be the true psychoneural equivalents of cognition. Just how distant is the connection is suggested by table 1.2, which lists some of the many gaps that must be leapt to link the brain image to cognitive activity.

In other words, despite many attempts to link fMRI images directly to cognitive processes, there remain serious gaps in the logic connecting cognition and its neural substrates. The illusion of directness is based more on the general ontological assumption that the brain is the seat of our minds rather than on any convincing empirical evidence.

Very recently, the robustness of the "→" (i.e., "which is assumed to lead to") between steps has itself has been challenged. The basic assumption in this chain of logic has been that the fMRI image, known to be sensitive to changes in blood oxygenation (the blood oxygen level dependence, or BOLD), is also closely enough related to the neural activity to be used as a measure of that neural activity. A few researchers have begun to question this most basic assumption. For example, in a recent research report Maier et al. (2008) considered a pervasive discrepancy in the neuroscientific literature. Previous research had shown that human fMRI signals were strongly correlated with a subjective suppression of a visual stimulus, whereas neurophysiological activity from the monkey's brain was not under what seemed to be nearly identical stimulus situation. To unravel this discrepancy Maier and his colleagues compared two situations (no perception due to the real absence of a visual

Table 1.2
Inferential steps from cognition to fMRI

Cognitive processes are encoded by patterns of local field potentials (synaptic activity) →
Increased glucose (?) metabolism →
Increased oxygen demand →
Increased oxygenated blood flow →
Decreased deoxygenated blood level →
Changed fMRI signature

Where "→" means "which is assumed to lead to."

stimulus and no perception due to cognitively suppressed vision) and discovered that the fMRI signals did not always match the neural signals. They put it very succinctly in their concluding comments:"Our results demonstrate that the very same signals that correlate strongly with the BOLD signal in one context (physical stimulus removal) fail to do so in another (perceptual suppression)" (p. 1197).

Furthermore, Sirotin and Das (2009) also showed that the hemodynamic activity reflected in the BOLD measure may not be as closely related to the neural activity as it has generally been assumed. These researchers used an optical method of measuring the blood volume and its level of oxygenation at the same time that neural activity was recorded. The neural activity was picked up by electrodes that recorded both multiunit records and local field potentials. Their results indicated that the blood volume and oxygenation measures seemed to be composed of two different signals—one that was correlated with the neural activity during on and off visual stimulation and another that was apparently unrelated to whether or not a stimulating light was on. They attributed this to anticipation on the part of the animal to the subsequent onset of a stimulus. This result suggests that the blood volume and oxygenation levels are not always related to the induced neural activity.[20] The very important conclusion of this study was to disassociate the blood measures and the neural measures at least in the context of this visual experiment. The authors concluded: "These results raise the further possibility that there may be other, hitherto uncovered exceptions to the assumption that hæmodynamic signals uniformly imply equivalent underlying neuronal activity" (p. 478).

Finally, even some of the most committed pioneers in the use of fMRI (Bartels, Logothetis, & Moutoussis, 2008) have now concluded that the measurements provided by this device do not reflect the cumulated spiking activity of neurons in the brain. Therefore they cannot be used to test for specific neuronal sensitivities such as directional sensitivities. They noted that ". . . most [fMRI] studies fail to convincingly demonstrate the directional sensitivity of its neurons" (p. 451.) Unfortunately we do not know to what property of the brain these images do reflect. Bartels and colleagues suggested that it may provide a "complementary" measure of brain activity but one whose relation to cellular neurophysiology is yet to be established.

The importance of all of these studies cannot be overestimated. Since the fMRI can be dissociated to at least some degree and in some contexts from the neural activity, the most fundamental premise of the enterprise—fMRI signals represent blood levels correlated with neural activity—is called into question. At the very least this is another variable that must be explored and that may help to explain the wide variability of responses observed in this kind of cognitive neuroscience.

These studies have been carried out in the sensory pathways, and all involve some kind of subjective variable (e.g., perceptual suppression and/or anticipation). Indeed it is with these complex, high-level cognitive states that the BOLD measure may fail most completely. It is the fact that these high-level cognitive variables, which most clearly characterize the enormous enthusiasm for brain imaging work these days, most demand our critical attention. It is important, therefore, to constantly ask—are we dealing with a distant epiphenomenon—a sign—or are we dealing with a valid measure—a code—of the cognitive phenomenon under study? The current status of brain imaging technique as it is used by so many cognitive neuroscientists these days does not yet provide an answer to the fundamental question of directness.

1.5.5   The Timescale Difference

In addition to the problems of measurement validity and directness, there is also a massive discrepancy between the time course of fMRI responses and our cognitive processes. This discrepancy raises additional questions about the meaning of these seductive brain images. Our thoughts seem to function at what appear to be millisecond timescales as do the responses of individual neurons. For example we are able to discriminate between two sequential visual stimuli when the interval is as little as 10 msec. As another example retinal disparities can be processed to produce the experience of stereoscopic depth with stimulus exposures of only a few microseconds.

However, since the metabolic processes (such as oxygen depletion) on which fMRI images are based take much larger fractions of a second—several hundred milliseconds to several seconds—it is obvious that the timescale of cognition and of the hemodynamic processes underlying fMRI brain images are not directly comparable. This, too, adds to the discrepancies and suggests that any attempt to use the brain image as a simple measure of cognitive activity is fraught with serious technical as well as conceptual difficulties.

1.5.6   Variability

Major problems with fMRI data are the variability and lack of reliability of the data gathered when brain images are recorded. Experiments vary; individuals vary; and, especially when data are pooled from a number of subjects, the cumulative results vary considerably. The reasons behind this variability are themselves varied. Obviously many factors that are not adequately controlled impact on the idiosyncratic results from this type of research. Furthermore there are technical reasons that transcend the problem of control. The lack of precision in the definition of the cognitive process under examination itself contributes greatly to the variability of answers to what seem to be even the most straightforward research questions. Maitra (2009) performed a useful service when he discussed some of the technical sources of variability in brain images. In this article he provided fresh empirical evidence that "identified regions of activation can vary from one replication to another" (p. 88). This variability is evident not only in the intrasubject results but also is evidenced between sequential slices of the scans for experiments as simple as measurement of the brain responses to voluntary finger movement. Maitra included the following technical sources of this variability in his discussion (p. 88):

1. The delay in the BOLD response relative to the cognitive process under investigation.
2. Cardiac and respiratory movements of the subject.
3. Voluntary, involuntary, and/or stimulated correlated motion during scans.
4. Scanner variability.
5. Signal difference between activated and control or resting states are small, typically on the order of 1–5%.
6. Subpixel motions can induce large apparent signal changes and result in false positives.

The problem of intersubject variability has also been dealt with extensively in the work of Miller and his colleagues (see, e.g., Miller et al., 2002; and Miller & Van Horn, 2007), who have noted that the individual data are very stable if the same subject is tested at long intervals (such as 6 months). Miller et al. (2002) argued, therefore, that "Exclusive reliance on group analysis may be to the detriment of understanding the underlying cognitive nature of brain activations" (p. 1200).

The problem of variability has not gone unnoticed, and many authors have written on various aspects of it. Many techniques have been suggested to control if not regulate the sources of variability; however there is still no comprehensive way to avoid the most significant sources of variability. Much of the variability is accounted for by psychological and physiological-anatomical factors over which even the most rigorous experimental protocols or stable hardware would not be able to overcome. Sutton et al. (2008), for example, estimate that these physiological-anatomical, stimulus-control issues account for 10 times the amount of variance introduced by the imaging equipment itself.

A result of this innate biological variability of brain images, as well as variable measurements, is that data are noisy, and many, if not most, data-based conclusions may be less than robust. Pooling based on noisy data permits a virtually unlimited number of misleading conclusions to be drawn. Indeed there is always the possibility that even the most fundamental and widely accepted conclusions may be wisps of our imagination or of randomness rather than solid, evidence-driven scientific conclusions. In a world of small and variable experimental outcomes, there are insufficient constraints to theory development. It is not just a matter of reliability, however, but also a matter of a simple lack of consistency. One does not have to do a statistical test to observe the contradictory nature of many of the results that are discussed in this book.

1.5.7 Statistical Errors

Many of the tests of activation in a typical fMRI are based on complex statistical tests that are subject to a number of subtle interpretive errors. Some of these errors are well known and have been a scourge to psychology for years. For example, Rosenthal (1979) summarized what has come to be called the "file drawer problem," otherwise known as "publication bias" (Rothstein, Sutton, & Borenstein, 2005). Rosenthal noted that there is a significant bias in scholarly publications that are dependent on significance tests resulting from the fact that only those experiments whose results arise to the $p < 0.05$ criterion are typically published. On the other hand, a larger number of studies that don't quite make this criterion level are simply cast aside and not submitted or accepted for publication. The problem is that there is a tendency for Type I (false positive) errors to be committed in published reports that are not counterbalanced by the publication of the essentially negative results of those experiments whose findings did not make the 0.05 criterion. Spurious conclusions and theories, therefore, can easily become a part of the corpus of psychological "knowledge."[21] Current investigators such as Nickerson (2000) and Killeen (2005) are among those becoming increasingly aware of the problems associated with significance testing. The statistical problem is exacerbated as the problem has grown in complexity as more and more subtle analyses are carried out by brain image researchers.

However even such simple statistical errors as inappropriately dividing two groups by some obvious factor (e.g., gender) can pollute the experiments of the best-intentioned investigators. Ihnen, Church, Petersen, and Schlaggar (2009) have recently shown how insidious and dangerous such a procedure may be. They were studying gender differences in language processing—a phenomenon that had been repeatedly, but inconsistently, reported by earlier studies. When Ihnen and colleagues carried out the usual basic experiment (dividing their subjects by gender and then using fMRIs to measure the response of a number of identified activation areas), substantial differences between the locations of brain activations were observed for men and women. However when they randomly grouped the men and women into two groups, thus presumably washing out the gender differences, "a similar number of statistically significant regions of 'group difference' in the task associated BOLD signal" were observed (p. 1020). Ihnen et al. (2009) then concluded that,

. . . these results suggest that one should be cautious when interpreting studies that purport to have identified regions of difference between groups, whether those groups are divided by sex or any other criterion. In particular, generalization or replication of a result in independent data sets is necessary for establishing conclusive support for any hypothesis about differences in brain function between groups. (p. 1020)

This kind of result demonstrates the need for experiments in which the various combinations of studies are permuted to avoid erroneous conclusions. However, even more important is its message that brain image localizations associated with experimental conditions may be illusory and not accurate statements of brain region functionality.

As we proceed in discussing the various topics in this book, the inconsistency of many other reports of brain activity and specific cognitive processes becomes obvious. This may at least partially be explained in the terms of the artifact highlighted by Ihnen, Church, Petersen, and Schlagger's important contribution. The need for totally independent replication and the desirability of permutation analyses of any study of brain imaging are becoming increasingly evident.

If such a simple process as selecting into which group subjects are grouped can produce spurious results, then one can easily understand how a complex data analysis protocol might lead to subtler but even more profound misunderstandings. The following example, taken from the work of Newman, Greco, and Lee (2009), illustrates the complexity of the current levels of analysis used in modern imaging studies and the potential for artifacts that are inherent in such analyses.

The data were analyzed using statistical parametric mapping (SPM2 from the Wellcome Department of Cognitive Neurology, London). Images were corrected for slice acquisition timing, and resampled to $2 \times 2 \times 2$ mm voxels. Images were subsequently smoothed in the spatial domain with a Gaussian filter of 8 mm at full width at half maximum. The data were also high-pass filtered with 1/128 Hz cutoff frequency to remove low-frequency signals (e.g., linear drifts). The images were motion-corrected, and the motion parameters were incorporated in the design estimation. The EPI data were normalized to the Montreal Neurological Institute (MNI) EPI template. At the individual level, statistical analysis was performed on each participant's data by using the general linear model and Gaussian random field theory as implemented in SPM2. Each event (trial) was convolved with a canonical hemodynamic response function and entered as a regressor in the model. Although there were two phases for each trial (plan and execute), only one regressor that encompassed both phases was used in this analysis. (p. 131)

It is important to stress that in this instance I am not challenging the details of this particular analysis nor any of the conclusions drawn by Newman, Greco, and Lee: I am using it merely as an illustration of the complexity of the analysis techniques now being used in the brain imaging field. Nevertheless the depth of this kind of analysis should at least warn us of the potential for uncritically accepting some really extraordinary findings.

A further demonstration of the virtual certainty that even simple statistical artifacts can distort the seemingly most direct conclusions drawn from the raw data is made clear in the work of Vul, Harris, Winkielman, and Pashler (2009) in their meta-review[22] of fMRI work in the emerging field of social neuroscience. They reviewed 54 articles that had shown what they believed demonstrated "implausibly high correlations" between fMRI images and measures of personality and emotion. They pointed out that correlations between two sets of data are constrained by the reliability of the data sets. Following Nunnally (1970) this constraint can be expressed as:

$$r_{\text{observed A, observed B}} = r_{A,B} * \text{sqrt (reliability}_A * \text{reliability}_B) \tag{1.1}$$

where $r_{\text{observed A, observed B}}$ is the "true" strength of the correlation between A and B, $r_{A,B}$ is the observed relation between A and B, and reliability$_A$ and reliability$_B$ are the reliabilities of the data sets A and B, respectively.

Vul and his colleagues then referred to the literature to get estimates of the reliability of personality tests and concluded that a range of 0.7 and 0.8 was the best that could be expected. There were few data available that could be used to estimate fMRI reliability, but on the basis of a modest amount of information, it was estimated that ". . . fMRI measures computed at the voxel level will not often have reliabilities greater than about .7" (p. 275).

Given the lack of reproducibility shown by meta-studies of fMRI research that I discuss in later chapters, even this estimate seems quite optimistic.

Based on this analysis of both the behavioral and fMRI reliabilities, Vul and colleagues estimated that even in the case that there was no measurement error (i.e., $r_{A,B} = 1.0$) then the highest plausible correlation between the social or personality tests and fMRI measures would be

$$\text{sqrt } (.8 * .7) = .74 \tag{1.2}$$

However when they reviewed the literature, they discovered that a substantial portion of the reported experiments were producing correlation coefficients well above .74. After carefully analyzing the 54 articles in their survey, they concluded that "Over half of the investigators in this area used methods that are guaranteed to offer greatly inflated estimates of correlations. . . . These procedures turned out to be associated with the great majority of the correlations in the literature that struck us as impossibly high" (p. 285).

What was the statistical error that led to these spurious or "voodoo" correlations? According to Vul and colleagues, there was one major factor—the use of a threshold criterion for selecting activated voxels in the fMRI images. That is, only those voxel scores that were above a threshold activity value were correlated with the full range of the behavioral tests. This procedure led to correlating two measures that were not independent of each other, thus producing spuriously high correlations. Such a procedure, they noted, could actually produce positive correlations out of "pure noise." How prevalent this error is throughout current cognitive neuroscience, Vul and colleagues (2009) could not say. However, they believed that it is likely that it is widespread. This is a very important finding just because it attacks the problem at its most basic level—the statistical validity of the empirical data itself.

For obvious reasons, the article of Vul et al. (2009) was met with an extraordinary amount of controversy. If they were correct, then a substantial portion of the scientific literature on the use of fMRI in cognitive neuroscience would have been questionable if not downright susceptible to rejection. Interest was so intense that prepublication copies of the article drew extensive comment. Eventually, an entire section of the journal *Perspectives on Psychological Science* was devoted to arguments both supporting and challenging their criticism. Of the seven contributors to this interesting discussion, four took a middle position agreeing with the main point but considering it to be a well-known argument, two took highly controversial positions, and one not only agreed but said that the problem was far worse than had been suggested by the authors. I deal in turn with the two most contentious responses; one critical of the work of Vul and his colleagues and one that argued they had not gone far enough.

The most spirited rebuttal to the argument put forward by Vul and his co-workers was made by Lieberman, Berkman, and Wager (2009). Their argument is based on what they believe are "misconceptions" on the part of Vul and his colleagues. First they argued that the frail methods criticized actually are not often used in this field, that the Vul et al data collection method (a survey) was incomplete and misleading, and finally that a reanalysis of those data does not support the argument that the results were fallacious.[23]

To the contrary, Yarkoni (2009) not only supported the conclusions drawn by Vul and his colleagues but asserted that the conclusions should have been "even worse" than Vul and colleagues had suggested. Yarkoni, however, did differ with Vul's group when he attributed the problem to "the pernicious combination of small sample size and stringent alpha-correction levels" (p. 294).

In a follow-up article Vul and Kanwisher (2010) extended this critique of the statistical analyses used by many researchers who routinely and somewhat naively use statistical analyses of fMRI data. They reemphasized the fact that a powerful and ubiquitous "selection bias" exists, for example, when information is "thresholded" leading to wide-spread misrepresentation of the findings of this class of cognitive neuroscience experiments. Vul and Kanwisher (in press) characterized a selection bias as simply a poor sample—they considered the sample used not fully representative of the total population. They pointed out that this error is so common that "of the eight papers in a special issue of NeuroImage [one of the leading journals committed to brain imaging], five contained variants of this error." How serious is this problem? Vul and Kanwisher stated that "in some cases (Summerfield et al., 2006), the researchers may have produced their main significant result out of nothing."

My feeling is that the most important contribution of Vul and Kanwisher's extraordinary article is their analyses of why interpretive statistical errors in fMRI studies of cognition are so common. I quote their comments in full here.

There are three circumstances of neuroimaging that put the field at high risk. First, fMRI researchers work with massively multidimensional datasets, in which only a subset of dimensions contain information that may be relevant to the experiment. This situation encourages researchers to select some subset of the data for analysis, thus to use non-independent selection criteria. Second, fMRI analyses are complicated, involving many steps and transformations before the final statistics may be computed, resulting in confusion (and thus a diminished ability to identify such errors) not only on the part of the researchers themselves, but also on the part of the reviewers. Finally, fMRI research usually asks binary qualitative, not quantitative questions—data are presented as binary values (significant or not significant) further veiling any biases that may lie behind the biases.

Another recent article by Kriegeskorte, Simmons, Bellgowan, and Baker (2009) also developed the idea that there are profound difficulties in the analysis of both single-cell recordings and brain images. The source of these difficulties, they argued, is the inadequate and improper selection of the responses to be analyzed. They note, "In neuroimaging an example of [inappropriate] selection is the definition of a region of interest (ROI) by means of a statistical mapping that highlights voxels that are more strongly active during one condition than another. In single-cell recording, an example of [inappropriate] selection is the restriction of the analysis to neurons with certain response properties" (p. 535).[24]

The problem is that all too often the same data are used, first, for selection, and second, for analysis—a process Kriegeskorte and his colleagues refer to as "double dipping." In agreement with Vul and his colleagues they argued that such a process can lead to mistaken conclusions based essentially on the nonindependent selection of data: essentially selecting a region of interest because it responded in an experimental condition and then using that same region of interest to prove the point. To demonstrate this procedure, Kriegeskorte and his colleagues (2009) analyzed a sample experiment that showed that a significant difference could found between visual stimuli. They then repeated the experiment with random data known to not differ between the two conditions and discovered that the same analysis "also suggested high decoding accuracies, significantly above chance" (p. 537).

Kreigeskorte and colleagues (2009) did not intend to nor did they invalidate all of the 134 papers[25] they reviewed in which they believe there was some sort of "double dipping." Some, they concluded, might have been correct in their conclusions despite the statistical error. However, they did show that there was a pervasive problem throughout the neurosciences with this kind of misuse of sampling statistics. They concluded by suggesting a strategy for avoiding this kind of inadvertent double use of the same data; this strategy is presented in figure 1.1.

Vul and Kriegeskorte and their colleagues deserve unending commendation for their important contribution to what have become inappropriate interpretations of brain images and cognitive processes in both the lay and scientific literature.

A profoundly disconcerting fact is that this statistical problem was anticipated almost 60 years ago by Cureton (1950). In a recent conference, Vul called our attention to an underappreciated article in which Cureton showed that data known to be random can be manipulated to produce spuriously high correlations. Cureton summed it up quite well when he argued that

The moral of this story, I think, is clear. When a validity coefficient is computed from the same data used in making an item analysis, this coefficient cannot be interpreted uncritically. And, contrary to many statements in the literature, it cannot be interpreted "with caution" either. There is one clear interpretation for all such validity coefficients. This interpretation is—"Baloney!" (p. 96)

Just how pervasive is the problem highlighted by the Cureton, Vul, and Kriegskorte interpretations is yet to be determined. The proportion of articles reported to be defective in this manner suggests that it should lead to a radical reevaluation of the meaning of the entire brain imaging enterprise.

One strategy, which is regularly used in an effort to reconcile some of these differences, is to go beyond the individual experiment by pooling the results of many experiments. This is the technique of meta-analysis or meta-review in which a group of what are purported to be similar or related experiments are jointly examined. The idea in a meta-review is that summarizing a large pool of data may provide a more accurate estimate of the properties of the mind-brain relation under study than may be possible with the small sample sizes typical of individual experiments.

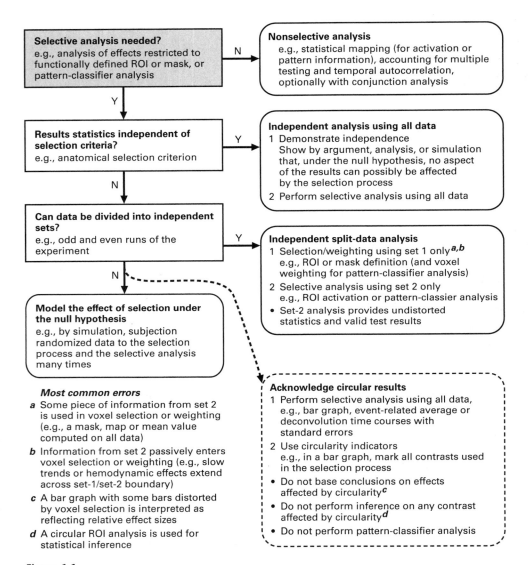

Selective analysis needed?
e.g., analysis of effects restricted to functionally defined ROI or mask, or pattern-classifier analysis

N →

Nonselective analysis
e.g., statistical mapping (for activation or pattern information), accounting for multiple testing and temporal autocorrelation, optionally with conjunction analysis

Y ↓

Results statistics independent of selection criteria?
e.g., anatomical selection criterion

Y →

Independent analysis using all data
1 Demonstrate independence
  Show by argument, analysis, or simulation that, under the null hypothesis, no aspect of the results can possibly be affected by the selection process
2 Perform selective analysis using all data

N ↓

Can data be divided into independent sets?
e.g., odd and even runs of the experiment

Y →

Independent split-data analysis
1 Selection/weighting using set 1 only[a,b]
  e.g., ROI or mask definition (and voxel weighting for pattern-classifier analysis)
2 Selective analysis using set 2 only
  e.g., ROI activation or pattern-classier analysis
• Set-2 analysis provides undistorted statistics and valid test results

N ↓

Model the effect of selection under the null hypothesis
e.g., by simulation, subjection randomized data to the selection process and the selective analysis many times

Most common errors
a Some piece of information from set 2 is used in voxel selection or weighting (e.g., a mask, map or mean value computed on all data)
b Information from set 2 passively enters voxel selection or weighting (e.g., slow trends or hemodynamic effects extend across set-1/set-2 boundary)
c A bar graph with some bars distorted by voxel selection is interpreted as reflecting relative effect sizes
d A circular ROI analysis is used for statistical inference

Acknowledge circular results
1 Perform selective analysis using all data, e.g., bar graph, event-related average or deconvolution time courses with standard errors
2 Use circularity indicators
  e.g., in a bar graph, mark all contrasts used in the selection process
• Do not base conclusions on effects affected by circularity[c]
• Do not perform inference on any contrast affected by circularity[d]
• Do not perform pattern-classifier analysis

Figure 1.1
A policy flow chart to avoid double dipping.
From Kriegeskorte, Simmons, Bellgowan, & Bake, 2009, with the permission of *Nature Neuroscience*.

Unfortunately, the usual result of a straightforward meta-review is to increase the variability. Most meta-studies show that the activated regions are more broadly distributed than indicated by the results of individual experiments. Rather then converging, meta-studies typically are dispersive in allocating brain regions to cognitive processes. Compelling pictorial evidence for this assertion can found in the meta-reviews carried out by Cabeza and Nyberg (2000), Turkeltaub, Eden, Jones, and Seffiro (2002), Laird et al. (2005), and Neumann, Derfuss, and Von Cramon (2005).

Meta-reviews of the kind mentioned here are increasingly strong evidence for the broad distribution of brain activations. Furthermore, they also are concrete evidence of the very large amount of variation and the lack of replicability among the individual studies that were collected for the meta-review itself. Experiments purporting to be analyzing the same cognitive process indentify activation sites that often are not even overlapping from one study to the next. Clearly the brain is more complicated than we think, or the entire brain imaging enterprise is deeply flawed for methodological reasons of which we are only now becoming aware. It is disappointing that so little attention has been paid to both the content and the significance of these meta-studies and the implications these meta-studies have for the entire imaging program.

A good summary of the problems encountered when the meta-study approach is followed has been provided in an article by Phan, Wager, Taylor, and Liberzon (2002) in which they themselves carried out a meta-study of emotion-driven brain imaging. According to them, the identified problems include:

1. The past and current literature in this field may bias investigators to search for particular behavior-brain region associations rather than to cast their research nets broadly.
2. Experimental protocols differ from one experiment to another so profoundly that it is difficult to assert that two or more experiments are really comparable.
3. The subtraction method, so widely used in brain imaging, is deeply flawed. It "does not identify all the regions that are involved . . . but only those that show a significant difference between the target and reference condition" (Abstracted and paraphrased from Phan et al. 2002.)

In particular reference to their meta-review, Phan et al. also listed the following problems—all of which can be generalized to any similar meta-study.

1. Classifying the variety of conditions is difficult and "somewhat arbitrary."
2. Not all relevant experiments may be included. Some may be intentionally excluded for reasons that are not valid such as arbitrary classification schemes.
3. Not all emotional or sensory stimulus conditions may be equally represented for practical rather than theoretical reasons.

(Above list was abstracted and paraphrased from Phan et al. 2002.) Whatever, the flaws of their meta-study, the empirical data they summarize are themselves compelling evidence for the some of the problems faced by brain imaging researchers. We do not yet know how devastating these challenging problems may turn out to be as the field matures. For the moment, however, caution seems to be the prudent course of action before we accept the validity of such new fields of inquiry as "social neuroscience," "neuroeconomics," or any of the other neologisms that have sprouted along with the emergence of the fMRI approach to cognitive neuroscience. Indeed, there are even more challenging issues that are only touched by these essentially statistical arguments. Conceptual issues such as the meaning of correlation or the conceptual basis of neuroreductionism itself are even more profound and very likely to rise to increased attention in the near future.

1.6   Some Useful Anatomy

In preparation for the many discussions to be presented in the remainder of this book, it is useful at this time to introduce several different ways with which we can organize the anatomy of the brain. The words used by various authors are not always the same and are not always very precise. Three different schemas are presented in two different figures as follows. First, a general scheme denoting the major lobes of the brain is presented in figure 1.2.

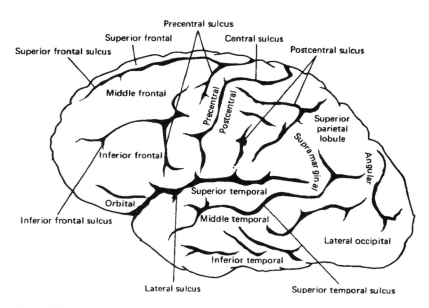

Figure 1.2
A lateral view of the human cerebrum indicating the major gyri and sulci.
From Robinson & Uttal, 1983.

Second, the study of brain anatomy has traditionally been organized in accord with the system proposed by Brodmann (1909/1999). His numbered system was based on criteria of neuronal shapes. Thus Brodmann's numbered areas originally had no special cognitive significance. Nevertheless it has been a mainstay in specifying which areas of the brain are activated or had been surgically removed for many years. The Brodmann system is shown in figure 1.3. This is the classic version of the original depiction by Brodmann a century ago. It is still widely used today.

A third three-dimensional coordinate system for standardizing brain locations based on topological distortions of the brain is increasingly being used. Talairach and Tournoux (1988) proposed such a system anchored to the location of the anterior and posterior commissures, the bands of fibers that (in addition to the great corpus callosum) connect the two halves of the brain. Using these two locations as a reference, they were able to develop a method for stretching an individual brain into something approaching a standard coordinate system that could in principle identify common brain regions. Although this was a step forward from the older anatomical location systems (and there are also new modifications of the original Talairach and Tournoux system), there are still many uncertainties and limitations as the brain is stretched and distorted to fit this "standard coordinate system."

With this preliminary information in hand, we can now consider the role of a number of anatomically specific brain regions in the representation of cognitive processes.

1.7   A Preview of Forthcoming Conclusions

Despite the undeniable fact that imaging techniques are among the most important scientific and medical developments of all time for the study of anatomy and physiology, their application to the problems of cognitive psychology, both theoretical and practical, remains problematic. In the past few years there has been increasing discussion of the lack of rigor exhibited in the flood of research reports now appearing in numbers that may approach tens of thousands a year. Articles in prestigious journals such as *Nature* (Editorial, 2007), *Science* (Miller, 2008a, 2008b), popular magazines such as *Scientific American* (Schermer, 2008), in scholarly journals such as *Trends in Cognitive Science* (Poldrack, 2006), as well as in books (Uttal, 2001, 2009a, 2009b) have begun to raise questions about the limits of the brain imaging approach to the study of cognitive processes. An immeasurable, but significant, portion of the field is now best considered to be exploratory and preliminary. As a result the flood of new observations and suggestive relations being presented almost every day in both professional and lay publications should be critically examined. The rigor of many of these reports has been increasingly challenged by skeptical reanalyses of the empirical findings and their interpretations. Unfortunately there has been a shortage of this kind of critical analysis to match the abundance of hyperbole currently characterizing the field.

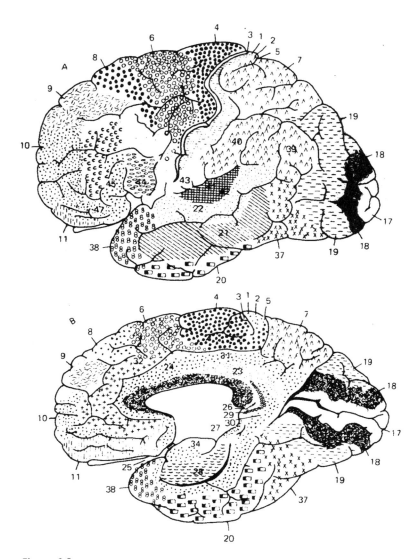

Figure 1.3
The Brodmann regions.
From Uttal, 1973, after Brodmann's, 1909, original drawing.

The empirical facts we encounter in the rest of this book should raise our awareness of the actual complexity of the mind-brain system. As such, they emphasize the increasing difficulty and ambiguity of the scientific situation rather than clarify the nature of the mind-brain relation. The brain probably should not now be considered to be an aggregate of isolated or isolatable components located in a particular place but, rather, as a dynamically changing four-dimensional (x, y, z, t), network of interconnecting and interacting components of vaguely defined, redundant, and overlapping functions and, thus, ever-changing spatial limits. No longer is the crutch for simplifying research designs offered by the neophrenological idea of the localized representation of cognitive faculties (either singly or as the separable components of a "system") available to us as a means of simplifying and organizing our findings. It is now increasingly apparent that brain images at the very least reflect the fact that vast regions of the brain, if not all of it, are involved in even the simplest cognitive processes.

Along with our increasing appreciation of the complexity of both the brain and the mind has come an appreciation of the difficulty of analyzing systems as complex as these. Two recent expressions of this new view of complexity (Foote, 2007; Binder, 2008) express this concern in different ways. For example Foote points out that "the seemingly 'deterministic' nature of such foundations may belie their ultimate intricacy and unpredictability" (p. 412), and Binder points out the extreme "frustration" that can arise out of the virtually unanalyzable behavior of complex systems. Not only are some of the problems mathematically intractable, but the problems of even evaluating the nature of their complexity and asking the correct questions can be overwhelming.

The point is—cognitive neuroscience, despite considerable ballyhoo, does not yet have the tools with which to deal with an intricately complex system such as the brain. Much less is it able to link the subtleties of behavior such as intent and perception with that level of neural complexity. Of particular concern are the unjustifiably strong conclusions drawn from noisy data, a characteristic of much of the current research. A close examination of the experimental protocols of a variety of publications is not encouraging; many studies are of low statistical power depending on only a few subjects and are rarely replicated to the extent that is desirable in such a new field of inquiry. Others produce data that are so variable from subject to subject that robust general conclusions are hard to establish. Various kinds of statistical manipulations may appear to define particular prototypical response patterns; however, given their individual variability, all must be considered skeptically.[26]

The basic problem is that this field is too rich and too unconstrained by either the dimensions of the brain responses or of the possible cognitive states to be adequately controlled or measured. As a result there are too many opportunities to try something "novel" or to inadvertently apply questionable statistical procedures. The inevitable outcome is that this phase of cognitive neuroscience shares with psychology in general a lack of specific, universal theory; both remain aggregations of isolated findings in which results have pyramided to evermore inclusive theoretical interpretations rather than follow a systematic science.

What this all means is that the MRI and the EEG are blunt instruments—epistemological sledge hammers—when it comes to understanding or even representing the detailed neuronal network mechanisms that actually underlie cognitive processes. They are techniques that operate at the wrong level of analysis; where we need information about the patterns of microscopic neuronal activity to understand something like learning, we only have available measures that pool all of the truly salient microscopic information into an unanalyzable compound. It may not be too severe a criticism to point out that whatever signs or biomarkers of cognitive activity may ultimately emerge from brain imaging studies, the whole enterprise is theoretically sterile because of this disconnect between the level at which we observe (molar chunks of the brain) and the level at which mind is actually instantiated (the details of the neuronal network). A logical conclusion of this argument is that any hope for practical applications that assume that we will be able to "read the mind" or use these tools as "biomarkers" for either normal or dysfunctional mental processes is unlikely to be realized.

If the macroscopic methods (e.g., fMRI and EEG) provided some additional information that could be of use to behavioral scientists that was not available by any other means, even these limitations would be acceptable. However if one's task is to measure, control, and predict behavioral, cognitive, or mental activities there is, in fact, another better and more direct means of getting much more high-quality information of the kind we need—the behavioral measurements themselves. Given the preliminary, noisy, and low predictive power of the current state of brain imaging and EEG data, my judgment is that the current effort to replace even poorly defined behavioral measures with "neuroscientific" measures would be a substantial misdirection of effort and resources. Little in predictive power would be added to solving the behavioral problems at hand by using these kinds of macroscopic methodologies. It is questionable what even the best neuroscientific knowledge adds to a robust, behaviorally oriented, psychology. Indeed, it may be that the entire current emphasis on imaging has detoured and obstructed psychological science from its main goals. The point is that a psychology without neuroscience may not only be feasible but preferable to the hyperbole of the current chaotic neuroscientific Zeitgeist.

Although no one can predict the future and as remarkable as are its achievements in terms of anatomy and physiology, at present brain imaging is a deeply flawed approach to the study of cognitive processes. This is not to deny the fact that if the optimistic expectations of this new field of cognitive neuroscience are achieved, they might have some role as biomarkers, indicators, or correlates (i.e., signs) of mental activity. However, at present, despite the large number of publications in this field, neuroscientific approaches in general have not come close to the precision of behavioral indicators in predicting human performance or determining the nature of a cognitive state. In short, a purely psychological approach, probably one based on behavioral rather the mentalist foundations, might be a better path to understanding the way our minds work.

This, then, provides a preamble to the main work of this book—an analysis of what neuroscience and psychology have contributed to each other. So far I have dealt mainly with generalities and technical criticisms. Now, I turn to a discussion of the specific empirical findings that have been forthcoming over the years for several of the traditional specialized fields of psychological research. My strategy is to present this material by discussing three topics for each of these standard psychological areas that serve as a primitive taxonomy of psychology. First I consider the purely psychological and behavioral concerns that will later play important roles in guiding the neuroscientific discussion. It is only in this context that the neurophysiological literature becomes meaningful, especially with regard to the inadequacy of the definitions and control of most of the cognitive processes with which this book is concerned. The second stage of discussion reviews the traditional neuroscience—work that was done prior to the advent of the imaging systems. Third, and finally, I consider what brain imaging has brought to modern cognitive neuroscience in the last two decades or so.

Although some neuroscientists may find the psychology portions a bit tedious and the psychologists may be equally challenged by the technical neurophysiology, this strategy is absolutely necessary. Cognitive neuroscience is truly both cognitive and neuroscientific! Both approaches are necessary, and neither is sufficient to make sense ultimately of what we all agree is the greatest scientific issue of all—how does the brain make the mind?

2 Sensation

2.1 Introduction

I now turn to the first topics in this review of cognitive neuroscience—sensation and perception. This pair of topics is characterized by the mental and neural responses to well-defined physical stimuli. Unlike the study of higher-order cognitive processes such as attention, it is relatively easy to control the stimulus conditions in sensory research. Furthermore, it is logically much simpler to evaluate the effect of such stimuli since a sensory experience is typically anchored to well-defined physical dimensions and units.

For reasons that have more to do with the sheer bulk of the material that has been published in this field than with any difference in substance between sensation and perception, I have chosen to separate this material into two chapters, one emphasizing "sensory" and the other emphasizing "perceptual" topics. The arbitrariness of this dichotomy should be obvious as many regions of overlap can easily be seen. The two chapters will, however, have two different themes. The emphasis in this chapter is on peripheral processes, whereas the next chapter concentrates more on comparisons between central neural processes and cognition.

To set the stage for the discussion in these two chapters on sensory and perceptual neuroscience, four very different research topics may be distinguished within the general problem area discussed: (1) sensory coding; (2) psychophysics; (3) a set of more complex responses we generically refer to as perceptual; and (4) actual neural-psychophysical comparisons.

2.1.1 Sensory Coding

Sensory coding is a study of the neural responses or "languages" that are used by the nervous system to transmit information from the receptors to the central nervous system. It is a purely neurophysiological enterprise and does not require any cognitive participation on the part of the subject; indeed with few exceptions, sensory coding research is carried out on animal preparations. The prototypical question asked is—what are the neural responses to specific properties of the physical stimulus? Sensory coding research, therefore, is not really a subdivision of *cognitive* neuroscience; instead it is a purely neuroscientific enterprise with only distant empirical and conceptual links to evoked mental activity.

Although much has been learned about these processes and much of sensory coding neuroscience has been useful in providing heuristics in understanding some of the more cognitive, perceptual, or psychophysical phenomena, coding studies operate in a considerably different context than do the more cognitive processes. In the main, sensory coding studies do not speak to the problems of the transforms between either stimuli or neural responses, on the one hand, and cognitive responses, on the other. Such relations can only be studied by comparing neural responses with cognitive processes, a research enterprise that is technically quite different and unfortunately much less frequently implemented. With the exception of a few experimental protocols based on fortuitous anatomical "accidents," most current explorations of sensory mechanisms involve secondary correlations or analogies rather than direct empirical comparisons of experience and neural activity carried out on the same preparation at the same time. A few of these exceptional studies are discussed later in this chapter.

Therefore, the neuroscientific study of sensory coding (I am referring here specifically to the transmission languages used by the peripheral nervous system to convey information from the receptors to the brain) does not close the theoretical gap between the physical stimulus and the experiential response. The reasons for this are fourfold. First, the perceptual experiences can only infrequently be directly compared to the neurophysiological codes. It is not possible to predict from even the most robust coding finding result what will be the psychological response.[1]

Second, since the relevant psychological responses—the experiences or qualia—are not directly measurable, we have to use carefully controlled procedures—psychophysical methods—to determine what the relation is between the stimuli and the experience. There is great uncertainty about many of the measures of experience that are made in such experiments. In any event, this is not done in the classical sensory coding experiment.

Third, the sensory codes are often surprisingly different from one stage of neural processing to the next; indeed a different code may be used at every level of the ascending pathway.

Fourth, stimulus-neural code-psychological comparisons, when they are done, typically demonstrate that there are nonlinear relations among the physics of a stimulus and our estimates of both the experience and the parameters of the neural code. Sensory coding findings, therefore, are incomplete in that they do not account for all of the neural and cognitive transformations that occur between stimulus and experience.

Despite these difficulties there is no question that sensory coding research is by far the most developed and consistent field of the neurosciences broadly construed. Nevertheless, its successes can be misleading. So much has been learned about sensory coding that it is often uncritically assumed that we have an equally complete understanding of higher levels of cognitive processing by the nervous system. This, as we see, is not the case.

2.1.2 Psychophysics

The second of the four aspects of sensation and perception research—psychophysics—has its own scientific culture and practitioners. The goal in this arena is to establish some relations between the attributes of physical stimuli and the most immediate properties of the psychological response—what philosophers refer to as the *qualia*. This approach, contrary to the sensory coding approach, skips entirely over all aspects of the neurophysiology; it is purely a psychological enterprise. The prototypical psychophysical experiment compares variations in the stimulus with psychophysical responses just as the archetypical coding study compares stimulus properties with neural responses.

The major complication faced by the psychophysicist is the need to limit the subject's responses to those that minimize the impact of higher-level cognitive processes. This is necessary because experiments purported to examine the straightforward relation between a subjective response such as the magnitude of a sensation and the amplitude of a stimulus can be seriously distorted by expectations, sequence effects, meaning, and other "judgmental" or "cognitive factors." For this reason, a highly circumscribed array of methods has been developed to constrain responses to simple "yes-no" or "same-different" statements. Since there are no means of determining the details of the neural codes in purely psychophysical experiments (beyond speculative inferences or analogies with neuroscientific studies), psychophysical studies have little to say about the neuroscience of phenomenological experience.

Furthermore, measures of the psychophysical and neurophysiological responses do not always agree. We must be vigilant not to confuse or conflate our understanding of transmission codes with the immensely more difficult problem of determining how brain mechanisms produce cognitive experiences. Nevertheless, psychophysical findings exert a profound heuristic influence on thinking in cognitive neuroscience by informing us about the functional relations between stimuli and responses.

2.1.3 Perceptual Processing

The third aspect of sensory and perceptual research concerns interactive and judgmental responses we refer to as perceptual. The prototypical experiment in this category requires that the subject be provided with an ambiguous stimulus and then directed to introspectively report what was the elicited experience. Geometrical or visual illusions, failures of perception, surface color and lightness, grouping, and similar discrepancies between the physical stimulus and the cognitive response are all typical studies in the field of human perception. This aspect, like psychophysics, is a part of cognitive science but not of cognitive neuroscience. Perception, to the limited degree that it can be distinguished from sensation is discussed in the next chapter.

The task of determining the high-level neural processes that are the psychoneural equivalents of what we refer to as perceptual phenomena remains recalcitrant notwithstanding the advent of the brain imaging systems. Not only are the neuronal mechanisms vastly more complicated, but the essence of these interpretative phenomena is to be found in the discrepancies, not the correspondences, between the stimuli and the cognitive response. With all due regard to those who may have proposed ingenious and creative explanations to such phenomena as illusions or change blindness, there are no acceptable neural theories of them. It is for this reason that the topic of perception is better handled in a separate chapter.

2.1.4   Neural and Experiential Comparisons

The fourth topic is the true embodiment of cognitive neuroscience. It is concerned with the comparison of neural responses of all kinds with the sensory and perceptual experiences. This is the main theme of this book. Research of this kind may involve the measurement of peripheral nerve responses (discussed mainly in this chapter) as well as those of the brain (discussed mainly in the next chapter).

Figure 2.1 diagrammatically represents the four approaches to the study of sensory and perceptual topics.

It is obvious from the outset that these four topics—sensory coding, simple sensory psychophysical responses, complex perceptual responses, and neural-experience comparisons—represent vastly different challenges to psychologists both in method and interpretation.

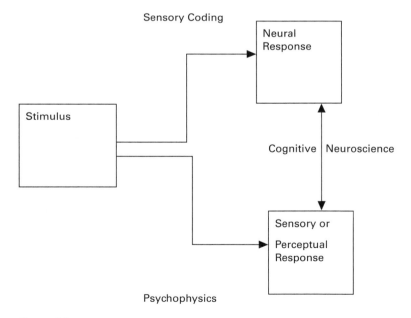

Figure 2.1
A conceptual map showing the relations among sensory coding, psychophysics, and cognitive neuroscience.

The relative success of research in the sensory coding domain has inspired many to look for equivalently simple neural answers to questions involving more complex perceptual processes. Alas, the simple, straightforward, and conceptually simple logical organization of the peripheral nervous system is lost when we begin to deal with such subtle and nebulous experiences as illusions (i.e., discrepancies between the stimulus and the experience). No longer are the responses, covert that they are, linked only to the physical parameters of the stimulus; no longer are the causal influences restricted to the stimulus alone; no longer are the salient responses localized to well-defined peripheral anatomical structures; no longer do we have well-developed methods that allow us to measure the critical neural activity; and, most important, no longer do we have any means of directly measuring, or, for that matter, adequately controlling the responses of interest—the awarenesses—the experiences themselves.

2.2 The Neurophysiology of Sensory Coding

Sensory coding neuroscience has been one of the great success stories in neuroscience, whereas the study of perception confronts many of the same difficulties in establishing the neural mechanisms faced by other high level cognitive processes. Why this should be the case is easy to discern. Sensory coding, a patently neuroscientific enterprise (although not a cognitive one) is characterized by the task of determining the peripheral neural codes or languages that are used to convey information from the receptors to the brain.[2] This has proven to be an eminently obtainable goal. Empirical technologies are available, and the biological concepts involved are relatively straightforward. Sensory coding studies are also graced by a tight relation between the physical measures of stimuli and the relatively simple arrangement and relatively easily accessible nature of the peripheral sensory pathways. The conceptual logic of the required experimental designs, therefore, is relatively simple; information flows mainly in one direction from the peripheral receptors to the central portions of the nervous system. With only a few exceptions, this centripetal or afferent flow accounts for almost everything we need to know about the sensory code.

Another advantage enjoyed in sensory coding research is that the salient questions asked can be answered with well developed technologies such as microelectrodes, electronic amplifiers, and oscilloscopes. The answers to sensory coding questions are largely to be found in the actions and activities of individual neurons and whole nerves whose sensitivities vary with the properties of the stimuli in a coherent, consistent, and predictable manner.

Best of all, the issue of localization does not arise at the macroscopic level—the anatomy of the neurons that convey the sensory codes is arranged so that there is no issue about what part of the peripheral nervous system is involved in carrying out their necessary functions—the optic nerve responses are not confused with the those of the acoustic nerve, which is anatomically quite distinct. Most important is the fact that the transmission properties of the peripheral nervous system are rarely confused with the representation properties of the central nervous system where neural activity becomes experience.

The salient coding information is to be found in the peripheral and anatomically segregated components of the nervous system—the receptors, the well known sensory tracts, and the earliest stages or primary receiving areas of the central nervous system. From this perspective, there is comparatively little difficulty in defining what it is that we want to measure and where it is. The overlap, redundancy, multimodality, and interchangeable functions of the brain make any comparable task for the brain much more complicated.

Sensory coding researchers are driven by some fundamental questions that remain as valid today as they were decades ago. What has changed is that we now have much better answers to some of these questions than we could have then anticipated. The range of issues faced by sensory coding theorists can be summarized in the following list (adapted and updated from Uttal, 1973, pp. 11–13):

1. What are the properties of the most efficient stimulus for each of the sensory modalities? That is, what is (in an older terminology) the adequate stimulus? For example the eye is tuned to respond maximally to electromagnetic energy varying between approximately 400 and 760 nm. Its adequate stimulus, therefore, is defined as this spectral band.
2. How is the physical stimulus energy passed through the nonneural portions of the receptors to the transducers—the neurons that are able to convert the raw physical energy of the stimulus to the biochemical reactions that are neural activity? For example light is attenuated and focused by the optical elements of the eye.
3. How does the transduction process lead to the generation of neuronal responses? For example the inner ear changes mechanical energy into neural energy by means of specialized cells in which the bending of certain cilia leads to the generation of neuroelectric responses in the cell membrane.
4. What dimension of the neural response at each stage of the ascending pathway is the salient code for which dimension of the stimulus? This is the heart of the neural coding problem.
5. How does coded information pass from one neuron to the next at a synapse, and what changes, if any, in the code occur at such junctions? Do the codes stay the same from neuron to neuron?
6. Ultimately, the cognitive neuroscience question one would like to answer is—what is the neural code for each sensory or perceptual experience? However, it is unlikely that we can answer this question for two reasons: (a) the codes used by the neuronal network that becomes "experience" are too complicated to be analyzed; and (b) we have no direct way to measure inaccessible cognitive processes so that they can be directly compared to the codes.

Two initial tasks are required to begin the evaluation of the sensory codes used to represent properties of the stimulus. The first is to specify what are the parameters, dimensions, or attributes of the physical stimulus. The second is to determine the possible or candidate codes—that is, the plausible and possible dimensions of neural activity. What is being asked here in the second question is—what are the observed dimensions of the neural response that could conceivably co-vary with the dimensions of the stimulus?

It has been useful to deal with the coding problem by seeking the commonalities of all of the sensory modalities rather than in terms of vision, hearing, somatosensation, taste, and smell in isolation. To implement this approach, I developed the matrix of physical stimulus properties and the candidate codes shown in table 2.1.

The task of sensory coding theory from the point of view of this matrix is to carry out the necessary experiments to make entries in it associating a given stimulus parameter with a particular candidate neural code. It must be appreciated that this matrix will have to be replicated for each level of the neural chain since the code is likely to be transformed from one level to the next. The code used by a receptor may not be (and we now know that it is not) the same for each successive neuron in the ascending pathway.

The most important contribution of this chart, however, is to highlight a very important generality. That generality is that there is no a priori reason that the candidate neural code need be dimensionally isomorphic to the stimulus parameter. For example, stimulus intensity need not be encoded by a simple quantitative dimension. Thus the amplitude (a purely quantitative attribute) of the stimulus may be encoded by a number of different candidate codes. These possible codes include the number of activated units, a temporal variable such as the frequency of neuronal responses or even the place that is activated. Furthermore, there are some stimulus attributes, for example the wavelength of light, that cannot be encoded isomorphically—the timescales of the electromagnetic oscillation and the maximum frequency of neural action potentials are so discrepant that the stimulus wavelength must be encoded in some other way. Evolution provided a wonderful alternative means of handling this problem—using differences in place (different kinds of retinal receptors) to distinguish the different electromagnetic frequencies that constitute the adequate stimulus for vision. Typically, such neural codes utilize a comparison of activities in various places to encode the properties of a qualitative stimulus parameter such as wavelength.

Despite its apparent complexity, the matrix shown in figure 2.1 is a very incomplete expression of the possible variations that might be encountered in a search to authenticate the use of particular candidate codes. For example the five nominal categories of temporally dependent candidate codes listed in this matrix do not begin to represent the full range of possible ways in which the frequency attributes of the neural response could be used to convey information about the stimulus. Cariani (2004) has expanded on the concept of temporal encoding by listing a large number of ways in which temporal fluctuations in the pattern of spike action potentials can represent stimulus properties. His proposed modes of temporal encoding are shown in figure 2.2 for single channels (A–J) as well as for several

Table 2.1

Matrix of stimulus dimensions and candidate neural codes

			Neural Response Dimensions (The Candidate Codes)			
			Place	Topographic Pattern	Number of Activated Units	Neural Event Amplitude
Common Sensory Dimensions		Quality				
		Quantity				
	Temoral Parameters	Relative Temporal Order				
		Temporal Acuity				
		Duration				
	Spatial Parameters	Spatial Localization				
		Spatial Interaction and Patterns				

From Uttal (1973).

multichannel or combination modes (K). Furthermore the five different modes of encoding involving multiple neurons particularize the concept of temporal comparisons between two (or more) places only hinted at in figure 2.2

Sensory coding research has been one of the mainstays of neurophysiology, not only because of the anchor provided by the physical stimuli, but also because of the relatively easy access to sensory neurons themselves in both human and animal preparations. These two simplifying factors seem to offer a wonderful opportunity to study the properties of the peripheral nervous system and have, in a few cases, provided a set of empirical findings as well as a manageable foundation for extrapolative interpretations. In the discussion that follows, I have divided the field of sensory coding research into two historical epochs—the first characterized mainly by research in the neurophysiological and neuroanatomic laboratories and the second in which theoretical, especially mathematic probability, studies elaborated on those preceding deterministic empirical results.

Neural Response Dimensions (The Candidate Codes)				
Temporal Parameters				Temporal Comparison Between Two Places
Frequency	Frequency Macrofluctuations	Frequency Macrofluctuations	Derived Statistical Measures	

2.2.1 A Brief History of Sensory Coding Research

The Early Neuroscientific History of Sensory Research

The earliest work in which specific associations were made between sensory experiences and brain mechanisms probably can be dated to the Renaissance and specifically to the work of Andreas Vesalius (1514–1565), one of the greatest anatomists of all time. Vesalius was among the first to ascribe mental activity to the solid portions of the brain. In doing so he overcame the dominant contemporary view that ventricular fluids constituted the "mind-stuff." At about this same time another key idea was intuitively proposed by Jean Fernel (1497–1558). He suggested that the dorsal and ventral nerves entering and leaving the spinal cord differed in their respective functions. For reasons that are inexplicable in terms of the limited technology of the time, Fernel correctly argued the dorsal roots were sensory (conveying information from receptors into the spinal cord) and the ventral roots were motor (conveying

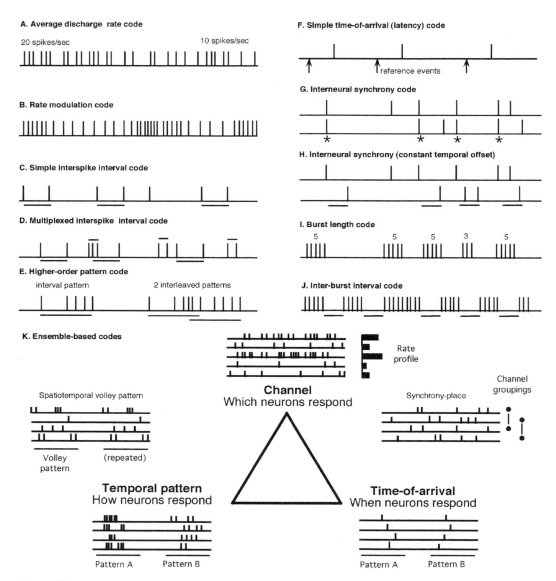

Figure 2.2

A sample of the many pulse interval codes that can be used to encode cognitive processes. These are candidate sensory codes; each needs to be tested to determine if it actually conveys usable neural information.

From Cariani (2004), reprinted with permission © 2004 IEEE.

signals from the spinal cord to the muscles of the body). This intuition was not confirmed until discoveries by Charles Bell (1774–1842) and Francois Magendie (1783–1855) two centuries later.

Fernel was also one of the first to suggest that, although the brain itself was more homogeneous than not, different regions might have different functions. This idea gained additional support from the subsequent discovery of what were supposed to be highly circumscribed "speech" regions in the brain by Pierre Broca (1824–1880) and Carl Wernicke (1848–1905) as well as what appeared to be regions specific to motor functions by Gustav Fritsch (1838–1891) and Edward Hitzig (1838–1907).

During the eighteenth and nineteenth centuries, a vigorous debate was carried on between "holists" (who argued that the brain was an undifferentiated mass) and those who believed that there were specialized regions for different mental processes or faculties as cognitive abilities were known then. The protagonists in this great debate included the leading phrenologists Franz Gall (1758–1828) and Johan Spurzheim (1776–1832), who assigned a host of curious psychological properties to different brain (and skull) regions, on the one side, and some of the greatest neurologists of the time such as Pierre Flourens (1794–1867), who supported the holist position, on the other. Gall and Spurzheim had an enormous cult following. Flourens, on the other hand, was a highly respected neurologist. It turned out that the phrenologists eventually won the day, not in terms of their specific assertions about the bumps on the skull, but in terms of their support for the general idea of localization of function on the brain. As I have discussed a number of times in this book, the localization principle dominated subsequent theory in cognitive neuroscience and still holds considerable influence today. However, its time may have passed as distributed mechanisms emerge as a more likely model of brain function.

Over the years, specific sensory functions were assigned to particular regions of the brain. Bartolomeo Panizza (1785–1867) and Hermann Munk (1821–1894) were probably among the first to assign the occipital area of the brain to vision. Hearing regions were mapped by Woolsey (1961) and shown to be located on the superior portion of the temporal lobe. Somatosensory regions located just posterior to the great central sulcus of the human brain were explored by Penfield and Rasmussen (1950).

Based on the localization idea, many regions in the brain have been associated with specific sensory and motor functions. Our interest at this point however is on what have traditionally been designated the classic primary sensory projection regions of the brain. There are several main strategies that have been used over the years to identify the sensory areas. The original method was to determine the sensory dysfunctions that resulted from brain injuries. Later, others used experimental surgery to determine the sensory functions of particular areas of the brain. If blindness or deafness or some other sensory defect resulted from a lesion, then the brain area was assumed to be the appropriate sensory region. Neuroanatomists simply traced the paths of the sensory nerves to particular regions of the brain. With the advent of more modern equipment it became possible to stimulate the peripheral sensory nerves with natural or electrical stimuli and measure the locations on the brain that responded with event-related potentials (ERPs) or even EEGs.

Based on an array of such discoveries, over the years the idea of localized primary receiving areas of the various sensory modalities became some of the most widely accepted concepts of cognitive neuroscience.

It is now appreciated that this simple conceptual model does not completely reflect the true complexity of the brain regions involved in vision, for example, and probably not the arrangement of the other sensory and motor areas as well. The initial theory of visual system organization has been supplemented in contemporary theory with the much more complete chart of the rhesus monkey visual brain areas provided by Felleman and Van Essen (1991) shown in figure 2.3. Each of these regions (some are on the temporal gyrus and some on the parietal lobe) is supposed to have a different function. Before we too glibly assign these same regions to the study of the human visual brain, it must be remembered that the corresponding or analogous human areas have not yet been fully identified.

Other visually responsive regions are now known to be scattered about the temporal, the parietal, and depending upon one's psychological taxonomy, well forward onto the frontal lobe. Similarly, the auditory regions of the brain are now thought to be more widely distributed than the just on the superior temporal lobe. Broad swaths of the frontal and parietal lobes of the brain now seem also to play a role in hearing. Even the traditional somatosensory area located on the postcentral parietal region seems to be supplemented by the regions in the frontal cortex (Hagen, Zald, Thornton, & Pardo, 2002). A full map of the auditory system, prepared by Kaas (2004), is shown in figure 2.4.

The important thing about these charts, as Kaas (2004) so eloquently points out, is that they are not yet empirically authenticated to the extent that is popularly assumed; instead they are theories based on an incomplete sample of available, but limited, empirical data. In his words, diagrams of this kind "tend to give the impression that we largely know the organization of such systems. . . . Some of the features of such diagrams are well supported by evidence, while others are not" (p. 207).

Speaking specifically of the diagram proposed by Felleman and Van Essen, Kaas points out that these visual scientists had gone to great lengths to indicate where the evidence was strong and where it was weak for not only the existence of these centers but also for the nature of the connections shown in their "theory." As an example, Kaas notes that Felleman and Van Essen had pointed out that few of the 32 "visual areas" had actually been "well established" (p. 208).

It is in this context of imaginative uncertainty that all brain imaging studies have to be taken with a grain of salt. Not only are they searching for what may originally only have been hypothetical components only weakly suggested by empirical findings, but the whole idea of a network of functionally isolated components may be deeply flawed. A softer kind of regional specialization in which there may be no boundaries or specific functions of a

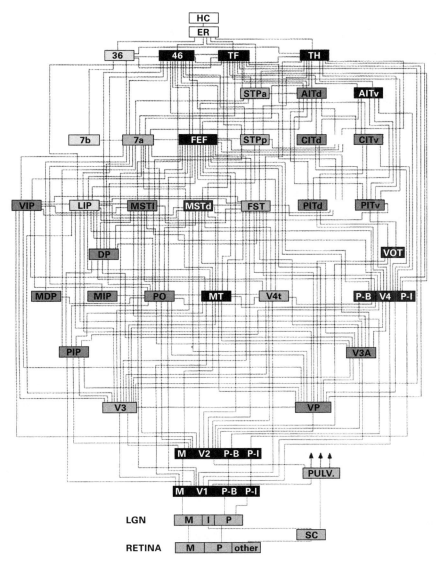

Figure 2.3
A theory of the organization of the peripheral visual system. The particular regions and pathways are not important. The key point made by this and all other similar charts throughout this book is the nature of the complex interactions among multiple brain loci in the encoding of cognitive processes. From Van Essen, Anderson, and Felleman (1992), reprinted with permission of AAAS.

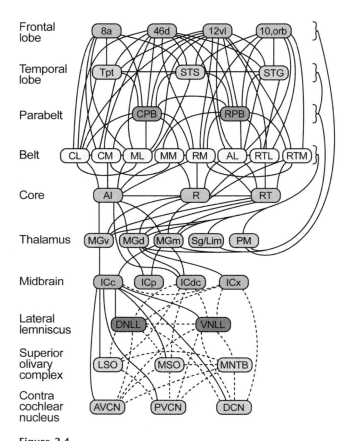

Figure 2.4
A theory of the organization of the peripheral auditory system.
From Jon H. Kaas (2004), *Cortex*, 40(1), 207–208, reprinted with the permission of Elsevier Science and Technology Journals.

brain region may be much closer to reality. Nevertheless brain imaging has an enormous potential for tracing out the functional anatomy of the sensory brain and adding substance to the sometimes fragile hypotheses implicit in such diagrams.

Findings like these can, thus, be interpreted in a number of different ways. What cannot be denied, however, is the trend toward increasing realization of the widespread distribution of brain regions involved in any sensory processing. It is also clear that a multifunctional role is played by what had hitherto been considered to be regions of the brain that previously had been thought to have unique and well-defined functions. In such a context it becomes increasingly difficult to either assign to these sensory regions any single function or limited localization. Furthermore, considering that each of these regions is probably a part of a system of interacting regions, several of which may receive sensory messages directly and indirectly, the task of identifying both their role and the extent to which they participate in perceptual experience becomes much more complicated. Indeed, it may be mathematically impossible to analyze either the hierarchical priority or the specific role of an individual component in such a heavily interconnected system.

It is becoming increasingly clear that functional specialization is rarely, if ever, complete even for the sensory and motor regions. Recent research (e.g., Foxe, Morocz, Murray, Higgins, Javitt, & Schroeder, 2000; Ghazanfar & Schroeder, 2006) has shown that the primary sensory areas of the cerebrum are often involved in other sensory activities other than the one traditionally assigned. A more complete discussion of polysensory neurons in levels as low as the superior colliculus and as high as the cerebrum is available in an interesting book by Stein and Meredith (1993). In the superior colliculus, which is conventionally considered to be a visual center, Stein and Meredith propose that the "bulk of the neurons" (p. 173) are polysensory. They argue, therefore, that the sensory projection areas are not as pristine as conventional theory suggests. Instead, from early on in the brainstem, auditory, somatosensory, and visual messages from the receptors tend to merge and thus to produce overlapping maps at all levels of the afferent pathways.

It is nevertheless clear that despite this declining view of the unimodal role of the various regions of the brain, the idea of localization of function still has a powerful hold on thinking in cognitive neuroscience. Its compelling, seductive, and persistent influence can readily be detected in the next historical phase of sensory neuroscience—that which I refer to as the empirical-deterministic era.

The Empirical-Deterministic Era

The ability of the sensory nervous system to encode stimulus information was of considerable interest to physiologists as early as the nineteenth century. The great polymath, Herman v. Helmholtz (1850a, 1850b), for example, made an excellent estimate of the speed of neural conduction using a string galvanometer. Another of the most important discoveries—the refractory period (the immediate period of insensitivity following a neural response) was made with another primitive device called a capillary galvanometer by Gotch and Burch (1899). Both of these results were done on whole nerves, and both depended on the availability of these primitive kinds of recording technology.[3]

Subsequent sensory coding research depended on key technical developments that were capable of measuring the details of the responses of single neurons to sensory stimuli. These included the development of sensitive electrodes that could pick up the extremely low-voltage signals generated by neurons and highly sensitive recoding and display equipment. Some of these developments came to fruition as early as the 1920s. Adrian (1926) was among the first to use electronic amplifiers to record whole-nerve responses. Among the first studies of individual nerve fibers in animals were the experiments reported by Adrian and Bronk (1929) on motor neurons.

The field burgeoned in the 1930s—a period that many would consider to have been the golden age of neurophysiology. It was in this period that investigators such as Erlanger and Gasser (1937), Gasser and Grundfest (1939), and Hodgkin (1937) made their fundamental discoveries about the nature of neuronal conduction. Much of this work was facilitated by the initial replacement of the various forms of electrometers by the cathode ray oscilloscope, a device that somewhat surprisingly had been around since the late nineteenth century in primitive forms.[4]

It was also at about this time that the first specific studies of coded responses were made. Adrian and Mathews (1927) studying the eye of an eel demonstrated changes in the response of the optic nerve over the course of a prolonged stimulus. This may have been the first demonstration of neural accommodation, an important idea that strongly indicated that the sensory codes might not be constant but could differ over time. Subsequently Graham and Hartline (1935) observed the response of a single optic nerve fiber from the eye of a horseshoe crab to a flash of colored light and demonstrated that the response was a burst of action potentials whose numbers varied with the wavelength of the stimulating light.

From the 1930s on many investigators successfully studied sensory coding in a variety of animals using what were relatively highly sensitive probes, high-gain amplifiers, and hugely efficient display and data-processing technologies. Specific functional relations were being plotted between stimuli and the coded responses of individual neurons. In 1948, for example, Hodgkin was able to electrically stimulate crab sensory neurons and charted the increase in frequency that occurred in parallel with increases in the intensity of an electrical stimulus. The problem was not as simple as the stimulus intensity-neuronal frequency response relation might have initially suggested, however. Hartline (1938) had observed that different neurons responded with different temporal patterns of response to what were believed to be identical stimuli. For example some of the neurons in the vertebrate eye responded mainly to the onset of stimulation, some solely to the offset, and some to both the onset and the offset. This suggested that some of these neurons were only responding to changes in the stimulus condition, a property we now call high-pass filtering. He attributed this to the way these neurons were interconnected with others.

Another similar complication inhibiting the establishment of simple functional relations had been observed in the pioneering experiments carried out by Galambos and Davis (1943). They determined that the neurons in the acoustic nerve were tuned to relatively narrow, but differing, frequency bands of acoustic energy. This work set the stage for the place theories of hearing that were to dominate later years. An equally important contribution was the work of Kuffler (1953) who discovered that the properties of the stimulus that could activate a neuron were not homogenous—different parts of the "receptive field" of a neuron could have different sensitivities depending on where the stimulus was positioned. These were important developments because they opened the theoretical door to much more complicated candidate codes (e.g., relative amounts of activity in spatially distributed regions of the brain) than had been suggested by earlier experiments. It also added to the argument that even in the peripheral nervous system, individual neurons were influenced by their neighbors.

Indeed, the idea of using a spatial pattern for the representation of a wide variety of other stimulus properties became widespread in the decades to follow. All sensory modalities are now believed to use spatiotemporal patterning to represent stimulus qualitative differences rather than simple labeled line codes. One of the most important studies of this type of coding was to be found in the work of Tunturi (1952) who showed that acoustic stimulus frequency and intensity were encoded by a two-dimensional array of locations on the primary auditory cortex of a dog.[5]

If there was any aspect of this research that remained constant throughout this initial era of sensory coding research, it was the use of simple stimuli—flashes, clicks, frequency components, and other simple one-dimensional stimuli. Such simple stimuli were almost universally used in this early stage, and they were, as we now have begun to appreciate, actually quite misleading about the true complexity of the neural codes for sensory transmission. The modern era that followed saw a quite different trend in which much more complex and multiple stimuli dominated sensory coding research. We discovered once again that the nervous system was full of tricks that strained our models and understanding to their limits.

By midcentury it was becoming clear that individual neurons were exquisitely sensitive to specific spatiotemporal attributes of a stimulus even when they were unresponsive to substantial amounts of the raw physical energy of their adequate stimulus. This type of sensitivity thus represented a finely tuned place code for different spatiotemporal stimulus patterns. That is, different neurons responded best to different aspects of the stimulus pattern.

The works of Lettvin, Maturana, McCulloch, and Pitts (1959) and Hubel and Wiesel (1959) are considered to be milestones in this new perspective on sensory coding. Both of these iconic experiments showed that neurons in the visual system of the frog and the cat, respectively, were relatively insensitive to visual stimuli unless the stimuli had a particular pattern of shape and movement. Thus, a diffuse illumination of the visual scene or a stationary spot of light produced no response; however, if an appropriately shaped object moved in a particular direction across the receptive field of a neuron, a vigorous response would ensue.

Hubel and Wiesel (1965) made an important conceptual contribution by pointing out that there was progressively more specific encoding by neurons in the visual pathway as one moved more centrally in the system. For example relatively low-level cells responded to shapes with preferred direction of movement and particular locations, whereas higher-order neurons required much more specific stimulus shapes such as edges, corners, and tongues of a particular size. The emerging view was that there was progressive convergence of inputs providing increasingly more specific sensitivities to stimulus properties on the part of different neurons.

This notion of a hierarchy of effective stimuli types had a profound effect on thinking in later years. Many psychologists who were not themselves carrying out neurophysiological work adopted this kind of conceptual neurophysiology as the basis of theories of perception. The culmination of the idea of progressive convergence on more and more specific cell sensitivities was Konorski's (1967) theory of "gnostic" neurons in which single or a few neurons might encode complex thoughts and perceptions. This kind of metaphorical thinking linking what were only marginally related neurophysiological properties to cognitive processes has become less and less frequent in recent years.[6]

An especially influential study of the well-organized array of the receptor neurons of the horseshoe crab eye was reported by Hartline and Ratliff (1957). Their most important discovery was the nature of the reciprocal inhibition produced by lateral connections in this primitive animal's compound eye. This regularity of the receptors and the lateral interconnections among the neurons emanating from the receptors was influential in setting off a string of theoretical models in the years that followed. Furthermore, many would argue, this seminal experiment was the point of transition between the predominantly empirical studies of sensory coding and the theoretical approach of recent years. Computer models of Hartline and Ratliff's work were the precursors of many modern trends in computational neurobiology. As we also see shortly, the process of lateral inhibition became a model of virtually all kinds of contrast and edge effects.

In order to overcome some of the constraints imposed by either overly simplistic stimuli or too complex real-world scenes, about this time a number of researchers (e.g., Campbell & Robson, 1968) began to use the sinusoidal components of Fourier-analyzed images as stimuli. These patterns had the advantage of being two-dimensional but still were limited with regard to their ability to activate some of the more subtle coding sensitivities of sensory pathway neurons. This type of stimulus led to a speculative model composed of hypothetical frequency-sensitive neurons that ignored many other properties of the visual system. Ultimately, empirical support for the specific presence of frequency space analyzers in the visual system also seemed to evaporate. An important lesson of this episode was that mathematical models, like behavior, are also neutral with regard to underlying neural mechanisms.

The Modern Probabilistic Era

The profound changes that occurred with the publication of the classic papers of the preceding empirical-deterministic era revolutionized thinking about the sensory encoding of stimulus attributes in later decades. Many studies like those described in the previous section, as well a host of other purely neurophysiological investigations, have continued in a number of laboratories. However to a surprising degree there has been a conceptual shift in sensory coding research. Now that we have more or less exploited the use of simple stimuli and have begun to understand their multidimensional nature, the field has undergone a major metamorphosis. A considerable portion of attention to the problem of sensory coding has currently been diverted to the cellular biochemistry and genetics of the problem—topics that are outside of the purview of this book. To a considerable additional degree, however, the thrust of research has become much more theoretical and formal in a mathematical sense. Building on the empirical results of the past few decades, a substantial number of leading-edge researchers have dropped their microelectrodes and have turned to their computers to explore sensory coding. The emphasis is now on such topics as neural response variability, coding efficiency and optimization, and the impact of response sensitivities on coding. There has also been increased interest in such topics as scene analysis in order to more completely and more precisely define the true nature of real-world stimuli to which it has become obvious that the nervous system has evolved some remarkable and highly specialized sensitivities.

The fact that multiple and simultaneous dimensions of a stimulus simultaneously and collectively determine the neural responses (as suggested by the work of such pioneering neurophysiologists as Hartline, Lettvin, Hubel, and their co-workers) has now become a main theme in sensory coding research. No longer is the response of a neuron assumed to be determined by the simple properties of a single stimulus dimension; instead the "real-world" scene (or some abstraction of it) has now replaced a flash of light, a click of sound, or a touch of applied pressure as the stimulus of choice. Not only have neural responses been shown to be determined by multiple properties of the incoming stimulus, but it has also become clear that high-level brain activity could be projected downward in the efferent direction to modulate the direct effects of the stimulus. Sensory coding had come of age in a world of complex, multivariate stimuli and equally complex system responses.

The abundance of information coming into our sensory systems at any point of time and how we deal with it also became concerns. What contribution do the coding mechanisms make in filtering out the huge amount of information constantly impinging on our receptors? What relation does such information reduction have to the cognitive processes of attention and the kind of filtering that goes on at all levels of the brain?

To anticipate a bit, the general result of this new direction in sensory coding research, not surprisingly, was that things are not as simple as even the most prescient pioneers of sensory coding research could possibly have appreciated. The result of this increased awareness of the complexity of the sensory system was to stimulate a substantial increase in the use of statistics and mathematics—a development that had been an anathema to many old-line neurophysiologists. Despite their protestations the field has moved on to consider the impact of novel analytic techniques on sensory coding theory. It is becoming increasingly accepted, furthermore, that our nervous systems have evolved in a way that is dependent on the statistical rather than deterministic aspects of stimuli. Furthermore, simple concepts suggesting that the basic attributes of a stimulus such as quality or quantity were all that matters have to be replaced with the idea that the effects of the multiple parameters of the stimulus must combine in complex and often probabilistic ways.[7] To not accept such a transition in thinking would seriously underestimate the complexity of the sensory coding process.

A further problem in developing an understanding of sensory coding processes is that the individual neurons are only able to carry a small amount of the information that is present in a real-world scene. Adding to this difficulty has been the emerging realization that our sensory neurons are relatively variable in their response patterns. Given this variability, if one deals with single neurons, it seems almost impossible to imagine how complex information could be represented in as precise a manner as seems necessary for the precision of our sensory experiences.

The problem then arises—given the multiple influences that affect coding and the high degree of variability in neuronal responses, what is an efficient, if not optimal, code that the nervous system can use to represent the real world? The task ahead for sensory coding theorists can be succinctly stated—how does the nervous system convey the maximum amount of information given the properties of real-world stimuli and its own response limitations? To answer this specific question we must understand both the statistics of real-world images and the nature of the neural responses they produce. We then must compare them to determine if the nervous system is operating at near optimal levels or, at least in some more restricted sense, at a reasonably efficient level.

To begin to answer such questions we have to be able to produce complex, multidimensional, real-world stimuli in a more quantitative way than simply presenting a picture or complex sound such as orchestral music to the eye or ear, respectively. This specification of the parameters of a complex stimulus is necessary to sort out the salient codes from the irrelevant signs. To make any progress in this direction, it is necessary to seek the common attributes of many real-world scenes in order to determine those to which the sensory system is responding.

The search for the common attributes of real-world scenes (and thus what is the essential sensory information to be encoded) is now considered to be a statistical problem in which common regularities are sought in what at first may seem to be quite different images. Geisler (2008), in a comprehensive review of natural scene analysis developments, made the case for a statistical, multidimensional approach to real-world stimuli when he said:

Our often-veridical perceptions of the world give the impression of a deterministic connection between perception and environment; however, this is largely an illusion. Most perceptual capabilities depend upon combining many very different sources of stimulus information, each of which is only probabilistically predictive of the task the organism is trying to perform. (p. 168)

How, then, can natural images be represented in a manner that permits us to determine if the sensory nervous system is optimally or efficiently encoding real-world scenes? Simoncelli and Olshausen (2001) and Smith (2006) have reviewed a number of the methods that have been used to represent such stimuli. In general, they point out that the task is to develop the empirical statistics of a set of images that are presumed to have common properties. One of the most basic techniques these researchers described is principal component analysis, a mathematical technique closely related to the factor analysis method familiar to psychologists. Both of these methods seek to reduce what are clearly highly redundant data in a real-world image to a sparse number of dimensions that carry the major portion of the critical information (i.e., account for the major portion of the variance) in a pattern. It is assumed, although not altogether proven, that the sensory system is using a similar or closely related process if the responses follow the same pattern as predicted by the principal component analysis. In other words, how does the nervous system extract the richest information dimensions and ignore those dimensions that convey little information. An important underlying assumption of this approach is that once we have identified the salient parameters, factors, or components of real-world stimuli, we will have a pretty good idea of the way the nervous system processes the same information *because* it is "logical" that it would have evolved to optimally respond to those properties.

There are many methods of real-world stimulus representation. One is to use autocorrelation of the image as the statistic of choice. The autocorrelation emphasizes the relations between nearby regions, dropping off with increasing distance between compared regions unless the function is cyclic. In that case, the autocorrelation function itself may display cyclic components.[8]

Another well-established method is to develop an analog of Fourier analysis in which the real-world image is reduced to a set of two-dimensional basis functions similar to the sinusoidal functions of a true Fourier analysis. These basis functions, which themselves may be a set of small two-dimensional patterns, may bear a great deal of similarity to the well known response function or tuning curves of individual neurons and, thus, have a certain face validity as being likely optimum or, at least, efficient sensory codes. Both have been described as exhibiting "Mexican hat" shapes.

Geisler (2008) has expanded this basic set of statistical image transformations by noting the following additional transformations that can be used to extract the salient aspects of complex real-world stimuli. He prefers to deal with a hierarchy of stimulus complexity starting with such simple parameters as the contrast levels of an image and varying up to its most complex spatiotemporal, multidimensional aspects. In table 2.2, drawn from his work, are shown the various stimulus dimensions and the statistics that he believes are most appropriate to represent the key information conveyed.

It should be noted that none of these functions has been fully vetted. We still have not come close to determining the "optimum" code. In Geisler's (2008) words: "It is difficult to know ahead of time which specific statistics will prove most informative for understanding vision. At this time, progress is being made by selecting statistics based on intuition, historical precedence, and mathematical tractability" (p. 173).

Despite the intrinsic difficulty of solving the problem of the optimal codes for real biological systems, a number of theoreticians have suggested a variety of specific neural coding schemes. One of the earliest was the idea of sparse or single neuron coding of complex

Table 2.2
Statistic of choice for various stimulus dimensions

Stimulus dimension	Statistic of choice
Luminance and contrast	Luminance at each pixel divided by average luminance
Color	Principal component analysis
Spatial structure	Fourier amplitude spectrum or spatial autocorrelation
Range	Plot of height against horizontal distance
Spatiotemporal structure	Simultaneous plots of spatial frequency and temporal frequency plots

After Geisler (2008).

stimuli proposed by Konorski (1967) and Barlow (1972) that has been reinvigorated by such researchers as Olshausen and Feld (2004); Rozell, Johnson, Baraniuk, and Olshausen (2008); and Bowers (2009).[9] The basic idea in sparse coding is that the optimal stimulus for a neuron becomes progressively more complex as one ascends the sensory pathway until single cells in the cortex are able to represent very complex ideas such as faces or even philosophical concepts.

Shannon information capacity rules similar to those used for designing optimum codes for signal transmission have also been used by such investigators as Lewi, Butera, and Paninski (2007). In information theory the task is to define a system of multisymbol "words" that will optimize the information transmission given the characteristics of the message.[10] Another approach was the use of Green and Swets's (1974) signal detection theory by Grewe, Weckstrom, Egelhaaf, and Warzecha (2007). Additional samples of the many efficient or optimal codes that have been proposed for sensory systems can be found in Smith's (2006) comprehensive dissertation.

These functions all attempt to do what sensory scientists should have been doing for years; that is to reduce complex stimuli such as real world scenes to a set of salient common cues rather than depending on intuition of what it should be. As Geisler (2008) noted, this is comparable to the reduction done by a spectrophotometer in visual studies when white light is reduced to a set of critical components. Without such a reduction it would be impossible to understand the receptor properties of the eye.

Statistical models of real-world images, therefore, reduce a complex, multifaceted stimulus to a much smaller set of salient and common dimensions or attributes. However, these transformations of the stimulus tell us nothing about what the nervous response actually is; all they can really do is to tell us how the nervous system *should be designed* to optimize the transformation of this kind of reduced stimulus. To go further than that requires the actual study of appropriate sensory systems to determine if such systems appear to be efficiently, or better optimally, encoding the information inherent in a complex, real-world stimulus. The next step, therefore, would be to examine the neurophysiological or psychophysical properties of the nervous system and behavior and see if information is efficiently or optimally encoding the real world scene in the manner predicted. This is something that should be relatively easily done in the peripheral sensory nervous system, but it is immensely more complicated at higher levels where neurocognitive interactions become so complex that it is likely to be impossible to ever determine the actual efficiency of their coding schemes.

It is difficult enough to determine whether a neuron is behaving efficiently for even a limited and well-defined complex real-world stimulus such as contrast. The difficulty is somewhat ameliorated by the fact that different aspects of a visual stimulus are conveyed along different neural pathways (Livingstone & Hubel, 1988). Thus, it is possible to compare a stimulus parameter with a response in a neuron that has only a limited range of functions. Notwithstanding specific situations, it must be remembered, as a number of investigators in this field have repeatedly pointed out, this is a very difficult task and may be intractable without using some potent simplifying assumptions or taking advantage of special neural situations such as the regular array of receptors in the horseshoe crab eye.

Neurophysiological laboratory studies exploring peripheral sensory coding mechanisms continue to be carried out by a number of workers. In general, the task is to determine if the parameter of the stimulus (often summarized by a particular statistic and identified as an optimal stimulus for that parameter) produces the largest neural response. In other words does the observed optimal sensitivity of neurons or tracts agree with the calculated optimal properties of the stimulus? If not, attention is redirected to other statistics, and the determination of which one produces the most robust response must be sought elsewhere.

By comparing reduced versions of many real-world images (i.e., optimum representations), the common attributes, both theoretical and neurophysiological, can be identified and an appreciation developed of what an optimal nervous system would have to do to convey the rich, but concentrated, information. Indeed, convergence between idealized real-world stimulus components and the neurophysiological properties of neurons would be compelling evidence that neurons have evolved to best represent the external world and justification for our ability to define "optimal codes."

The advantage of formally predetermining an efficient or optimal code over a simple, exhaustive search is that it acts as a guide to what a neuron should be doing (based on the hypothesis that a neuron will evolve to do what it should do). A simple exhaustive search could easily overlook the optimal stimulus for a neuron, however, if it is subtle and not initially included among the plausible possibilities. At that point simple luck would have to play a large part in finding the best code.[11] Statistical studies of the optimal properties of a stimulus can, thus, provide guidance for the experimenter—guidance that was not available prior to this emphasis on defining optimal stimulus properties in a formal quantitative manner.

Of course simply defining this goal does not make it an easy task. Many of the authors working in this field have pointed out that the task as described here is intrinsically difficult; indeed it may be NP-hard (i.e., intractable of solution in a finite amount of time) according to Smith and Lewicki (2006). The difficulties of trying to analyze the functions of an inter-acting network of neurons in the sensory pathways, although not as severe as those of the analogous task of dealing with the neural mechanisms of higher-level cognitive processes, are still profound. Furthermore the nonlinear nature of even the simplest sensory neural mechanisms adds considerable difficulty to defining their properties with what is necessarily still a linear mathematical approach. Noise and the variability of individual neurons also introduce serious obstacles.Obviously there are many technical problems that require that we deal with populations rather than individual neurons, always a technically challenging aspect of neurophysiological research. Although investigators are still exploring many of these ideas, there is at present no standard, universally agreed-upon method for measuring the efficiency of a code.

Difficulties such as these are paralleled by other challenges. Grewe et al. (2007), for example, point out that: ". . . different measures applied to the same data can yield different answers to the same question" (p. 6). This problem is going to be especially relevant when we consider brain imaging.

Nevertheless the payoff would be substantial in understanding the relation between nervous activity and sensation if we could succeed in this quest. The most significant con-tribution of this work currently is to provide an alternative organizational theme to the hit-and-miss history of sensory coding research in past years.

As I previously noted in this present discussion there is an interesting a priori assumption built into the logic of the search for optimal codes in sensory mechanisms. Although we cannot be sure until further empirical evidence is available, it seems logical that the sensory system has evolved to optimally respond to whatever are the optimum coding properties of real-world stimuli. Unfortunately this part of this new research paradigm—testing optimal codes for stimuli in neurophysiological paradigms has not yet matured. Only a few studies actually respond to the challenges of specifically testing stimuli deemed to be optimally encoded in neurophysiological preparations. Furthermore some of this work has failed to show the anticipated correspondences. Among the few examples that I have been able to uncover that at least partially accomplish this task is the work of Machens et al. (2005). They carried out neurophysiological studies on grasshopper auditory neurons and discov-ered that the response of the neurons ". . . was not matched to the statistics of stimuli per se, but rather to a weighted ensemble of natural stimuli, where the different behavioral relevance determines their relative weight in the ensemble. . . ." (p. 454). Thus there was a discrepancy between what some investigators had previously thought, a discrepancy that only became obvious when the codes of this animal's auditory system were compared with the theoretically determined optimum encodings.

The approach, nevertheless, has worked on occasion. Neurophysiological findings from the zebra finch obtained in an experiment carried out by Hsu et al. (2004) showed that there was a close correspondence between the properties of synthetic song-like sounds and the response at low levels of the nervous system regardless of whether or not they had the statistical properties of real songs—no agreement here of optimal and irrelevant codes—anything went! At higher levels, however, the sounds that did not have the statistical properties of the finch's natural songs did not activate the neurons to the same extent as did the more natural coded songs. This result suggests that the convergence of the stimulus and neural sensitivities, probably as a result of evolutionary processes, does seem to hold, at least at high levels of the nervous system.

Nevertheless sensory coding research has much going for it in terms of relative simplicity compared to higher-level cognitive processes. The sensory nerves and primary receiving areas are especially accessible; there is a predominantly one-way flow of information; and the task of determining the transmission codes for well-defined physical stimuli is much less challenging than the task of determining the neural states of such free-floating processes as attention or the neural mechanism associated with whatever it is that we mean by the word "perception."

All in all, strategies to determine efficient codes can provide some suggestions and heuristics about how the nervous system works. How far this strategy can go in triggering new explanations of sensory coding is yet to be determined.

In summary, although much of the work in sensory coding research nowadays has shifted to mathematical models of what are efficient, if not optimal, codes for real-world stimuli, this work remains in large part isolated from human perceptual phenomena. Thus it is, if we are to make a strong judgment, only an indirect contributor to cognitive neuroscience—a science tasked with comparing neural with mental or cognitive responses.

2.3 Psychophysics

In the previous section I considered the field of sensory coding and noted that despite some wonderful progress in its own domain, it was essentially neutral to the problems of *cognitive* neuroscience. The reason for this neutrality is that sensory coding researchers deal with the relation between stimuli (even real-world, spatiotemporally patterned scenes of substantial complexity) and the coding language used by the peripheral nervous system to convey the properties of these stimuli to the interpretive sections of the central nervous system. It is only there that the transmitted information becomes experience and awareness. Unless behavioral experiments are either carried out simultaneously or later compared, sensory coding research of the kind described in the previous section is intrinsically unable to bridge the gap between experience and neural activity.

Determining the relation between neural responses and some measurable aspects of our experience, perception, or cognition, however, is a completely different task. It is not always the case that this discrepancy between what is truly cognitive neuroscience and what is purely neuroscience is appreciated. This oversight is exacerbated by the fact that, for the reasons I have already mentioned (e.g., well-defined stimuli, simplicity, and predominantly afferent directionality), a considerable amount of progress has been made in the neurophysiology of sensory coding mechanisms. Unfortunately that success does not directly transfer to the more complicated neural mechanism that represents our higher-level cognitive processes.

I now consider another form of psychological research that also finesses the great question of cognitive neuroscience when it asks—how are the properties of the stimulus related to the sensory response? This domain is well known as "psychophysics"; indeed, it is the simplified prototype of all purely psychological or cognitive research in which the experimenter varies the properties of the stimulus and observes the evoked behavior. Such an approach eschews direct examination of the underlying neural mechanisms (although there is a long tradition of seeking metaphors and correspondences from what are often only weakly linked neurophysiological experiments). The critical intellectual barrier to both neuro- and cognitive reductionism in this case is the underdetermination of the behavioral report; a multitude of alternative possible underlying mechanisms are possible when all you have to work with are behavioral observations and speculative inference.

Psychophysics is traditionally defined as the science studying the relation between stimuli and the more or less immediate responses to them. The emphasis has always been on relatively simple responses of the kind we refer to as "sensory" as opposed to the connotation encompassed by the words "perceptual" or "cognitive." The powerful advantages of the psychophysical approach are its tight anchor to physical stimuli and the relatively immediate perceptual responses to them. By immediate responses I refer to answers to such questions as: Did you sense anything? How much stronger does that stimulus seem to be than this one? Are these two stimuli the same or different?[12] It does not usually refer to such processes as "thinking," "problem solving," "learning," or "attention." Of course, this is a matter of emphasis more than substance.

An alternative definition of psychophysics (other than the study of such immediate stimulus-response relations) refers to the methods used to study sensory processes. Psychophysical methods are highly refined attempts to minimize intrusion from high-level cognitive processes so that as pure a measure of the relation between the stimulus and the immediate response as possible can be obtained. Although this is a sensory science, it is not a cognitive neuroscience; I, therefore, leave further discussion of the powerful methods and notable achievements of psychophysics to others.

2.4 Cognitive Neuroscience of Sensation

In the previous sections, I have tried to distinguish among several areas of sensory and perceptual research. First I discussed the purely physiological literature concerned with neural coding and then followed with a brief comment on psychophysics. The argument being made in both of these cases was that there was little that could be identified as *cognitive neuroscience* in these traditional and well-developed fields. It is only when direct comparisons are made between neural activity and psychophysical processes that a true cognitive neuroscience of sensation or perception can be claimed to exist. In general such comparisons are far more difficult to implement than they may at first seem. Many technical and ethical problems have been encountered in the past when investigators attempted to carry out neurophysiological studies on introspective human beings. What was more often done in the search for experiential-neurophysiological correspondences was to carry out neurophysiological experiments separately from the psychophysical ones and subsequently to search for analogous or isomorphic responses among the respective findings. The usual difficulties of species differences, a diverse set of alternative explanations, the likelihood that one will find support for almost any hypothesis in the varied and complex activities of the nervous system, underdetermined responses, and potentially misleading analogs hold in such situations.

The history of sensory neuroscience and sensory psychophysics, therefore, has largely run on parallel, but separate, tracks over the years. One can only look on with amazement and pride at the enormous range of accomplishments in each of these fields. Sensory neurophysiology and anatomy are, for the reasons suggested earlier, among the best-known fields of modern neuroscience. A comprehensive review of the field can be found in many different handbooks and references, not the least impressive of which is Kandel, Schwartz, and Jessell's (1991) *Principles of Neural Science*. Chapter after chapter presents detailed evidence for the neurophysiology of all of the senses. In recent years we have added much to this corpus of knowledge by explicating the biochemistry of many of the molecular actions that account for transduction and transmission as well as the genetic factors that control the development of the sensory system.

Similarly, psychologists have a long history of studying the experiential results of stimulating the sensory nervous system with physical energies and patterns of all kinds. In these psychophysical experiments human observers report what they experience as the parameters of the stimuli are changed. However, no robust information about the internal structure is obtainable from psychophysical experiments of this kind. Nevertheless, we know easily as much about these overall psychophysical responses as we do about the neurophysiology of the organs and cells that connect us to the outside world.

Mixing these two domains (neuroscience and psychophysics) of well-developed knowledge to produce a true "cognitive neuroscience" of sensation is a much more difficult task. Some would even argue that prior to the development of the brain imaging devices, it was not possible. It was only in the rarest circumstances that such a goal could be achieved with any degree of scientific rigor. Accomplishing such a task ideally requires that both the neurophysiological and the psychophysical responses be acquired as simultaneously as possible and that both be the product of the same well-controlled stimulus. It is also desirable that, whenever possible, both parts of the comparison should be made on the same experimental animal and that the animal of choice be the human.

In the past, relatively noninvasive techniques for measuring human neural activity were routinely used including EEGs, ERPs, and electroretinograms (ERGs). In a few exceptional cases, as I shortly describe, peripheral nerve responses have provided a somewhat more invasive and promising, albeit somewhat disappointing, entre into human cognitive neuroscience. Virtually all of these techniques, however, suffer from being the sum or accumulation of many individual neuronal responses. Unfortunately such cumulative responses obscure the level at which the detailed coding of the sensory message is most likely carried out—the interplay of individual neurons.

The near-simultaneous capture of both neurophysiological and human psychophysical responses produced by the same stimulus being so challenging, it had almost always been the case that such comparisons were made between different preparations—the neurophysiological work carried out on animals and the psychophysical results obtained from humans. The comparisons were, therefore, indirect and did not meet the stricter standards of a robust cognitive neuroscience experiment. Indeed the comparison was almost always carried out on the basis of analogical thinking—a procedure that left the door open to conceptual errors not too different than those produced by purely verbal models.

One example of how analogical thinking can lead erstwhile sensory cognitive neuroscientists astray is to be found in a proposed neuroscientific model of a well-known perceptual phenomenon known as *simultaneous contrast*; a phenomenon first reported by Chevreul (1839). Simultaneous contrast is the different phenomenal appearance of a constant lightness field when it is surrounded by a dark field and a light field respectively as shown in figure 2.5.[13]

This phenomenon has been explained by several different neurophysiological theories including lateral inhibitory interaction (the kind that produces Mach band edge effects) and on-off fields in the visual cortex. Both of these putative "explanations," however, are deeply flawed by the superficial nature of the analogies being drawn and the fact that the responses in the two domains simply do not correspond in magnitude or extant. For example the neural mechanisms invoked to explain simultaneous contrast are highly localized (i.e., they produce narrow edge effects) whereas Chevreul's simultaneous contrast phenomenon is uniform across the entire contrasted field.

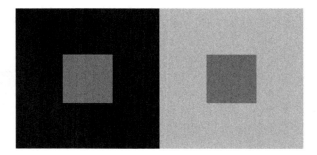

Figure 2.5
The simultaneous contrast illusion first described by Chevreul (1839).

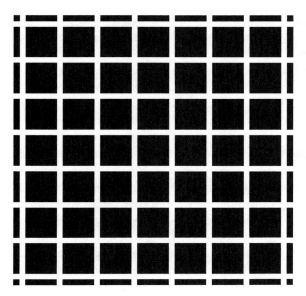

Figure 2.6
The Hermann grid illusion first described by Hermann (1870).

A closer analogy exists between the Hermann grid phenomena (Hermann, 1870) shown in figure 2.6 and possible neural interactions. The Hermann grid illusion is manifested by very small regions of fleeting gray spots at the intersection of the blocks. Despite the fact that this illusion is very different than the simultaneous contrast phenomenon in both extent and duration, it, too, is often identified with simultaneous contrast (e.g., by Spillmann, 1994) rather than to the center-surround (Mexican hat) shape of receptive fields (for example, by Baumgartner, 1960) with which it does share some common attributes.

This internal inconsistency between the phenomenon and the neurophysiological observation as well as between two quite different phenomena illustrates the dangers of reasoning by analogy. Indeed in recent years a new point of view has emerged that suggests that such superficially simple visual illusions as simultaneous contrast may actually be mediated by much higher levels of neurocognitive processes (Lotto & Purves, 2000) that are determined by our past visual experiences rather than the simple geometrical relations of the stimulus.

Despite these arguments against casual analogizing of neurophysiological data and psychophysical reports, a number of my colleagues have argued that such reasoning is supportable and productive. A comprehensive discussion of the ways in which psychophysics might be conjoined to neurophysiological studies has been presented by Spillmann and Ehrenstein (1996) and Spillmann (2009), who argue that psychophysical results can inform us about their underlying neural mechanisms, an argument with which I strongly disagree. They drew from a wide-ranging set of psychophysical data and what appear to them to be analogous neurophysiological findings to explain everything up to and including phenomena as complex as the Gestalt laws of perception. Notwithstanding the substantial scholarship that went into this study, it is important to point out that it is almost entirely based on analogous reasoning—similarities or perceived isomorphisms of neural and sensory responses observed in two very different experimental contexts.

The major criticism that I highlight in this and all of the related work to be discussed in this section is that these analogous relations are often selected from among a huge array of other potential neural responses that might have been measured. There is so much going on in the nervous system that it is almost impossible not to find some support for virtually any hypothesis about neural coding or representation. Furthermore many of the analogs drawn between psychophysical and neural results are less close than they may seem at first glance. Some seemingly simple processes turn out to be far more complex than initially thought and ultimately are found to involve high-level cognitive processes. One example is the well-known phenomenon of meta-contrast[14]; what appears to be a simple suppression of information by neighboring stimuli turns out to be recoverable in forced choice experiments.

The largest proportion of the neural studies cited by Spillman and Ehrenstein (1996) involved microelectrode experiments carried out on animals. As discussed elsewhere (Uttal, 2005), the very narrow perspective of the microelectrode technology makes results obtained with this technique particularly susceptible to misinterpretation. It seems unlikely that one can go from such detailed local observations to explanation of such global phenomena as Gestalt grouping by invoking single-cell responses as Spillman and Ehrenstein have suggested. This is much too large a logical and empirical leap from the microscopic to the macroscopic. Such overly simplistic explanations illustrate the problems involved in cross-species comparison and the need for simultaneous experiments carried out on the human.

In the discussion that follows I concentrate on the limited corpus of experiments in which the neural and psychophysical responses were recorded from humans. In doing so, it becomes clear that achieving the experimental ideal is not going to be easy—the major problem being the rarity of appropriate and accessible neural responses from humans.

In the section that follows I discuss a number of interesting comparisons between sensory neural responses and human psychophysical responses. In general the results have been disappointing in elucidating the codes used by the peripheral nervous system.

2.4.1 The Traditional Period of Sensory Neuroscience

To go beyond reasoning by analogy to robust evidence that a particular candidate code represents a particular sensory function requires that at the very least we record both the psychophysical and the neural responses to the same stimulus from the same animal at nearly the same time as possible. To whatever extent anatomy and ethics make it possible, it is also desirable to make that animal the human. Here the instructions are conveyed easily and unambiguously, and the meaning of the psychophysical responses is relatively unmistakable. Although the historical record makes it clear that even human subjects may not be able to carry out all of the instructions of the experimenter, at least the possibility is enhanced that a meaningful comparison can be made. Of course this ideal situation is not always possible, and the few experiments that have met these ideal criteria are often fraught with unexpected complications and uncertainties arising from the medical condition of an injured patient. Nevertheless there is a kind of face validity of this experimental paradigm that is not possible with animal comparisons.

Surprisingly, because of a few anatomical curiosities in the physical accessibility of the various sensory nerves, human experimental designs approximating the ideal are occasionally available to the intrepid experimenter. The somatosensory nerves, the auditory nerves, and even the chorda tympani (which conveys taste information to the brain) have all been subject to controlled stimulation and near simultaneous recording of both electrophysiological and psychophysical responses. The optic, acoustic, or vestibular nerves are far less easy to access directly except in the most challenging surgical procedures where coordinated psychophysical experiments would be inadvisable. Nevertheless some progress has been made by using indirect neuroelectric methods such as the ERG or brainstem responses or even direct measurements of accessible peripheral nerves. However, as we see when we examine the data of a few exemplar experiments, even when the idealized protocols can be used, simple and consistent answers to some basic questions have not been forthcoming.

A major factor in the limited success of any of these cognitive neuroscience experiments is the type of neurophysiological recording that is used. Since we are reasonably confident that the key coded information conveyed along these nerves is dependent on the response patterns among individual neurons, it would seem desirable to stimulate and record at the single-cell level. However, this is not always possible; an alternative is to use the pooled activity of many neurons picked up by large extracellular electrodes. Unfortunately there remains a great deal of uncertainty about both the origins of these compound responses and how much the pooled responses obscure the true sensory codes, which are more likely based on the activity of individual neurons.

Somatosensation

Among the first studies that directly compared sensory experiences and the relevant peripheral neural coding responses in humans were those carried out in my laboratory (Uttal, 1959, 1960a, 1960b) on somatosensory neurons.[15] The purpose of these experiments was to compare the perceived magnitude of a stimulus both with the physical magnitude of the stimulus and the amplitude of the compound neural response recorded from the ulnar nerve in the arm. This was truly a cognitive neuroscience experiment closely approximating the ideal experiment in which psychophysical and neurophysiological data were recorded from the same subjects under as nearly identical conditions as possible. The guiding hypothesis was that the perceived magnitude would follow the amplitude of the neural response, which itself would be dependent on the timing relations among these compound amplitudes.

In both experiments the procedure was essentially the same. Electrical pulse stimuli in pairs or triplets were presented to the ulnar nerve at the wrist. These stimuli produced compound action potentials that were recorded by high-gain amplifiers from a superficial portion of this same nerve near the elbow. At the same time psychophysical estimates were made by the subjects of the perceived intensity of the stimulus.

The key factor in these experiments was that the refractory period of the earlier responses affected the amplitude of the subsequent compound action potential when two or three stimuli were presented in close temporal order. Thus, if a later stimulus was presented in the "shadow" of a previous one, the response to the later stimulus would be attenuated. Furthermore, it was also proposed that the magnitude of the perceived experience would essentially follow the cumulative amplitude of all of the neural responses.

Indeed, the results of these experiments supported these predictions. The psychophysical response did not follow the cumulative amplitude of the two or three stimulus pulses but did follow the amplitude of the refractory period-modified compound neural responses. One possible code for subjective magnitude, therefore, was demonstrated in this case to be the sum of the amplitudes of the modified neural responses. Of course other codes might be at work at the microscopic level of individual neurons where the normal transduction mechanism created other patterns of response.

This general technique was developed further by Desmedt and Cheron (1980). Stimulating at the fingers, they were able to record at six points ranging from the wrist to the spinal root along the nerves of the arm. Thus they were able to track the course of the transmitted response from the wrist until the point at which the median nerve entered the spinal cord over a path that was as long as 80 cm.[16] This provided the opportunity to make measures of conduction velocity and also served as a useful diagnostic tool to study various kinds of neuropathies.

. Although there are substantial advantages to using electrical shock (e.g., the timing can be exquisitely controlled) there is a compelling argument that it would be preferable to use natural touch or tickle stimuli to study the normal somatosensory receptor-generated responses. Unfortunately, when one is concerned with peripheral nerves, the absence of the kind of neuronal synchronization artificially produced by electrical stimuli makes the responses of individual neurons all but undetectable percutaneously with the large electrodes routinely used. Such a handicap can be overcome if the nerves could be directly accessed with microelectrodes penetrating the skin.

During the 1960s and 1970s, with the development of robust metal microelectrodes, such an approach became possible, and a few researchers, mostly in Scandinavia, began to study human neural reactions to both natural and electrical stimuli in surgical or quasi-surgical preparations. Hensel and Boman (1960), for example, pioneered this approach by using touch and temperature to elicit responses from both single neurons and bundles of neurons.

They surgically isolated individual somatosensory neuron fibers (i.e., axons) in the radial nerve of the arm from human participants and recorded both compound and single-neuron responses. Although experimental surgery on humans of this kind is not likely to pass vetting by today's institutional review boards, their work opened the door to the possibility of examining single-neuron responses at the level of analysis that most likely represents the foundation for sensory encoding. They showed that there was a systematic monotonically increasing relation between the frequency of action potentials in a single neuron and the force applied to the skin. They also reported that some single neurons were able to respond to both temperature and pressure stimuli.

Unfortunately their work was almost devoid of any coordinated psychophysical measures. The one exception was that they alluded, almost in passing, to the fact that threshold stimulus capable of producing a response in a mechanosensitive fiber was about the same as the threshold reported psychophysically.[17]

Other more successful efforts to take psychophysical advantage of the accessibility of the somatosensory nerves in the limbs were made by Ochoa and Torebjork (1983). Rather than using the heroic surgical procedures of Hensel and Bowman, they chose to impale single neurons in the median and ulnar nerves with a microelectrode passed through the skin to the nerve. The use of a microelectrode permitted them to record the activity from a single neuron and to compare the neural and psychophysical responses to electrical stimulation also introduced through the microelectrode. Using this technique, Ochoa and Torebjork (1983) were able to show that even a single neuron was capable of conveying information that could be classified in terms of quality and localization. Repetitive stimulation of the neuron (presumably an axon of a receptor in the skin), for example, would result in a sensation of "tapping" or "flutter." However the sensory experience was always quite different than that obtained with natural mechanical stimuli applied to the receptors in the skin. Ochoa and Torebjork attributed this difference to the unnatural situation in which only a single fiber was being activated rather than a population of many neuronal responses.

With regard to sensory magnitudes, Ochoa and Torebjork (1983) somewhat surprisingly reported that increasing the frequency of the electrical stimuli to a single neuron did not produce a comparable change in the magnitude of the experience reported by the subject. This result runs counter to the widely accepted idea that neuronal frequency should encode the magnitude of the psychophysical response, but does support the alternative idea that psychological magnitude estimates are encoded by recruiting many neurons.

Different qualities of sensation, furthermore, were found by Ochoa and Torebjork (1983) to be associated with different areas of the skin. This finding supported the theory that individual neurons, although bundled together into a compound nerve, were individually associated with a specific kind of receptor unit and, thus, a specific kind of sensory quality. But results were varied; some units produced only a sensation of pressure with no sensitivity to the temporal sequence of the stimulus; no neuron ever produced a sense of pain or itch—responses that may also depend on a pattern population of responses; and a number of other activated units did not seem to produce any reported sensation according to these researchers. The superficial simplicity of their experimental design in this case belies the actually complexity the coding processes in these first-order neurons.

In a follow-up study from the same laboratory Lundberg, Jorum, Holm, and Torebjork (1992) studied the same problem using much the same technique and found equally contradictory results for individual small pain fibers. In this study the amplitude of pain did increase with stimulus frequency, however, even more so for irregular patterns than for irregular ones. This discrepancy may be due to a difference in the size of the sampled neurons with pain and touch possibly requiring different codes. A fairly recent review of somesthetic psychophysics and a bit of related neurophysiological work on humans can be found in Craig and Rollman (1999).

In the twenty-first century this kind of heroic invasive electrophysiological work on humans has diminished. In its place has been a considerable amount of work in which evoked brain potentials were recorded by averaging a number of noisy responses. Pioneering studies of this kind were carried out by Goff, Rosner, and Allison (1962), Rosner and Goff (1967), and Beck and Rosner (1968). They compared the evoked brain potential (or the event-related potential [ERP] as it is currently known) with psychophysical judgments and showed that at the high cerebral level at which the experience was encoded there were discrepancies between the ERP and psychophysical measures. Other work in this field has been carried out by Allison, McCarthy, Wood, Darcey, et al. (1989a) and Allison, McCarthy, Wood, Williamson, and Spencer (1989b) in which the goal was to distinguish between brain regions that produced short-latency responses and long-latency responses respectively. The literature on ERPs is immense and has been appropriately summarized in a major book by Regan (1989).

Taste

As just discussed, the radial, medial, and ulnar nerves of the arm are unusually accessible because of their anatomical location and the relatively long and exposed distance they run from the periphery of the body to their spinal roots. This is an anatomical curiosity that created an unusual opportunity for stimulating and recording along the elongated path of the great somesthetic axons. This anomaly in accessibility, however, is not unique. Almost as accessible is the chorda tympani, a nerve that innervates the portions of the tongue and carries information about taste to the central nervous system. This nerve is accessible because it runs through the middle ear and thus is exposed during auditory surgery, for example to free the stapes from bony impediments to its movement. Experiments of this kind are still difficult to carry out on conscious human subjects in the surgical theater; however in a few isolated cases near simultaneous psychophysical and neurophysiological experiments of the ideal kind described here have been carried out. Most of these experiments have been directed at the determination of the codes for subjective magnitude. The reason for this is that there are some special conceptual and logical problems that arise when one attempts to make value judgments about the quality of the experience generated by taste and other stimuli. Erickson (2008), for example, pointed out that the language we use can, for a variety of reasons, dominate the judgments that are made about how sensory quality is reported. He notes that our theories of taste are almost universal in proposing that there exist four separate tastes (sweet, sour, salty, bitter). This idea is so prevalent in our culture that any attempt to carry out an experiment to determine what are the "basic" tastes[18] will be highly confounded by a subject's prior experience with these four words.

In general, this caveat holds for all of the other senses. Should we ask a subject to name or define a color, for example, we are faced with a host of previous experiences that shape and limit the kind of responses that may be obtained and that may mislead us from an objective analysis of the salient codes. This is a classic instance of "cognitive penetration" influencing and confusing what were hoped to be pristine "sensory" topics.

The point is that the psychophysical judgments obtained even in the best simultaneous psychophysical-neurophysiological experiments are going to represent something quite different in kind than the more "objective" neurophysiological measurements. Cognitive neuroscientific research on taste quality is particularly vulnerable to this kind of contamination as described by Erickson (2008). It is a hopeful sign, therefore, to note that from the outset such experiments concentrated on magnitude judgments—a dimension that is much less influenced by cognitive penetration than are judgments of quality.

Separate electrophysiological and psychophysical studies of taste using animals have a relatively long modern history. Pfaffmann (1941) was among the first to study neural responses to taste stimuli in the chorda tympani (which innervates the front of the tongue) and the glossopharyngeal (which innervates the back of the tongue) nerves. These experiments showed that by far the majority of single fibers were responsive to more than one of the traditional quartet of taste stimuli. In a separate experiment (Pfaffmann, 1969), he studied the preference of experimental animals such as the squirrel monkey for different kinds of sugars and drew analogies between the neural and behavioral responses.

The pioneering taste study using human subjects, however, was reported by Borg, Diamant, Strom, and Zotterman (1967). They used the pooled action potentials of the chorda tympani as the source of their physiological measure and compared it to judgments of the amplitude of the taste responses that were generated by applying citric acid, salt (NaCl), or sucrose solutions separately to the tongue. Two patients, being operated on for ossification of the stapes, were asked to judge the intensity of the sensation produced when the tongue was stimulated with various concentrations of any one of these chemicals while the pooled neural response from the chorda tympani were recorded.

The general results of their experiments indicated that the psychophysical functions and the neural responses were all monotonic functions of the concentration of the taste stimuli. When plotted on log-log paper, the functional relations among the three chemicals and the neural responses were all characterized by power functions, although each with a different exponent. The exponent for citric acid was always less than 1 while the exponents of sucrose and salt were always equal to or greater than 1. They also noted that exponents for the neural responses were always comparable to the subjective ones for the same substances.[19]

Recent replications of this kind of experiment have been relatively rare. Somewhat similar studies have been carried out by Dimant, Oakley, Stroem, Wells, and Zotterman (1985) and by Oakley (1985), all of whom also compared responses of the chorda tympani and psychophysical judgments of amplitude. Oakley (1985) reported that the psychophysical and pooled neural responses generally agreed but only when the comparisons were for the same taste substance. Cross-sensory comparisons did not agree. Another interesting fact was that the responses to combinations of citric acid and sucrose together were less than to the sum of the two presented individually. This hints at a kind of reciprocal inhibitory interaction among the taste receptors similar to those previously reported in other sensory modalities. Somewhat less directly this finding also supports the idea of interneuron comparisons as a code for sensory quality.

Since the 1980s most work on the neurophysiology of taste has been carried out on laboratory animals and, thus, few direct comparisons of the kind carried out on humans by these pioneering Scandinavian investigators have been published recently.

Audition

Study of the complexities of the psychophysical responses to acoustic stimuli has been an extremely active field for over a century dating from at least Helmholtz's time (Helmholtz, 1863/1954). Reviews such as those by Hirsch and Watson (1996) provide at least a partial view of the breadth of this field. Auditory theory seeking to explain these psychophysical data has also been a major topic throughout this period; Helmholtz's resonance or tuned fiber theory competed with and eventually was replaced by Bekesy's (1960) standing-wave model.

Although single-fiber studies in experimental animals have been possible for many years (e.g., Galambos & Davis, 1943), it is far more difficult to access the auditory nerve fibers directly in humans, arising as they do deep within the bony vaults of the skull. The opportunity to carry out the kind of ideal experiment on the human auditory system in the ideal manner I suggested earlier is possible only in certain highly specialized situations and generally involves compound action potentials in which the responses of many neurons are pooled together into a composite response.

One way in which this can be done is to use an averaging computer to detect the very small signals on the scalp that have been associated with the response of the brainstem to acoustic stimuli. Pioneering studies of this kind were carried out by such researchers as Jewett, Romano, and Williston (1970). Although it is extremely difficult to measure the responses of individual fibers in the human acoustic nerve and its successive centers, it is possible to detect cumulative measures of activity at what are believed to be a number of places along the auditory pathway. The response produced by this method, designated as the auditory brain response (ABR) or the auditory evoked response, has been used to determine if an infant can hear (e.g., Sininger, Abadala, & Cone-Wesson, 1997) as well as in predicting the suitability of a patient for a cochlear implant.[20] Furthermore this noninvasive technique is believed to be sensitive enough to track the integrity of the auditory pathway all the way from the acoustic nerve to the cerebrum. Thus, it may add a great deal of specificity to the study of the possible levels of auditory transmission failure that could be the underlying cause of a psychophysically detected deafness.

A number of investigators have noted that there is a discrepancy between auditory thresholds measured psychophysically and the threshold response of neurons in the auditory pathway. In general, one of the great disappointments of comparisons of this sort has been the discrepancies between the two values. For example, Stoodley, Hill, Stein, and Bishop (2006) found that dyslexics showed abnormal ERPs even when they had compensated sufficiently to overcome many of their verbal problems. Similarly Pfingst (1988) reported that animal thresholds compared well with patients who had been treated with cochlear implants but not well with people with normal hearing. The reasons for this discrepancy may be that the cochlear implants use of electrical stimulation bypassed some of the very sensitive receptor properties. Other investigators have limited their conclusions to showing that deficits in hearing are linked to gross disturbances of the auditory nervous system at a particular level of processing rather than attempting to compare specific sensitivities or discriminabilities.

A major problem with the ABR as far as it is used to track responses throughout the acoustic pathway, however, is that it is the cumulative response not only of a number of neurons at each level but most likely the summation of near simultaneous responses from several levels of afferent processing. This multiple nature of the origins of the ABR is reflected in the complex nature of the signal as shown in figure 2.7.

Chiappa (1990) and Stelmack, Knott, and Beauchamp (2003) have all suggested that the wave component marked I is a result of activity in the auditory nerve; wave component III is a result of activity in the lower pons; and wave component V is due to activity in either the lateral lemniscus or the inferior colliculus (or both). Even later signals associated with the auditory cortex and the frontal lobes of the brain have also been reported.

Despite some residual uncertainty in assigning particular levels of the brainstem to each of these voltage excursions, this technique has, nevertheless, been used by researchers to carry out an approximation to the ideal cognitive neuroscience protocol proposed earlier. Werner, Folsom, Manci, and Syapin (2001), for example, compared ABR measurements with psychophysical thresholds for detecting a gap in a train of acoustic stimuli. They reported that a gap in the neural response, the ABR, was usually substantially shorter than the shortest gap that could be detected psychophysically—a somewhat surprising result.

Stelmack et al. (2003) carried out a similar experiment to see if auditory nerve conduction speeds were correlated with intelligence—a highly suspect hypothesis originally suggested

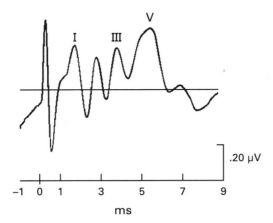

Figure 2.7
An averaged auditory evoked potential (AEP).
From Stelmach, Knott, and Beauchamp (2003), reprinted with the permission of Elsevier Science and Technology Journals.

by Ertl and Shafer (1969). Their results, to the degree they were just not an experimental or sampling artifact, indicated that not only was this hypothesis incorrect but that any slight correlation was negative—the slower the conduction speed, the higher the intelligence score.

There are several possible placements of the electrode used to pick up the ABR. Recording electrodes can be placed in the ear canal itself (in which case the signal is referred to as an electrocochleogram). This alternate placement probably produces an ABR that is more heavily weighted by the responses of the receptors in the inner ear as well as the auditory nerve responses than by higher levels of the auditory brainstem system. Such a placement is, therefore, especially useful in detecting peripheral receptor and nerve damage. Placing the recording electrodes on the skull, however, enhances the brainstem and cerebral responses to acoustic stimuli.

Vision
Although the optic nerve from the back of the eyes to the brainstem is accessible only in the most extreme surgical procedures, it is possible to noninvasively record a measure comparable to some of the compound action potentials just described. One electrophysiological response—the ERG—is detectable when an electrode is placed on the cornea; however, its signal strength is also so low that it can only be seen when it is averaged over multiple stimulus presentations. The procedure was first described by Armington (1974). The ERG is believed to be a cumulated measure of all of the neurons in the retina—rods, cones,

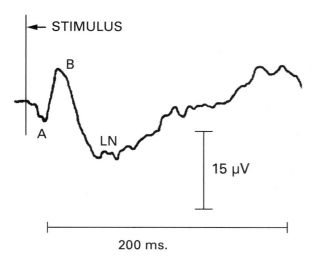

Figure 2.8
A typical electroretinogram.
Courtesy of the late Dr. John C. Armington.

amacrine, and horizontal cells. A typical ERG is shown in figure 2.8. The exact shape of the ERG will vary depending on the conditions of stimulation.

The various components of the ERG have been associated with the different neuronal components of the retina. The early component (the A wave in figure 2.8) was thought to be predominantly the result of the receptor cells; the B wave was mainly attributed to the horizontal and amacrine cells; and the late waves, it was thought, may be a result of activity in the pigment epithelium. Changes in any of the constituent waveforms substantially depend on the stimulus conditions. Because of the variation of the response with variations in the stimulus, the ERG has proven to be useful in determining a large number of pathological conditions in the eye.

Since the visual stimulus has so many different parameters that can be manipulated (e.g., intensity, wavelength, spatial locus, and so on) and the retina can exist in different states (e.g., those associated with dark adaptation), the opportunities for comparing this response with psychophysical data are extremely varied.

One of the most basic comparisons is between the absolute visual thresholds measured with the ERG and psychophysical methods respectively. Sieving and Nino (1988) carried out such a comparison for the most sensitive receptors of the retina—the rods—by dark-adapting the eye. They discovered that the psychophysical threshold was considerably lower than the threshold for a measurable ERG. Considering that the rod or scotopic threshold is very low (perhaps as low as a single quantum as demonstrated by Hecht, Shaler, & Pirenne,

1942 and Sakitt, 1972), this is hardly surprising; the ERG on the other hand is detectable only when a sufficiently large number of retinal neurons is activated.

A similar discrepancy between the human ERG and the effect of background light was reported by Frishman, Reddy, and Robson (1996). They found that the amount of background light that was necessary to produce a measurable decrement in the ERG under dim light conditions was five times higher than the psychophysical threshold.

The human ERG has also been compared with the contrast sensitivity function (i.e., the ability to detect a repetitive grating with minimal contrast) of the human eye by Peachey and Seiple (1987). Again there were discrepancies between the ERG sensitivity function and the psychophysical one. The ERG measure exhibited maximum contrast sensitivity at a lower frequency than did the psychophysical functions.

2.5   Interim Summary

The determination of the neural codes used by the sensory system to convey information from the receptors to the central nervous system represents one of the crown jewels of cognitive neuroscience. We know far more about the neuronal responses involved in these transmission processes than any other area of cognitive neuroscience. For decades investigators have been able to take advantage of the tight links and relative conceptual simplicity of the afferent pathways to unimpeachably determine the relation between the parameters of physical stimuli and the generated neurophysiological responses. Stimulus quality, quantity, and the temporal and spatial attributes of a stimulus have been directly shown to produce highly specific responses in peripheral nerves as well as the early stages of the receiving areas of the brainstem and cerebrum.

Similarly, a highly developed psychophysical methodology has also made it possible for psychologists to show well-developed patterns of relations among stimuli and simple judgments of the nature, amplitude, location, and time of occurrence of the resulting experiences.

Where we have been less successful is in carrying out true cognitive neuroscience experiments in which human subjects report the effects of stimuli while neurophysiological measures are taken.[21] It initially seemed that in those few instances in which the neural responses could be directly compared to psychophysical judgments would be a powerful means of fulfilling the meaning of a true cognitive neuroscience and, thus, open the door to a deep understanding of the coding processes involved in human sensation. For a number of reasons, this possibility has not been fulfilled to the degree that had been expected or hoped.

Typically, the neural responses studied in humans are compound potentials that are composed of the sum of many individual neuronal responses. The result is that specific sensory coding mechanisms of individual neurons are obscured in the pooling process. Furthermore there have been relatively few robust correlations of the neural and psychophysical responses that constituted the outcome of the ideal comparison experimental protocol in which human psychophysical and electrophysiological responses were compared as nearly simultaneously as possible. What is more usual are the many inconsistencies between the results obtained with the two types of measurement. For those interested in decoding the sensory nervous system, this has been a vast disappointment.

Because of such disappointments and the rise of other techniques to obtain objective measures of neural responses, interest in these compound potentials as a research tool for the study of sensory coding in humans has cooled over the last two decades. Current applications of this technique are mainly in the field of diagnostic medicine. Even then the tests are mainly used to simply evaluate the binary integrity of the auditory, visual, or somatosensory pathways—to determine are they conducting normally or not? In retrospect, little has been added to what we learned from animal models in which the psychophysical information was minimal.

Looking back over this chapter, it is clear to me that the class of experiments that I have designated as "sensory" have been mainly attacked with neurophysiological techniques. As a result these studies dip deeply into the temporal domain simply because of the high time resolution available with both macroscopic and microscopic measurement tools. It should be noted that this is a different outcome than the class of studies attacked with brain imaging devices in which the emphasis has been on spatial dimensions.

The following statements summarize the discussion in this chapter.

1. We distinguish between sensory and perceptual topics mainly as a convenience due to the huge amount of data available. The only other criterion of import is that sensory coding topics are mainly concerned with peripheral neural responses and perceptual ones are mainly concerned with central nervous responses.
2. Sensory codes are now known to be different at successive levels of the nervous system. There is no unique sensory code.
3. Sensory codes may be nonlinearly related to the stimulus and to the subjective experience.
4. Sensory coding phenomena and psychophysics are not directly linked by common postulates or robust demonstrations. Therefore, conceptual bonds between the two are mainly based on isomorphic analogies—a questionable approach.
5. Not all neurophysiological responses associated with stimulus dimensions are *codes*. Some may be concomitant, but irrelevant, *signs* that convey no information.
6. Structural maps of the sensory areas of the brain are best considered as speculative theories rather than proven maps.
7. It is now appreciated that the primary sensory receiving areas of the brain also respond to other high-level centrifugal signals. Thus, their supposedly unique sensory responses are influenced to an unknown degree by higher-level cognitive processes. However these centrifugal signals may be superimposed on topological maps (e.g., retinotopy and tonotopy) that have long been known to characterize the sensory areas.

8. Sensory mechanisms also self-modify transmitted information by means of such processes as lateral inhibitory interaction or feedback.

9. Sensory mechanisms are now known to be more sensitive to particular spatiotemporal patterns than to the raw energy content of a stimulus.

10. Sensory codes are now known to be especially sensitive to the probabilistic nature of stimulus patterns, particularly when we are dealing with real life stimuli such as pictures. The initial peripheral codes may be embedded in or be subsets of the probability sensitivity that actually characterizes the optimum response of a neuron.

11. A major goal of moderm sensory coding research is to determine if a neuron is encoding information efficiently. From an evolutionary perspective, it seems likely that it is, but it is not yet certain that this is the case. Unfortunately different methods produce different answers to this fundamental question.

12. Psychophysics is not neuroscience.

13. Psychophysical findings are neutral with regard to neural mechanisms.

14. Psychophysical research methods (in which relations between stimuli and experience are pursued) are aimed at controlling cognitive penetration into our judgments.

15. True cognitive neuroscience experiments in which sensations and neurophysiology are directly compared are relatively rare and depend on anatomical accidents in which neurons are superficial or accessible. However little supplementary knowledge beyond that available from animal studies has actually resulted from such studies. The reasons were varied but disappointing. One possibility is that experimental control of the adequate stimulus was never quite equal to that provided by nature. Another is that most of these studies involved compound action potentials rather than individual neuron responses, the actual level of salient sensory codes. Interest in such studies has flagged especially under the impact of the brain imaging devices that promised "direct" recordings of brain activity.

3 Perception

3.1 Introduction

For almost a century and a half, neuroscientists had been attempting to define which areas of the brain serve as the primary and immediate receiving areas for the several perceptual modalities. It is here, it has generally been assumed, that the transition from sensory information transmission begins to change to the representation of perceptual experiences. And it is to this latter topic—perception—mainly concerned with central nervous mechanisms (as opposed to those peripheral ones emphasized in the previous chapter) to which I now turn.

Over the years it has been difficult to distinguish between the meanings of the words *sensation* and *perception*. In some circles sensory research has been characterized as the study of the more immediate stimulus-determined responses. Indeed this is the source of the great advantage that sensory research has had over other kinds of cognitive experiments— the responses are closely linked to the precisely controlled and well-known properties of physical stimuli. It is the general congruity of the simplest of "Class A" responses (see note 12 of chapter 2) and the properties of the stimulus that has made sensory experiments so well defined and conceptually simple and the science so stable and relatively noncontentious. A sensory experiment, either phenomenological or physiological, succeeds to the degree that it can be shown to have a functional relation to a stimulus. We make every effort to minimize cognitive penetration by the use of simple binary type (i.e., yes–no) responses on the part of the subject. Functional agreement is taken for granted in sensory experiments.

The class of experiments that we designate as perceptual, however, is based on a different conceptual foundation. In general perceptual experiments dote on the discrepancies rather than the congruities between the phenomenological response and the stimulus; the prototype of a "perceptual" experiment is one in which the response is discrepant with the stimuli because of some "interpretation" or "cognitive penetration" that alters the "simple" sensory relation. The classic example of such an experimental category is the visual illusion—a phenomenon in which the perceived experience does not match the stimulus. Indeed in some cases the perceptual responses may be totally discrepant with the stimulus: that which is straight may appear curved; the hue may depend more on the surround than on the wavelength of the stimulus; or that which is stationary may appear to be moving. Clearly, however, the dividing line between sensation and perception is a fuzzy one, and several of the topics considered in the previous chapter could well be placed in this one and vice-versa.

Why perceptual discrepancies such as illusions occur is probably best attributed to the influence of higher-order cognitive influences on and misinterpretations of the incoming sensory information. These high-level cognitive influences may be short term (such as momentary figural aftereffects based on preconditioning) or long term (based on interpretations due to a lifetime of experience leading to stereotypy and prejudgments). Efforts to make the distinction based on where the critical causal events occur may also be useful in this context (as I did in Uttal, 1981). For example the trichromacy of vision is largely explained by the absorptive properties of the retinal receptors, whereas the size-distance illusion (incontestably a perceptual phenomenon) is largely thought to depend on higher-level cognitive processes.

The distinction between the two kinds of explanation, of course, is not always made as sharply as I make it here. Sensory and perceptual phenomena, furthermore, are often simply pooled together without critical examination of the fundamental conceptual differences between them. However, if one examines the range of perceptual topics to which brain imaging has been applied, it becomes clearer what is included in the rubric of "perceptual" research. For example the following topics are among the many usually included under their rubric of perceptual topics:

- Object recognition
- Face recognition
- Space and motion perception
- Illusions
- Change blindness
- Mirror neurons

3.2   The Imaging Epoch of Perceptual Cognitive Neuroscience

3.2.1   Prologue

In the previous chapter I considered four different approaches to the study of sensory and perceptual processes. First I considered the purely neuroscientific studies of the neural responses to physical stimuli—sensory coding. Then I turned to the purely behavioral studies of how people respond to the same physical stimuli—psychophysics. My argument was that neither of these two methodologies was actually an example of cognitive neuroscience. The third approach was also psychological; it challenged the perceptual system with ambiguous stimuli and then concentrated on observations of how these ambiguities were perceptually resolved.

The fourth approach, which is truly both cognitive and neuroscientific but rarely achieved, was to actually compare neural responses with attendant psychophysical responses in the same organism—ideally the human. It was only by means of this approach, I argued, that we could rise above the limitations, incompleteness, and indirectness of the first two approaches in our search for understanding of how the brain produces the mind.

The hope was that by carrying out simultaneous studies of neural and psychophysical responses on humans we would be able to determine answers to some of the most profound questions of mind-brain relations. For a number of reasons (including ethical constraints on experimentation on humans and idiosyncratic responses to both surgical interventions and traumatic injury), this idealized experimental protocol did not turn out to be as explanatorily fruitful as was originally hoped. It was hoped that by taking advantage of those few anatomical "accidents" in which peripheral nervous activities were accessible and measurable, we might converge on the ideal experimental protocol. However with only a few exceptions, the recorded neural responses were pooled or cumulative signals in which most of the subtle coding information was lost. Furthermore the results never seemed to be as informative as the designers of these neural-psychophysical investigators had hoped. Technical and procedural impediments always seemed to prevent clear-cut answers to what seemed to be even the simplest and best questions.

The alternative and unfortunately all too common strategy in this domain of cognitive neuroscience was to invoke what seemed to be related neurophysiological findings from model animal experiments as explanations. This kind of reasoning by analogy or seemingly isomorphic[1] functional relations was always subject to the limitations of interspecies comparison and a host of technical differences between the animal neurophysiological and the human psychophysical results.

Traumatic or experimental surgical manipulations of the human brain were equally unfruitful with clinical cases rarely having adequately defined lesions and usually having idiosyncratic behavioral results. With all of the clinical evidence, we still have not come very much further than the original pioneering studies that suggested where the primary projection sensory areas were located on the brain. The brain regions associated with higher-level cognitive processing still remain uncertain.

The revolution made possible by the introduction of brain imaging techniques promised to change almost everything, almost instantly. It seemed possible that we would be able to carry out experiments that were very close to the ideal protocol—simultaneous comparisons of psychophysical and neural responses on conscious, undamaged, and cooperating humans. This approach promised the opportunity to utilize a variety of elaborate stimuli and cognitive tasks that vastly exceeded those possible with animals and to collect information about brain localization that could resolve some of the classic uncertainties.

As a result of these high expectations, the classic approaches of psychophysics and sensory coding research have been supplemented to a substantial degree by brain imaging technologies emphasizing perceptual neuroscience. This is perhaps one of the most significant paradigm shifts in the history of physiological psychology. For example, nowadays sensory and perceptual researchers are far more likely to be seeking brain activations that correlate with processes such as recognition than seeking to redefine the extent of the primary visual cortex.

The impact of this new technology on cognitive neuroscience has been enormous. Within a couple of decades many of those who are interested in sensory function and who had depended on lesioning or stimulation methods simply dropped the tools and techniques with which they had worked for a lifetime and moved into the positron emission tomography (PET) or, more likely, the fMRI laboratory. Many others, whose work had been purely behavioral, psychological, or psychophysical in their previous research orientations, joined those who had been traditional physiological psychologists in this new environment. The most extreme version of the dream was that now that we could directly, as well as noninvasively, examine the mind-brain relationship including the study of perception, cognitive neuroscience would come of age. No longer would we be bound by the constraints of uncertain interspecies comparisons or ethical concerns preventing human experimental surgery. No longer would we be confined to a few iconic cases provided by accident or surgical necessity. Now we could apply all of the powerful statistical tools developed over the years to large samples of individuals.

Unfortunately these high hopes have not yet been fulfilled. Instead the study of cognitive and perceptual processes that had hitherto been so recalcitrant to understanding remains elusive. Why did this happen? One answer to this question is that although brain imaging techniques are extremely powerful, they have some severe limitations, and the field failed to take these limitations into account. Because they are relatively insensitive (i.e., they display high thresholds relative to the exquisite sensitivity of both the whole visual system and individual neurons) and cumulative (i.e., the details of individual neuronal responses are always obscured in the cumulative response), the goal of comparing brain image data and psychophysical thresholds remained unfulfilled.

What the brain imaging techniques do best is to provide an answer to the question of where on the brain activity is observed when a stimulus is presented.[2] Unfortunately empirical data are driving us in another direction in which the question of "where" may be becoming meaningless. The preponderance of modern brain imaging data, as we see throughout this book, suggests the wide distributions of brain activations to even the simplest stimuli.

Furthermore as Poldrack (2006) and Van Horn and Poldrack (2009) have repeatedly pointed out, we cannot reverse engineer the brain to determine what thought is being processed when a particular area of the brain is highlighted (see chapter 1).[3] The best we can do is to use patterns of activity to select among a prior set of alternatives. The most fundamental reason for this constraint is that brain imaging is operating at the wrong level of analysis. The accumulation of individual neuronal responses into (blood oxygen level dependent) BOLD signals washes out the detailed interactions of the great neuronal networks of the brain, and it is there, most likely, that the psychoneural equivalent of perception resides.

The main point of this prologue is that a brain image is highly limited in what it can say about the neuroscience of processes such as sensation and perception. It is not a panacea that will open the door to full understanding of the mind-brain problem any more than did any of the previous technological approaches. The brain's role in our mental life remains a hard nut to crack, despite the radical promises of many of the brain image aficionados.

With this cautionary prelude in hand, I now turn to a review of some of the more significant studies in which brain imaging techniques have been applied to perceptual problems. Once again I choose to organize the following discussion in terms of the sensory modalities, although in a somewhat different order than used in the preceding chapter.

3.2.2 Vision

There is no more appropriate place to start this discussion of fMRI studies of human visual perception then with a very important question asked and answered by Bartels, Logothetis, and Moutoussis (2008) concerning visual area V5 in the medial temporal gyrus of the brain. As they noted, based on a number of electrophysiological studies of single cells (e.g., Maunsell & Newsome, 1987), individual neurons in this area have long been thought to encode the motion of visual stimuli in a directionally sensitive manner. The question asked by Bartels and his colleagues was—is it possible to determine from fMRI images the properties of the individual neurons that make up this brain region? This question is so generally important to understanding the advantages and disadvantages of the fMRI technique that I choose to deal with it in detail at the beginning of this discussion.

To answer this question, Bartels, Logothetis, and Moutoussis reviewed and critiqued experiments that used two popular procedures. The first was the adaptation technique in which subjects were preconditioned with movement in one direction, and the diminished responses that resulted from this selective use were recorded. The second used "drifting gratings" for which the sensation of motion was very strong, but the physical stimulus was not explicit for motion. They ultimately concluded that both of these experimental protocols were deeply confounded; the findings from these experiments were highly sensitive to the attentional state of the subject, adding further to the uncertainty about what the fMRI measures had to say regarding the properties of the constituent neurons. It is, therefore, not possible, they concluded, to draw the conclusion that V5 contained directionally sensitive neurons in it from the fMRI data alone. The general implication of their work is that the cumulative nature of any fMRI signal prohibits its use as a means of establishing the nature and the properties of the neurons that contribute to it.

There were two main reasons for this outcome of their analysis according to Bartels, Logothetis, and Moutoussis. One was that the spatial resolution of the fMRI was not adequate to separate out the individual responses of the large number of neurons encompassed even within the boundaries of a single voxel—a volume that constitutes the current resolving power of the technique but that includes thousands of neurons. Thus, the results of a mixed bag of neuronal responses could cancel out any special sensitivity on the part of individual neurons. As we see later in this chapter this is exactly the flawed strategy used by a number of workers who attempt to reason from the whole to its parts.

The second reason, as Bartels, Logothetis, and Moutoussis (2008) also pointed out, is that an fMRI image may be the result of cumulating something quite different than the spike action potentials thought to be a key to neural coding of sensory processes. Instead, they argued that: "A key reason for this is that BOLD signal is not primarily driven by principal neuron spiking, but by the input and local processing of the area under investigation and that in some cases the two can be entirely dissociated" (p. 451). Bartels, Logothetis, and Moutoussis then went on to argue that, however different are the results obtained with traditional neurophysiological experiments and brain imaging techniques, these techniques should not be rejected entirely. Both are capable of adding some information—at least in the sensory domain where the experimental conditions are so much better controlled than in the domain of higher-level cognitive functions. They concluded their critical discussion by noting that although it is not possible to confirm that there are directionally sensitive neurons in V5, fMRI can be expected to be a "valuable methodology that provides complementary information" and "might be sufficient to formulate hypotheses" (p. 451). From the outset, therefore, the answer to the question—is there an fMRI measure of individual cellular sensitivities?—has to be a negative one. As we see later, many other investigators have not been as self-critical as were Bartels, Logothetis, and Moutoussis concerning the use of fMRI signals to describe the properties of individual neurons.

Regional Sensitivity

The literature on brain imaging studies of the location of visual system activations is extensive. A few examples in which fMRI systems were used to investigate stimulus produced neural responses to visual stimuli will help to clarify some of the main points and highlight some of the progress that has been made as well as some of the difficulties and limits of this approach.

An important question concerns the differences in the location of brain activations to different categories of stimuli. One of the most notable of these studies, which led to the discovery of what is now known as the fusiform face area (FFA), was reported by Kanwisher, McDermott, and Chun (1997). Support for the idea that this area was specifically if not uniquely sensitive to face stimuli came from observations that showed that the response was enhanced to intact faces compared to images containing scrambled parts of faces.

An often overlooked interpretation of their results, however, was that this area is not exclusively a face area. The FFA not only responds strongly to faces but also less vigorously to other classes of objects. Furthermore other brain regions have been shown to be involved in face stimuli processing by such workers as Haxby et al. (2001) and Hanson, Matsuka, and Haxby (2004). Despite suggestions like these that there are no unique regions for encoding visual processes and that virtually all such processes are widely distributed in the brain, many researchers using fMRI techniques have continued to search for localized areas in which such entities as faces are encoded.

A number of investigators have, thus, simply (and often naively) taken advantage of the main capability of brain imaging equipment to attempt to answer the question of where brain activity is evoked by various kinds of visual stimuli. For example Wilkinson et al. (2000) reported that radial and concentric gratings produced strong responses in V1, V4, and FFA unlike parallel gratings, which only differentially activated the V4 and FFA areas. Moving illusory contours were shown to produce activity in the primary visual cortex by Seghier et al. (2000).

Furthermore, Gauthier et al. (2002) associated superior parietal gyrus activity with mental rotation but not with object recognition. Likova, Tyler, and Wade (2003) reported that moving stereoscopic images induced activity in the medial temporal and medial superior temporal areas and virtually nowhere elsewhere.

A number of fMRI experiments have been carried out to map the components of the human visual system corresponding to those described by Felleman and Van Essen (1991) for rhesus monkeys. One of the earliest of these was the study by DeYoe et al. (1996) in which flickering checkerboards were used as the stimulus to produce cerebral activations. This technique produced evidence of six regions of the extrastriate cortex that were responsive to this kind of visual stimulus. Although there was considerable variability from subject to subject, these investigators did report reliable regional responses for their six subjects.

A more recent study also using fMRI techniques to map out the visual regions of the brain has been reported by Stiers, Peeters, Lagae, Van Hecke, and Sunaert (2006). In their work they used more realistic stimuli consisting of samples from one of three classes (1) photographs of common objects; (2) moving scenes; and (3) a single fixation dot used as a control. Building on earlier ideas that visual information leaves the primary projection area in two streams, one of which projects into the parietal area (the dorsal stream) and one of which projects into the temporal gyrus (the ventral stream), they reported the existence of 29 distinguishable regions of the human visual system responsive to what we call perceptual stimuli.[4] It is not clear from their analysis how closely their results fit with the Felleman and Van Essen (1991) model, but each of the two sets of regions observed by Stiers and his colleagues did seem to encode "distinguishable activations" according to them. Nine ventral (mainly occipital-temporal) regions were preferentially activated by passive viewing of objects, whereas the dorsal stream (mainly occipital-parietal) seemed to be most sensitive to moving stimuli.

There were of course substantial differences between subjects; not all subjects produced the same activation regions. Therefore, it was not possible for Stiers and his colleagues to link these 29 visual regions with the 30 or so that are otherwise believed to be present in the human being. Nor, for that matter, is it possible to define precise boundaries between these 29 regions (their extent being defined by arbitrary statistical criteria).

The complexity of the human visual system and the difficulty of rigorously defining the functional role of even the best demarcated brain region can be appreciated from studies like those of Kourtzi and Kanwisher (2000). These researchers showed that it was not only *real* motion but also *implied* motion that could activate some of the visually responsive regions. Using an fMRI method, they studied the activations in the medial and medial superior temporal gyrus and found that responses were enhanced when pictures of stationary objects that were obviously in motion (e.g., a running athlete) were compared to the lesser responses elicited when the object was apparently at rest (e.g., a picture of a person sitting in a chair). The suggestion from this kind of finding is that it is not just the physical aspects of the stimulus (i.e., real motion) but also the cognitive implications that drive the responses of neurons relatively early in the visual system. This suggests that very high-level interpretive mechanisms are also involved in what had hitherto been thought to be the more or less passive response of this "perceptual" system. The semantic meaning, the logical significance, or the implication of a static picture can produce responses that are far from the physical stimulus.

All of these studies make it clear that the visual nervous system is much more complex than our current models suggest. There is little agreement among the studies I have reviewed here on the exact location of what all agree are multiple areas, much less what are the perceptual functions encoded by each. Part of this inconsistency is due to experimental protocol reasons—too great a variety of stimuli are used and too few experiments are exactly replicated. Part results from differing statistical criteria for what constitutes activation as well as differences in the data analysis techniques. However, I believe that the most substantial source of disagreement is the simple fact that these visual brain regions are not driven solely by information flowing in the afferent direction. Even in the periphery, cognitive penetration is regularly observed—implied as well as actual stimuli can affect the responses of these regions. Therefore, the functions of a given area may shift almost momentarily given factors that are not controlled by the experimenter. Obviously not enough control is exerted on higher-order cognitive processes when what are touted as purely perceptual experiments are carried out.

Interactions of Visual Areas with Other Areas of the Brain

Kourtzi and Kanwisher's (2000) experiment is a good point to transition to another class of brain imaging studies of perceptual phenomena—those that suggest further that the process is not simple, but very complex and increasingly so as our knowledge expands. We are learning that many different regions of the brain are involved in what are even the simplest and most direct perceptual responses to visual stimuli. The point is that assignment of a particular sensitivity to a particular region of the brain may be a vast underestimate of the true functional complexity of even these most peripheral portions of the nervous system.

It had long been a basic postulate of cognitive neuroscience that the primary sensory projection areas of the brain were more or less passive responders to the physical (including spatiotemporal patterns) properties of the stimulus. This concept permeates many of the studies just discussed; differential sensitivity to stimulus properties was thought to be independent of the interactions that that area might have with other regions of the brain or with other cognitive states. We now know that this is an understatement; high-level brain regions can exert a strong influence on the most peripheral visual regions.

We also now appreciate that such cognitive states as attention may have a powerful influence on any number of different sensory and perceptual tests including such seemingly basic ones as determining absolute thresholds for subjective magnitude or motion. The neuroscientific question that arises, therefore, is—where is the effect of such high-level processes being mediated in the brain? Is the information passively ascending through the brain from the primary projection areas before being modified at high levels or, to the contrary, is the high-level activity being projected downward (centrifugally) to modulate the activity in even the most peripheral portions of the nervous system. As brain imaging studies proliferated, the hope was that answering this question would become both plausible and possible.

One of the first of the efforts to resolve this question was reported by Somers, Dale, Seiffert, and Tootell (1999). Using an fMRI procedure and controlling the attentive state of the subject by directing attention either toward or away from a visual stimulus projected on a rear projection screen, they generated brain images for both attentive and inattentive conditions. Although a number of different visual areas of the brain were shown to be influenced by the direction of attention, the most notable result of this experiment was the "robust" response of V1 when attention was directed at the stimulus. Somers and his colleagues concluded: "The overall view that emerges suggests that V1 is not simply a passive, image-processing front end, as is often assumed" (p. 1668).

Another early fMRI paper (Lumer & Rees, 1999) from the same time period examined the related question of which brain areas were involved in "subjective visual perception." The question attacked was related to but is not the same as the one concerned with the effect of attention previously discussed. Lumer and Rees were concerned with the broader question of what parts of the brain are required for perception—that is, conscious awareness. Their answer to that question, nevertheless, spoke directly to the problem of the interaction between different areas of the brain in cognition. What they discovered was that the system of brain regions that is involved in visual perception is very broad indeed. It included the frontal and parietal areas of the brain as well as the peristriate and striate areas.

Although this is not surprising, it does suggest that activation of much of the entire brain occurs when we are experiencing something as simple as the perception of a tangible and concrete physical object. It also suggests, albeit less strongly, that the lower levels of the visual system (V1, V2, V3, etc.) may not be sufficient to account for perceptual experience. At another level of discourse, it also raises questions about the true complexity of the nervous system and just how far we can go in potentially explaining it.

Recent studies very emphatically make the same point of broad distribution of brain activations in perception, albeit in a completely different manner. They suggest that there are multiple interconnections between distant regions of the cerebrum that may further impact on our ability to understand perceptual representation. Ruff et al. (2006) used a novel stimulus—transcranial magnetic stimulation—applied to a brain region known as the frontal eye field (FEF). (The FEF is a region of the prefrontal motor cortex known to be associated with the control of eye movements.) Using fMRI to measure the response of the visual cortices (V1-V4), Ruff et al. discovered that the FEF stimulation also affected the response of these early visual regions.

In a related experiment Bressler, Tang, Sylvester, Shulman, and Corbetta (2008) reported that both the FEF and a region around the interparietal sulcus enhanced the fMRI response of the visual cortex when the subject was "prepared" by focusing attention on one of two positions in a visual field. The effect was greater in later regions of the visual stream (e.g., V4) than in V1 and V2, but some subjects showed modulations of even V1 and V2.[5] All of these experiments and many others argue for widely distributed and heavily interacting nature of the brain in responding to what were hitherto considered to be relatively simple stimuli. Clearly high-level effects have powerful effects on even the earliest parts of the perceptual brain.

Perceptual Contents and the fMRI

One of the many important issues raised by the advent of brain imaging techniques is the hope that they will be able to measure or decode the contents of the mind. That is, we are now asking whether or not it is possible to determine what a person is "thinking" or "perceiving" from an fMRI image. For many of the reasons discussed in chapter 1, it seems unlikely that the details of complex cognitive processes such as attention, problem solving, or truth-telling can be extracted from the images produced by this kind of measurement. However, although it may be possible to distinguish in some rough manner what kind of perceptual activity is under way, discerning the details of our high-level thought processes with an fMRI seems more distant than travel to another star. Nevertheless, "reading the mind" is considered by many researchers to be the ultimate goal—the "holy grail" of fMRI studies. This section examines the progress that has been made and evaluates what I believe is the remote possibility that this kind of physiological measure might open an objective window into subjective experience.

The situation with perceptual phenomena, which involve interpretations of the sensory codes, is a much more ambiguous situation than are some of the seemingly simpler sensory processes. Starting in about the year 2000, a number of researchers began to ask if it was possible to attack the problem of inferring our perceptual experiences from fMRI data. Given that any number of studies had been published showing the different areas of the brain were differentially responsive to certain aspects of the stimulus, a logical next step would be to ask whether or not it might be possible to infer from the brain image produced by real-world images what was being perceived by the subject? If possible, this would be one of the most extraordinary developments in the two-decade-long history of the attempt to associate brain images and cognitive processes.[6]

At about this time a major conceptual change occurred in this kind of fMRI research that has been well captured in the publications of such workers as O'Toole et al. (2007) and Poldrack, Halchenko, and Hanson (2009). O'Toole and her colleagues pointed out that we are now asking a fundamentally different question than in the early years of fMRI brain imaging. Where we had previously been looking for localized regions associated with cognitive processes, the current task for some researchers is now becoming the quite different search for the answer to the question: "How reliably can patterns of brain activation indicate or predict the task in which the brain is engaged or the stimulus which the experimental subject is processing?" (p. 1736). Poldrack, Halchencko, and Hanson's (2009) formulation of this basic question is conceptually the same: "What task is the subject engaged in given the observed pattern of brain activity?" (p. 8). Curiously, the answer to these questions does not depend on robust knowledge accumulated from the search for localized functions—it is not essential that the location of the salient regions be known before they can be considered. This issue can be resolved on the fly, so to speak, if one takes into account activity widely dispersed around the brain. All that is necessary is that the brain activation pattern varies from one cognitive experience to another.

As impressive as this work is most of it depends on a prior set of responses that have been linked to the particular pattern of brain activations. This is a critical point in understanding the work to be described. These results do not mean that the percept is being reconstructed directly from the brain images; instead it allows us to use some unexpected differences in the pattern information to select forms from a "library" in much the same way that the Asian telegraph system used number codes to represent the 5,000 or so characters that could be transmitted. The number code itself contained none of the pictorial or semantic content of characters.[7]

Although the change from the search for localization to the inference of distinguishable perceptual experience would not be tantamount to "reading the mind," it would represent a major step forward toward discriminating cognitive processes from each other and open the door at least a little bit to achieving that "holy grail."

To appreciate the significance of this change in the direction that cognitive neuroscience has taken, it is useful to consider some of the studies that have led to it. A seminal study that played a large role in moving the question from speculation to laboratory investigation was the work of Ishai, Ungerleider, and Haxby (2000). These researchers were interested in comparing the fMRI responses of the brain to real stimuli and imagined ones. In setting the stage for this comparison they determined the response of various areas of the ventral temporal cortex to real stimuli including houses, faces, and chairs respectively. They found that the maximum responses to houses were observed in the medial fusiform gyrus, the maximum responses to faces were recorded from the lateral fusiform gyrus and the maximum responses to chairs were observed in the inferior temporal gyrus; all of which were regions of the temporal lobe. Comparable selectively sensitive regions, they reported, were also found in the occipital cortex.

An important aspect of their findings was that these sensitivities to real stimuli were not paralleled by any equivalent responses to imagined objects or faces. In empirical fact, imaging equivalent faces or objects produced activity in only a few of the many areas activated by real stimuli. However, a large number of other brain regions ranging from the cerebellum to the cingulate and the frontal lobes (not usually associated with vision) were activated. From these findings, they concluded that the imagined stimuli did not utilize the same regions of the visual system but, instead, invoked activity in regions devoted to higher-level cognitive skills. The suggestion in their findings, therefore, is that the differential fMRI responses they measured were following the *real physical stimulus* but not the *perceived experience*. One implication of this difference between real and imagined stimuli is that the early responses may not encode perception as much as transmission.

However the main impact of this work for the purposes of this discussion was to suggest the possibility that one could to a limited degree determine what was being "perceived" (if not "imagined") by examining the pattern of the fMRI images. At the least, Ishai and colleagues (2000b) showed that it was possible in the restricted case of determining which of the three stimulus types—houses, faces, and chairs—was being presented to the subject. It must be kept in mind, however, that each of the regions activated by each of the stimulus types, is not only associated with the particular type of stimulus used in this experiment but is also involved in many other perceptual and cognitive processes (including, to a lesser degree, the other object classes that had been studied in this experiment). Therefore attributing a particular perception to heightened activity in one of these temporal or occipital regions remains problematic even if this experiment showed that this or that region would be differentially activated by a particular class of stimuli. In any case their accomplishment was substantial; at the very least they were among the first to discriminate between broad classes of stimuli by means of the pattern of fMRI activations.

Over the last decade a considerable effort has been made to infer what kind of stimulus was being perceived from fMRI images. Some remarkable results have been forthcoming. During this time period a number of investigators proposed that the conventional analysis of fMRI signals in which correlations were shown between a stimulus and a particular place or places in the brain did not take full advantage of the power of the fMRI technique; much more information might be available if more complex multivariate analyses were utilized to tease out a richer store of data. This new approach essentially required that measurements be made of the pattern of activity among voxels that were widely distributed over and within the brain rather than concentrating on specific "signature" locales of activation. Carlson, Schacter, and He (2003), for example, had reanalyzed data obtained by Ishai, Ungerleider, Martin, Schouten, and Haxby (2000) and by Ishai, Ungerleider, and Haxby (2000) using linear discriminant analysis (LDA). Although the results were modest (typically one category of objects—houses, faces, or chairs—was discriminated from either one of the other two about 75% of the time), the results were better than could have been obtained with a simple univariate correlation. Again, there was no explicit inference of what the subject perceived, just a distinction drawn between the neural signals associated with classes of objects. Nevertheless the idea that a broad distribution of a group of activated regions, rather than a single area, could be more effective than a single area in suggesting what stimulus was being viewed was further encouraged.

The ability of an fMRI pattern analysis to determine what class of object was being viewed was significantly expanded by the work of Haxby and colleagues (2001). This group worked with eight different categories of visual stimuli and concentrated their attention on the ventral temporal cortex, a region long thought to be deeply involved in object vision. Again, it was possible to associate a specific pattern of responses with each of the stimulus categories. Indeed Haxby et al. (2001) were able to accomplish this identification even when activations in the area responding maximally to each of the stimulus categories were excluded from their analysis. This strongly supports the idea that there was no cryptic localization, and, in their words: "These results indicate that the representation of faces and objects in the ventral temporal cortex are widely distributed and overlapping" (p. 2425).

This study produced classification accuracies that were very high (70–100%). However, these were the results obtained from individual subjects, not comparisons between subjects, a much more complicated task.

Kriegskorte, Formisano, Sorger, and Goebel (2007) expanded this line of inquiry and showed that it was not just the ventral temporal cortex studied by Haxby and his colleagues, but also the FFA and the anterior inferotemporal cortex (aIT) that were involved in face recognition. They went to hypothesize that each of these two regions may have different functions—the FFA being responsible for detecting a face and the aIT for the recognition process. However, even more striking was their claim that the right aIT produced fMRI-patterned responses that could be used to distinguish between individual faces!

Cox and Savoy (2003), using a variety of multivariate methods, looked at data from even more widely distributed regions of the visual system. They had 10 different categories of stimulus objects so the task was more difficult than the simpler designs used by Ishai, Haxby, and Carlson and their respective colleagues. Cox and Savoy designed their experiment so that a subject was exposed to the stimulus set during a "training" period. The distributed responses to each of the stimuli were then taught to several different kinds of statistical pattern recognizers.[8] At a later time, the same subjects were exposed to the same stimuli, and the task of the pattern classifier program was to determine from the new images which of the stimuli had been presented.

The results of Cox and Savoy's experiments depended on whether the exemplars of each of the ten categories were the same or different in the training and test situations, the number of voxels incorporated into the analysis, and which pattern-recognition technique was being used. Under the best conditions (mainly using the linear support vector machine program) 97% accuracy was obtained. Most combinations of analysis method, stimuli, and voxel count, however, produced much lower recognition scores. However there was one design factor that mitigates the contribution this report and others like it might have made. Cox and Savoy (2003) set up sample reference signals for their analysis by pretraining their system and collecting a library of fMRI responses to their stimulus set. Thus the analysis programs simply had to seek the best match between the trained and test conditions. This is not the kind of robust procedure that would permit us to transfer this method to a new naïve subject. Separation of the training and test subjects would be an even more important accomplishment.

In addition to the methodological contribution and this newfound ability to use the fMRI to seemingly associate perceptual experiences and brain responses, another important aspect of all of these experiments was to further enhance the emerging consensus of distribution. That is, even the simplest percepts are encoded by multiple, distributed regions of the brain instead of single, unique locales. However, as noted earlier, there may be an even more substantial practical implication of this work; namely that the cumulative fMRI has much more information in it than had been previously thought. The new multivariate methods used by these investigators helped to extract more of that information and promised the ability to provide a possible means of associating fMRI responses with our perceptions.[9]

An important next step was made by Kamitani and Tong (2005) when they showed that fMRI images of the early visual areas (V1 and V2) could reliably be associated with a stimulus consisting of a set of eight oriented gratings *without training*.[10] This experiment used the statistical analysis of an ensemble of voxels, each of which was only a weak indicator, to produce a relatively robust estimate of stimulus orientation. Presumably this outcome resulted from the pooling of the responses of many individual orientation-selective neurons stimulated within the appropriate portion of the visual field. However as the signal rose through the visual pathway, according to Kamitani and Tong (2005), the fMRI signals showed progressively less orientation sensitivity. This tendency to lose the correlated signals in the higher reaches of the cerebrum (a result appearing several times in this research literature) raises the question—are the correlations between the fMRI image and the afferent sensory transmission codes or between the fMRI image and the neural apparatus of perception? If the former, then the hope of examining high-level cognitive processes with this approach remains remote.

A related study was reported by Thirion and colleagues (2006) in which they utilized the known fact that the retina is represented in visual areas of the brain in a retinotopic manner. That is, the spatial pattern of the retinal stimulus is replicated on early brain regions in a topological manner in which spatial relations are maintained. Using stimuli composed of sets of oriented Gabor patterns in a domino-like arrangement and then recording fMRIs, they could infer which arrangement was being perceived. This could be accomplished for a rather broad swath of visual regions as well as for voxels limited to V1.

The basic idea inherent in this experiment was that the fMRI was able to measure the spatial arrangements of brain responses and show that these were correlated with stimulus patterns which presumably evoked a particular perception. Correlations between the reconstructed brain images and the original stimulus patterns were in the range of 0.5 to 0.6 (random responses would be about 0.16). Thus, Thirion and his colleagues (2006) were also able to find a modest ability on the part of their analysis method to infer which pattern was being presented and presumably perceived on the basis of fMRI signals. Perhaps of even greater significance was that they were also able to discriminate among imagined patterns using the same procedure, a finding not reported in the earlier work.

All of these results are, from some points of view, still relatively ambiguous. First it remains unknown what the subject actually perceived. All that we really know is that early levels of the visual system (which may be more involved in information transmission than perceptual representation) did display a differential fMRI response to different stimuli. Many questions remain unanswered. For example—is it at the periphery that the conscious experience is manifested or instantiated, or is this simply a composite response of a population of neurons that collectively responds to stimuli with or without conscious experience? Furthermore, what is the significance of the fact that this orientation specificity declines as one ascends the visual pathway?

These questions were only partially answered in a supplementary experiment carried out by Kamitani and Tong and also reported in their 2005 article. Using an ambiguous grating as a stimulus, they showed that a subject produced orientation-distinguishable fMRI responses depending on the mental state, that is, which way the grating was perceived. Kamitani and Tong concluded that what a person perceived could be detected with orientation-sensitive fMRI signals. This suggests that the word "orientation" may have multiple meanings: (1) The Hubel and Wiesel sense of the sensitivity of individual neurons, and (2) the apparent or perceptual sense.

The application of statistical classifiers or pattern recognizers to the interpretation of fMRI images has had an enormous impact in the last few years. As I note earlier the main contribution is to tease out information to a degree that had not previously been thought to be possible. However, as O'Toole and colleagues (2007) point out in their thoughtful and comprehensive discussion of these statistical pattern classifiers, there are fundamental changes in our thinking when the problem is approached from this new point of view. No longer is the emphasis on the now seemingly quaint idea of identifying narrowly localized regions of the brain associated with modules of the mind. Instead, it is now possible to conceptualize the brain as a distributed system in which the overall response pattern rather than the individual locale is the significant dependent variable. Using this distributed concept and using a statistical approach in which many voxels of the brain are involved in the analyses, it is now being claimed that the cognitive processes involved in perception can be discriminated. Even for some of us skeptics there is a promise here that cannot be ignored.

The majority of applications of these new statistical pattern-processing algorithms to fMRI analysis have been in the area of visual perception and relatively low-level encoding. However the implicit promise that we may be able to actually use fMRI as a means of determining what the person is "thinking" or "perceiving" remains a tantalizing future goal. Ideally there would be enough commonality between the pattern of fMRI responses from different individuals to permit us to say what it was that a person perceived or, in the ultimate case, what a person was thinking at a much more complex level of cognitive activity.

It is vitally important in this context to appreciate that most of the work in this field carried out so far and that I have reviewed here deals with relatively low levels of visual information processing. Frequently the process fails, and the fMRI fails to distinguish between these relatively low-level sensory and perceptual states as activations from higher and higher levels of the brain are introduced into the analysis. Therefore, the possibility remains that what are really being measured are just the neural transmission codes that may or may not have a direct relation to more complex perceptual experiences. Thus we may not be reading the "cognitive mind" as much as using a new tool to study afferent neural codes.

Furthermore it is important to understand that these pattern classifiers are not by themselves any more direct measures of the mind than are the signals from an EEG or a microelectrode. What they represent is a powerful means of correlating a rather indirect measure of distributed neural responses with perceptual activity. *However, even the most highly correlated signals may be signs of perceptual experiences without being measures of the psychoneural equivalents for experience.*[11] It is quite likely that we will be able to get a general idea of what a subject's nervous system is doing as it passes information from receptors to high cortical levels without being able to make the fine distinction between the brain activations representing a cup of coffee or tea or between a lie and truthful expression.

This uncertainty sits as a major impediment at the frontier of current cognitive neuroscience that seeks to determine how brain activations correlate with potentially higher-order cognitive processes. It is where some of the most interesting and challenging (but possibly most misunderstood) work is currently being done. Among the most imaginative and provocative studies are those emerging from the laboratories of Marcel Just and Russell Poldrack. I now consider the accomplishments of each of their groups in turn. However, let us quickly summarize what the discussion so far has shown.

1. Some of the studies demonstrated that it is possible to distinguish among a relatively small number of exemplar visual stimuli or among a few classes of objects using a statistical pattern-recognition approach for the analysis of fMRI images.

2. The design of many of the studies is confounded by a confusion of what may be sensory transmission codes with the true psychoneural equivalents of perceptual phenomena.

3. Few of the studies examined the plausibility of this approach for the discrimination of high-level cognitive processes; all are studies of visual perception, either real or imagined.

4. Most of the studies so far reviewed used statistical measures that were based on a subject population that included the same subject or subjects in the standardization process who were subsequently tested. Little effort was made to determine the commonalities that might exist among subjects by testing other individuals who were not a part of the training group.

There have been two new developments that add considerable impact to this new approach to the analysis of fMRI activations. In the first Shinkareva and colleagues (2008) report that they overcame the obstacle of individual differences by showing that there are common fMRI features that permit identification of viewed objects by individuals who had not been part of the original training group. The second (Poldrack et al., 2009) carries this work forward to what is seemingly the impossible task of discriminating between high-level cognitive processes with fMRI activations. I now discuss each of these pioneering studies in turn.

The contribution by Shinkareva et al. (2008) could be an extraordinary step forward; if replicated and substantiated[12] it would mean that it is possible to use the fMRI signal to determine what an individual person, literally taken off the street, (not a part of the training sessions that set up the templates for the pattern-recognition process) was viewing. However small the set of items or processes to be discriminated, this would be a major accomplishment. Most previous work had almost entirely dealt with groups of subjects who were used in both the standardization and test groups. Furthermore if there is not some cryptic artifact, it could be fairly claimed that the precision of this technique was great enough to distinguish not just the class of stimulus objects but a substantial number of individual exemplar objects within a class. No longer would experiments be limited to distinguishing between categories such as houses and tools or among just a few objects within a category; instead Shinkareva and her colleagues claimed that it could be determined which of ten objects (five types of tools and five types of dwellings) was being viewed using the pattern-recognized fMRI data!

The design of this experiment involved two different experimental conditions, each of which involved combinations of objects and brain regions. First the ability to identify *individual* objects (exemplar identification) using whole-brain pattern-recognition procedures was compared to the use of only a single brain region. Then, the ability to identify which *class* (category identification) of object was studied for both whole-brain and single-region analyses.

An important part of the research reported by Shinkareva and her colleagues concerned which response areas of the brain were used in training the pattern recognizer. According to their report the best results were obtained when a number of different areas of the brain were involved in the training of the pattern-recognition algorithm. These included the following areas:

- Left inferior frontal
- Left inferior parietal
- Bilateral medial frontal
- Precentral
- Posterior cingulate
- Parahippocampal
- Cuneus
- Lingual
- Fusiform
- Superior parietal
- Superior temporal
- Middle temporal

When all of the regions were involved in the statistical analysis, object identification scores as high as 0.94 were obtained from one of their 12 subjects for a set of 10 objects. When single regions were used to identify the exemplar objects, the scores were considerably lower—0.77—for the same subject.

The less-challenging, two-alternative task of determining which class of stimulus (for which random responses levels would be 0.50) produced even higher identification scores using the whole-brain fMRI pattern recognizer. As with the exemplar identification, the highest scores (as high as 0.97) were obtained when the whole-brain records were analyzed, However, even single brain regions were able to produce class identifications with remarkably high accuracies (0.82–0.93).

As Shikareva and her colleagues (2008) pointed out, there are three main conclusions that can be drawn from this work. First, in agreement with most of the other studies discussed earlier, it is clear that whatever it is that is being measured by the fMRI procedure and the attendant analysis, it is a process that is distributed across broad reaches of the brain. Second, and even more important in the context of the limited reliability of the results from many other studies, is that the responses are sufficiently common from subject to subject that an individual can literally be taken off the street and exposed to one of these stimulus objects, and which of a small number of stimulus objects is being "seen" can be determined from a suitable analysis of the fMRI image. Finally, they drew the third conclusion that this can be accomplished without including the primary visual projection areas in the occipital cortex. Thus, the possibility of a conflation of transmission codes with perceptual neural equivalents is somewhat reduced.

Shikareva et al. (2008) qualified their conclusions by noting that given the pattern of results obtained in this experiment: "The category and exemplar classification accuracies when training across participants were on the average lower than when training within participants, indicating that a critical diagnostic portion of the neural representation of the categories and exemplars is still idiosyncratic to individual participants" (p. 8). Given this idiosyncrasy, the small number of objects and classes used in this experiment, and the variability in results, it is not yet clear just how far we can go in "reading the cognitive state of human beings" using this kind of procedure. However, there is no question that Shinkareva and her colleagues have made a major contribution in this study by showing that it is possible to train a statistical pattern recognizer on one set of subjects (within group comparisons) and then to extrapolate those criteria to other subjects who were not in the training group (across group comparisons). The relatively small size of the stimulus set (either two categories or 10 objects) makes any extrapolation to more complex cognitive processes than this predominantly perceptual response problematic. Nevertheless, this study and those others that I have previously reviewed in this section represent the germ of a technique that may allow us to eventually determine what a person is looking at in a way that was entirely unexpected until the last few years. However, all of the work reported so far in this section was limited to visual experiences and, thus, has the possibility of being confounded by sensory transmission processes rather than being dominated by perceptual ones. The next question, therefore, is—to what other cognitive processes can this approach be applied?

A potential answer to this question can be found in a recent study by Poldrack et al. (2009). They were also concerned with the use of the fMRI as a means of identifying the higher-order cognitive processes in which a person might be momentarily involved. They, also, used a statistical classifier to evaluate the distributed patterns of fMRI responses. However, their experiment was designed to determine what activation patterns occurred when their subjects were participating in one of eight different cognitive tasks, tasks whose complexity exceeded that of the perceptual studies already discussed. Herein lay the major contribution of their study; the eight cognitive tasks were not simple perceptual (i.e., visual) responses to different stimulus objects or classes of stimulus objects but relatively high-level cognitive tasks. Specifically, the eight tasks they claimed could be distinguished included these (from Poldrack et al., 2009):

1. Risky decision making
2. Probabilistic classification
3. Rhyme judgments on pseudowords
4. Working memory (tone counting)
5. 50/50 gain-loss gambling decisions
6. Living/nonliving decision on mirror-reversed words
7. Reading pseudowords aloud
8. Response inhibition

Poldrack and his colleagues carried out their experiment in the same "across subject" manner used by Shinkareva and her colleagues (2008). That is, the statistical pattern classifier utilized data from 130 people, and then the resulting classifications were tested on a single individual who had been excluded from the standardization process.

The reported ability of their fMRI pattern classifier to distinguish among these subtle cognitive tasks was impressive. Accuracies, as reported in a confusion matrix, for example, were highest for the probabilistic classification task (90%), whereas the worst identification score was for the rhyme judgment task (61%). (Chance levels, of course, were 16%.) Thus, there appear to be distinguishable fMRI signals associated with each of the cognitive tasks.

One caveat about this work remains unresolved. Despite the fact that the eight high-level cognitive tasks were supposed to be relatively free of possible confounding sensory transmission processes, Poldrack et al. (2009) did note that the elimination of confounding was not complete when they pointed out:

Substantial predictability was present in sensory cortices; given the fact that the different studies [the cognitive tasks] varied substantially in the visual stimulus characteristics and the presence of auditory stimuli, this was not surprising, and it suggested that the classification does not necessarily reflect the higher-order cognitive aspects of the task. However, a number of regions in the prefrontal cortex also showed substantial predictability, including the premotor and the anterior cingulate cortices. (p. 1366)

Thus, as acknowledged by the authors, the possibility remains that this work, virtually unique in this busy field in its concern with high-level cognitive skills (as opposed to sensory or perceptual ones), may nevertheless be contaminated by influential sensory transmission information. Whatever its limitations, this discrimination among cognitive tasks is an extraordinary development unanticipated by most of us. If replicated and substantiated, it would demand special attention by anyone interested in cognitive neuroscience.[13]

We can summarize our view of these stunning new experiments in the following comments.

1. The articles by Shinkareva and Poldrack, their colleagues, and the authors of the preparatory studies reviewed earlier in this section are major contributions. They raise possibilities that, frankly, were not expected prior these remarkable studies.

2. Because of the mathematical methods for evaluating the fMRI measures used in these studies, they add support to the argument that responses to even simple stimuli and tasks are widely distributed in the brain. It makes understandable why much of the older work looking for isolated regions or cutting out bits of the brain produced such variable and inconsistent findings.

3. Because of their importance and paradigm-shifting potential, it is vitally important that these studies be repeated and any possible artifacts identified. Poldrack and his colleagues (2009) have been particularly astute in pointing out that the sensory components of the brain's activities may be loading these results in subtle ways. The findings of these experiments may not be decoding the contents of consciousness as much as decoding sensory information transmission.

4. It is important to understand what has been done here. However important these findings are, they are theoretically neutral. That is, they do not provide any more detailed explanation of how the mind emerges from the brain than any other neuroscientific method. What they have done is find cumulative components of the fMRI signal that correlate with perceptual and cognitive processes. These indicators may be irrelevant biomarkers or "signs," however well they correlate with the perceptual experiences rather than psychoneurally equivalent "codes." What they are saying, in general, is that there are patterns that occur over the brain that allow us to distinguish to a limited degree among a few perceptual and cognitive processes. In other words the brain is doing something that is demonstrably different as it processes different percepts or other cognitive processes. The main problem is determining how far we can go in making these fMRI-based discriminations. Whatever the final outcome of this work, it is clear that there is more information in the fMRI images than had previously been thought.

5. Thus, while there may be more information in the fMRI activations than had previously been thought, these measures are more comparable to the measurement of the power being used by various components in a computer or the heat distribution than they are of the programs being executed. Therefore, although correlated, they actually are informationally neutral and tell us nothing about how the gap between the neural and mental is being crossed.

6. This is not "mind reading" in the popular sense. At best, these results suggest that the pattern of responses across the brain is different for different thoughts and percepts.

Despite the obvious excitement of these results, there are a number of other possible limitations on the meaning and importance of these findings. As just noted, the results may be theoretically and even anatomically meaningless. In a recent critical evaluation of this class of studies, Anderson and Oates (personal communication) pointed out that although it may have been possible to determine what a person might be looking at from a multi-voxel pattern analysis (MVPA) of the type used in this type of experiment, that success does not mean that it would be possible to work backward and specify what are the particular involved brain mechanisms. Anderson and Oates base their argument on the fact that these techniques are capable of identifying perceptual tasks from an analysis of the "most informative voxels." However, they point out that these voxels may change depending on the analysis method used. That is, different pattern analyzers may produce different anatomical response patterns. In other words, and this is critically important, *the actual locations activated and neural response patterns may depend as much or more on the analysis method used as on the stimuli or the organization of the brain.* Sample experiments carried out by Anderson and Oates with synthetic data showed that the most informative voxels changed from run to run. Thus it was a pattern of interaction among the selected voxels, not the particular voxels themselves, that was cueing the successful determination of what a person was viewing or thinking. Different runs and different pattern-recognition algorithms could have equally successful outcomes based on widely disparate locations and mechanisms for the voxels used in each of the pattern analyses.

The implication of their analysis led Anderson and Oates to conclude that, however successful they may be in extracting information about which stimulus was being presented or task being executed, it was not possible to specify what the involved brain mechanisms were that accounted for the related cognitive process. Furthermore, it was not possible to be assured that the person was consciously aware of the stimulus or task—it might be a preconscious processing of stimulus information. Anderson and Oates (personal communication) sum up their conclusions as follows: ". . . MVPA [multi-voxel pattern analysis] offers an exciting new way to investigate the operation of the brain by looking at the predictive value of (typically widely) distributed patterns of activity. The problematic inferences come in the attempt to reduce such patterns to local patterns of brain activity."

Thus, although useful in some practical sense, this form of analysis, like so many others, may be neutral with regard to the underlying neural mechanism. The ability to determine what a person is looking at or thinking about may be better conceptualized as a trick than as a major step forward in scientific analysis of the mind-brain problem. Thus it must be emphasized that the psychoneurally equivalent pattern of responses cannot be determined from this kind of MVPA; the reason for this is that the analysis method, although successful, may be using a different algorithm than the one actually used by the brain despite there being some "signs" of particular kinds of neural activity. In other words these signals may tell us what is happening but not how. What the analysis of Anderson and Oates does further suggest and support, however, is that whatever the brain mechanisms are that account for our cognitive processes, they are widely distributed and not localized on and within the brain.

The next step in this analysis was to deal with larger sets of alternatives than those reported by Poldrack and colleagues (2009), and the others who were successful in distinguishing among relatively small sets. In two notable studies Kay, Naselaris, Prenger, and Gallant (2008) and Naselaris, Prenger, Kay, Oliver, and Gallant (2009) reported progress in this direction. In the first of these two studies Kay and his colleagues reported that they were able to distinguish between the fMRI signatures recorded from V1, V2, and V3 of 120 different pictures. First, they examined the fMRI signals to a larger (1,750) library of natural images and measured the fMRI responses produced by each of a number of voxels. This established a training set. A representation of each picture was then formed based on the Fourier properties of the image in which spatial frequency and orientation information were summarized as a "predicted activity pattern" for each of many voxels that were associated with the presented picture. This provided a quantitative representation of the fMRI responses to each of the images.[14]

Then the smaller set of 120 novel images was presented. Based on similarities in the model's representations (i.e., the voxel patterns) between the images in the large training set and the small test set, the best-fitting picture could be selected (i.e., identified) from the

120 images. For thirteen repeated trials for a given picture, Kay and his colleagues (2008) report a correct identification score in the mid-90%, random performance being 0.8%. When only the fMRI signals from a single presentation were used, the identification performance was reduced to much lower values (51% and 32% for two subjects).

This was an impressive step forward, but it still depended on a training set of stimuli and recognizing pictures on the basis of an fMRI pattern analysis. Furthermore Kay et al. (2008) were basing their identification scores solely on the visual areas of the brain in which some semblance of retinotopic mapping presumably was retained. Thus, as they say "The problem is analogous to the classic 'pick a card, any card' magic trick" (p. 352). It is certainly impressive that novel stimuli were used; however, it would have been interesting to have been informed about the similarity of the images in the training and test sets.

The logic behind the contribution of Kay and his colleagues (2008), however complex the analysis and whatever increase in the number of items to be identified, is relatively straightforward. Representations were made in the Fourier domain of a set of stimuli, and these matched with stimuli that shared at least some properties of the training set. The task in psychological parlance is one of *recognition* or *identification*.

A far more difficult task for subjects in psychological experiments would be to *reconstruct* an image from its components. Given the statistical complexity of natural images, this is also a formidable task for a computer system as well as for a visual system for which information is limited to spatial representations and is devoid of semantic associations. The process of accomplishing this formidable task has been called "reverse retinotopy"—that is, "inferring the visual content of images from brain activation patterns" (p. 1104) by Thiron and colleagues (2006). A form of this kind of reconstruction has been accomplished by at least two groups of investigators. The first was by Thiron and his colleagues just mentioned, and the second was by Miyawaki et al. (2008). Again the logic is straightforward—the shape of simple geometrical forms is preserved enough in the early retinotopic regions of the visual system to support the inference that these simple contrast patterns such as squares, ×s, +s, and letters of the alphabet can be inferred from the pattern of spatially and topologically constant voxels. No prior set of images is required to reconstruct these simple shapes; and the salient voxels are limited to the visual areas that are retinotopically organized. This method depends solely on the preservation of the topology of the original stimulus pattern and the spatial resolvability of the spatial pattern. Nor, for that matter, is there any attempt to infer images on the basis of the semantic content. It may take some heavy mathematics to account for the topological distortions, but, once again, the logic is straightforward; examine the spatial pattern of the activated voxels, and infer the shape of the stimulus. Nor can one deny the formidable accomplishment of carrying out this kind of experiment or its robust empirical support of the notion that spatial information is retinotopically persevered in the early portion of the visual system. Although we have known this for many years, this is a major accomplishment.

A considerably more complex and far-reaching claim has been made by Naselaris, Prenger, Kay, Oliver, and Gallant (2009) in their laboratory's next publication that goes far beyond "reverse retinotopy." They report that they have been able to "reconstruct" not just retino-topically preserved simple visual patterns but complex natural scenes from nonisomorphic fMRI images. However, their meaning of reconstruction is considerably different from the conventional one in psychology. Learning psychologists such as McGeoch and Irion (1952) refer to reconstruction as a test method in which "The subject is given the parts of the original material, arranged in random order, and is asked to reconstruct the original order" (p. 23). The order may be in the form of the original temporal sequence, or it may be in the form of the spatial reorganization of the parts into the original pattern in the way a jig-saw puzzle is reconstructed. Naselaris and his colleagues (2009), however, define "recon-struction" quite differently. In their terminology, "Under the Bayesian frame work used here, a reconstruction is defined as the image that has the highest posterior probability of having evoked the measured response" (p. 902). Although this is a much more complex task (120 novel target images were tested after training with 1750 natural images) than that described in Kay et al. (2008), it still appears to be better described as a process of recognition, selec-tion, or identification of an image from a known library of alternatives rather than a recon-struction in either the psychological or the neuroscientific sense.

A further source of misunderstanding is the use by Naselaris and his colleagues (2009) of realistic complex visual scenes as the exemplars of outputs from their methods. These are not pictures that were directly reconstructed from the fMRI data but pictures produced by combining parts of pictures that were selected from the library of images, that is, the Bayesian priors on which the system was originally trained.

Despite these errors of presentation, one has to admire the accomplishments reported in this article. At the very least Naselaris and colleagues (2009) were able to select pictures from a much larger library than had hitherto been used. At the most they were able to show distinctive fMRI responses from a number of visual cortical areas (V1, V2, V3, V3A, V3B, V4, as well as the lateral and anterior occipital cortex) that could be used to identify images from the training set. What they did not do was to take fMRI images and directly plot from them pictures of the original stimuli; once again they selected pictures from their library based on the pattern of activations. This is not reconstruction per se; it is once again select-ing from a predetermined "deck of cards."

Nor can one credit their assertion that occipital and perioccipital regions encoded "semantic" information. Additional information was provided by these regions that helped to select images from the priors, but, it is not necessary to characterize it as "semantic" just because it did not come from the primary visual projection areas.

3.2.3 The Other Senses
Although most of the work in this burgeoning field of fMRI studies of perceptual processes has been aimed at studying the visual system, a number of researchers have used similar

methods in the study of other sensory modalities. I briefly mention in the material that follows a few such studies that have examined human brain images with fMRI techniques in order to provide a bit of an insight into what the state of the art is in these fields.

Audition

Because of the acoustic noise produced by fMRI devices themselves, especially echo-planar imaging (EPI) systems, there has been a much smaller number of research studies carried out on the auditory system than on the visual system. It is simply too noisy an environment to perform some of the relatively straightforward experiments available to vision researchers. Nevertheless, a few intrepid researchers have managed to carry out some auditory-imaging experiments by using novel techniques that work around or within gaps in the scanner noise, that wait for the scanner noise to conclude, or by using completely different technologies such as magnetoencephalography. (See Seifritz et al. [2006] for an example of one strategy of working around the scanner noise.)

Among the relatively few (compared to the expansive literature on vision) auditory studies using fMRI techniques are the reports by Altmann, Bledowski, Wibral, and Kaiser (2007) and Warren and Griffiths (2003). Both of these groups of researchers provided imaging support for the current theory that the auditory system seemed to have two different divisions for representing acoustic temporal pattern and spatial location, respectively. This idea was similar to the two pathways for vision in that it involved dorsal and lateral pathways (or streams) that only partially overlapped. The data seemed to support the idea that the frequency or pitch information was encoded in a set of brain regions other than those representing the neural codes for spatial localization. Acoustic frequency pattern changes mainly produced activations in the anterior portion of the temporal gyrus whereas spatial location seemed to drive activity in more posterior portions of the temporal gyrus according to Altmann and his colleagues (2007). Warren and Griffith (2003) found similar activation regions; specifically, temporal (i.e., pitch) changes activated regions around the superior temporal gyrus, and spatial changes produced activity in a parietotemporal region known as the *planum temporale*.

Lest we be tempted to assign the coding activities of these regions to auditory spatial and temporal signal processing alone, it must also be noted that these very same regions are also involved in the motor actions involved in vocalization as well as in working memory. Hickok, Buchsbaum, Humphries, and Muftuler (2003), for example, used fMRI techniques to show that nearly the same areas in the superior temporal or temporal-parietal areas that had been shown to be specific to pitch changes or spatial shifts also were activated when subjects were told to rehearse nonsense sentences or to hum piano tunes. These authors believed that this convergence of functions was an explanation for the auditory-motor interactions; however it is possible that they were actually recording a selected sample of responses of much more widely dispersed cerebral functions.

Furthermore, some recent fMRI studies (e.g., Eckert et al., 2008) have shown that the primary auditory and visual cortices may be directly interconnected both anatomically and functionally. A similar pattern of results has been reported in a situation in which somatosensory signals converge on a region originally thought to be auditory association cortex (Foxe et al., 2002). It seems increasingly clear that many regions of the brain are so heavily interconnected with others that have traditionally been associated with particular sensory modalities that any concept of regional specificity for perception has to be reexamined.

This is a very important point because it also strikes at the conceptual foundations of much of the research on brain regional specialization. The wide variety of functions that can produce a response in a given area suggests that any notion of a separate auditory, visual, somatosensory, or cognitive area should be discarded once one has moved past the primary sensory projection areas. Beyond that point, feedback of centrifugal signals may lead to involvement of other regions in determining the responses of even the primary receiving areas. The influence of attention, for example, on V1 has already been discussed in section 3.22.

Somatosensation

The somatosensory system has also been probed with fMRI techniques. In general the research has verified the conventionally accepted organization of somatotopic organization of the brain regions associated with the body senses. The primary somatosensory region, located on the contralateral postcentral region, and a bilateral secondary region respond to touch stimuli. Partial confirmation of the somatotopic mapping of the somatosensory "homunculus" has been provided by Ruben et al. (2006), who showed that electrical stimulation of the ring and middle finger of the hand activated slightly different regions of the primary somatosensory cortex in a region hitherto assigned to the hand.[15]

In addition to these "classic" somatosensory regions, Del Gratta et al. (2000) reported some other weakly responding areas that were also activated by electrical stimuli presented to the median nerve. These previous undetected regions were located on the ipsilateral side of the body in the frontal and parietal regions. These findings again reinforce the idea that far more regions of the brain are involved in perceiving stimuli than just the traditional "sensory areas."

Olfaction

Even less attention has been paid by practitioners of brain imaging when it comes to the other, so called minor, senses. In general fMRI measurements mainly confirmed what was already known about the regions of the brain associated with the olfactory modality. For example the olfactory system was studied in an early research project by Levy et al. (1997) in an effort to determine if the magnitude of the fMRI response could be quantitatively associated with the perceived strength of an odorous stimulus. Not unexpectedly they reported activations to some chemicals in widely distributed portions of the brain, including the orbitofrontal cortex, frontal, entorhinal frontal cortices, and the cingulate gyrus, as well as other regions of the limbic system. When subjective intensities were compared with the degree of activation, however, the most intense-smelling chemical stimulants did not produce the greatest degree of activation. Quantification of subjective intensities by fMRI signals, therefore, proved to be an elusive, if not impossible, task.

A more recent study of the olfactory brain using fMRI was carried out by Lombion et al. (2009). They were interested in distinguishing between olfactory and trigeminal brain activations to odorous stimuli. Most germane to our current discussion, however, was the very broad range of brain regions that were activated by olfactory stimuli including the frontal and entorhinal cortices, the amygdala, and the anterior insula. The actual distributions depended, somewhat surprisingly, on the duration of the stimulus. Those regions that did respond generally were inclusive of those that had previously been known.

In sum the main result of both of these studies was to involve broad regions of the brain in the encoding of olfactory information. Whether or not these brain activations also represent the experiential aspects of smell or are irrelevant artifacts, that is, signs, cannot be determined from these findings.

Gustation

A pair of studies of the gustatory system may provide a picture of the state of the art in this sensory modality. Both of these studies are mainly concerned with the identification of what were thought to be the primary projection regions for taste. Ogawa et al. (2005) explored the problem with fMRI techniques. They found that a number of brain areas were activated by applying salt to the tongue. Their fMRI activations showed that some of these olfactory regions were buried within the lateral sulcus of the brain by the operculum, an extended region at the intersection of the frontal, temporal, and parietal regions of the brain. The activated regions included some areas of the operculum itself, the embedded and infolded insula, and other regions buried within the Sylvan fissure. However these activations did not correspond to those obtained with other techniques such as magnetoencephalography.

Another study that attempted to determine if there were any differences between normal tasters and those with some kind of gustatory defect or ageusia was published by Hummel, Frasnelli, Gerber, and Hummel (2007). Although the major activated regions tended to be in roughly the same region, the results were inconsistent from subject to subject. Subjects with total ageusia still showed activations in some regions of the brain thought to be taste related. Indeed in some cases the responses in the brains of ageusic subjects were greater than normal. Individual differences were substantial. Not much help there either!

The study of the gustatory system, therefore, is at a much earlier stage of development than are studies of vision. The reasons are fairly obvious; except for the clinical specialist the topic is of limited interest compared to the amount of research attention aimed at visual studies. Furthermore, manipulation of the stimulus is difficult and limited to a few variations. However, by far the most important finding from these studies was that the gustatory system is far more complicated and interacts with far more different brain systems than previous work had suggested. Figure 3.1 shows a recent "theory" of gustatory system organization suggested by Jones, Fontanini, and Katz (2006). Although much less research has been done on this system than on the visual system, it is clear that even this "other sense" is encoded by an interactive complex of many different brain regions.

Vestibular Sensation

Finally, we must provide a brief mention of what is probably the most difficult sensory system to study with brain imaging techniques. The very nature of the stimulus—

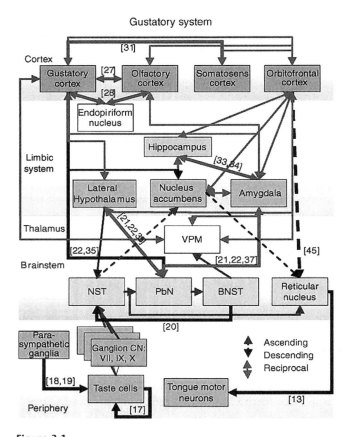

Figure 3.1
The organization of the gustatory system.
From Jones, Fontanni, & Katz (2006), reprinted with the permission of Elsevier Science and Technology Journals.

mechanical positioning and repositioning of the body—is contrary to the needs for stable body position when one is gathering the data necessary to compute an fMRI brain image. As a result alternative (nonadequate) techniques such as electrical or caloric stimulation were typically used when the brain components of the vestibular system were imaged. The fact that these alternative stimuli can also affect other sensory processes (for example cutaneous afferents) means that research of this kind is almost always conflated with somatosensory or thermal (i.e., caloric) sensitivities,

A further problem in studying the vestibular system is that our states of orientation, acceleration, and position are heavily impacted by other motor and sensory capacities. In addition the areas of the brain that have been associated with vestibular encoding are to be found in many of the same regions as those encoding gustation—surrounding the parietal operculum and within the central and Sylvan sulci.

Eickhoff, Weiss, Amunts, Fink, and Zilles (2006), using both cytoarchitectonic and fMRI mapping procedures, zeroed in on a particular area—a subregion of the parietal operculum known as OP2 on the right side of the body—as the primary projection area for vestibular sensation. They postulated that this region was the equivalent of the monkey's parieto-insular-vestibular cortex (PIVC), also a region located deep in that animal's Sylvan sulcus. They also noted that previous research had indicated that the monkey had a number of secondary regions that were responsive to vestibular stimuli scattered about the posterior frontal and the anterior parietal regions. Eickhoff and his colleagues (2006) also demonstrated fMRI activations in the regions surrounding OP2 that suggested that they may be homologous to these supplementary regions in the monkey. However, another area, OP1, was the only area that met all of the fMRI and cytoarchitectonic criteria to justify its designation as a "primary" projection area. Notably, both animal and human research indicated that this area does not carry out its function in isolation but, like the parts of so many other brain systems, is one of an integrated system of brain components. Nowhere is this more clearly indicated than in the discomfort of motion sickness, long known to be a result of a clash between visual and vestibular sensory stimuli.

Essentially similar results to the Eickhoff et al. (2006) findings were reported by Brandt and Dieterich (2006) at almost the same time. They, too, argued that the parieto-insular cortex in humans is the homolog of the PIVC in monkeys. However they added an interesting additional interpretation of why so many different investigators found so many different sensory sensitivities in this region. Their suggestion was that this region (OP2-the parieto-insular cortex) is not exclusively dedicated to vestibular sensation or, for that matter, any other sense that produces activations in this region. Instead they propose that it is a polysensory region to which a number of sensory modalities project. To speak of it as a "vestibular area" is simply a manifestation of ideas that should have long ago been rejected as being vestigially "phrenological."

It is important to appreciate that the literature on all of these perceptual processes is filled with many caveats, special conditions, and controversies about what regions of the brain are activated under what situations. Factors such as attention and experience, as well as stimulus or task conditions, can modulate the effect of any stimulus on brain images. It has, therefore, been extremely easy to find what appears to be conclusive evidence for virtually any hypothesis or, conversely, to rule out any seemingly plausible one. The basic fact is that we are, at best, still in a period of exploration seeking the basic facts of the brain organization of these sensory regions. The order that might be imposed by comprehensive theory is not yet with us.

3.3   Perceptual Processes

3.3.1   Recognition

The term "recognition" includes many different kinds of cognitive functions in which cognitive classifications are carried out. Recognition can be defined as the act of placing an unknown stimulus in a particular category. A form may be classified as a "hammer"; a face can be classified as "John"; or in some other way, a stimulus defined as a particular exemplar representing a class of objects. In the cognitive neuroscientific literature, object recognition is distinguished from face recognition and both are thought to be different than the recognition of spatial relationships. Indeed, the word "recognition" encompasses a very wide variety of acts, some of which differ so much from the others that it is unlikely that all forms of recognition have a common foundation either behaviorally or neurally.

Early work on recognition was predominantly a psychological research topic with only rare neuroscientific explorations being carried out. Some early extirpation studies used object recognition as a dependent variable, but the field really blossomed with the advent of the brain imaging technologies. When PET and fMRI techniques were applied to recognition, researchers reported that there appeared to be segregation in the brain pathways associated with each class of stimulus. Some of the earliest imaging work, for example, suggested that the object recognition and spatial location processes were encoded in different visual regions. Aguirre and D'Esposito (1997), for example, located spatial localization responses in the more dorsal portions of the brain including the parietal and premotor gyri. On the other hand the encoding of shape or form, which constituted the basis of object recognition, seemed to selectively activate the ventral region at the rear of the brain known as the lateral occipital complex (LOC) according to Grill-Spector, Kushnir, Edelman, Itzchak, and Malach (1998). Similarly, faces seemed to be separately encoded by activity that was concentrated in regions near the ventral occipital-parietal boundary including the area now known as the FFA discovered by Kanwisher, McDermott, and Chun (1997).

This multiple-locale hypothesis is a continuing theme in much of this work—the segregation of different properties of the stimulus into dorsal and lateral (or ventral) pathways (or streams) in accord with the distinction made between the different stimulus classifications made in the psychological literature.

Recent work using fMRI techniques to study recognition processes continues to indicate that the LOC plays an important role in the encoding of form. However the situation is far from being fully understood. Discrepancies occur between object recognition and object-directed grasping; the former can be seriously degraded without any reduction in the appropriate grasping of unrecognized objects (see James, Culham, Humphrey, Milner, & Goodale, 2003); yet, grasping is a process that seems to require prior recognition. Thus, what appears to be required as a prerequisite (form recognition) seems not to be necessary for the correct manipulation of that form. Obviously, covert and complex processes that remain completely unexplained are not explained by current neuroscientific theories of recognition.

Controversy also continues about what it is that the LOC actually encodes. Is it the contour or the shape; the outline or the surface; or indeed is it some much more subtle relational aspect of the stimulus? Indeed it does not seem to matter what the nature of the stimulus is—even incomplete objects can activate this area as noted by Grill-Spector, Kourtzi, and Kanwisher (2001) and by Schatpour, Molholm, Javitt, and Foxe (2006). In addition the responses are not stable—they vary with the familiarity of the stimulus objects or faces.

It is now becoming widely appreciated that there are some severe limitations in using fMRI techniques to study form recognition. Grill-Spector and Sayres (2008), for example, point out that the resolution of fMRI systems is not fine enough to study the neuronal encoding of faces and objects either at the level of neuronal networks or even in terms of the neural activity in some of the smaller regions purported to have localized recognition functions. Although Grill-Spector and Sayres offer some techniques that may help to alleviate the latter of these two problems, we must always keep in mind that we actually are answering a very gross kind of question—where is the maximum response produced for a given category of stimulus?—rather than unraveling the much more difficult question of how the neural circuitry encodes these complex cognitive processes. Furthermore none of this research speaks to the more fundamental issue of how these neural responses are transformed into recognition experiences. Nor, for that matter, is it yet clear that we have properly defined the psychological processes of recognition with a level of precision that permits us to consider their neural underpinnings.

The clinical situation is equally poorly understood.[16] Reports of agnosias (inability to recognize patterns) of all kinds (visual, auditory, and somatosensory) are widespread in the neuropsychological and neurological literature. However, even with the most modern imaging techniques, the variety of possible neurological causal mechanisms is so confusing that no generally accepted theory of their specific pathologies exists. It is now generally accepted in cognitive neuroscientific circles dealing with faulty face recognition (prosopagnosia), however, that there are several brain regions (the fusiform face area—FFA, the inferior occipital gyrus—IOF, and the anterior inferotemporal cortex—AIT) on the right side of the brain are involved in face recognition (Kanwisher et al., 1997).

Although some researchers have pointed to neural dysfunction in one or more of these areas as the correlate of prosopagnosia (for example, see the work of Kriegeskorte, Formisana, Sorger, & Goebel, 2007; Bentin, DeGutis, D'Esposito, & Robertson, 2007), a number of fMRI studies, including one by Avidan, Hasson, Malach, and Behrman (2005) have found normal activation levels in these areas even though patients were severely visually agnostic! Furthermore the neurological anomaly associated with prosopagnosia was the *absence* of a response in the targeted area when faces and non-face objects were compared, an inconsistent result that had been observed earlier by Kanwisher, McDermott, and Chun (1997) in the FFA. Thus, the evidence associating gross morphological and functional neuropathology with face recognition deficits remains equivocal.

A more balanced approach, it seems to me, is to contend that none of these areas is uniquely responsible (i.e., sufficient) for face recognition. For example it has been proposed by Rossion and colleagues (2003) and Hadjikhani and de Gelder (2002) that the FFA, IOF, and AIT systems, probably in conjunction with other brain areas involved in the acquisition of the visual input, must act as a coordinated system to account for normal face recognition. Once again the idea that a cognitive process is represented by a broadly distributed system of brain regions arises as the most plausible explanation—at this level of analysis.

3.3.2 Illusions

No other subfield of perceptual psychology has attracted the attention of the lay public over the years as much as has the phenomenon of visual illusions. It is, perhaps, in this field that psychologists have found more fame than any other. Many illusions have become eponymous—that is, named after their discoverer. Names such as Poggendorf, Hering, Neckar, Ebbinghaus, Benham, Müller, and Lyer, and many others would have been hidden within the confines of the academy despite their otherwise notable scientific accomplishments if it had not been for their discovery of a curious illusion. Visual, optical, or geometric illusions, as they have been called at different stages of psychological history, have entertained in salons since Victorian days, and they still amuse and perplex people in modern times. Books are still being regularly published about these phenomena, and new research is continually being carried out that uncovers new illusions or extends measurements about well-known ones. What has not appeared are cognitive neuroscientific theories of any consequence of these fascinating phenomena.

Illusions come in many kinds, and new ones are being invented all the time.[17] The best known are the visual ones in which shape, motion, lightness, and even hue are distorted by what remain mysterious mechanisms. Recently there has been special interest in the illusory contours first reported by Kaniza (1955). However, auditory illusions have also been discovered in recent years; the most famous one was reported by Shepard (1964a, 1964b). It has even been suggested that much of the charm of music is due to the illusions of auditory experience that it engenders.

Somatosensory illusions are also well known; if one pushes sideways with one's arm against a wall from a standing position, the subsequent illusion of induced motion is very compelling. Illusions in which the perceived weight varies with the size of an object have been a mainstay of research in this field since the nineteenth-century work of Charpentier (1891).

In recent years new technologies have given rise to new kinds of illusions. The "illusion" of being present at the site of a remotely controlled device—remote presence—has now become of importance to military and civilian operators of such devices. Phantom limb illusions are also a major orthopedic issue in a world where prosthetic limbs are now becoming more prevalent and more capable.

Another class of illusion concerns not only our ability to misperceive but not to perceive at all. Static situations of this type are referred to as the effects of camouflage while recently discovered dynamic ones are designated as "change blindness."

Despite this popularity and increasing application of what had hitherto been a curiosity, as I have just noted, there is a remarkable paucity of theoretical explanations of these phenomena. Almost all preceding theories were simply verbal associations with other illusions or post hoc "just so" descriptions based on past experiences and current expectations. Explanations have frequently been phrased in terms of maintaining figural goodness or constancy or some other such cognitive outcome that could be plausibly related to the illusion. However, none of these descriptive "explanations" really explains anything. The only explanation that came close to a neuroscientific theory of illusions was the concept of neurons that were "fatigued" due to prior conditioning, thus releasing the other side of an opponent system to produce an aftereffect, especially in color or motion.

With the advent of imaging techniques, however, some stalwart investigators have plunged ahead to look for neural explanations of these elusive perceptual phenomena. Before beginning my discussion of this work, however, it is important to point out that any explanation that is provided by brain imaging is of a very limited kind. The only thing that one can accomplish with a brain image is to identify the brain regions that might be involved in the phenomenon. Quantitative changes are rare indeed.

It is not possible, as I have noted several times in several different ways in this book, to specify anything about the actual computational mechanisms. There are major technological constraints on the extent to which even this kind of localization can be achieved for illusions simply because, despite their ubiquity and apparent simplicity, they represent a very high-level cognitive process in which distortions from the stimulus, rather than their congruities, are the signature response. Obviously high-level processes are involved in such distorted perceptual experiences. What they are, where they are, and how they work neurally, however, remain complete mysteries.

Furthermore brain images of illusions share with all brain images the fact an arbitrary threshold is usually specified to reduce image background "noise." This means that there inevitably will be some involved regions that are missed or ignored in any mapping of activated regions. Because of the high cognitive level at which they operate, it is highly unlikely that only a few restricted regions are participating in the elicitation of a visual illusion. In addition, however low a threshold may be set, it still will miss macroscopic areas that do not change between the experimental and control conditions despite major changes in the state of the microscopic underlying neuronal networks.

Finally there is the continuing problem of response variability; when one broadly examines the whole corpus of brain imaging research on visual illusions, it quickly becomes clear that there are no general conclusions yet to be drawn. Publications differ significantly from each other in assigning salience to particular areas in a way that precludes strong generalizations.

In the following paragraphs I draw a few examples from the extensive pool of research on visual illusions. The samples chosen should make it clear that the study of illusions with brain imaging devices is still in its infancy, at best, and hopeless, at worst.

Illusory contours are powerful and compelling phenomena and obviously involve the interpretation of suggestive cues that are not physically present in the raw stimulus. They create the perception of a boundary where there is no physical line of demarcation. Since the phenomenon is most likely to be based on a relatively high-level interpretation of the meaning of a stimulus, it is somewhat surprising that our research attention has been mainly directed by the data toward the earliest portions of the visual pathway rather than at some higher level where such cognitive processes might seem to be more appropriately instantiated. Neural responses to illusory contours have been reported as early as V1 and V2 with both single-cell and fMRI techniques.

Because of ambiguity and controversy in the results concerning which brain areas were involved in illusory contours, a recent study by Montaser-Kouhsari, Landy, Heeger, and Larsson (2007) used a new technique that depended on selective adaptation with stimuli that produced illusory contours and those that did not. When the adapting stimuli were aligned with the stimuli for the illusory contours, the fMRI responses in all of the responsive brain regions were smaller than when the adaptor and the illusory contour stimuli were at right angles to each other. This result was observed throughout the visual regions from V1 and V2 up to peristriate regions. An important result of this work was to show that the adaptation effect became stronger as measurements were made at progressively higher levels of the visual nervous system.[18] What happened at regions beyond the nominally visual areas was not discussed in their article.

Montaser-Kouhsari et al. (2007), however, acknowledged that their experimental paradigm was difficult to compare with either previous single-cell or fMRI work. They were very careful to call attention to the conceptual limits of this kind of research, as well as the difficulties with their own experimental design. These constraints included the following from Montaser-Kouhsari et al. (2007, pp. 2186 and 2194).

• The recorded overall increase in neural activity may not be the equivalent of contour processing (i.e., the increases may be signs, not codes).

- Previous studies measured the overall response, whereas their work measured differences to orientation sensitivity.
- There are likely to be strong attention and other cognitive penetration effects on illusory contours.
- Current theories generally argue that illusory contours are due to opponent mechanisms, not the amount of activity as measured by their procedure. Thus, their data do not support the prevailing consensus concerning the origins of the illusory contour phenomena.
- The stimuli used in the several studies Montaser-Kouhsari et al. cited differed from one experiment to the next. Thus variability in the results among the several studies should be expected.

A comprehensive and timely review of the state of fMRI research on the perception of illusory contours has been published by Seghier and Vuilleumier (2006). In their earlier support for the issues raised by Montaser-Kouhsari and colleagues, they discussed the "great diversity of findings across the studies" (p. 595). Basic questions such as where in the nervous system are the salient processes carried out still remain unanswered according to Seghier and Vuilleumier. The answers to the question of whether or not both V1 and V2 respond to illusory contours were almost evenly split. According to Seghier and Vuilleumier, experimental studies of the putative role of other higher level regions in representing the psychological phenomena provide answers that are wildly inconsistent. The only brain area that is mentioned in these reports with any frequency is the LOC, and then only in about half of the studies.

Clearly the data are not yet strong enough to answer some of the most basic neuroscientific questions concerning visual illusions even if one is limited to asking about only the involvement of various cerebral regions. Indeed the finding that regions like the LOC are involved in many other kinds of perceptual processes suggests that we may not have defined exactly what the salient perceptual properties of these famous illusions are.

Seghier and Vuilleumier (2006) also noted that not only are the data "diverse" but so, too, are the many theories that have been proposed to explain the perception of illusory contours. Most of the earlier theories were simply restatements of the phenomena, either in their own phenomenological terms or in terms of what seemed to be related illusions. Of course none of the early theories spoke with neuroscientific authority prior to the electrophysiological and imaging revolutions of the past few years. It seems that none of them yet has any robust support from the brain imaging data. Indeed any hope of discriminating among alternative psychological theories of illusory contours is forlorn; none of them has any neurological postulates that can be examined with brain imaging devices.[19]

The general difficulties in relating neural responses to perceptual responses are manifold, as we have just discussed. At its most fundamental and relevant level, any putative solution to the problem requires that we know how a complex network of neurons transforms its activities into conscious experience, knowledge that is neither available from brain images nor any other neuroscientific technique.

In summary, although a number of researchers (22 published reports according to Seghier and Vuilleumier's list) have attempted to apply various kinds of brain recording and imaging techniques to study illusory contours, the results still remain idiosyncratic and inconsistent from study to study. The reasons for this variability include the following:

• Diversity of brain recording techniques. Seghier and Vuilleumier (2006) note that of the 22 studies, only 10 used fMRI or PET techniques.
• Difference in statistical methods used for data analysis: of the eight fMRI studies, Seghier and Vuilleumier (2006) noted that each had used a different means of analyzing the data.
• Poor control of individual differences or cognitive penetration due to such factors as attention.
• Diversity of the stimuli used. There are a large number of stimuli producing illusory contours. No standard "fruit fly" has been agreed on with which to compare results from different laboratories.

Classic geometric, optical, or visual illusions (other than illusory contours) provide another example of the many difficulties in pinning down the neural correlates, if not mechanisms, of our perceptual experiences. Some of the most famous have been subjected to brain imaging including the apparent-size illusion, the Müller-Lyer, and the McCullough contingent aftereffect illusions. For reasons that are not clear but may have something to do with the difficulties tabulated previously, interest in this application of brain imaging seemed to have flagged during the last decade—only a few reports followed up on this application of fMRI techniques to the study of perceptual phenomena. Brief mention of at least a few of these recent studies of brain responses to these illusions may be useful, however, to round out our discussion.

The apparent-size illusion is a misperception of the size of an object when there are other cues to distance such as those in visual convergence. Murray, Boyaci, and Kersten (2006), in one of the few recent papers on this topic, compared fMRI images and subjective reports about the apparent size of objects. Their result was that activations associated with perceived size were observed in V1, the primary projection region for the visual sense. The effect they observed was a parallel increase in the size of the fMRI activation in area V1 that seemed to be correlated with apparent object size. This was surprising because illusions of this sort have long been thought to be interpretations carried out by complex and high-level processes rather than in what many consider to be distortions occurring in the early stages of the transmission pathway. Murray et al. explained their result, somewhat inadequately and without further evidence, as a distortion in the retinotopic map.

Among the most familiar optical or geometrical illusions is the Müller-Lyer phenomenon—the misjudgment of line length depending on the direction of the "arrow wings" or "fins." In another relatively rare recent excursion into brain imaging and visual illusions, Weidner and Fink (2007) explored what they believed were the "neural mechanisms underlying the Müller-Lyer illusion." Once again this meant that they found responses in the

LOC and the IOC that responded in a manner that was analogous to the perceptual illusion when they varied the angle and number of the fins in the display. On the basis of such a comparison they concluded that "the neural processes underlying the Müller-Lyer illusion are likely to occur in the occipital cortex . . ." and, furthermore, that ". . . the right SPC [i.e., the superior parietal cortex] contributes to the processing of the Müller-Lyer line length illusion" (p. 882). Their assignment of this compelling illusion to the higher levels of the cortex is consistent with interpretive theories of illusion but inconsistent with the study of Murray et al. (2006), which argues a much more peripheral site for this kind of illusion.

Unfortunately, no quantitative data were provided by Wiedner and Fink to support the contention that the activated areas "show a signal increase with an increasing illusion magnitude" (p. 881). Thus the major finding of this study was merely to suggest that responses in these two areas (the LOC and the SPC) were correlated with the phenomenology of this illusion. It is difficult to understand how this qualitative result led the authors to so strongly assign the Müller-Lyer illusion to these regions. It is also somewhat difficult to understand how such a phenomenon could activate only the areas they mentioned; it is more likely that other, widely distributed, activations were submerged by a relatively high threshold.

Another significant study was carried out on one of the most famous illusory phenomena in this expansive and popular psychological literature. Barnes and colleagues (1999) examined the fMRI correlates of McCollough's (1965) study of contingent color aftereffects. The McCollough effect demonstrated that the perceived color of a stimulus not only depended on the previous color to which a subject had been conditioned but also on the orientation of the colored lines in the conditioning stimulus. The dependence (i.e., contingency) on the interaction of the spatial and the chromatic aspects of this illusion made it one of the most notable of modern discoveries in visual perception. A number of authors have shown that the effect cannot be explained by simple neuronal fatigue of the color receptors since the illusory aftereffect persists for many months after the conditioning period as long as the illusion is not tested (Jones & Holding, 1975). Thus the McCollough effect must be influenced by some high-level cognitive processes that are unlikely to be explained solely by peripheral neural effects but may be more akin to learning. Barnes and his colleagues (1999) provided support for this supposition by showing that fMRI activations were observed in the ventrolateral prefrontal cortex, the left insula, as well as in anterior fusiform cortex, but not in V4 or V1, areas that others have suggested were presumably activated by simple color aftereffects as well by the other illusions we have discussed here.

Why the McCollough illusion might differ from other kinds of illusory perception in terms of activated regions can be partially explained by the difference in stimulus conditions. However the absence of low-level visual responses clashes strongly with the results from other closely related phenomena. Either the McCollough effect is not a typical illusion or there is some major conceptual error in the logic underlying these experiments on illusory phenomena. Perhaps this inconsistency and modern technology's inability to corral it are the reasons that interest in pursuing visual illusions with brain imaging techniques has ebbed in recent years.

Another fascinating behavioral observation concerning the limits of our visual system is change or attentional blindness (Grimes, 1996; Simons & Levin, 1997; Rensink, O'Regan, & Clark, 1997). The terminology inherent in the phrase "change blindness" reflects the fact that there may be substantial changes in the stimulus environment that go completely unperceived if the scene is even momentarily obscured or interrupted. The classic example of change blindness is the reduced ability to note that one person behind a counter was substituted for another if the scene was momentarily obscured by an object being carried in front of the counter during the personnel changeover. The obscuration, on the other hand, may be very brief—an eye blink or a gap in an otherwise continuous motion picture. Simple tests show that massive changes in the scene become invisible unless attention is specifically directed at the changing region or component. Needless to say such a peculiar and interesting visual effect quickly was subjected to the fMRI treatment.

The first attempt to study change blindness with fMRI techniques was reported by Beck, Rees, Frith, and Lavie (2001). Their experiment presented two pictures of places or faces separated by a brief interval to subjects while they were also carrying out a letter-detection task. The subject's task was both to say if a target letter was present and also if there had been any change in the two pictorial presentations; the letter-detection task was merely a ploy to control the subjects' attention—away from the changing parts of the picture. Beck and his colleagues (2001) reported fMRI activations for two conditions—one in which change was detected and the other in which the subjects did not detect the change. The former condition, in which the change was detected, activated the parietal lobe, the dorso-lateral prefrontal cortex, and the fusiform lobe. The latter condition in which the change was undetected showed activations in the lingual lobe, the inferior frontal lobe, as well as the fusiform lobe.

A completely different picture of the brain responses to change blindness–inducing stimuli was reported by Pessoa and Ungerleider (2004). They suggested that the effects reported by Beck and her colleagues were artifacts based on inadequate control of the subject's attentional state. Pessoa and Ungerleider also suggested that the Beck et al. technique of comparing correct and incorrect responses confounded the experimental design and led to contaminated results. Pessoa and Ungerleider, therefore, designed their experiment in an effort to overcome this difficulty by comparing only correct detections with incorrect rejections—both of which involved making a positive response. Furthermore they did not use the auxiliary letter-detection task—subjects were simply directed to hold a presented stimulus in short-term memory for six seconds; then a comparison stimulus was presented to determine if any changes had been detected.

What Pessoa and Ungerleider (2004) found was that the subject's response that there had been a change (i.e., either a correct hit or a false alarm) produced similar widespread fMRI activations throughout the brain including the inferior temporal, interparietal, precuneus, superior, inferior, and medial frontal, and pulvinar regions as well as the cerebellum. On the other hand when subjects reported that there had been no change when there was (a miss), few of these regions were activated to any significant degree. The implication of this finding was that the recorded brain activations were encoding the subject's "yes" or "no" responses rather than the change blindness phenomenon itself!

The pattern of results reported by Pessoa and Ungerleider (2004) suggests how easy it is to mistake the actual condition or state being measured with fMRI techniques for the phenomenon under study. It also illustrates how easily a cryptic confound can distort not only the data but their meaning. Here, too, there seems to have been a diminution of interest in the effort to find neural correlates of change blindness as the difficulties and complexities as well as the potential for misunderstanding became apparent.

3.3.3 Mirror Neurons

Each year or so another fascinating perceptual phenomenon leaps into the collective consciousness of the cognitive neuroscientific community. Although of legitimate interest as behavioral phenomena, the effort to find neural correlates with existing technologies is often fruitless and wasteful. Usually psychological phenomena inform or suggest to the neuroscientific research community what would be an interesting project to pursue. In a few cases, however, the flow of ideas is in the opposite direction. One of these exceptional cases concerns what have come to be called mirror neurons. Mirror neurons were discovered in the early 1990s in the laboratory of Rizzolatti at the University of Parma in Italy (di Pellegrino, Fadiga, Fogassi, Gallese, & Rizzolatti, 1992; Gallese, Fadiga, Fogassi, & Rizzolatti, 1996; Rizzolatti, Fadiga, Gallese, & Fogassi, 1996). The initial observation was straightforward. Some of the neurons impaled with microelectrodes in a smallish region of the prefrontal motor cortex known as F5 were found to be activated not only when a monkey performed some grasping action but also when it saw another monkey or even the experimenter perform the same grasping action. The action by the other monkey or the experimenter had to be significant and complete; that is, there had to be an object being grasped, not just a hand movement; a pantomime would not activate this type of neuron. However, even if the visual pathway from the arm to the object was partially occluded in a way that did not lose its significance, the action activated the mirror neurons (Umiltà et al., 2001). Even more recent work (Ferrari, Gallese, Rizzolatti, & Fogassi, 2003) reported that the mouth can also be the salient effector for activating mirror neurons located in another equally small region of the inferior parietal cortex. These neurons have also been shown to be activated by both executed and observed motor actions and, on this basis, identified as putative mirror neurons.

Not all of the mouth or hand cells in their respective regions are mirror neurons. Of those that were, the mouth cells could be associated with either eating or communication but not both. On the other hand the neurons responding to the grasping hand were not sensitive to the properties of the grasped object and seemed to be very unselective in that quite different stimulus conditions would activate them. It seemed as if the symbolic action of grasping an object was the key factor, not the particular hand, arm, or object. As noted earlier, even an occluded scene that implied the process of grasping activated these neurons. Whether this is the result of convergence from visual and motor neurons or selection on the part of the cell itself is unknown.

In summary, there are neurons in the monkey's brain that appear to be responsive to specific complex and meaningful "effector processes" whether performed by or observed by the monkey. These mirror neurons are reputed to provide a neural basis for learning motor responses or, more cognitively, in the vocabulary that has become associated with this work, "action understanding."[20] According to Hickok (2008), they are a modern example of and conceptually consistent with well-known motor theories of thinking and perception.[21]

The next important point to be made here as I review the empirical foundations of mirror neuron research is that, unless someone has managed to evade all of the ethical, technical, and procedural limitations imposed on human brain research, *no complementary research has yet been carried out that convincingly demonstrates the existence of mirror neurons in the human brain with microelectrodes or any other technique operating at the neuronal level.*[22] Instead, a number of investigators have turned to the tools they have available to study the macroscopic properties of the human brain, specifically modern brain imaging techniques such as the fMRI. For example brain activations tentatively associated with mirror neurons have been reported by Chong, Cunnington, Williams, Kanwisher, and Mattingley (2008); Buccino et al. (2004); Iacoboni et al. (1999); Puce, Allison, Bentin, Gore, and McCarthy (1998), among many others. The net result of brain imaging studies on mirror neurons is that activations purportedly associated with mirror neurons are often found in the inferior frontal and the superior and inferior parietal cortices but that lesser activations are found in many other brain regions. Whether or not these regions are directly comparable to the monkey's inferior parietal and ventral premotor regions remains problematical.

This work remains very controversial, however. The most comprehensive meta-review of studies that sought some evidence of mirror neurons in the human brain by imaging techniques was carried out by Turella, Pierno, Tubaldi, and Castiello (2009). They reviewed 33 PET and FMRI studies that claimed to produce evidence of mirror neurons in humans. The criterion used by Turella and colleagues was that an experiment was deemed to be supportive of the hypothesis that mirror neurons (or even a system of mirror neurons) were present in the human brain if activated regions responded to both observation of a motor response and activation of it. Of the 33 studies, only 5 met this criterion. Even this remaining group was inconsistent in suggesting which brain areas were activated by both observation and execution. They concluded the analysis with the following statement. "Put together, the above studies do not provide consistent evidence in favor of "mirror" type of activity with the frontal and parietal complex as found in monkeys" (p. 15).

Since robust single-cell recording work has not been carried out on humans and the fMRI measures cumulative activity of many neurons in what are typically many different areas of the brain, the idea of a single-cell correlate of this kind of either executed or observed behavior has begun to be replaced with the idea of a "mirror neuron system." That is, the conceptual basis and vocabulary of this work changed slowly from one in which the individual neuron was paramount to the notion of an assemblage of brain regions that collectively carried out the representation of such processes. This is a significant switch and illustrates the dangerous role of analogy in much of cognitive neuroscience. Stimulated by a fortuitous discovery of a particular kind of polysensory neuron, investigators in the field at first theorized that this neuron had broad behavioral effects. Then when it was deemed impossible to carry out the necessary microelectrode studies on humans, the theory of a highly localized "mirror neuron" changed from a single-cell explanation to a completely different neuroscientific model—one invoking broadly distributed regions of the brain.

The only thing the two approaches have in common, beyond their name, is that both are putative neural explanations of some of the most molar kinds of human behavior. Each is in substantial conflict with the most basic attributes of the other. Furthermore both are inadequate as explanatory theories of that molar behavior. Let us put aside for the moment the "mirror neuron system" approach and consider the frailties of the original hypothesis— namely that the mirror neuron is the basis of much of human behavior.

From the very beginning of mirror neuron research, some theoreticians have speculated that mirror neurons might play a profound role in some very important human activities. The list is long and impressive including the following traits:

- Action understanding
- Altruism
- Art appreciation
- Autism
- Empathy
- Evolution of speech
- Gender differences
- Ideomotor control (automatic movement without explicit decisions)
- Imitation
- Marriage relations
- Mental illness
- Mind reading
- Morality
- Motor theories of learning, perception, and thought
- Perception of other's minds and behavior
- Self-awareness
- Social cognition

- Social interactions
- Speech perception
- Sports team activities

One must question the logic of the huge leap from activities of single neurons to such complex behaviors as the social interaction of bridge players, a hypothesis that, if it has not already made the headlines, almost certainly will soon enough. Even if we ignore for the moment all of the challenging technical and empirical details faced by the mirror neuron hypothesis, a number of questions arise: Are the properties of these highly specialized single cells a reasonable explanation of these social and interpersonal behaviors? Does a single neuron or class of neurons have the power to control the behavior of groups of individuals and regulate such complex human passions as altruism or empathy? The answers to these questions are that the role of mirror neurons remains highly speculative and increasingly controversial.

From the outset it should have been noted that mirror neuron theory is a further development of a theoretical approach to cognitive neuroscience that has reduced support in recent years—the "single-cell" theory. I have discussed this approach in detail in Uttal (2005) and will not recapitulate that argument here. It is sufficient to point out that the main argument against single-cell theories is that they are all so incomplete. They are based on the behavior of one or a very few of perhaps 10^{10} neurons and ignore the activity of the entire multitude of the unstudied neurons. In such a situation it is highly likely that further exploration would find other equally interesting cells with equivalent or opposing properties IF one looked for them. The social nature of science is such that once an interesting and iconic discovery like that of the mirror neuron is made, research attention is directed to that type of neuron alone. Furthermore, since there are so many neurons, it is also probable that we would find many others of equal interest but quite different functions. The residual question is—which ones of this huge number of neurons will control behavior at any moment. The most likely answer to this question is both "none" and "all." No single cell can control behavior and all, many, or most may be involved. Behavior is governed by the network state of millions, if not billions, of neurons working collaboratively.

The point is that the fortuitous discovery of a class of cells like mirror neurons that behave in a manner that is roughly analogous to complex social behavior is not a strong argument that these neurons are the psychoneural equivalent of behaviors as conceptually distinct as empathy, for example. It is a form of reasoning by analogy that is as incorrect as that stimulated by many other observed correlations between these two vastly distant levels of discourse. Furthermore as pointed out by Dinstein, Thomas, Behrmann, and Heeger (2008), although considerable work has been done on the physiology of mirror neurons, no studies have shown them to be directly involved either in the behavior of either the monkeys in which they were discovered or in that of humans.

This kind of logical or philosophical argument aside, there are also a number of technical, empirical, and other interpretative reasons why much of the exaggeration concerning mirror neurons should be considered to be over the top and why a reconsideration of what these mirror neurons really mean is in order. Is the hyperbole extreme in this case? The range of applications to which they have been applied certainly suggests that this is the case. Any arguments that "mirror neurons are the fruit fly for all of cognitive neuroscience" suggest that much too much has been made of what may be an interesting and important demonstration of a new class of polyfunctional neurons.

Currently, a number of investigators have begun to raise serious questions about these extreme generalizations to human behavior from these observations of monkey neuron behavior. The overall problem is that macaque monkeys do not exhibit many of the behaviors (e.g., imitation) supposedly encoded by mirror neurons, and mirror neurons have not been unequivocally shown to be related to either animal or human behavior.[23]

One of the most important classes of criticisms of this or any other cognitive neuroscientific hypothesis concerns the robustness of the empirical data. Putting aside the absence of evidence for single-cell mirror neurons in humans, the evidence for even macroscopic patterns of "mirror" activity from brain imaging is also, as we have seen, fragile and questionable. One of the reasons for this uncertainty is that much of this work is based on the idea that mirror neurons can be selectively adapted by preconditioning. Dinstein et al. (2008) have also pointed out that the adaptation technique (which they otherwise favor) may be flawed because of the pooling of responses that may come from cells sensitive to movement and observation respectively rather than from a single "mirror neuron." They conclude their essay with the following admonition. "Mirror neurons are exceptionally interesting neurons, which may underlie certain social capabilities in both animals and humans. However, the study of mirror neurons and the 'human mirror system' in particular has been characterized by much speculation and relatively little hard evidence" (p. R17).[24]

In this same context Lingnau, Gesierich, and Caramazza (2009) reported that their adaptation experiments using fMRI did not support the existence of mirror neurons in humans. They came to this conclusion based on the fact that no adaptation of the fMRI activations occurred when their subjects "first executed and then observed" a motor response. The critical condition in their experiment is one in which execution of a motor act should have degraded the activations obtained during observation of that motor act. Their results did not show any such outcome. Therefore, they concluded that there is no evidence for mirror neurons in humans. Of course, one can criticize the entire approach of using fMRI imaging techniques to ask questions about the responsiveness of individual cells, but even if one should accept the validity of this approach, Lingnau et al.'s (2009) findings do not provide any support for the existence of mirror neurons in the human. The importance of this finding for the entire mirror neuron movement is well summed up by them:

Despite the lack of evidence for a mirror neuron system in humans, mirror neurons have been claimed to be involved in a variety of cognitive functions including empathy, mind reading, and the development of language. . . . Such claims would be undermined if we failed to find evidence for the involvement of mirror neurons in action understanding. (p. 9925)

One of the most extreme leaps of logic in this situation was the suggestion by a number of investigators (e.g., Fecteau, Lepage, & Theoret, 2006) that mirror neuron dysfunction in humans was associated with autism. An empirical refutation of this hypothesis was presented by Dinstein and colleagues (2010). Using fMRI techniques they showed that autistic and normal subjects not only exhibited the same pattern of activations during both observation and execution but that their adaptive responses were the same. Thus autism and the macroscopic fMRI responses were disassociated, thereby rejecting the suggestion that dysfunctional mirror neurons accounted for the behavioral disorder. This empirical evidence, of course, is not totally convincing given the frailties of brain imaging, but, beyond the data, it suggests that some of the logic behind associating behavior and neural responses may have been faulty.

A commentator of the mirror neuron hyperbola is Gopnik (2007) who discussed the "myth of the mirror neuron." Writing in an essay on the topic, she noted that mirror neurons have much of the same misleading charm that the left brain/right brain theory did in the 1960s and are likely to persist in the popular literature far longer than in the attention of researchers. Gopnik lists four misconceptions concerning the theoretical extrapolation from mirror neurons to human behavior that I now paraphrase. These four misconceptions, in her opinion, are the foundation of much of the unwarranted excitement during the past two decades in theoretical leaps from the interesting and solid neurophysiological research on multimodal "mirror neurons" to social interactions (2007).

1. We cannot generalize from animals to humans, especially when we are leaping from single neurons to some global behavior like language or empathy.
2. We cannot assume that brain structure is innate. Mirror properties might result from experience and be different in animals and humans.
3. We cannot tell anything about neurons from fMRI signals.
4. Single cells cannot encode complex kinds of behavior. Vast networks of different kinds of neurons represent and control both simple and complex behavior.

Perhaps the most comprehensive criticism of mirror neuron theory was published by Hickok (2008). In this eloquent and elegant critique, he dealt with the basic problem of their existence. Hickok did this by asking—are these mirror neurons really encoding such an elusive concept as action understanding?

Hickok's compelling argument against the role of these mirror neurons in encoding "action understanding" is eightfold. His eight arguments included these:[25]

1. There is no evidence in monkeys that mirror neurons support action understanding (p. 1231). [Comment: Research has not shown a disruption of related behavior when F5 is lesioned.]
2. Action understanding can be achieved via nonmirror neuron mechanisms (p. 1233). [Comment: Hickok points to neurons in the superior temporal region that seem to encode actions in a more "sophisticated" manner than do F5 neurons.]

3. M1 contains mirror neurons (p. 1233). [Comment: Primary motor neurons seem to have mirror properties suggesting that they also may encode future movements. Thus there may be nothing special about these visual-motor neurons in F5.]

4. The relation between macaque mirror neurons and the "mirror system" in humans is either nonparallel or undetermined (p. 1234). [Comment: The logic connecting mirror neurons in macaque and the mirror system in humans is deeply flawed, and the empirical evidence is nonexistent. The analogies between the two do not support a common homologically sound explanation for the two sets of data that come from very different levels of analysis.]

5. Action understanding in humans dissociates from neurophysiological indices of the human "mirror system" (p. 1235). [Comment: The speculative idea of a human "mirror system" has not been connected to the behavior of action understanding. Indeed, some research actually shows that the two are not related.]

6. Action understanding and action production dissociate (p. 1236). [Comment: Research at the behavioral level dissociates action production (e.g., raising the arm) from the ability to recognize which of two arm movements may have been made.]

7. Damage to the inferior frontal gyrus (BA 44/6—the purported human analog to the monkey's F5 region) is not clinically correlated with action understanding deficits (p. 1237).

8. Generalization of the mirror system to speech fails on empirical grounds (p. 1238). [Comment: Motor theories of speech have largely been abandoned because current data do not support any association between speech production and speech understanding.]

Hickok (2008) concludes his astute critique of the mirror theory of action understanding with the following comment: "Unfortunately, more than 10 years after their discovery, little progress has been made in understanding the function of mirror neurons. I submit that this is a direct result of an overemphasis on the action understanding theory, which has distracted the field away from investigating other possible (and potentially equally important) functions" (p. 1241).

I would go even further than that. I am convinced that much of the problem lies at the fundamental level at which attempts are being made to explain high-level cognitive or behavioral functions by means of neurophysiological properties of single cells or even of patterns of activation observed with brain imaging devices. This difficulty is exacerbated by the fact that our psychological descriptions are necessarily so vague that it is not usually clear what behavior it is that we are comparing with the neural data. Thus theory is inadequately constrained, and any vague similarity between the response of any available neuron and a behavior is loosely interpreted as an "explanation" for that behavior. In retrospect it seems that the explanation of altruism or empathy in terms of the activity of a neuron that happens to be sensitive to both motor and sensory properties is an unsupportable extrapolation—not only in this context of mirror neurons but also to any form of neuroreductive psychology in general.

Nothing I say here is intended to diminish the interest and excitement that the research on either mirror neurons in neurophysiology or social behavior in psychology should properly generate. Even the most severe critics of the mirror neuron–action understanding hypothesis do not reject the scientific value of the neurophysiological studies. There is an enormous amount we can learn from studies of these two levels of activity. However, it has been the historical case that extrapolative leaps from one level to the other rarely persist beyond the first few years of the neurophysiological discoveries. One example was the extension of the very important work on feature-sensitive neurons in the visual system to object recognition. Hubel and Wiesel's neurophysiological work deserved the Nobel Prize. The extensions of it to human perceptual processes did not!

Finally in this brief and selective review of the perceptual literature, we can once again turn to the meta-review carried out by Cabeza and Nyberg (2000). One of their divisions of cognitive processes was perception, which they subdivided into three categories relevant to the present discussion—object, face, and space/motion perception. Without going into the details of their review, it is sufficient to note that experiments evaluating the brain imaging findings showed that whereas everyone reported occipital and temporal activations for these three categories, most (but not all) also showed substantial frontal and parietal imaging responses. Thus even for this class of activity that is so heavily loaded with visual implications, there was substantial high-level and widely distributed activity generated. Even more surprising, however, was the inconsistency of the responses from these high-level (i.e., frontal and parietal) regions among the reports Cabeza and Nyberg reviewed.

What this all means is yet to be determined. It is clear, however, that the simplistic assertion that activation of a particular region of the brain is tantamount to that region being the site or among the sites representing a particular cognitive process is highly questionable.

In addition to the various technical, empirical, and statistical problems that underlie this kind of research, there are a number of logical and conceptual flaws permeating the entire program of neuroreductionism. Among the most prominent is that the fact that the absence of changes in an fMRI signal is not determinative of absence of changes in the computational state of the participating neuronal network. No difference in an fMRI signal may obscure the fact that the underlying neural network has undergone massive reconfigurations. Similarly, activation does not necessarily mean relevance despite observed correlations. There are many indirect routes by means of which a region may change its state of activation without any participation in the perceptual process under study. The argument for broad distribution is made strongly when one examines a broad swath of research and raises one's attention from the individual finding to the overall pattern of research findings.

Most of all, however, is the fact that the empirical data seem so idiosyncratic and so elusive of generalization. Some illusions show correlated activations in V1; others do not. Slight changes in the experimental design create major, inconsistent changes in the pattern of neural responses measured by fMRI techniques. There is, as yet, no sign on the horizon of how this noisy and idiosyncratic data will eventually be rationalized.

This then brings us to the end of our review of the modern brain imaging studies of perceptual processes. We now turn to a summary of the general ideas emerging from these findings.

3.4   Interim Summary

This chapter has dealt with a range of topics that probably do not differ in kind from the sensory ones considered in the previous chapter. However, there are two main points of emphasis that allow us to distinguish between the two topics. The first is that the theories and interpretations of perceptual phenomena are directed more at central brain mechanisms, whereas sensory topics are mainly associated with peripheral and early portions of the nervous system, particularly with the transmission codes used to convey information from the receptors. As we have seen, the depth of understanding of sensory coding mechanisms is so great that the explanatory mechanisms are actually more factual than speculative. On the other hand, perceptual theories are far less well understood and often nonexistent for some for the most familiar phenomena.

The second difference has to do with the emphasis placed on the experiential measurements. Specifically, sensory measurements are aimed at constraining the stimuli and phenomenal responses in a way that minimizes any differences between them. Thus sensory research is aimed at demonstrating the similarities, if not the congruence, between input and experience. The connotation and thus the experimental emphasis in perceptual research, on the contrary, are on measuring the differences, the discrepancies, between the stimuli and the experience. Although perceptual experiences have a much lower level of explanation, our main effort in studying them is to describe how poorly the experiential responses fit the stimuli and, in particular, how the responses deal with ambiguous stimuli.

It is clear that few theories of perceptual phenomena are robust; most often they depend on superficial isomorphic similarities in the data recorded from animal preparations and do not always agree even in the analogical sense. Simple explanatory models based on single-cell neurophysiological data are deeply flawed for this reason. The advent of brain imaging devices has not ameliorated the generality of this conclusion; few new insights have emerged that help us to understand from the neurophysiological point of view what are actually extremely complex processes.

A major failing in perceptual theorizing is the attempt to leap from observations of the properties of single neurons to much more molar or global properties of human individual psychology or, in some extreme cases, to social situations. The best current example of unwarranted extrapolation from single-cell responses to a variety of social needs and ills is to be found in the logically unsupportable theoretical leaps stimulated by the discovery of "mirror neurons."

The application of brain imaging techniques to the study of perception has been relatively fruitless. Findings have generally confirmed that the various sensory modalities initially project to what were known to be the primary receiving areas. In some cases improved maps of these projection regions became available. However, the more complex the perceptual phenomena studied, the more inconsistent were the imaging data. As with so many other topics considered in this book, the major findings in recent years have indicated that perceptual responses are much more widely distributed over the brain than had previously been thought. By the time we get to processes such as recognition, the complexity of the involved nervous system becomes evident, and there is as yet no robust neurophysiological explanation of perceptual phenomena.

The following specific comments help to summarize the current view of the cognitive neuroscience of perception.

1. Because of the tighter anchors to physical stimuli the quality of the brain imaging research in the area of sensory phenomena is much better than the often confusing and inconsistent results obtained when studying phenomena we collectively classify as perceptual.

2. Throughout this chapter there is a prevailing indication that many of the data obtained in perceptual neuroscience experiments are idiosyncratic, contradictory, and inconsistent. Different researchers working in the same problem area report dramatically different results. This is probably due to the complexity of the brain subsystems and the way the system actually encodes perceptual phenomena. The persistent question is—is this complexity analyzable, or does it represent an intractable problem to which current macroscopic methods are incapable of responding?

3. Traditional ideas of special roles for restricted areas of the brain must be reevaluated. There is no evidence of any unique role for any brain region in perceptual encoding or in any other domain of cognitive neuroscience. All brain regions, including the "primary projection areas" of the brain have been shown to be multimodal and multifunctional in one situation or another. It must not be overlooked that the heavy emphasis on vision in this chapter may obscure the fact that many of these same visual areas have also been reported to be activated or influenced by other cognitive tasks such as memory or attention. The overall pattern of evidence rejects the idea that there are areas exclusively associated solely with perception.

4. There is an emerging awareness that many of these multifunctional brain regions contribute collectively and interactively to the representation of a stimulus or a task. Perception is heavily penetrated by other powerful cognitive processes. Whatever this phrase means neurophysiologically, psychologically what we perceive is heavily determined by previous experiences and prejudgments. The anatomical analog of this psychological statement is probably reflected in the many interconnections between widely distributed areas of the brain.

5. The brain's response to what we have designated as perceptual stimuli is always widely, if not universally, dispersed. It is not only technically but conceptually very difficult to isolate any portion of the brain and consider its function independently of the "many" others that are typically involved. The controversy then revolves around the specific meaning of the word "many." Is it possible that virtually all of the brain is involved in virtually all cognitive processes? In other words, just how distributed are the brain responses to any mental activity? Can we truly isolate either individual areas or complete systems from other portions of the brain?

6. It is not possible to go from fMRI images to the properties of single cells. Too much information is lost by the pooling process to argue from the whole to the parts. The only possible exception is in the peripheral (including the early receiving areas of the cerebrum) situations where a large number of cells share a common orientation. Even then it is only the properties of the group that can be defined.

7. Although most detailed information about the state of the neural network is lost in brain imaging experiments, there is still some residual information left to distinguish between a modest number of alternative stimuli. However, this is not a matter of reconstructing the mental contents but, rather, of using these residual signals as a means of choosing among a set of stimuli in much the same way that a magician can determine which card was selected from a deck.

8. A problem with such analyses is that the specific residual brain signals vary depending on the analytical technique used to define them. Different analysis techniques and different patterns of the residual response may work equally well to make the discriminations.

9. It is not clear if these interesting experiments distinguish between the stimulus properties themselves or the perceived properties of the stimulus. If the former, this accomplishment may be dependent on the maintenance of the topological properties of the stimulus. If the later, the effect may be attributable to the residual information that is maintained after the activities of the neuronal network are pooled.

10. Research findings on particular perceptual processes such as face or form recognition, remain controversial and inconsistent.

11. Clinical evidence remains variable and idiosyncratic. There has been little, if any, success in finding neurophysiological explanations for illusions in any sensory modality. Single-neuron explanations founder on the problems faced by any analogical argument as well as the discrepancies between the phenomena and the neural responses. Brain imaging studies of illusions still have not risen to the level of "good science" because of the great variability of the reported responses. The real success in the study of illusions has been in the discovery of new perceptual phenomena, with one extraordinary example being change blindness.

12. In general we still have no satisfying models of perceptual phenomena at any level of neurophysiological analysis. Like all other cognitive processes, percepts seem to be represented by activity of such great complexity and wide distribution that none of our available research tools is able to unravel their function.

4 Emotion and Affect

4.1 Introduction

The psychological study of learning is enhanced by its advantage of having very simple and quantifiable independent variables—the number of trials or the passage of time—and solid behavioral dependent variables—the changes in behavior that result from manipulation of those independent variables. The psychological study of sensory and perceptual processes enjoys the advantage of being solidly anchored to the parameters of the physical stimulus world in a similar way. The study of emotions, however, is one of those subfields of psychology that are beset by some of the most fundamental barriers to understanding cognitive processes. Like attention, the target of this field of research is an inaccessible mental state that is only loosely linked to stimuli, behavioral outcomes, or neural mechanisms. Actors can feign emotional states, and well-controlled individuals can modulate or regularize their emotions by consciously recalibrating their interpretations of the affective meaning of an aversive stimulus. As a result of this inaccessibility and their lack of robust anchors to both stimuli and behavior, emotions, although profoundly important in human life, remain relatively inscrutable and immune to definition, understanding, measurement, and neuroreductionist analyses.

Indeed it is extremely difficult even to define what we mean by an emotion. Dictionaries fail, as they do with all other mental states, to provide a compelling definition that is not circular or empty. For example, my computer dictionary says that an emotion is "a heightened feeling" or "agitation caused by strong feelings." The former is an inaccessible mental state; the latter has an archaic and arbitrary connotation for exactly the same sort of mental state it attempts to define.[1] Neither provides a satisfactory definition for this elusive cognitive process.

Clearly the key word in all of these definitions is "feeling"—an equally ineffable term whose own definition remains obscure and vague. For example, "feeling" is circularly defined as an "emotional experience" (once one gets past its alternative use in the field of somatosensation).

The closely related term "affect" also frequently arises in discussions of emotion. This term suggests that we can separate the mental "feelings" from the physiological and behavioral aspects of emotion; affect tends to be used as the purely psychological aspect of an emotion. Affect is a word that describes the impact of the raw "experience" or "qualia" of that which is felt as an emotional experience. It is distinguished from the physiological responses that may accompany, or from some points of view, be the source of our affective feeling, that is, our emotions. The term "absence of affect" is often used synonymously with a lack of emotion.

Clearly defining emotion is a daunting task. Even as eminent a personage as Charles Darwin who wrote what is probably the most famous book on emotions (Darwin, 1872) finessed the problem and never clearly defined "emotions." In its place he distinguished among emotions, thought, and sensations, but he never grappled with the issue of what they were or what were their underlying mechanisms.

William James (1890) in his effort to answer the question—what is an emotion?—suggested that emotions are just perceptual responses of physiological changes that happen in our bodies. In his words:

Our natural way of thinking about these coarser emotions is that the mental perception of some fact excites mental affection called the emotion, and that this latter state of mind gives rise to bodily expression. My theory, on the contrary, is that the bodily changes follow directly the perception of the exciting fact, and that our feeling of the same changes as they occur IS the emotion. (vol. II, p. 449)

This idea, which has come down to us as the James-Lange theory of emotion (more about this later), was for him only valid for those emotions that were associated with some kind of bodily or behavioral responses. Emotions such as enjoying music or observing the beauty of an art object that might not evoke measureable physiological responses were not a part of James's theory of emotional responses. This exclusion was quite a major simplification and made possible his theory by limiting the study of emotion to that associated with observable behavior; however, it does not serve our need for a complete and precise definition of the term very well.

Furthermore James's answer is not a definition in the sense a good taxonomist would desire. It simply finesses the issue of definition by relating one cognitive process—emotion—with another—perception—without really defining either. This is a familiar strategy in psychology; because the targets of our interest are inaccessible and can at best only be assayed by indirect methods such as experimentation or introspection, there are few barriers that prevent us from freewheeling speculation about what emotion might be.

Although one may hope for crisp and operational definitions, it is much easier to concentrate on the connotations (i.e., the symbolic meanings) rather than on the more precise denotations. The result is that one is likely to encounter extended philosophical discussions of all of the implications, theories, and behavioral accompaniments of the inner "feelings" that are inferred to be the essence of emotional responses. Many of the discussions of what is an emotion, therefore, tend to simply wander off in circular arguments and in the end accept the common sense notion of "intense" but "irrational" conscious experiences as the essence of what we mean by emotion.

Some investigators simply avoid the issue of definition and assume that the subject matter is well enough understood that they can finesse the issue entirely and simply use common-sense definitions. Behaviorists do not seek any definition of fear or any other cognitive state; their strategy is simply to observe a class of "agitated" behaviors that are different than "normal" behavior. They try to link such responses with the stimulus situations that have some positive or negative affective implications and that produce erratic or unusual behavior. From this point of view we might include in the behaviorist family Charles Darwin. In his influential book on the topic, *The Expression of Emotion in Man and Animals* (1872), he adopted the strategy of describing the *expression* of emotional behavior without making any effort to define the term.

Others have sought to understand emotions in terms of the environmental stimuli that induce them. Both of these strategies exemplify the fact that consensual agreement without precise definition characterizes the psychological study of emotions. All of this has significant practical implications in the cognitive neuroscience of emotion by loosening our control over the independent variables in an experiment. The net result of avoiding or confusing what is being manipulated is to produce results that are even more variable and unreplicable than is the norm in cognitive neuroscience research.

Still others adopt whatever is the current metaphor guiding psychology in general. For example Cosmides and Tooby (2000) see emotions as computer-like programs that control and organize what otherwise would be a chaotic confusion of competing localized and psychological faculties or modules. To them ". . . a superordinate program is needed that coordinates these components, snapping each into the right configuration at the right time. Emotions are such programs" (p. 93). The experimental evidence for the existence of these "programs" being so elusive, this is hardly a good foundation on which to build a cognitive neuroscience of emotion.

An analytic approach to achieving an understanding of what we mean by "emotion" is to define a set of basic emotional states from which all of the others presumably could be produced by a process of compounding or mixing. The stimulus for developing this metaphor is, of course, color mixing; a process in which a few basic stimulus parameters can be used to generate the full range of millions of possible color experiences. Thus from the basic "emotional" prototypes would be formed the entire gamut of distinguishable emotions that were tabulated in even a moderately inclusive list. Examples of this approach are to be found in the works of philosophers such as Spinoza as well as more contemporary psychologists as McDougall (1926), Plutchik (1991, 1997), and Panksepp (1982, 1998).[2] Spinoza, for example, postulated that there were only three basic emotions—desire, pleasure, and pain— from which all others were created by mixtures, and mixtures of mixtures, of these three. A notable modern example of this set of basic "emotions" can be found in the work of Plutchik, who suggested that eight basic emotions, their opposites, and their paired combinations account for the full range of emotional phenomena. His eight basic emotions included joy, acceptance, fear, surprise, sadness, disgust, anger, and anticipation.

This approach, in which a set of basic emotions is invoked, has been severely criticized by a number of psychologists including Ortony and Turner (1990). Their criticism is summed up in the following statement: "Thus, the view that there exist basic emotions out of which all other emotions are built, and in terms of which they can be explained, is questioned, raising the possibility that this position is an article of faith rather than an empirically or theoretically defensible basis for the conduct of emotion research" (p. 315). For that matter can we be sure that an "emotion" or any of these putative basic components is actually a distinguishable psychobiological reality? Or, to the contrary, are they merely different psychological manifestations of some indivisible mental "feeling" or reaction of our autonomic system. Furthermore, in the same vein as with so many other mental activities, might such terms merely be reified names for phenomena (or groups of phenomena) that we are incorrectly inferring from observations of behavior?

In our search for the denotation of the word "emotion," can we really expect to distinguish emotions from such closely related cognitive processes as attention or perception with which they may be profoundly entangled? Or, to make a further stab at defining them, are emotions merely another set of properties of a more inclusive holistic entity we call mind? That such a "property" list approach is the actual nature of emotion has been proposed by LeDoux (2002). If he is correct, then how do we go about measuring the putative properties of "emotional experience"? Questions like these challenge researchers interested in emotion as well as any psychologist who seeks to explore any of the other mysteries of the mind.

In one of the most direct and eloquent assaults on the meaning of the word "emotion," Kagan (2007) suggested that the search may be fruitless. He noted that ". . . the answers offered [to the question of what is emotion] are riddled with ambiguity and do not enjoy the more consensual, transparent meanings of such concepts as velocity and heat" (p. 1).

The father of modern emotional neuroscience—James W. Papez—suggested in 1937 the following dichotomous meaning of the word emotion:

The term "emotion" as commonly used implies two conditions: a way of acting and a way of feeling. The former is designated as emotional expression; the latter, as emotional experience or subjective feeling. The experiments of Bard have demonstrated that emotional expression depends on the integrative action of the hypothalamus. . . . For subjective emotional experience, however, the participation of the cortex is essential. (p. 726)

The problem of definition of emotion, then, remains a continuing one; certainly the chaotic accumulation of findings from the large number of recent studies on emotion does not allow such a simple conclusion as was proposed by Papez. *The Handbook of Emotions* (2000), one of the most authoritative collections of articles in this field, never really comes to grips with a satisfactory definition; most of the contributing authors agree that its lack of precise definition is a formidable obstacle to the field. In the place of a robust denotative definition, many investigators look on emotion as a variable that may be used to study other forms of behavior. Emotion, thus, is typically embedded in studies of affective language, clinical dysfunction, gender differences, or various cognitive processes. Even feelings as patently emotional as love or fear are often evaluated in terms of interpersonal interactions rather than as the response of particular brain regions.

It should be obvious by this point that any proffered definition of emotion is going to be as elusive and contentious as that of any other mental activity. Emotions are private experiences that can be only weakly inferred from introspection or behavior but that cannot be directly measured. Nevertheless philosophical and psychological research on emotion has been extensive throughout history and, with the advent of brain imaging, continues well into the present time.[3]

What is incontestable is that emotional responses are subjective experiences that have roots in the nervous system and that serve numerous useful adaptive roles, many of which are deeply involved in maintaining or improving the life of the individual. As such, they are at least a useful adjunct to higher-level cognitive processes if not just another one of them. Whatever a subjective emotion is, it is clear that emotional behavior evolved early on in the development of vertebrate life. It serves protective, defensive, and reproductive functions. Without such responses we might not have evolved—their adaptive advantage is so profound.

The study of emotion can also be attacked from the undiluted point of view of neuroscience. Much of our nervous system is dedicated to the perpetuation and protection of our personal existence and genetic heritage. Thus, stimuli that produce both pleasant and unpleasant feelings can be studied by recording the responses of various parts of the body in stressful situations. To do so, however, eschews the otherwise ubiquitous agreement that emotions are conscious experiences first and foremost. Additional assumptions have to be made; for example, it must be assumed that behavior is tightly linked to mental states; that mental states are closely enough linked to brain states; and that brain states are closely enough linked to physiological responses of other parts of the body to justify linking bodily responses directly to what we call emotional states.

Thus it is clear that the study of emotions has constituted a large part of modern psychological science and will probably continue to do so in the new era of brain imaging. Although it is not possible to image the subjective state of an "emotion," it is conceivable that we will be able to image some of the correlated states of the brain during emotional responses. This chapter is dedicated to examining the degree to which this promise has been achieved.

4.2   A History of Scientific Research on Emotions

The question of how we do research on such an indefinable, inaccessible, and immeasurable mental process as perceived emotion has conflicted psychology throughout its history. Prior to the emergence of scientific psychology in the nineteenth century, philosophers and theologians had already considered emotions a topic of deep concern. All agreed that emotions are important aspects of human existence and have sought explanations of inter-personal values and ethics that have guided and will continue to guide human social inter-actions. Other scholars and artists see emotions as the "spice of our mental lives." How drab a novel or a play would be if it did not invoke passions of love or fear; how easy it is to control people's behavior by appealing to or manipulating their emotions. For millennia these two truisms have either implicitly or explicitly guided our political and economic behavior as well as our entertainments.

It is difficult to avoid finding concerns with the nature of emotions in the most distant documents of human thought. Fellous and Hudlicka maintain an Internet page tracing the historical outline of the history of emotions entitled The Emotion Home Page (accessible at http://emotion.nsma.arizona.edu/emotion.html) that lists the many philosophers, theo-logians, and scientists who have concerned themselves with the problem of emotion over the millennia. Although many of them use archaic terminology or invoke concepts that have long been rejected (e.g., "fear arises from brain overheating" [Hippocrates] or "pleasure and pain result from blood aeration" [Diogenes]), it is clear that there has been a deep concern with emotions, however difficult it has been to define them, that has persisted throughout human history.

Fellous and Hudlicka organized the history of the field in a fascinating and informative way. The overall impression that one gets, however, from perusing their list is that there was little progress in the scientific study and understanding of the nature of emotions until the nineteenth century, when two important developments occurred. The first development was the scientific observation of emotional changes that occurred with brain injuries; the second was the availability of physiological measuring instruments that permitted us for the first time to correlate behavioral and neurobiological states. It must be remembered that this relatively modern neuroscientific approach does not resolve many of the enigmas sur-rounding emotions and emotional behavior. Before we deal with the neuroscientific study of emotions, we must briefly consider some of the vast amount of purely behavioral research that has been done in this field.

4.3   Emotions and Behavior

It is worthwhile to begin by at least briefly introducing some of the difficulties facing the kind of empirical research on emotions that has occupied experimental psychology through-out its history. This is useful to set the stage for the subsequent neuroscientific discussion in later sections.

The psychological study of emotions is beset by a number of problems that transcend those of definition I already introduced. First and foremost are the practical problems of controlling the stimuli driving emotions and emotionally rooted behavior in even the best-designed experimental protocols. Although some emotions may be controlled with verbal instructions or simple reward schedules, the control of more complex or hazardous emotional reactions can easily violate the ethical and legal standards now guiding human research. For reasons such as these, much of the research on emotion had until recently been carried out on animals or depended on the fortuitous and idiosyncratic nature of clinical cases. This situation, as the reader should appreciate full well by now, has changed considerably with the advent of brain imaging systems.

The control of emotion as an independent variable in an experiment using human subjects is fraught with practical uncertainties, procedural difficulties, and ethical constraints. How does one go about producing the emotion of fear in a responsible way? Imagine placing a person who exhibited strong emotional reaction to heights (acrophobia) at the top of a ladder. Even showing such a person a picture of the Grand Canyon might induce strong fearful reactions that violate experimental proprieties. Although these are extremes, such stimulus situations are regularly approximated in any laboratory situation that seeks to produce and control negative emotions in humans. Similar ethical questions arise when one seeks to manipulate positive emotions such as those associated with sex.

There are many other complications to research on emotions including methodological problems that interfere with clear-cut conclusions from even the best-designed empirical investigations. In an earlier work (Uttal, 2001) I noted the following difficulties that inhibited understanding of cognitive neuroscientific findings even when an experiment might have been deemed to have been successful (abstracted from Uttal, 2001, p. 153):

- Inadequate definition of the boundaries of brain regions.
- Difficulty in isolating a lesion to the region under investigation.
- System complexity due to the high level of interconnectivity including feedback, feed forward, redundant coding in more than a single region, massive parallelicity, the interplay of excitatory and inhibitory modules, and finally the multiple roles of single brain regions.
- Variable and idiosyncratic data from human brain injuries.
- The fact that, in the main, only behavioral deficits could be localized by lesion methods. In the final analysis all that can be done is to show that behavior is changed from the norm after a brain lesion.
- The effects of inadvertently cutting fiber tracts passing near or under the lesioned nuclei were often misinterpreted as functions of the lesioned region.
- Recovery of function.

A further complication is that emotions fluctuate rapidly in time; therefore, it is frequently difficult to stably maintain the emotional experiences that supposedly result from manipulation of emotional stimuli. Paper-and-pencil tests are incapable of measuring these momentary fluctuations. Although they may have some use to clinicians in determining long-term chronic emotional conditions, they are virtually useless in the kind of high-speed emotional reactions in situations that require quick flight or fight responses.

Furthermore, emotions are subject to cognitive penetration (i.e., to modification by high-level cognitive processes) and thus may either mask or cognitively enhance behavior that we would associate with emotional situations. People can, thus, both simulate emotional responses and inhibit true emotionality. Indeed, the cognitive penetration may be so extreme that it may not be possible to distinguish between cognition and emotion in an operational sense.

Despite these difficulties many distinguished psychological researchers have attempted in one way or another to study emotions, or perhaps more usually, the effects of emotions on other forms of behavior. This is possible because emotion remains one of many psychological imponderables that can be attacked from many different directions; social, cognitive, clinical, and neuroscientific psychologists each approach the problem from a distinctly different conceptual position. Whereas all may share a commitment to the scientific empirical method, the tools that each uses and the intellectual contexts in which each implants his or her own research may be quite different.

In many cases research on emotions is really on the effect of emotions—poorly defined though they may be—on such psychological issues as development, personality, expressions, and social interactions. Needless to say, emotions also play an important role outside of psychology per se. Emotions are a well appreciated part in studies of economics, politics, sociology, and certainly in our interpretations of history itself. Although emotions do not fossilize, there is a continuing effort in archeology to infer from those artifacts and tissues that do, what was the emotional behavior of peoples who long ago departed from the scene. Modern evolutionary psychologists also suggest that they have a special insight into emotional behavior.[4]

Many other scientists attacked the problem of emotions from a psychological or behavioral point of view. Among the most notable was the work of Charles Bell on the expression of the emotions (like Descartes, he called them passions). Bell had already achieved considerable fame for his neuroanatomical discoveries of the different roles of the dorsal and ventral spinal roots (see section 2.2.1). Bell's (1824) book was in many ways a precursor of Darwin's (1872) much more famous tome on the *Expression* of emotions. Both books are extremely interesting because their authors shared a behaviorist approach in which they concentrated entirely on the expression of emotions and explicitly eschewed study of what both agreed were the underlying and unobservable physiological processes that accompanied the feelings and the behavior. At that time, insufficient knowledge of the organization of the nervous system was available to provide the foundation for the neuroscientific theories that were to emerge later.

The behavioral and psychological literature on emotions is enormous and diverse because of its widespread connection to so many other psychological issues and topics. Both experimental and theoretical literatures are extensive. It would be impossible, therefore, to attempt an exhaustive review of the huge diversity of psychological studies that involve emotion in one way or another. Suffice to say that psychology has made a major commitment to the study of this pervasive and influential aspect of human mentation. Our attention is now directed to what has become the newest development in the study of emotion, the application of neuroscientific knowledge and techniques in the search for this elusive process.

4.4   The Search for Emotions in the Brain

Despite the difficulty in defining what an emotion is, there has been a considerable amount of research on the biological bases of the topic. However, this research has not been continuous throughout the last century. According to LeDoux (2000), although the study of emotions was vigorously pursued during the early part of the twentieth century (mainly by means of experimental surgery on animals), interest in it waned in the latter part of the century. He attributes this to the rise of cognitive psychology, the subjectivity of emotions compared to thinking, as well as to a misunderstanding that the simple identification of an emotion-related brain system by Papez constituted a "final" solution to the problem of the brain mechanisms of emotions.[5] LeDoux argued, however, that this ebbing of interest is changing. He suggested that both the linking of the limbic system to higher cortical regions and the association of emotional and learning processes suggest that both fields may add something to their respective studies by considering results from the other. LeDoux's argument that the inhibitory effect on our thinking of the limbic system as an emotional center could be overcome if we turned to specific combinations of emotions and learning, one example of which was "fear conditioning."

Whatever the particular model, the important point is that cognitive neuroscientists currently believe that a widely distributed system of brain components ranging from the brainstem to the highest levels of the cerebrum are involved in the subjective states we call emotions. A further assumption widely accepted these days is that emotion invokes activity in parts of the limbic system, in particular the components known collectively as the Papez circuit. How we got to this point is discussed in the remainder of this chapter.

4.4.1   The Early Stage

As usual, it is not exactly certain when brain-based research into emotions and theories first began to replace philosophical and humanistic speculations. It is not unlikely that even the most primitive humans appreciated that their bodily responses both controlled and reflected feelings and emotions. Emotions produce (or are produced by) obvious bodily signs. Shortness of breath, flushing, clammy skin, as well as more subtle indicators as pupillary dilation have, over the years, all been commonly associated with the subjective states of emotion, and all are overtly obvious to even the most casual observer.

In less ancient times, the survival of patients with traumatic injuries offered an opportunity to discern how the brain might be involved in emotional expression. Perhaps the most famous iconic case was that of Phineas Gage, a railroad worker, who had the unfortunate experience of having a tamping rod blown through his frontal lobes by a premature explosion in 1848.The changes in his personality (a generic term for the emotional and cognitive factors that describe a person's social responses) were reported by the physician (Harlow, 1868) who attended to him both during the accident and over the years as he recovered. Harlow's description of Gage's behavioral changes following the accident is one of the classic items in the literature of emotional behavior.

Gage was fitful, irreverent, indulging at times in the grossest profanity (which was not previously his custom), manifesting but little deference for his fellows, impatient of restraint or advice when it conflicts with his desires, at times pertinaciously obstinate, yet capricious and vacillating, devising many plans of future operations, which are no sooner arranged than they are abandoned in turn for others appearing more feasible. A child in his intellectual capacity and manifestations, he has the animal passions of a strong man. Previous to his injury, although untrained in the schools, he possessed a well-balanced mind, and was looked upon by those who knew him as a shrewd, smart businessman, very energetic and persistent in executing all his plans of operation. In this regard his mind was radically changed, so decidedly that his friends and acquaintances said he was "no longer Gage." (Harlow, 1868)

The attribution of Gage's emotional changes to this traumatic brain injury was hardly the first to suggest that the brain was deeply involved in the processing of emotional behavior. However, Harlow may have been one of the first to make what was to become the archetypical connection between the frontal lobes and the control of emotional behavior. He presciently concluded that the frontal lobes acted as an inhibitor of other regions, whereas other regions of the brain acted as activators or exciters of emotional behavior.

The relation among bodily (specifically autonomic) functions was formalized in one of the most persistent and consensual theories of psychological research by William James (1842–1910) and Carl Lange (1834–1900).[6] These two proposed what is now known as the James-Lange theory of emotion. In their view, in which external stimuli directly elicit responses in the organs of the body, an "emotion" *is* the perception of these physiological responses. The essence of their theory is that the autonomic responses came first, only then to be followed by the perception of these bodily responses.

An alternative theory proposed by Walter Cannon (1871–1945) and Philip Bard (1898–1977) offered a contrary view that argued that it was our perception of the external emotion-evoking stimuli that led to the subsequent activation of the somatic responses. Other theories of subjective emotional responses build on this same distinction. Some modern theories (for example, Lazarus, 1966; Schacter & Singer, 1962) give priority to the physiological response but require some kind of a cognitive interpretation before the subjective emotional experience develops.

Since the classic debate between these two approaches was joined, there have been numerous attempts to explain the causal sequence of the relation between our perceptions of emotion and our bodily responses. It was in the 1930s that the stage was set for much more specific and general neuroscientific theories of emotions. A major step was made when the limbic system, a collection of brain structures located within and below the lower edge of the cerebrum, was associated with a cluster of psychological processes, some of which were the emotions. Although the specific role and even extent of the limbic system has been questioned, it is still considered by most cognitive neuroscientists (led by McLean, 1949) to represent a cohesive subsystem of the brain, both anatomically and functionally. The limbic system incorporates some cerebral and some brainstem structures. It is now known to be heavily involved in a substantial number of cognitive and emotional functions. A more complete discussion of the various components of the limbic system can be found in another of my books (Uttal, 2009a).

Of particular interest in the present discussion is the role of a subset of the limbic system components and some additional cortical regions that have been specifically associated with emotion—the Papez (1937) circuit. Although coextensive with much of the rest of the limbic system, the functions of the Papez network of interacting regions seem to be deeply, if not solely, involved in the regulation and control of emotional behavior through their ability to regulate endocrine and autonomic mechanisms.

Papez's original paper is still well worth reading despite being over 70 years old. He was primarily an anatomist, and much of his article deals with the interconnections of a number of brainstem and cerebral regions that he argued, by virtue of one of those great intuitive leaps in cognitive neuroscience history, were *collectively* the brain instantiations of emotional experiences and behavior. There was no one center that had priority (the hippocampus played a central and participatory role, but not a commanding one); intrusions of one kind or another into any portion of the circuit could produce emotional behavior.

Papez appreciated early on, by virtue of his anatomical training, the nature of the two-way connections between the various components he considered to be parts of his "emotional circuit." He was one of the first to acknowledge that earlier work, which had concentrated on the role of individual centers, might well be misleading by falsely suggesting a kind of localization of different kinds of emotional mental modules. Instead, he proposed that this cluster of centers and "their interconnections constitute a harmonious mechanism which may elaborate the functions of central emotion, as well as participate in emotional expression" (p. 743). Although, he went on to support the archaic idea that the "seat of consciousness is located somewhere near the midline [of the brain]" (p. 743), there is no denying that Papez had an enormous impact in modern theory about what constitutes the neural basis of emotion. A traditional version of the Papez circuit is illustrated in figure 4.1.[7]

Papez identified the particular structures that were involved in his emotional circuit on the basis of some of the pioneering work that had been done by earlier physiologists. Goltz (1892), for example, had long ago come to the same conclusion as had Harlow (1868) (on the basis of the Phineas Gage case) that the cerebrum was an inhibitor of emotional behavior. This conclusion was forthcoming from Goltz's research in which the entire cerebrum had been removed from a dog. The animal survived but was continuously aggressive, that is, hyperemotional.

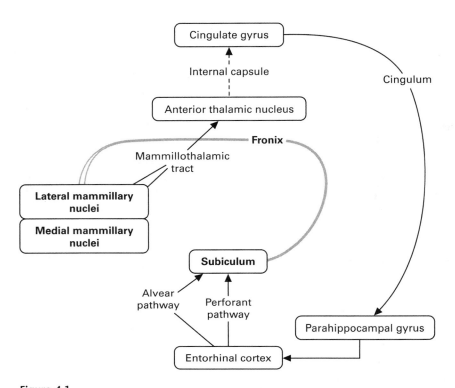

Figure 4.1
An early version of the Papez circuit.
From Wikipedia article entitled "Papez Circuit" and used with the permission of their Creative Commons
License Grant.

Goltz's work had been followed up by the investigations of Bard (1928) and Ranson
(1934), who had both suggested that the hypothalamus was the portion of the brain that
produced aggressive behavior when released from cerebral inhibition. Penfield (1933), on
the other hand, had shown a more general involvement of brainstem and limbic structures
in the representation of emotion. Papez, as an anatomist, however, had mainly been influenced by the anatomy of the tracts that seemed to interconnect these and other structures
that he and other anatomists had so painstakingly mapped out. Subsequent work by such
investigators as Kluver and Bucy (1939) added the idea that temporal lobe regions such as
the amygdala were also deeply involved in emotional behavior.

During the next few years a series of studies was carried out that selectively removed
portions of the brains of cats and dogs. These experiments produced a theory of the organization of the brain that still has some currency these days. The hypothalamus, in particular, was thought to play a central role in organizing hyperemotional responses. However,

the results were very ambiguous. Removal of parts of the hypothalamus led to responses that were considered to be parts of a full-blown rage reaction. Electrical stimulation of the hypothalamus produced an animal with persistent rage responses. Thus, either removal or stimulation (activation or deactivation) of the hypothalamus seemed to produce the same effect—rage, (i.e., hyperemotional behavior). If the cerebrum was removed, unconstrained and persistent hyperemotional states were released in most cases. Bard and Mountcastle (1947) summarized the role of the cerebral cortex as an inhibitor of emotional behavior in a now classic review.

It is important not to overlook the now obvious fact that a very large portion of the brain's structures are involved in the modern view of the extent of the Papez circuit. However deeply involved any center may be in controlling emotional responses, each has also been associated with other cognitive and bodily functions. Therefore inclusion in this list of components of the Papez circuit does not mean that this is the sole function or purpose of a given structure. We have already seen how the hippocampus and the amygdala, for example, are as deeply involved in spatial and learning processes as in emotional ones. The thalamus, now considered to be a part of the Papez circuit, is also well known to be a pathway for sensory information. Indeed many of the very same regions enumerated by Papez had sensory functions. For example, many of the same centers he included in his circuit were originally thought to be associated with olfaction and/or olfactory memory. Finally, to emphasize this point, the frontal lobes are known to play many other cognitive roles.

Subsequent to Papez's theoretical contribution, other similar theories have contested for the center stage in theories of the brain mechanisms of emotion. LeDoux (1987), for example, has downplayed the role of the hippocampus highlighted by Papez in favor of the contribution of the amygdala. However, all such theories of the physiological basis of emotion share many comparable features, most notably the idea that a combination of regions must cooperate to produce balanced and adaptive emotional experience and behavior.

We must also keep in mind the high probability that the various components of the Papez and LeDoux circuits are so heavily interconnected with other portions of the brain that it is likely to be extremely difficult to determine at what point an emotional response may be initiated and what role they may play in other cognitive functions. Distinguishing between contradictory theories (such as the James-Lange or the Cannon-Bard types or between the Papez and LeDoux approaches) may, therefore, be impossible in principle.

As I noted earlier, the components that make up the emotion-regulating circuits of the brain have varied from time to time.[8] Currently, the Papez circuit is not only considered to be made up of a subset of the limbic system components but also to involve at least three areas of the cerebral cortex. Specifically, the Papez circuit is now considered to consist of a loop of the components on the following list.

- The hippocampus and the amygdala
- The mammillary bodies
- The anterior thalamus
- The cingulate cortex
- The parahippocampal gyrus
- The entorhinal cortex
- The hypothalamus
- The septal nuclei
- The frontal cortex

I use this list and figure 4.1 to organize the research findings that I now consider to have occurred in the intermediate stage of neuroscientific studies of emotional behavior.

4.4.2 The Intermediate Stage

The intermediate stage of brain research on emotions is characterized by the use of a number of the standard research techniques that have long played important roles in the study of the brain. These included surgical lesioning of particular brain regions, electrical stimulation and recording, and the insertion of neurologically active chemicals—in particular, several of the identified synaptic transmitter substances. A major problem with much of this stage of research was the uncertainty of the extent of some of the surgical interventions. As physiological psychology became increasingly committed to the idea that the brain was divided into separate functional units, the identification of these units became a more and more important activity in cognitive neuroscience. However many questions remained. What were the boundaries of brain regions? How precise were the experimental lesions? Did they, or did they not have distinguishable roles in mediating emotional activity? Much of the surgical work prior to the turn of the twenty-first century was directed at answering these questions; unfortunately many doubts remain concerning what were often uncritically accepted answers to them.

Similarly, it is not always certain just what kind of current spread there may have been when electrical stimuli were used or when a transmitter substance such as serotonin was injected into the brain. Practical difficulties such as these make much of the research conducted during this period equivocal at best and downright erroneous at worst. Nevertheless, these traditional techniques provided the conceptual foundations on which many of the later brain imaging studies were based. I now present a sampling of this kind of research in which attempts were made to determine the role of the various components of the Papez circuit in emotional activity.

The Hippocampus and the Amygdala

The hippocampus, which is generally thought to be a collection or complex of functionally differentiable regions, appears to be involved not only in emotional behavior but also in learning, particularly in consolidation of short-term to long-term memory. I have already discussed its additional role in providing a locus for a spatial model of the environment proposed by O'Keefe and Nadel (1978). Thus, the hippocampus, like all other components of the Papez circuit, seems to have a diversity of functions; different investigators see it playing out these different roles depending on their specialized research interests. To Papez, it was one of the central, if not the central, components of his circuitous system, with others being the hypothalamus and the anterior thalamus. The hippocampal role in emotion is especially ambiguous because electrical stimulation of ventral regions produces aggressive reactions in cats, whereas the same stimulus applied to the dorsal hippocampus inhibited this kind of emotional activity (Siegel & Flynn, 1968).

The hippocampus is also located adjacent to the amygdala. Given the imprecision of surgical lesions and the uncontrolled spread of electrical stimuli, the roles of these two centers in regulating emotion are often difficult to separate. The fact that both regions have both memory and emotional functions supports the common-sense notion that we remember emotional experience better than those not involving strong feelings.

Laboratory research on the roles of the hippocampus and the amygdala, therefore, has often been intertwined. Lesions of one affect one kind of emotional learning and of the other often produce different effects. For example Phillips and LeDoux (1992) demonstrated that lesions of the amygdala affected both classical cue conditioning and learning of the context of a noxious experience. However, when the hippocampus was surgically damaged, only the classical cue conditioning was affected. Separating the roles of the two regions can be very difficult.

Others however have parsed the system in a different manner. Adolphs, Trannel, Damasio, and Damasio, (1994), for example assigned the experience of fear to the amygdala and have suggested that it acted in concert with the medial frontal region of the brain to instantiate this strong emotion. On the other hand, the processing of the fear-provoking stimulus was mainly mediated by the hippocampus in conjunction with the lateral frontal region according to them. A further complication arises from the fact that two brain regions—the hippocampus and the amygdala—are heavily interconnected. This provides an anatomical basis for their joint effects, especially when "emotions meet memory" (Phelps, 2004, p. 201).

Clearly the intricacies of the interaction of these two regions are complex and not fully understood, and there are probably many alternative ways in which this system could be conceptualized. The most persistent problem is that we really have no way of measuring what an animal, or for that matter, a human is experiencing during emotional behavior.

The Mammillary Bodies
The mammillary bodies also seem to have dual roles. In addition to their place as an integral part of the Papez circuit, they also seem to play a role in recognition memory. Research suggests that their role in regulating emotion is predominantly excitatory. For example,

Santacana, Pelaez, and Tejedor (1972) have demonstrated that if the mammillary bodies were bilaterally excised, emotional behavior diminished in experimental rats. Of course we cannot know exactly to what the effect is due. Is it merely a matter of a break in the Papez circuit, or do these structures actually stimulate emotional responses by means of their own activity?

The Anterior Thalamus

The thalamus is a complex structure with many distinguishable functional regions. The lateral geniculate body of the thalamus, for example, is one of the main transmission junctions in the visual pathway. One of the main problems with evaluating the role of the thalamus in emotional responses is that the elicited responses depend not only on the stimulus but also the social structure of the community from which the experimental animals were selected. For example Delgado (1966) showed that electrical stimulation of the same region of the thalamus could produce either aggressive or submissive behavior of monkeys depending on the social rank of the animal! It is now thought that the thalamus does not itself encode any emotional responses but acts mainly as a transmission pathway for emotion-evoking stimuli. The reasons behind the contradictory results produced by social status remain unclear. At the least it does seem to suggest a very high-level cognitive input into whatever mechanism is actually encoding emotional experience and behavior.

The Cingulate Cortex

The cingulate cortex was originally included as a part of the Papez circuit. However its many connections with other parts of the brain and the many sensory, motor, and autonomic processes have made it something of an enigma. Indeed many of the early results seemed to differ from species to species even for what were thought to be homologous lesions. For example Kennard (1955) demonstrated that bilateral lesioning of the cingulate cortex produced a number of bizarre motor changes in the behavior of a cat as well as an increased propensity toward rage responses. This finding, however, contradicted the results reported by Glees, Cole, Whitty, and Cairns (1950), who excised the anterior cingulate region bilaterally in monkeys and found a marked reduction in fear reactions—the animals seemed tamer and less "shy" of their handlers and displayed "increased restlessness and hyperactivity."

A human study of the effect of surgical lesions in the cingulate carried out by Tow and Whitty (1953) demonstrated quite a different pattern of results. Patients with this kind of lesion seemed to have relatively minor personality changes, seeming to be virtually normal. This was in contrast to the substantial effects of the cingulate operation on monkeys and cats and with the substantial changes in personality and emotionality that occurred following frontal lobe surgery.

The uncertainty of the role of the cingulate cortex is further compounded by the fact that different parts of this region may have different functions. Vogt, Finch, and Olson

(1992) reported that while the anterior region of the cingulate cortex is involved in emotional control, the posterior region has only sensory functions. Bush, Luu, and Posner (2000) also reported a variety of functions of the anterior cingulate lobe; they described it as having a wide variety of specialized regions controlling many emotional, cognitive, and other functions.

The problem of how to define and then partition the various centers of the cingulate cortex becomes a major one. One possibility is that these observed functional differences in different areas of the cingulate do not have any biological reality; rather this organ may be indivisible, and any effort to subdivide it may be another vestige of the all too persistent assumption of localized function that has dominated recent theory. In its place we may have to substitute quite a different assumption—namely that the cingulate cortex and the other portions of the Papez circuit are general-purpose structures that serve different roles in different contexts in different animals.

A further consideration of this problem raises another interesting possibility. That is that the psychological processes are so poorly defined that we cannot accurately distinguish between such terms as "cognition" and "emotion." McNaughton (1997) eloquently summed up this problem in the context of his concern with hippocampal research when he said:

Cognition and emotion, since they are distinct terms, might be expected to refer to quite distinct entities. . . . From a Darwinian point of view, however, they must at least be synergistic. Emotion, far from being something that interferes with rational action, must be something that results in adaptive responding (and, hence, in a sense, rational responding) at least under phylogentically frequent circumstance. (p. 603)

The implication of this well-articulated point is that the entire goal of assigning artificially divided cognitive functions to localized regions of the brain may be an ill-chosen quest. The multimodal role of virtually all brain regions, the arbitrary modularity of cognitive processes, the variability of response, and the interactions at the mental and behavioral levels all argue, to the contrary, that the brain operates in a much more distributed and interactive manner than current theories suggest.

In addition to the specific conceptual issues mentioned here, the history of cingulate research reminds us of the general problem of species differences. Highly suggestive results from animals as closely related to us as monkeys do not necessarily transfer to comparable conclusions for human beings. Nor do the results from cats correspond to those obtained from monkeys.

The Parahippocampal Gyrus

Surrounding the hippocampus is the parahippocampal gyrus. Because of its spatial relation to the hippocampus it has been difficult to distinguish the functions of the two regions within the context of emotionality and the Papez circuit. One curious finding is that the parahippocampal gyrus seems especially sensitive to pleasant and unpleasant music. Patients with parahippocampal lesions reported that dissonant music was not unpleasant, a report completely contrary to normal controls (Gosselin et al. 2006).

The Entorhinal Cortex

The entorhinal cortex is located at the anterior end of the temporal lobe and, like other components of the Papez circuit, seems to have roles in both emotion and learning. It has been proposed that this is due to its high degree of connectivity with the hippocampus and the amygdala (Amaral, 1992). However, the entorhinal cortex is heavily connected to many other sensory and motor regions of the brain as well (Freeman, 2000). Research on the role of the entorhinal cortex in emotion generally results in erratic findings that are not easy to classify. Aggression is not affected by lesions there; both defensive and affiliation responses to humans were affected in some animals but not in others (Meunier, Cirilli, & Bachevalier, 2006).

In addition to these original components of the Papez circuit, the following regions have also been added over the years;

The Hypothalamus

The hypothalamus, another important part of the diencephalon, has a curious role in emotion research. It was one of the first regions to be investigated by such researchers as Goltz (1892) and Woodworth and Sherrington (1904) all of whom showed that decerebrate animals exhibited a high degree of emotional responses even when barely stimulated. This finding seemed to fit in with the emerging consensus that the cerebral cortices restrained the highly emotional responses elicited by the activity in the hypothalamic nuclei. However, in an important article on the subject, Masserman (1941) considered the question of the role of the hypothalamus in emotion and came to the conclusion that interpretations of the role of this structure ". . . stress[ed] unduly the role of the hypothalamus in the connotative and emotional aspects of behavior" (p. 20). His arguments were both empirical and theoretical including the fact that human clinical data did not support the idea of a direct link between the hypothalamus and the experience of emotion.

At the time of Masserman's research, some investigators believed that the hypothalamus played a major role in eliciting both autonomic and hormonal responses to threatening stimuli; however many questioned whether or not it was directly involved in the experience of emotion. By the 1950s, however, more and more investigators (for example, Nakao, 1958) were conclusively establishing that stimulation of various parts of the hypothalamus produced highly emotional responses including abnormal sexual, eating, and drinking behaviors.

However, the role of the hypothalamus has always been uncertain. For example, Adams (2006) pointed out that:

Many studies elicit attack behavior by electrical and chemical stimulation of the hypothalamus, but there are problems in interpreting the results. Behavioral results of stimulation are contradictory to the results of neural activity during similar naturally occurring behavior. Neural activity in the hypothalamus has been found to be either unchanged in activity or inhibited during defense in cats evoked by the attack of another cat, even though electrical stimulation through the barrel of the electrode could often produce affective defense behavior. . . . Furthermore, the nature of the attack behavior elicited in the hypothalamus by electrical and chemical stimulation is ambiguous. . . . A more recent review (Kruk et al., 1998)[9] provides a detailed analysis of the "equivocal outcome of such attempts to classify hypothalamic aggression into the motivational categories of offense and defense. . . . One reason for the ambiguity of stimulation results may be the close proximity in the hypothalamus of cell bodies and axons involved in offense and defense motivational systems at several levels. . . . Another source of paradoxical results may be local inhibitory circuits such as those found in the central gray matter where single neurons are inhibited by nearby electrical stimulation. (p. 310)

Much the same can be said about most of the other centers involved in the Papez circuit. The consensus view today is that the hypothalamus is deeply involved in evoking bodily responses involved in emotion; however its role in encoding the mental experience remains obscure.

The Septal Nuclei

The septal nuclei are buried deep within the cerebrum and are heavily connected with other portions of the Papez circuit. Their anatomical connection with these other regions suggested that they, too, might be deeply involved in emotional behavior. Surgical lesions of the septal nuclei carried out by such investigators as Spiegel, Miller, and Oppenheimer (1930) and Brady and Nauta (1953) resulted in animals that had heightened emotional reactivity and a proclivity to respond to unexpected stimuli with exaggerated startle responses. A comprehensive review of the role of the septal nuclei in experimental animal surgery as well as its possible contribution to mental illness has been published by Sheehan, Chambers, and Russell (2004). They suggested that the septum plays a regulating and coordinating role of the activity of the many other structures involved in emotion.

The Frontal Cortex

Finally, we turn to a part of the brain that was not originally a part of Papez formulation, but whose involvement in so many aspects of our mental lives made it inevitable that it would be implicated in the control of emotion as well as virtually everything else. Indeed, the iconic case of Phineas Gage, like so many examples of this kind of anecdotal result, immediately sets the tone of many years of research to follow. Gage's changes in behavior and personality were so profound that it has long been taken for granted that damage to the frontal lobes would cause emotional changes as well as problems with other cognitive functions such as planning and personality.

Currently the emotional functions of the prefrontal cortex are often assigned to the orbital and the medial regions. The lateral areas, on the other hand, are supposed to be dealing with temporal organization of a wide variety of high-level cognitive skills (Butter,

Snyder, & McDonald, 1970; Fuster, 2001.) However, the large number of different cognitive functions that are influenced by the frontal lobes makes it extremely difficult to assign any particular role to any particular location on it. A further difficulty with the study of the frontal cortex is that animals obviously do not represent good models of human function; they do not have either the anatomical or behavioral complexity of the human organ. This is especially true with regard to the frontal cortex's role in emotion where it is not at all certain that "emotional" *behavior* in a lower animal represents the same thing as "emotional" *feelings* in humans.

Any emotional contribution of the orbital and medial prefrontal lobes is currently supported by the anatomy of the connecting tracts in the brain; we now know that the frontal lobes are heavily interconnected with the other portions of the Papez circuit including the amygdala, the hippocampus, and the hypothalamus as well as to virtually every other region of the brain (Damasio & Anderson, 2003). This interconnectivity is probably the reason that so many different functions have been attributed to the frontal lobes and why damage to the frontal lobes may produce such a variety of effects including perceptual, learning, language, decision making, humor, as well as all things emotional.

Two excellent reviews of the role of the frontal cortex in general with some commentary on the specific effects on affect and emotion can be found in Fuster (1989) and Stuss and Benson (1986) with the latter dealing more with the psychological impact than the former. Stuss and Benson point out that any conclusions drawn are "highly dependent on the definitions used" and that "altered personality based on brain damage may be quite different in different individuals" (p. 135). The best they could do then was to restate the classic result on decerebrate animals—to a certain degree, the frontal cortex "appear[s] to be important for emotional control" (p. 135). However, damage there is equally as likely to produce apathy rather than uncontrolled emotionality as the ill-advised psychiatric adventure into frontal lobotomies so clearly demonstrated.

What can we glean from this hodgepodge of findings? First, many of the interventions into many parts of the brain produce changes (either excitatory or inhibitory) in emotional behavior (including autonomic responses) that are difficult to characterize given our current vague vocabulary. Surgical lesions or electrical stimuli of a given area either enhance or diminish emotional activity, but the nature of these emotional changes is difficult to categorize. It is, therefore, difficult to determine whether the effect of a particular lesion was simply to violate the circularity of the Papez circuit as a whole or had a specialized effect on a particular part of it. Of course, not all of the lesions produced exactly the same response, but given the influence of environmental, stimulus, and experiential factors, and the uncertainty of the extent of experimental lesions, it is often difficult to determine the function of a particular region. Thus, it is not only difficult to control the independent variable in an experiment on emotion, but it is also uncertain what the measurements of the dependent variable mean.

There is one further issue that should be raised again at this point. Throughout the history of neuroscience, there has been a strong impulse to divide the brain into components. The cytoarchitectonic bases of the Brodmann areas notwithstanding, there are no sharp dividing lines between the putative regions of the brain. The gross anatomical structure of the brain also is more or less indeterminate with regions barely separated and defined by what is generally agreed to be the more or less random divisions of the sulci. Thus, there is a strong tendency to attach functional differences to a protrusion or location that may seem to be structurally separate from the rest of the brain, but that is actually quite close topologically.

This effort to assign unique functions to arbitrarily defined brain regions acts in concert with the equally strong impulse to arbitrarily modularize cognitive processes including emotion. If one stands back a bit, however, and observes the empirical fact that major portions of the brain are involved in everything, including emotion and emotional behavior and that behavioral results of a lesion to any part of the Papez circuit are difficult to describe, one from another, then the question lurking at the boundary of our attention is—do these centers, nuclei, and regions really have as different assignable properties or functions as has been traditionally thought? If the answer to this rhetorical question is negative, then much of the research in cognitive neuroscience in the past century or so was ill-directed and led us away from rather than toward understanding of this remarkable organ—the brain. The only ameliorating thing that can be said in this case is that we did what we could do when we could not do what we should have done.

Given the confused state of brain research on emotion, we now must ask: Will the new brain imaging techniques provide a way out of this morass of confusing data and irreconcilable findings? This is the subject posed in the next section of this chapter.

4.4.3 The Current Stage—Brain Imaging

With the advent of modern brain imaging techniques, many investigators thought that the door to understanding how emotions are encoded in the brain was finally going to be opened. Certainly, the amount of research in this field immediately blossomed; in its path psychologists hoped that some of the classic debates (e.g., between the James-Lange and Cannon-Bard theories) could now be resolved. However, many of the usual obstacles to understanding exactly what brain images mean and what is their relation to cognitive processes remained intact as this experimental program moved ahead. Repeatability and reliability of the early results, as usual, remained a major concern. However the overarching problem in dealing with emotions remains the intransigence of defining and controlling the "emotional" stimulus or independent variable. It is instructive to consider this latter issue (stimulus or task control) before beginning our review of the imaging literature.

The context in which emotions were to be studied by imaging techniques was set by a number of pioneering studies. Important preparatory investigations of what can be considered to be emotional responses had been carried out by such pioneers as Olds and Milner (1954) and Olds and Olds (1963). Their work involved direct electrical stimuli of the amygdala and the septum of rats. The behavioral result of this stimulation was a continuing stream of responses by the rats in an apparent effort to repeatedly elicit the brain stimulation.[10] It was inferred from this finding that these regions had some sort of a positive hedonic valence or pleasure associated with them, and they could be considered to be localized pleasure centers. Thus was the idea that there may well be specific locations in the brain that encoded such positive emotions as "pleasure" reinforced.[11] Nevertheless, this kind of experiment is terribly confounded; the repetitive responses may be due not to the fact that they "felt good" to the rat but, rather, that a motor response was continuously being activated by the stimuli. However influential and solid the experimental findings may be, Olds' work remains subject to many different interpretations.

Some Pioneering fMRI Studies

The earliest experiments with fMRI techniques were also plagued by the same kind of uncertainty. Breiter and Rosen (1999), for example, used this technique to determine which areas of the brain responded to the "pleasurable" feeling induced by infused cocaine. A number of different brain areas including some of those in the Papez circuit responded. The activated regions included the amygdala that had been targeted by the Olds work as well as many others. However, the value of their work was mitigated by their acknowledged report of a great deal of variability both at the individual level and when the findings from different groups of subjects were pooled.

The next step in this chain of research on emotions was to use the emotions themselves (rather than electrical stimuli or infused drugs) as stimuli. Among the most exotic of these studies was the attempt to find the neural correlates of "love." Notwithstanding the difficulty in defining such a concept psychologically, researchers such as Bartels and Zeki (2000, 2004) and Fisher, Aron, and Brown (2005) attempted to measure fMRI activations to both maternal and romantic love. Bartels and Zeki's (2000) first experiment used pictures of loved ones as stimuli and recorded both increases and decreases in activations compared to those produced by pictures of casual acquaintances. Increases were observed in the insula, cingulate, caudate, and putamen, whereas decreases were observed in the prefrontal, parietal, and temporal lobes. The uncertainties of using a picture of a "loved one" versus a "casual acquaintance" are obvious; who really knew what emotional experiences were associated with pictures of "casual" acquaintances. It is sufficient to note that the differential responses to this kind of stimulus were reported to be widely distributed over the brain in these studies.

Aron and colleagues (2005) carried out a similar study of romantic love. Their results, however, did not correspond to those obtained in the Bartels and Zeki (2000) experiment. This discrepancy raised once again the issue of replicability as well as the uncertainty of what was actually being stimulated with such stimuli as those supposed to be infused with "romantic love." Two important generalizations emerged from this work. First, widely distributed portions of the brain responded to these photographic stimuli. Second, the results of even as straightforward experiments of this kind did not produce reliable activations.

Bartels and Zeki (2004) followed up their original experiment with a study of maternal love. Their technique in this case was to show pictures to mothers of both their own babies and age-matched babies who were not their own. The results of this experiment were more complex. Bartels and Zeki reported that 15 brain areas were increasingly activated, and 14 were increasingly deactivated when the mothers observed their own offspring compared to the other children. However, the regions of the brain showing either decreased or increased activations to maternal "love" did not correspond to those that changed during romantic "love." Obviously this kind of simplistic interpretation of what is meant by love (or, for that matter, any other kind of emotion) leaves much to be desired.

Emotion being so vaguely defined, a great deal of leeway and variation in the effects of stimuli are conceptually possible and to be expected. What is clear is that the mind-brain relation is much more complicated than we had thought, and words such as "love" may disguise a complex of emotional and cognitive processes that are not well denoted by such simplistic terms.

Contemporary fMRI Studies of Emotion

In the last several years a substantial number of different kinds of emotion have been studied using fMRI techniques. In the pages that follow I review a small sample of these recent studies and then draw from them whatever common features may be extracted from the reported brain activations. In preview, I note that great distribution and diversity characterizes the extent of these brain responses to what are collectively incorporated within the rubric of "emotion." Furthermore I show how this distribution and diversity are strong indicators that many, if not all, portions of the brain are involved in almost any emotional process.

Phan, Wager, Taylor, and Liberzon (2002) performed a useful service by summarizing much of the work that has been done on emotions prior to 2002 using PET and fMRI methods. They carried out a meta-review of 55 experimental reports in which 761 activation peaks were reported. They concluded from this meta-review (p. 331) that:

1. The medial prefrontal cortex has a general role in emotional processing.
2. Fear specifically engaged the amygdala.
3. Sadness was associated with activity in the subcallosal cingulate.
4. Emotional induction by visual stimuli activated the visual cortex and the amygdala.
5. Induction by emotional recall/imagery recruited the anterior cingulate and insula.
6. Emotional tasks with cognitive demand also involved the anterior cingulate and insula.

However, the correlations were not strong. The general tone of all of these experiments was summed up by Phan and his colleagues (2002) as follows: "No specific brain region was consistently activated in the majority of the studies, across individual emotions and induction methods, suggesting that no single brain region is commonly activated by all emotional tasks. . . . no region was activated in over 50% of all studies" (p. 335).[12] Phan and his colleagues (2002) were thoughtful in pointing out the difficulties and limitations in drawing such conclusions by means of a meta-review as well as from individual studies. They noted, first, that there was a tendency to underreport activations from regions that had not had a long history of research in the field. Second, "non-uniform" experiments differed in the degree to which they can be compared. Third, they also alluded to the difficulties associated with the subtraction method adding to our continuing concern with this issue. Fourth, they pointed out that the various stimulus conditions are not always well defined, are arbitrary, and not always reproducible. Fifth, not all types of emotionally loaded stimuli were used in their analysis (only happy, fearful, angry, sad, and disgust-inducing stimuli were used) a factor that they noted reduced the statistical power of the experiments.

An examination of their summary chart of the raw data (their fig. 2A on p. 338) shows that most of the brain regions in which activations were observed were activated to at least some modest degree by most of the emotional categories of stimuli. Despite the wide distribution of activation they observed throughout this meta-review, Phan and his colleagues (2002) came to the seemingly inconsistent conclusion ". . . that separate brain regions are involved in different aspects of emotion" (p. 331). This conclusion runs counter not only to their own data but also to the main thrust of more recent work in which broad regions of activation are shown for virtually all emotional stimuli; regional specialization at this level of emotional analysis, therefore, seems unlikely.[13]

Like all of the other traditionally defined nuclei and centers of the brain, the amygdala has also been divided into different subnuclei that are posited to have different functions. Three different regions have been described: (1) the laterobasal group (LB): (2) the centromedial group (CM): and (3) the superficial group (SF). Using music as a stimulus (because of its assumed emotional impact), Ball and colleagues (2007) provided some initial fMRI evidence that these three different regions respond differently to different classes of stimuli and tasks. For example, the LB seemed to respond more than the other two regions to music that was considered to be "pleasant," whereas the other two groups seemed to respond more to "unpleasant" musical selections.

Costafreda, Brammer, David, and Fu (2008), updating the work of Phan and his colleagues, have taken on the daunting task of reviewing 385 recent PET and fMRI studies of the amygdala's role in processing emotional stimuli. Despite the many difficulties in imaging the relatively small amygdala, a surprisingly large number of studies have been carried out to determine its role in emotions as well as a few to explore the interaction of emotions and learning. Costafreda and his colleagues point out that many different factors of the experimental protocol influence amygdalar response. These include such practical details as instructions to the subjects, the type of emotion, the stimulus modality, and whether or not a conditioned stimulus had previously been associated with an aversive unconditioned stimulus. Furthermore the type of imaging system used to make the measurements also impacted on the obtained results as did use of language or masking as part of the experimental protocol. The important point to draw from the meta-analysis carried out by Costafreda and his colleagues (2008) is that it would be extremely easy to confound the results of even a well-designed experiment with an effect produced by a totally cryptic and uncontrolled variable.

These results on the impact of emotions on learning are particularly germane to the present discussion. One general conclusion of the Costafreda et al. study (2008) was that the amygdala is especially sensitive to the valence of the stimulus. That is, the amygdala is activated more by aversive than by positive stimuli.[14] In general, they conclude that one of the strongest factors in determining whether or not the amygdala will be activated in an fMRI monitored task is the negative emotional impact of the learning situation.

Costafreda and colleagues (2008) performed an exceptionally useful service by also pointing out some of the difficulties in carrying out a meta-analysis of such a varied collection of experiments. Specifically they note the following sources of artifacts:

• The published data accumulated for their meta-analysis is often of limited quality.
• Only peak levels of activations are reported.
• Data are often pooled in a way that obscures the individual responses.
• The amygdala is relatively small, and yet earlier work suggests that different portions of it have different functions. The resolution of imaging does not permit such fine distinctions.
• The amygdala is part of a complex system of brain parts, and its influence on that system could be seriously misunderstood.

Furthermore, they state: "Some of the conclusions in our study are based on a limited number of experiments. In our view this is an inescapable consequence of the methodological heterogeneity between functional neuroimaging studies. It is rarely the case that a study is identically replicated" (p. 66).

We continue with some recent studies of the effect of various kinds of emotions on fMRI images to see if we can flesh out the current state of the field. In the past few years brain image responses have been recorded to music, voices, and social situations that are purported to produce emotional experiences. Johnstone, van Reekum, Oakes, and Davidson (2006), for example, studied the joint effect of angry and happy vocalizations presented with simultaneous visual stimuli (standardized pictures expressing anger or happiness drawn from the Karolinska image set of Lundqvist, Flykt, and Ohman, 1998). Their results indicated that the responses to happy voices were strongest in the right and left middle temporal gyri and the right inferior frontal gyrus and were stronger than the responses to angry stimuli. In the left middle temporal gyrus, however, enhanced activation required simultaneous stimulation with a happy face. However, the effects became less intense when the subjects were told to attend to either a happy or an angry face—attending to a happy face increased the response to a happy vocalization. Other regions such as the insula and the amygdala were involved in complex ways depending on to what the subject was attending.

As Johnstone and his colleagues point out, these experiments are confounded by the acoustic properties of happy and angry vocalizations. It is possible, they noted, that these results may be due to the physical properties of angry and happy speech respectively. This is a major problem for any experiment on emotions in which the stimulus must be introduced through a sensory modality—what is the cause of the response, the stimulus or the conveyed emotion-inducing message?

Music also has strong emotional overtones. Although it is conceptually very difficult to compare music associated with pleasant memories with music associated with unpleasant memories—that is a matter of personal history—it is possible to approximate differences between what we might call "pleasant" and "unpleasant" music. How well this analogy mimics positive or negative emotional responses is problematic, but the technique is relatively simple even if the conceptualization of the problem is not. Pleasant (consonant, familiar, etc.) music could be changed into unpleasant "music" by taking some classic and presumably pleasant music and distorting it by shifting the pitch of the musical notes. Such a comparison was carried out by Koelsch, Fritz, von Cramon, Muller, and Friederici (2006). These investigators argued that, although pitch shifted, the original and the distorted versions had the same rhythm and melody and thus would be identical in terms of their sensory properties; by their logic, the original version would sound consonant, and the distorted one would sound dissonant. Koelsch et al. further assumed that the consonant (original) music would be pleasant and the distorted (pitch-shifted) would be unpleasant. Their goal was to determine if the emotional pleasantness or unpleasantness of the two forms of music would produce different patterns of brain activation as measured with fMRI procedures.

The results of Koelsch and his colleague's (2006) experiment indicated that different patterns of activations were produced by the "pleasant" and "unpleasant" music respectively. Pleasant, (consonant, original music) predominantly produced greater activations than did unpleasant (dissonant, pitch-shifted music) in a number of brain regions including "the inferior frontal gyrus, Brodmann's areas 44, 45, and 46, the anterior superior insula, the ventral striatum, Heschl's gyrus, and the Rolandic operculum" (p. 239). Unpleasant music, on the other hand, predominantly produced greater activations than did pleasant music in "the amygdala, hippocampus, parahippocampal gyrus, and temporal lobes" (p. 248).

Koelsch and his colleagues (2006) speculated on the basis of cognate research that some of these regions may have other functions (e.g., mirror-function mechanisms or premotor preparation mechanisms for vocalization) beyond the representation of emotional "pleasantness" or "unpleasantness." They suggested, further, that attentional processes might also modulate the results. However, nothing in their experiment directly supported these speculations. What their contribution does make clear is that the brain mechanisms of music appreciation and the attendant emotional experiences are widely distributed throughout the brain.

Further evidence of the breadth of the brain's response has been provided by Garrett and Maddock (2006). They compared the activations produced by emotionally aversive pictures with those produced by emotionally neutral pictures. Activations were observed throughout the brain, primarily the occipital, temporal, fusiform, and parahippocampal gyri, but including as well many other brain regions including the cerebellum, amygdala, hippocampus, thalamus, hypothalamus, caudate, and putamen. Because of the uncertain logical chain and problematical nature of what is an emotional stimulus, any attribution of emotions to particular brain regions remains uncertain.

On the Dimensionality of Emotions

Studies like these raise several important questions. Among the most important is—is emotion a constellation of relatively separate components that are encoded in different portions of the brain? Such a hypothesis is based on the longstanding psychological analysis of emotions as having different properties or aspects. Russell (1980), for example, applied factor analysis to the study of emotions and produced eight different factors that he believed represented the following dimensions of affect—pleasure, excitement, arousal, distress, displeasure, depression, sleepiness, and relaxation. An alternative classification scheme is based on the work of Kurt Lewin (1938) who introduced the idea of the valence of an emotional stimulus—namely that a stimulus could exert either a positive attractiveness or a negative repulsion. Modeling his work after the field theories of relativistic physics, Lewin further suggested that the emotional experience could be graded in intensity depending on our previous experience with that emotion-evoking stimulus. To these two dimensions has been added a third (usually that of recognition, the necessity for the stimulus object to be identified) to complete a three-dimensional characterization of an emotional experience.[15]

The question of whether these three putative dimensions of emotion—valence, intensity, and recognition—were represented in the brain in different regions was studied by Grimm and colleagues (2006). These investigators used pictures[16] that had been scaled for their emotional impact on valence intensity and "dominance," the latter presumably involving recognition in some way that was not defined. Their experimental design was surprising because the activations studied were limited mainly to the prefrontal cortex, a region that is almost certainly going to be activated by many other cognitive processes associated with viewing pictures, making decisions, or controlling events of one kind or another, as well as its involvement in emotion. It essentially ignored the rest of the Papez circuit, now generally agreed to be involved in the neural representation of emotion.

The findings reported by Grimm and her colleagues (2006) were equally surprising because they found that the three dimensions of emotional experience seemed to be reflected in different regions of the frontal cortex. Specifically, valence correlated with activations in the ventromedial prefrontal cortex, intensity with activations in the ventrolateral prefrontal cortex, and recognition with activations in perigenual anterior cingulate cortex. Although we do not know from their work what was going on in the rest of the brain, specifically the other portions of the Papez circuit, this specialization of the dimensional properties or parameters of an emotion does not make sense. Instead it seems to have represented a coincident association of the psychological model of modular cognitive processes with a few activated regions. What is probably being reflected here is the action of a network of distributed cortical loci that are parts of a much more complicated interacting system than the compartmentalization suggested by the work of Grimm and her colleagues.

Grimm and her colleagues (2006), to their credit, also pointed to some of the difficulties and limitations of this kind of work. For example, whatever findings they obtained with "emotional pictures" had to be heavily loaded with the personal life experiences of the subjects who participated in their experiments. Thus, cognitive and memorial influences should have been but could not really be controlled. They noted, furthermore, that the stimuli used in this experiment to induce emotional experiences probably also induced cognitive processes. Therefore the prefrontal cortex response is going to be contaminated by responses that are not purely emotional in any sense of the word.

Just how badly this kind of experiment is confounded cannot be determined. However, it seems clear that attribution of the three hypothetical properties of an emotional experience suggested by earlier psychological concepts to particular parts of a specific part of the brain strains credulity.[17] Most of all, the concluding statement by Grimm and her colleagues (2006) that "our findings indicate a segregated representation of distinct emotion dimensions in prefrontal cortex" (p. 338) probably underestimates the true extent of the distribution of emotional activity throughout the brain.

Gender Differences

One secondary suggestion of the report by Grimm et al. (2006) was that there were no gender differences in this kind of task. Thus is raised a question of considerable interest to many—are the brains of men and women organized in the same or different manner? Given the many anecdotal tales of differences in behavior, this is a question of some interest.

The same year as the paper of Grimm et al. was published, another report in the same journal by Hofer and colleagues (2006) considered the problem of gender differences. Specifically, they reported that:

When subtracting the activation values of men from those of women, suprathreshold positive signal changes were detected in the right posterior cingulate, the left putamen and the left cerebellum during positive mood induction, and in bilateral superior temporal gyri and cerebellar vermis during negative mood induction. The subtraction of activation values of women from those of men yielded no significant differences. (p. 854)

Obviously, there is a great difference between the findings from these two studies, some of which can be attributed to experimental design: Grimm and her colleagues (2006) concentrated on the prefrontal cortex, and Hofer and his colleagues threw their net more broadly; Hofer et al. found responses as far removed from the prefrontal areas as the cerebellum. It is clear, however, that the Grimm et al. (2006) results present only a partial and potentially misleading answer to the question of gender differences. Hofer et al. (2006), although a much more comprehensive survey, certainly did not support the conclusion of no differences. Could it be that there are no gender differences in the frontal lobes but that there are in other regions of the brain? Unfortunately, the results presented so far do not lead us to an answer to this question.

The differences between the designs of these two experiments, however, only partially account for the observed differences in their results about gender differences. Despite the fact that most studies find some gender differences in brain activations, there is still no conclusive answer to this basic question forthcoming from them mainly because of a plethora of uncontrolled factors in the experimental protocols. Hofer and his colleagues add to the list of those factors that might be involved in creating this chaotic situation. They specifically pointed out that "neither personality traits nor smoking behavior, which are known factors in influencing brain activation and differ between gender, were assessed in our study participants" (p. 857). Obviously, these two factors are only a small sample of a much longer list of properties that are not controlled in any brain imaging study but especially in those dealing with the complex problem of gender differences.

Unfortunately, there are not even enough consistencies or overlap between the two studies with regard to the frontal lobes that might help us answer this question. Grimm and her colleagues' findings of the substantial activity in the frontal lobes are not reflected in the Hofer et al. data. Hofer et al. (2006) report that positive emotions that produce enhanced responses in both men and women only differ in the right posterior cingulate, the left putamen (a part of the basal ganglia), and the left cerebellum.[18] There are, therefore, few common points of comparison.

Recent work does not tend to clarify this matter. A new experiment on gender differences has been reported by McRae, Oschsner, Mauss, Gabrielli, and Gross (2008). The protocol was different enough in this study that no direct comparisons can be made with either the Grimm et al. (2006) or the Hofer et al. (2006) results; nevertheless, the McRae et al. experiment now to be discussed involves gender effects in emotional responding, albeit in a novel way. McRae and her colleagues studied the brain responses of men and women while they were tasked to (cognitively) suppress their emotional reaction to negative affect pictures using a familiar clinical psychology technique called "regulation." Regulation or self-regulation, as used in their experiment, is a process by means of which the emotional impact of a strongly negative stimulus can be downgraded by conscious (i.e., cognitive) effort. It is assumed that this is accomplished by using an implicit cognitive process during which a negative stimulus is reframed in a more positive context.

Although no behavioral differences were found between men and women in this experiment, fMRI recordings did produce substantial brain differences between the genders as they carried out this regularization process.[19] Specifically McRae et al. (2008, p. 143) reported that, "[c]ompared with women, men showed (a) lesser increases in prefrontal regions that are associated with reappraisal [the result of regulation], (b) greater decreases in the amygdala, which is associated with emotional responding, and (c) lesser engagement of the ventral striatal regions, which are associated with reward processing." Note that the two experiments did not implicate the same regions of the brain in their respective searches for the brain mechanism of emotions. This is characteristic of this entire field of research.

The initial conclusion one is likely to draw from these observations is that men and women apparently have different neural mechanisms for emotions and emotional control. However, this conclusion may be inappropriate. McRae and her colleagues (2008) explained these findings not in terms of emotions but, rather, in terms of the cognitive processes that are invoked to moderate the negative emotional impact of the pictures. They argued that women and men differ in their regularization strategies, with men using more effortful cognitive strategies and women balancing negative emotions with positive ones. Of course these are post hoc explanations sampled from a universe of plausible explanations, none of which can be accepted or rejected on the basis of fMRI image data alone.

Other researchers (e.g., Schmidt et al., 2009), however, report no brain activation gender differences in other cognitive tasks such as the N-back test. Thus, there is a question concerning what, if anything, even those brain regions that had been associated with emotion had to do with emotion per se. Once again, this illustrates the extreme difficulty in disentangling or parsing the many mental activities that are involved in what are often considered to be simple if not unitary mental processes.

Although a preponderance of the fMRI studies of gender differences seems to report evidence that the sexes are different, many of the experiments either report different regions or describe broadly distributed regional activations that include almost everything in the brain. If there are gender differences, it seems likely that they will be very difficult to assign to particular regions of the brain. Equally uncertain are the effects of growing up in different social environments and the effect of such early life experiences on the cognitive strategies, rather than the specific brain mechanisms, that are used by men and women in dealing with emotion. Furthermore, the variety of stimuli used (e.g., pictures, bad smells, mental calculation demands, etc.) in different experiments adds uncertainty to the interpretation of the results. The need for a standard experimental protocol—a cognitive neuroscientific "fruit fly"—is, once again, highlighted.[20]

The question of brain mechanism gender differences, therefore, remains under dispute. The contribution of this study and the others mentioned is not their speculative explanations but the lack of exact replicability and substantial lack of reliability regarding the involved brain regions that may or may not be involved in gender differences. In large part this is due to the uncontrolled nature of the stimuli and tasks we use to invoke emotional experience. However, it may also be due to the fact that we are not asking the right questions. Clearly there is a need for psychology to more robustly define our mental processes; however, this is a need that may not be possible to meet. In its place, therefore, we have "just so" stories of what lies underneath publically observable behavior and how they may relate to a wildly diverse set of brain images.

Aggression

Of all of the emotions, perhaps none has such a profound effect on the smooth functioning of our society than that of rageful aggression, anger, and the behavioral acting out of our fears and resentments. If we would be able to determine what the brain mechanisms of aggression are, it would be an enormous boon to society; it might, perhaps, permit us to intervene to reduce what appears to be senseless aggression. Even if intervention were not possible, it would be a benefit to understanding the roots of dysfunctional behavior. Unfortunately, despite some popular and professional beliefs that we understand the neural causes of aggression, a review of the current literature suggests that no "biomarker" yet exists that can predict aggression or that would permit us to control what is often violent criminal behavior.

There is a rich history of animal research on aggression, and I considered some of it in earlier sections of this chapter. Human aggression is studied using two main strategies—case studies of individuals and statistical studies of groups of subjects who either have common behavioral patterns or brain injuries. Both of these approaches have now begun to use brain imaging techniques in the search for the underlying neural factors involved in aggression. However the recent use of devices such as the fMRI has not brought us much closer to an understanding of how the brain regulates aggression—no one has been able to show any unique association between any aspect of brain activity and aggressive behavior.

The use of fMRI to study individual cases of human brain damage is clouded by the idiosyncrasies of the lesions done to individual brains whether resulting from therapeutic surgery or trauma. Individual brains differ enough that even the most precise surgical procedure leaves residual uncertainty about the extent of the lesion. The evidence coming from trauma is even less certain, with accidents being notoriously unspecific about what brain regions are damaged. Nevertheless, given the ethical restrictions on human experimentation, case studies remain a major medium of research in the field of aggression.

The problem is further compounded by the fact that measurement of aggression remains more of an art than a quantified science. By this statement I mean it is extremely difficult to measure the magnitude of aggression. Much of the work in this field is of a binary nature—a person or an animal is aggressive or not. This dichotomy is not served well by the fact that aggression may be situationally determined by the environment, context, or social interactions. "Neuropsychological tests" (which are actually tests of current and predicted behavior and cognitive competency and have little to do with the neural foundations of aggression nowadays) are appreciated by all to be unreliable and of questionable validity.[21] Furthermore, like other kinds of emotional behavior, aggression is difficult to define, and there is no consensus on what we mean by the term.[22]

A number of recent meta-reviews of the literature have failed to find any consistent and particular pattern of brain activity that can be associated with aggression. For example, speaking of the frequent association of aggression with the frontal lobes, Kandel and Freed (1989), Brower and Price (2001), and Bufkin and Luttrell (2005) all agreed that the relation is poorly understood and typically misinterpreted by investigators interested in it.

The typical result in this field was that weak positive correlations were found between specific brain activity and aggression (e.g., Tateno, Jorge, & Robinson, 2003); this is hardly the stuff of robust science. Kandel and Freed summarized their review by noting that "evidence for the association between specifically violent criminal behavior and frontal lobe dysfunction is weak at best" (p. 410).

Bufkin and Luttrell's study is of particular interest in the present context because it was a summary of brain imaging studies of aggression. After reviewing 17 imaging studies, they came to the conclusion that it was a system of brain structures, rather than any single region, that was responsible for aggressive behavior. Unfortunately, both decreases and increases in activations were associated with increased aggressiveness. It is instructive to list the brain regions that seemed to one or more of the 17 studies to be abnormal in aggressive patients.

Regions Involved in Aggression
(*N* = number of times mentioned)

- Amygdala (2)
- Anterior frontal (1)
- Anterior medial frontal (2)
- Anterior temporal (1)
- Anteromedial frontal (1)
- Bilateral prefrontal (1)
- Dorsolateral frontal (1)
- Frontal (1)
- Hippocampus (1)
- Inferior temporal (1)
- Lateral prefrontal (2)
- Left anterior temporal
- Left basal ganglia (1)
- Left frontal (1)
- Left frontal gray matter (2)
- Left temporal (4)
- Medial prefrontal (2)
- Medial frontal (1)
- Medial temporal (1)
- Orbitofrontal (2)
- Parietal (1)

- Posterior parietal (1)
- Prefrontal (2)
- Prefrontal gray matter (1)
- Right orbitofrontal (1)
- Right parietal (1)
- Right prefrontal (1)
- Right subcortical (1)
- Right superior parietal(1)
- Right temporal (1)
- Superior frontal (1)
- Temporal (2)
- Thalamus(1)

In other words, pretty much the whole brain!

In addition, the following general (i.e., distributed) abnormalities were reported in at least one of the original papers.

- Generalized hypometabolism
- Generalized lowered autonomic activities
- Generalized MRI abnormalities
- Generalized white matter abnormalities

Basically, these experiments suggest that the regions that are associated with emotional activity by imaging experiments tend to differ from study to study. The strongest conclusion is that much or even most of the brain is involved in emotional activity just as much or even most of the brain is involved in many other cognitive processes. Whatever differences that may be observed from study to study are the result of either the special conditions of each experiment, the thresholds and emphases placed on certain responses by the investigators, or the variable neurobiology of the brain itself.

4.5 Interim Conclusions

The study of the brain correlates of emotion, like those of any other cognitive process, is beset with a number of basic difficulties. Perhaps the biggest impediment to progress in this field is the extreme difficulty of defining (and thus controlling) emotion and emotional phenomena. Inadequate and circular definitions that have perplexed psychologists for years are injudiciously used as independent variables in experiments. Thus, it is often difficult to evaluate the significance of the dependent results. There is also a continuing problem with definitions not being adequately exclusive in parsing out other cognitive processes that are almost always simultaneously activated. Whatever arbitrary definitions are used, it is impossible to functionally isolate emotions from other cognitive processes. This is something that plagues virtually all contemporary cognitive neuroscience research.

The following list presents a few general conclusions that emerge from this review of emotional neuroscience.

1. Emotional responses can often occur separate from behavioral ones. Thus, like many other mental processes, emotions are not directly accessible to experimental assay techniques.

2. Similarly, introspective reports of emotional reactions can be heavily influenced (i.e., cognitively penetrated) by the needs of the individual and thus may not correspond to what is actually being perceived.

3. Both the conventional and imaging studies of emotion are heavily confounded by the use of ill-defined and arbitrary psychological constructs. It is, for example, still debated whether an emotion is a unitary cognitive process or a constellation of interacting processes.

4. The control of emotion-producing stimuli is a difficult problem for researchers in this field. Ethical, experiential, as well as practical problems abound when an experimenter tries to evoke a standard kind of emotion. The task is complicated by the intensely personal nature of emotion-provoking stimuli for individuals.

5. Conventional lesion studies of emotion (an approach that dominated the 1900s) are now appreciated to be inconclusive with the same brain areas often either exciting or inhibiting emotional behavior under slightly different conditions.

6. Virtually any set of emotional conditions (or for that matter any set of cognitive conditions) will show differences in their respective brain images.

7. The empirical literature on brain correlates of emotion is wildly inconsistent with virtually every part of the brain showing some activity correlated with some aspect of emotional behavior. Those experiments that do report a few limited areas are usually in conflict with each other.

8. The one inescapable empirical fact is that emotions are encoded by widely distributed activity in the brain. The emerging conclusion is that many parts of the brain, well beyond the boundaries of the Papez circuit, are involved in emotion. Although it is certain that it is conceptually correct, the idea behind the Papez circuit is probably an incomplete statement of the brain regions actually involved in emotional experience.

9. Not all of this distributed activity is directly related to the affective aspects of the stimulus. It may be psychobiologically impossible to parse an emotion from the sensory or perceptual signals that conveyed the emotional message and the cognitive ones that interpreted that message. Similarly, it is difficult to distinguish between an "emotional response" and any of the evoked motor responses that may accompany the emotional response.

10. Many regions of the brain have been the targets of cognitive neuroscience research on emotions using a variety of techniques. Many of these regions have been assigned some emotional function; however, there is little consensus about what is the actual role of a particular region. It is likely that the entire brain operates in a coordinated fashion,

complexly interconnected, so that much of the research on individual components is misleading and inconclusive. This problem is exacerbated by the poor definition of the anatomical boundaries of the various regions as well as possible species differences.

11. Modern brain imaging studies have only partially been able to ameliorate the empirical and interpretative problems in the neuroscientific studies of emotion. There are substantial individual and group differences reported; it is problematical whether these variations are due to procedural matters or reflect true neurophysiological differences.

12. Correlations drawn between brain activations and emotional situations are relatively modest. No single area was shown to be consistently associated with emotion. Many different areas responded in one situation or another. Meta-studies show that many different factors of the stimulus world influence the obtained brain images. A multitude of artifacts and confounds permeate this whole body of work.

13. Different investigators using different assumptions about the dimensions and components of emotion report different regions associated with each of their "emotional components." Unfortunately, none of the systems seems to produce any agreement with any other.

14. Data on gender differences remain controversial and inconsistent for both data and societal reasons. Although there are a number of activation-pattern differences between men and women, it is uncertain what these mean.

15. If there is any uniformity in the conclusions drawn by imaging research, it is that the frontal lobes are heavily involved in emotional behavior. However the frontal lobes are heavily involved in almost all cognitive processes, and it is not certain what role they are playing in emotion per se.

16. Brain imaging studies of human aggressive behavior demonstrate only weak correlations between aggressive (particular criminal) and the pattern of brain activations. Virtually every brain region has been connected by one study or another to aggressive behavior. Distinguishing between the genetic and experiential foundations of aggression also remains an unresolved problem.

5   Learning and Memory

5.1   Introduction

Learning is a generic term for a diverse number of different cognitive processes. Its simplest and broadest definition can be encapsulated as: learning is a change in the state of a system produced by experience and reflected in behavior. Learning must be distinguished from similar behavioral changes produced by growth, maturation, or development, each of which can mimic the effects of experience. Obviously this diffuse term includes an enormous array of behavioral changes ranging from psychomotor skills such as learning to ride a bicycle to learning one's multiplication tables to learning how to think logically. That which we call learning comes in many guises.

Learning is closely related to but must also be distinguished from the closely related and sometimes misused false synonym—memory. Memory refers to the states, conditions, images, or traces produced by the learning protocol that record what was learned. The word memory may also refer to the medium or place in which the new experiential information is actually stored. It is often referred to as the "engram" following the suggestion originally made by Semon (1921) and later made famous by Lashley (1950). To both of them the engram was the physical, physiological, or neural change that occurred when learning took place; it was the actual embodiment of the stored information. Although there have been many suggestions about what the engram might be physiologically, its actual nature remains one of the great mysteries of modern cognitive neuroscience. Hypotheses ranging from synaptic growth to neurochemical changes in the transmitters or their receptor sites to reorganizations of the microscopic neuronal network have all been forthcoming. In actuality, however, despite a substantial body of research aimed at identifying it, where and what the engram is remains as much a mystery as the great question of how the brain produces the mind discussed in chapter 1.[1]

The nature of the engram is also closely related to the problem of whether or not mental processes (including learning) are localized. Disputes have raged for years about the degree to which memory is dispersed throughout the brain. The most famous study of memory is now generally assumed to be incorrect. Lashley (1950), working with rats, was never able to show any specific regions that distinctively affected his experimental results. Instead, after a series of experiments that lasted over 30 years, his general result was that it was the amount of tissue removed, not the particular brain tissue that accounted for most of the observed decline in learning ability. He referred to this distributed ability to store information as "equipotentiality"—the idea that all or most brain areas participated in or were capable of participating in the storage of experiential information. The theory of equipotentiality ran counter to almost all of the thinking about localized function in cognitive neuroscience then as well as now. Currently, it has not even been possible to resolve this issue of where the engram is stored, much less to define its physiological nature in other than a few model preparations and for simple protective responses that seem to be almost reflexive.

No matter how unsuccessful the search for the engram—the physiological trace of learning—has been, learning studies have constituted a dominant, if not the dominant, activity of experimental psychology over the years. Behavioral studies of learning have the tremendous advantage of having precisely defined input conditions (e.g., how many training trials were used?) and equally precise performance measures (e.g., how did the observed behavior change?). However, as noted in chapter 1, response measures are underdetermined—it is possible for the experimenter to conjure up an enormous number of hypothetical constructs or theories of what was going on inside the mind-brain to explain behavior.

As noted, learning comes in many different types, some of which appear to be the result of very simple neuronal changes and some of which appear to be inscrutably complex. Classical conditioning and habituation, demonstrated in simple model preparations such as *Aplysia californica* (a marine gastropod mollusk) anchor one end of the complexity spectrum while learning of complex processes such as mathematics and physics or learning to recite a poem are examples of changes going on at the other end.

To further complicate the matter, two behaviors that may superficially appear to represent the same kind of learning may not involve the same mechanisms in different species. One can look on with amazement at the studies of habituation in *Aplysia* carried out by Castellucci, Carew, and Kandel (1978). However elegant, it is not clear that the neural mechanisms producing this animal's behavior are the same as those producing the analogous behavior in humans. Analogous behavior is not robust evidence that homologous neural mechanisms are at work.

The deeper one goes into the study of learning, especially that of humans, the more and more intricate, multidimensional, and ubiquitous it seems. Should we ever be able to resolve the learning problem, it is likely that the door to understanding the general mind–body problem would also be opened. Both goals currently, however, seem far beyond the power of our research protocols.

Another important aspect of learning research is that it has such wide applicability to human affairs. Learning results are applicable over an enormous range of activities that are important to human society. These activities range from training athletes to determining optimal strategies to helping children profit from schooling to the training of operators to use complex tools to the improvement of military leaders. Learning obviously is such a ubiquitous part of our society and of human behavior that the kind of behavioral change implied is believed by many to be essential for maintaining human society. Some would thus argue that our profound and extraordinary ability to modify our behavior beyond reflexive and other innate responses may lie at the core of the advantage that our species has enjoyed over 150,000 years of its evolutionary history.

Studies of learning, for this and many other reasons, proliferated during the heyday of behavioral psychology and continue to play important roles in modern cognitive psychology. It is not too much of an exaggeration to say that there are more learning studies in psychology than in any other subfield of this science. Although it is difficult to say absolutely, it is probable that tens of thousands of research reports are published every year concerned with learning, educational techniques, and cognate topics.

My goal in this chapter is to deal with several aspects of learning in order to produce a snapshot of where learning research has been, where it is now, and what the cognitive neuroscience study of learning has done to tell us where it might go in the future. The various topics to be discussed are the following ones:

- A history of learning research
- A taxonomy of learning types
- Review of a sample of the empirical literature over three stages of neuroscientific studies of learning

I then draw some interim conclusions about the state of current cognitive neuroscientific research in learning.

5.2 A History of Learning Research

There are three main themes that reverberate down through the history of psychological studies of learning and memory. Since the earliest classic Greek times when matters of this kind were first considered as a part of the natural world, philosophers and scholars asked (1) How do new experiences become a part of (or influence) our mental life? (2) What is the nature of the memory that is stored after an experience (e.g., is it symbolically or pictorially represented)? and (3) How do we access those memories at some later time? Although I have phrased these questions in the terminology of learning, it should be obvious that these questions were at the heart of the great epistemological issues of classic times; they can as easily be rephrased in that alternative framework as questions of how we acquire knowledge.

Early on, led by Thales of Miletus (ca. 620?–540? BCE), Greek thought came for the first time to be characterized by a naturalism that may be interpreted more as a physics of the mind and body than as a psychology. Questions were asked such as what was the nature of the material of which the mind was made? Fire, water, and other less tangible substances were invoked to explain the relations between the mind and the body. Although the materialism was primitive, the important thing was that it was about this time that supernatural explanations began to be replaced by the glimmerings of naturalist ones.

This naturalist period in which efforts were made to explain the mind lasted up to the time of Socrates (469–399 BCE) and Plato (428–348 BCE). Rather than trying to understand the structure of the mind, both of the great philosophers emphasized ethics and morality as opposed to seeking our place in the natural world. The origin of what can be considered to be more scientific protopsychologies came with the emergence of Aristotle (384–322 BCE), Plato's most illustrious student, as the prototypical model of a modern naturalistically oriented philosopher–scientist.

Aristotle and Plato differed in many ways in their philosophies and approaches to the study of human nature; most germane to our present discussion was the difference between their respective theories of learning and memory. Plato saw learning and recall as a process of recollection of previously recorded images called eidola.[2] Eidola were more or less direct and exact copies of sensory experiences that were recorded in some unknown way by the body. That is, we learn simply by recording experiences in memory. Once so stored, according to the Platonic model, we could recollect the previously experienced information almost as if one were looking through a book of pictures. Plato's interpretation of these pictures was that they were essentially complete reproductions and required little further processing. Herein lie the roots of the rationalism that was to characterize much of later psychology.

Aristotle's views were quite different. He proposed that learning occurred as the result of the connection or combination of many previous experiences into a progressively improved and persistent state. The memories were not even poor spatially congruent copies; instead, they were symbolically recorded states that represented, but did not copy, the incoming information. Complex ideas were built up by concatenating simpler ideas rather than by recalling isomorphic eidola. His ideas thus anticipated the development of the empiricist school of thought and foretold the heavy emphasis on associationism that was to become such an important part of psychological thinking in the future.

Aristotle also made many other insightful and practical contributions to the way we think about learning. He was a strong proponent of learning by doing and emphasized the importance of repetitive practice. It was by these procedures that each learning trial added more information to a cumulative representation.

Among Aristotle's most important and persistent contributions was his suggestion that there were certain properties of stimuli that enhanced the probability that associations would be made and increased the probability that they would be bonded together into an ever-improving representation of previous experiences. In other words, Aristotle was enunciating specific rules of learning. He was probably the first to suggest that the progressive improvement in an ability to perform was due to the degree to which successive sensory experiences were alike (similar), contiguous (occurring together in time), or contrasted with previous knowledge. These three rules of efficient learning have persisted down to the present time and can be found at the root of many current theories and applied practices intended to improve learning.

Not the least of Aristotle's gifts to psychology, as well as to all of the other sciences, was his dedication to the role of experimentation as a step forward from the purely speculative role on which most previous philosophers had based their search for knowledge. Aristotle, therefore, deserves additional credit for bridging the idea of natural science first enunciated by Thales across the gap that was represented by the humanism of the Socratic and Platonic systems.

From the time of the classic Greek philosophers until the sixteenth century, learning per se seems to have taken on a secondary role. Throughout the late Middle Ages much of the emphasis in philosophical thinking was aimed at problems of religion and ontology rather than applied or theoretical epistemology. Many philosophers were concerned about problems such as the nature of universals and only indirectly, if at all, considered problems that we might consider to be preliminary theories of learning per se. A few scholars such as William of Ockham (1285–1349) wrote about the relation of words and their meanings as well as the relations between particulars and universals. Ockham also vigorously supported the empirical approach to learning to the extent that he also believed, as did Aristotle, that experience was the primary source of knowledge. However, little was done at this time to study the particulars of how knowledge was generated by that experience. The experimental approach to the study of learning was many centuries ahead.

It is hard to find, therefore, specific positions on the questions of how we learn during this period. It was not until the time of René Descartes (1596–1650) that the epistemological problem of acquiring and storing information once again became a major scientific interest. The contemporary subject matter of learning was characterized by what was by that time becoming a critical, but slightly derivative, issue—is our acquisition of knowledge accomplished by rationalist or empiricist processes? Extreme rationalists argued that there were certain innate ideas that could not be learned by experience. The extreme empiricists, on the other hand, argued that all knowledge had to be achieved through experience as introduced through the senses. Although one of the major contributors to the development of scientific method, Descartes has mainly been considered to be a rationalist who assumed that logic based on innate ideas was the foundation of our understanding of the nature of the world we live in.

The antithesis to the rationalist hypothesis was empiricism. Empiricism, both as the doorway to knowledge and as a method, found its renaissance in the works of Francis Bacon (1561–1626) and Thomas Hobbes (1588–1679). Bacon was instrumental in reestablishing the Aristotelian ideal that science can best be served through the medium of experimentation, thus helping to break the moribund chain of speculative thought that had dominated much of the world of philosophy and theology for so many centuries.[3]

It is from Hobbes's work, however, that many authorities agree that most of modern experimental psychological research on learning really takes it origins. Hobbes bridged the gap between Cartesian rationalism[4] and modern empiricism by asserting that all mental processes were actually "matter in motion." In other words, he argued that the processes of the mind could be dealt with in the same way as any other natural phenomenon and that they followed certain basic laws, which may or not be the same as the laws of physics. Although Hobbes's work was mainly framed in terms of the political and social levels of human interaction, he clearly was arguing that there were forces at work, comparable to (and possibly included within) those in the physical world, that drove and motivated human behavior. A major implication of this line of thinking was that human behavior could be considered to be the results of real events and forces introduced through the senses and processed by the brain. Thus, they were susceptible to scientific examination in much the same sense as were animals or machines.[5] Hobbes argued that this susceptibility to orderly scientific examination of human nature held true for both animals and men.

Hobbes and Bacon are important in this brief history of learning because they reemphasized Aristotle's argument that human knowledge is dependent on the senses and thus is linked to the physical world by measurable quantities. That is, since all knowledge comes through the senses, it is possible to examine the acquisition of knowledge by manipulating the stimulus world and observing behavior; in other words, we can pursue how knowledge is acquired by carrying out experiments that determine how our behavior changes as a result of the manipulation of the sensory environment. This was a profound change from the rationalist, religious, and philosophical doctrines that we could solve the human mystery by speculation alone.

With this basic idea in hand, a whole new approach to studying human behavior, including learning, emerged in the form of what is now known as British empiricism. In a very true sense, the modern scientific study of human knowledge acquisition (i.e., learning) that had hitherto been attacked solely from the philosopher's armchair can be dated from the time of this period of transition. Methods provided by Aristotle, Ockham, and Hobbes, (among numerous others) were mature enough to be applied to scientific research on the dynamics of human behavior. Although the original motivation behind this research was still mainly philosophical (i.e., to resolve what were fundamentally epistemological problems such as the rationalism-empiricism debate or the innateness of ideas), the situation evolved into modern psychological studies of the dynamics of learning for its own sake. What had hitherto been speculative epistemology now took on a totally different strategic direction—scientific, empirical studies of how we learn. It should not be overlooked, however, that the assumptions and problems behind modern experimental psychology's study of learning are much the same as some of those that date from Aristotle's time. Indeed, it is not too much of a stretch to say that all of modern experimental psychology is really only applied epistemology. Whatever the approach, the problems tackled when we study learning are, at their most basic roots, attempts to fill in the details of how we gain knowledge from the world.

The most specific expression of this new empiricism can be seen in the work of the British and Scottish schools of the seventeenth century. The intellectual leader of this harbinger of modern scientific psychology was John Locke (1632–1704). Although Locke, like Hobbes and Descartes, was interested in a broad range of topics, it is his epistemological ideas that are relevant to this current discussion.

Locke was not only the first but the archetype of modern empiricism in the Aristotelian tradition. He is most famous to psychology students of all vintages as the originator of the idea of the tabula rasa—a blank slate. The most extreme version of this idea is that humans are born with absolutely no knowledge and that everything they subsequently know is acquired through experience and interaction with the external environment. Although there are no innate ideas from his perspective, Locke did acknowledge that some of the raw sensory inputs had to be processed, manipulated, or combined by built-in intellectual processes to determine their subsequent influence. He was extremely specific about the nature of associationism, using the word frequently in his great work *An Essay Concerning Human Understanding* (Locke, 1690/1995). Some consider this to have been the most important "textbook" of psychology (among other topics) since Aristotle's *de Anima*.[6]

Locke stimulated the development of the school of British empiricism, profoundly influencing others such as David Hume (1711–1776) and John Stuart Mill (1806–1873). Whatever historical trail one follows, it is clear that the major contributors to our current thinking about the way in which we achieve knowledge are Aristotle, Hobbes, and Locke, each of whom in turn initiated a major change in the most basic assumptions and orientations of psychological research. They and their successors shared a common approach, an approach that was to become the foundation of modern studies of learning. The essence of this empiricist tradition is that we mainly learn as a result of experiences and interactions with our environment and to only a limited degree by any innate "ideas." This perspective dominated well into modern times. However, evolutionary and genetic developments that could not have been conceived of by Aristotle and his successors may ultimately change our views. Two postulates—the dominance of experience and its corollary—this experience comes to us in bits and pieces and must be associated with other bits and pieces—defines the most basic foundations of modern learning theory as well as much of the rest of modern psychological science.

It was under the influence of these two postulates that modern psychological research on learning began to evolve. Although the earliest studies in psychological science were what we would nowadays refer to as psychophysical, perceptual, or sensory, it did not take long for studies of learning to proliferate. Indeed, learning studies dominated the next century of psychological thinking as suggested by the propositions and content of the "schools" of psychology popular in the twentieth century. Although there were many differences in their respective doctrines, the commonalities of their approaches and the overlap of their basic principles concerning learning often made it difficult to distinguish among them.

There was, however, one great advantage of learning research for those who desired to emulate the "harder sciences." Learning studies only required specification of the environmental stimuli and recording of the changes in behavior. Changes in behavior associated with experience were, by definition, learning, and experience could be precisely regulated; it was not necessary to draw inferences about the internal processes. The drawing of inferences and the development of reductive theories could come later, if they were to come at all.

Nowhere is the task of organizing what became a bewildering and overlapping collection of different theoretical and practical approaches better developed than in the still classic history of psychology by Marx and Hillix (1963). They suggested a taxonomy of modern psychological systems that was distilled down to the following categories: [7]

- Structuralism
- Functionalism
- Associationism
- Behaviorism

All of these systems of psychological thinking ultimately grew out of the empiricist traditions of the philosophers who preceded them. Regardless of the details of their respective points of view, each was mainly intended to search out the answers to questions of how we learn. Each of these systems was also founded on the assumption that the human mind can be studied by experimental procedures that did not differ in kind from those available to physicists or chemists. Indeed, structuralists such as W. Wundt (1832–1920) and E. B. Titchener (1867–1927) dealt with psychological phenomena almost as if they were chemical compounds: Their goal was to search out the elements of these compound experiences. This extreme elementalism was difficult to sustain in light of the complex interactions among our thoughts. However, the proximal causes of the eventual demise of structuralism were ultimately based on the shortfalls of their chosen method—introspection. What remains of this line of thought is a sometimes extreme elementalism, an intellectual precursor of the cognitive modularity, on which many cognitive theories are still based.

Associationists such as Vladimir Bekhterev (1857–1927) and Edwin R. Guthrie (1886–1959) were even more empirical in the classic sense if one can quantify the degree to which such a principle is adhered to by its proponents. They epitomized the great idea that we learn, not by logic or innate ideas, but by virtue of the flow of information into our senses and the combination or association of this flow of discrete events into meaningful patterns. The associationists' persistent contribution was preserving the classic traditions exemplified by ideas of the British empiricists.

Functionalists such as William James (1842–1910) and Edward L. Thorndike (1874–1949), although less interested in learning per se and more interested in determining how things worked, were still highly empiricist in the sense that they also believed that sensory stimuli were most important in determining our behavior. Their emphasis in the study of learning was on determining the nature of the parts from which a useful process might develop.

Thorndike's work not only bridged the nineteenth and twentieth centuries, but he was also active well into the twentieth century. Originally interested in animal learning, his magnum opus is considered to be *Animal Intelligence: An Experimental Study of the Associative Process in Animals* (Thorndike, 1898) in which he sought to distinguish between insightful and associative learning. However, his later work continued on in such diverse fields as developmental psychology and the psychology of arithmetic until his death. Thorndike was also the formulator of three general laws of associative learning that also had enormous influence on his successors—effect, recency, and practice.

• The Law of Effect: Associations are strengthened when the performance has a positive effect.
• The Law of Recency: The most recent association determines the next responses.
• The Law of Practice: Responses are increased in probability and strength as a result of repetition.

Each of these laws also had its converse. For example, the Law of Effect was paralleled by the statement that associations were weakened if the performance had an unproductive outcome.

Behaviorists, under the influence of J. B. Watson (1878–1958) and B. F. Skinner (1904–1990), were perhaps the most specifically interested in learning. For them the goal of studying mental chemistry that had so dominated the thinking of Wundt and Titchener was simply not achievable for the reasons of first-person privacy and inaccessibility. They argued that these barriers to understanding could not be overcome with the introspective method. Instead, Watson and Skinner proposed that we should concentrate on the observable behavior of animals and humans and ignore the intervening mechanisms that could not be directly measured. As a result of such arguments, much of modern behaviorism is based on the idea that the task of psychology is the determination of the rules of good learning that lay between the stimulus and the responses.

The most obvious challenge to the associationist and empiricist traditions is Gestaltism or holism—the approach to the psychology of learning that says that how we learn depends on the overall organization of an idea rather than the elements that make up wholes. Born out the German school that included M. Werthheimer (1880–1943), W. Kohler (1887–1967), and K. Koffka (1886–1941), Gestalt psychology's approach to learning was that organization and arrangement (and our interpretive reconstructions of them) played a much more important role than simple association of an aggregate of quasi-independent parts.

The transition between the nineteenth and twentieth century also saw many important developments in the study of learning. One milestone was the work of Hermann Ebbinghaus (1850–1909), an early associationist who was one of the first to specifically study memory and learning using what was essentially a modern paradigm. His classic work entitled *Memory: A Contribution to Experimental Psychology* (Ebbinghaus, 1885/1964) first introduced several of the main research tools, for example the "nonsense syllable," which are still used today by investigators interested in learning.

Another bridging personality from the associationist tradition was Ivan Pavlov (1849–1936), a Russian physiologist who had been studying the digestive system. In a fortuitous observation Pavlov discovered that his dogs were anticipating the arrival of a stimulus (food) by a learning process that he called "conditioning" (which established responses called "conditioned reflexes") and that has come down to us as what we now call "classical conditioning." Pavlov's interpretation was that by pairing a novel and otherwise neutral stimulus (the conditioned stimulus, or CS—for example, a well timed whistle) with a naturally occurring stimulus (the unconditioned stimulus or UCS—food for example), the CS would come to elicit the natural response or reflex to the UCS—salivation in this case—even in the absence of the UCS (i.e., salivating to the whistle alone). The pairing that matters is between the CS and the UCS, although the link between the CS and the unconditioned response (UCR) is what is established by doing so. The UCR in response to the CS alone is then called the CR (conditioned response or reflex). The critical time difference is between the CS and the UCS; for most classical conditioning situations, timing is optimal when the CS precedes the UCS by about 500 milliseconds. Trained as a biological scientist, Pavlov was one of the first researchers to study this form of learning with precise, well-controlled, experimental procedures. Although Pavlov's work was published in numerous obscure scientific articles, his work was not summarized in the form of a book until a 1927 translation of his work (Pavlov, 1927/1960).

As psychological research emerged in the nineteenth and twentieth centuries, learning became one of the earliest topics to which neuroscientific techniques were applied. I now turn to another fundamental issue—the complexity of types of learning and the difficulties that are involved in defining those types.

5.3   A Taxonomy of Learning Types

In the last half century the explicit role of the various schools of psychology has significantly diminished. The differences between them are now considered to be more interpretive than substantial and represent little more than the emphases of their respective approaches. In the place of schools of thought has arisen a diverse methodology aimed at evaluating a host of different kinds of problems associated with learning and a large number of different kinds of learning and memory research protocols. Technological research developments and new research methodologies have pushed philosophical discussions of such topics as the controversy between innate and empirical sources of knowledge to the periphery of current psychological science.[8]

With this brief preamble in place, we now consider the variety of different types of learning on which research has been carried out over the years. I must alert my readers at this point that there is a major conflation of the vocabulary we use in the study of learning and memory. Many authors use "memory" as the target of their research. However, in point of fact, they often are studying and reporting the parameters of the experiment—how manipulations of the learning experience affect behavior without saying anything about the memory trace. In the discussion that follows, I simply use the two words—learning and memory—as representing experimental designs in which operational designators define the parameters of the experimental protocol (learning) on the one hand and inferences about how the information might be stored (memory) on the other. It should not be misunderstood that this is the only conflation in this field. Studies of forgetting—the decline in performance as a result of either the simple passage of time or as a result of intervening learning—also are part and parcel of research into the nature of the learning paradigm.

The situation is even further complicated by the fact that the process of retrieving a memory in the form of some utterance or some measured behavior is also sometimes confused with the words memory and learning. In point of fact, no learning-memory-retrieval experiment can ever be carried out in which one factor is isolated from the other two. The only way to test what was learned, what was stored, or what can be recalled is to carry out an experiment in which all three aspects of the learning process are involved, if not considered. One or another may be emphasized in any given "learning" experiment, but by its very nature, each of the three different experimental designs must involve the other two.

The picture is even further complicated by the variety of retrieval methods that can be used to access stored information. The three prototypical methods are the following ones:

• Recall: The participant in a memory experiment is asked to retrieve a memorized item without cues of any kind.
• Recognition: The participant in a memory experiment is asked to say whether certain information has been presented previously or not.
• Reconstruction: The participant in an experiment is asked to reconstruct an object or cognitive structure from a set of parts or ideational components.

It is well known that an experimenter's choice of retrieval methods can strongly affect empirical results, and in turn, one's theoretical orientation.

There are a number of other obfuscations and confusions inherent in the vocabulary used in the study of learning. Current cognitive psychology distinguishes between sensory, short-term, medium-term, and long-term learning, on the one hand, and memory, on the other. This is an extension of an idea that has been present in experimental psychology since the time of William James (James, 1890). Its modern instantiation was reinvigorated by the well-known study of Peterson and Peterson (1959) that suggested that there were two separate neurobiological mechanisms of memory—long-term and short-term. The idea was formulated into what has come to be widely accepted as the standard model of memory by Atkinson and Shiffrin (1968). To this basic model have been added other components that have been circulating in the scientific literature from time to time. These additions include other subdivisions such as sensory storage (Sperling, 1960) and medium-term memory (e.g., Melcher, 2001.)[9] It must be noted, however, that each of these memory classifications is associated with a specific experimental procedure chosen from among many possible kinds. It thus becomes problematic whether these constructs are distinct psychobiological entities or just manifestations of the measurement method used.

Whatever they are, an enormous variety of learning types have been assayed over the years by researchers in this field. Indeed, the main problem in developing a taxonomy of memory or learning types is that there are a virtually unlimited number of procedures that can be used to evaluate one form or another of learning. Unfortunately, no one has yet put together anything that approaches either a universal theory or a taxonomy of learning types that is based on basic cladistic principles.

Thus, while the concept of "short-term" memories being "consolidated" in serial order into "long-term" memories has wide currency these days, researchers like McGaugh (2000) have pointed out that alternate schema are possible. He noted, for example, that short- and long-term memory might be independent processes mediated by parallel and independent pathways. The important point being made here is that all of these systems of learning types are themselves primitive theories that are far more speculative than is usually appreciated.

Despite these uncertainties, the influence of behavioral classifications of learning that have been offered by such researchers as Endel Tulving and Daniel L. Schacter on neuroscientific thinking and research protocols has been of the highest importance. Just as the work of Linnaeus and Mendeleev broke the dams on biological and chemical understanding, respectively, Tulving and Schacter's classification system has provided a working framework for virtually all current neuroscientific studies of learning. It is not likely that their system will remain unchanged as the years go by; however, at the moment, it dictates the design of a substantial portion of cognitive neuroscience research protocols. We now search for the correlates of such constructs as "episodic memory" or "procedural learning" instead of vaguely defined generalities as "learning." Nevertheless, it must not be overlooked that their contribution is devoid of specific empirical links from cognitive modules to brain mechanisms.

Specifically, Tulving (1972) and Schacter and Tulving (1994) proposed a typology of learning and memory that included the following components:[10]

1. Long-term memory, which may last for a person's lifetime, and consists of two types:
• Declarative memory that consists of memories we can talk about (i.e., declare). It, in turn, consists of two subtypes:

Episodic memory: Memories of special events specific to our individual past experiences.

Semantic memory: General knowledge of the world that is not a part of our personal experience.

- Nondeclarative or procedural memory that consists of such motor skills as riding a bicycle, playing a piano, and various kinds of conditioning.

2. Short-term or working memory in which we actively manipulate information (current or retrieved) and possibly prepare it for long-term storage. Short-term memory seems to last for minutes rather than hours but is constantly refreshed by a presumptive process called rehearsal.

3. Sensory memory, which involves very short-term retention of sensory signals briefly exposed to our sense organs. These are remembered in what may be considered to be their raw physical form, as echoes or quickly fading images. Sensory memory is also referred to as "iconic storage."

4. Priming, which is the effect of a previously presented stimulus to enhance or inhibit the recall of a memory.

Sensory memory is akin to a persistent visual image that must be read out before it fades in less than a second. Short-term, or as it is sometimes known—working memory—is the relatively brief preservation of information for at most a few seconds. The phrase medium-term memory refers to the results of a few unusual experiments that seem neither to involve short- or long-term memories but to reflect an intermediate form in which information is temporarily stored in preparation for consolidation into long-term memory. Long-term memory refers to information that may have been stored for decades if not a lifetime.

Other forms of memory that may last for a lifetime may or may not be the same as that indicated by the traditional use of the term "long-term memory." Bahrick (1983), for example, carried out an experiment in which he measured the effect of very long periods of time—up to 46 years—on forgetting by asking people to describe their recollections of the spatial arrangement of the city (Delaware, Ohio) in which they had spent their college years. He then compared these recollections with those of new students as well as physical maps of the original Delaware environment.

Although there were many possible confounds (such as the number of times that an alumnus had visited Delaware in the intervening years), there were some measures (such as the free recall of the order of campus landmarks) confirming that some people retained information over their entire lifetimes. His experiments showed that although there were progressive declines in accuracy over the 46-year period, subjects were still performing at nearly a 50% level of accuracy on memory tests. This extraordinary experiment demonstrated that at least parts of long-term memory are virtually permanent over a person's lifetime. The question then arises, is it necessary to invoke an "ultra-long-term memory?" Or, the contrary, are these just different measures of some universal long-term memory?

Table 5.1
A typology of learning

Working memory	Episodic memory retrieval	Procedural memory
• Verbal/numeric	• Verbal	• Conditioning
• Object	• Nonverbal	• Classical
• Spatial	• Retrieval success	• Instrumental
• Problem solving	• Retrieval effort	• Skill learning—motor
Semantic memory retrieval	• Retrieval mode	• Skill learning—nonmotor
• Categorization	• Context memory	
• Generation	Priming	
Episodic memory encoding	• Perceptual	
• Verbal	• Conceptual	
• Object		
• Spatial		

After Cabeza & Nyberg (2000).

Another comprehensive classification of learning and memory has been implicitly presented by Cabeza and Nyberg (2000). They carried out a pioneering meta-study of 275 experimental reports that compared brain images and cognitive processes.[11] In doing so they actually provided a taxonomy of learning. Their major categories were very similar to those of Tulving and Schacter, but they broke them down into finer subcategories that are useful for the present discussion. Their subcategories are shown in table 5.1.

The degree of redundancy in this list is not clear but must be high. Whether or not each of these terms actually denotes a separable neural mechanism or cognitive process is one of the pillars of the contentious current debate on modularity and localization. Although this is a convenient taxonomy capable of organizing our research protocols, it may be that each of these types of "learning" is actually only a stage in or a synonym for a part of a more inclusive and continuous process. In other words the actual process may be such that the boundaries between each of these "memories" or types of "learning" may be arbitrary, if not artificial, and that the biology of learning may actually be organized in an entirely different way. I remind my readers that initial definitions of each of these types come from psychology, not from neuroscience.

Traditional psychological research on learning has many different parameters that are only hinted at in these lists. For example, research has been carried out on the following topics:

• Age differences
• Autobiographical memory
• Aversive learning
• Category learning

- Coding processes
- Delayed response learning
- Developmental stages in learning
- Discrimination learning
- Emotional learning
- Encoding
- Everyday memory
- Expertise
- Explicit and implicit learning
- Conditioned fear
- Context-specific versus invariant memories
- Forgetting
- Generalization and transfer of training
- Habit formation
- Habituation
- Imprinting
- Incidental learning
- Individual differences in learning
- Knowledge
- Language learning
- Memory capacity
- Metamemory
- Object discrimination learning
- Paired associate learning
- Perceptual learning
- Preference learning
- Problem-solving learning
- Recognition memory
- Reinforcement
- Reminiscence
- Reward learning
- Rote learning
- Sensitization
- Sensory discrimination learning
- Serial learning
- Transfer of training
- Verbal learning

These are all in addition to a host of specific subject matters such as learning arithmetic, bicycle riding, or any number of other tasks that an army of learning researchers may have studied over the years. In addition, a large number of independent variables defined by experimental protocols have been manipulated in order to determine their effect on an equally diverse set of dependent variables. Within this context of types, most studies of learning and memory mainly have been directed at determining the nature of various rules and parameters involved in the coding, storage, and retrieval processes.

It is important for me to point out that the huge corpus of findings from psychological experiments has been extremely informative and useful in many different contexts. It represents a substantial and useful body of knowledge of the nature of human behavior. Within the constraints of experimental variability, inadvertent errors in design (especially pay attention to the work of Vul, Harris, Winkielman, and Pashler, 2009 and Vul and Kanwisher, 2010 discussed in chapter 1) or, rarely, intentional deception, I have enormous confidence that most of these studies are measuring real behavioral properties of the learning process. Our science and our society have benefitted greatly from the effort and skill that the many students of learning have applied to the studies. The flip side, however, is that these experiments may be totally neutral and cannot tell us anything about the inner cognitive and neural mechanisms that account for this behavior.

It does not take too deep an analysis of the literature, therefore, to appreciate that, beyond the behavioral aspects of stimulus manipulation and response measurement, attempts to explain the internal cognitive and neural mechanisms of learning and memory storage remain controversial and ill-understood. Many of the problems that were of interest in the first half of the twentieth century remain unresolved. Reductive explanation is still filled with the same controversies and debates that dominated during that period concerning both the cognitive and neural understructure. Phrases such as "remain fascinating riddles," "many of the details remain unknown," and "much research is yet to be done" permeate any report that purports to connect the behavioral data to neural mechanisms.

The reasons for this high degree of (and quite appropriate) uncertainty and caution are manifold. First, there is enormous variability in the findings emerging from even the best-designed cognitive neuroscience experiments and relatively few replications. Second, the absence of a definitive taxonomy of definitions (based on formal cladistic rules) of the various types of learning amplifies the complexity and thus the inscrutability of this research field. Third, there are so many facets to the problem of how the brain encodes learning and memory that most studies generally remain isolated and unrelated to others. Fourth and most important of all, however, is that all putative extrapolations from behavioral to neuroscientific mechanism are vastly underdetermined inferences from data that do not provide the logical or empirical constraints necessary to draw robust conclusions. As a result, there is a myriad of hypothetical cognitive constructs and many less-than-robust theories of learning. No matter how deep one goes into the list of learning types, it is difficult to be sure that what one is studying is really different than that studied by another investigator.

Nevertheless reductive theories of learning abound; they range from hypothetical cognitive modules to less-than-robustly supported neural mechanisms. Each of these theoretical approaches has its own properties and approaches; cognitive theories tend to infer from the behavioral data, whereas neural theories seek out correlations between neural and behavioral observations. This brings us to the crux of this chapter—the empirical literature in which brain and cognitive processes are compared.

5.4   The Search for Learning and Memory in the Brain

Since the Renaissance, when the brain was finally acknowledged to be the organ of the mind, cognitive neuroscientists and their predecessors have sought to understand the relation between the neural and mental domains. There were many critical steps that had to be made to arrive at the level of current understanding. These steps involved some of the greatest luminaries of human history. Leonardo da Vinci (1452–1519), for example, studied the anatomy of the brain with ingenious methods among which was the lost wax method, a technique he borrowed from jewelry makers to determine the anatomy of the cerebral ventricles. Leonardo believed it was the ventricles, the fluid filled spaces within the brain, that embodied the mind. Shortly thereafter, Andreas Vesalius (1514–1564) carried out a set of monumental dissections of the nervous system that were to guide neuroanatomists for centuries. A major outcome of his dissections was the shift in attention from the ventricles to the solid portions of the brain. Rene Descartes (1596–1650), for example, speculated that it was the pineal gland at which the mind and the body interacted.

The next centuries saw the flourishing of neuroanatomy with such great names as Thomas Willis (1622–1675), Emanuel Swedenborg (1688–1772), Francisco Gennari (1750–1795), and Francois Magendie (1783–1855). In even more recent times, the work of Gustave Fritsch (1838–1927) and Eduard Hitzig (1838–1907), Herman Munk (1839–1912), and David Ferrier (1843–1928) provided the empirical foundations for the prevailing idea that specific behavior functions were located in specific regions of the brain.[12]

Learning, however, remained a cryptic terra incognita during much of this period. By the twentieth century however, new techniques, particularly in surgery and the ability to maintain animals in severely acute conditions, as well as the burgeoning psychological base of knowledge about learning, made it possible to conceptualize a new approach to the study of the brain correlates of learning—controlled lesioning of the brain. This brings us to the modern period of cognitive neuroscience—a period that I divide into three distinguishable stages, early intermediate, and current; each characterized by a specific research approach to the study of the brain mechanisms of learning.

5.4.1   The Early Stage

By the 1950s, when I was in graduate school, the search for the neuroanatomical correlates of learning was heavily committed to the controlled lesioning techniques. That is, an animal was trained (either prior to or following brain surgery), and efforts were then made to determine the effect of a surgical lesion on learning, storage, or retrieval processes. The performance of a surgically lesioned animal was compared to one for which there had been no surgical intervention beyond the much-desired, but not always honored, "sham operation."[13] The main topics studied were: (1) sensory learning—in which the animal had to make some discrimination between two or more aspects of some stimulus material; (2) precursors of cognitive processing generically referred to as problem solving; (3) a search for the neural locus of classical conditioning.

Sensory learning was exemplified by behavioral changes in an animal's ability to distinguish between two lights of different intensity with experience and following surgical brain interventions. Problem solving was exemplified by the ability of an animal to learn a path through a maze, a task offering the animal a reward for successful behavior. The search for neural correlates of Pavlov's great discovery of classical conditioning typically involved the transection of sensory and motor tracts to determine if, for example, the unconditioned response was required for this kind of conditioning.

The sensory discrimination experiments had one great advantage that drove many researchers to pursue this paradigm. It was fairly well known by then where the primary receiving areas where incoming sensory information was first encoded and represented. Of course, this was also the source of a considerable artifact (among many others of procedure and methodology) in this work. It was very difficult to distinguish between a lack of sensory information (e.g., blindness) and a subtler inability to learn.[14] Nevertheless, this attempt to relate sensory areas to learning and discrimination was the main theme of many researchers during this early modern stage. For example, Settlage (1939) studied the effect of the removal of the visual cortex on visual discriminations and found that even after a complete removal of the visual area of one side of the monkey brain, after a recovery period, the animal was able to learn visual discriminations to an almost normal degree. Settlage attributed this recovery to the animal's learning to selectively fixate within the remaining visual field.

Visual cortical damage was also used by Kluver (1937) to show that some simple kinds of discrimination learning were possible even if the animal was functionally blind. On the other hand, more complex forms of visual learning involving spatial perception were completely obliterated by removal of the visual cortex.

These experiments, so typical of their time, reflect some of the many problems faced when one carries out this kind of research. There is an inherent difficulty in distinguishing among the various involved factors and processes—sensing, learning, relearning, retrieval, species of animal used, recovery of functions, ambiguity of the cues being used, etc. that are all involved in the task chosen.

The search for the locus of classical conditioning was in large part aimed at determining the influence of surgical interventions of the spinal cord and sensory pathways. A number of classical conditioning studies were also carried out on dogs and cats that had been more or less completely decorticated (e.g., Culler & Mettler, 1934). These investigators reported that some kinds of simple conditioning could be established in such animals thus suggesting that some unknown subcortical portions of the nervous system could mediate learning.

Shurrager and Culler (1940) later investigated whether the spinal cord in acute dogs could support classical conditioning and reported that it did. On the other hand other workers such as Kellogg, Deese, Pronko, and Feinberg (1947), working with chronic preparations, did not find spinal conditioning. No modern experiments have yet definitively resolved this controversy, and it has largely fallen off the table of active research questions. Contradictory results of this kind permeated much of the research using controlled extirpation methods and still do. An important general conclusion one can draw from these inconsistent findings is that slight changes in methodology can produce major changes in experimental outcomes.

This was also the time at which the central idea—equipotentiality—of Karl S. Lashley's (1890–1958) 30-year-long research program (summarized in Lashley, 1950) began to be heavily criticized. Much of Lashley's experimental work had been carried out on the rat, and a major argument against his theory was that the rat is "different" from other mammals. In its place, the idea of modules of learning represented by localized regions of brain tissue became the dominant guiding assumption among most learning theorists.

Another research method popular for the study of memory at that time was the delayed response test; especially famous examples were reported by Jacobsen (1936) and Jacobsen and Elder (1936). They showed that selective removal of the frontal lobes destroyed an animal's ability to remember where an object had been placed if it was prohibited from responding for a period of time after the stimulus was displayed.[15] Although it was initially assumed that this result was due to a failure to translate information from working to long-term memory, Finan (1939, 1942) definitively showed that it was not a memory defect. What then could account for the animal's failure to perform on the delayed response test? A possible answer was that the animal had not been paying attention during the preparatory phase of the test and therefore had nothing to store in memory.

Modern investigations and theories continue to perpetuate the controversy about what parts of the nervous system are necessary for conditioning to occur. One of the most contentious of these issues is whether or not conscious awareness is necessary for classical conditioning to occur. There is little agreement on this matter, the residual disagreement being accentuated by the importance of its implications. Should conscious awareness be required for classical conditioning in humans, a pathway to evaluating whether there is any consciousness in a behaviorally unresponsive patient would be opened. Such a test, however, would require that the necessity of awareness be established for conditioned responses.

At the present time, this issue has not been resolved, and thus, any argument that classical conditioning can be used to determine conscious awareness in vegetative or "locked in" states is premature. Nevertheless, some investigators (e.g., Bekinschtein et al., 2009) have uncritically accepted the questionable association between conditioning and awareness (and, thus, its clinical utility) as their justification for ascribing consciousness to vegetative patients. Much is yet to be learned about this relationship, and, for the moment, the value of such classical conditioning as a test for consciousness remains minimal.

This is only the briefest of summaries of this important early stage of research on the physiological counterparts of learning. Many other researchers studied many other learning processes using the surgical lesioning procedure. The impression that one gets from reviewing the accomplishments of this early stage, however, is that many questions were being asked, but few robust, unambiguous, and uncontroversial answers were being uncovered.

Many of the experiments were directed at problems involving the role of the cerebral cortex in learning for eminently practical reasons. Surgery was relatively easy on the surface of the cerebrum; learning could be precisely measured; and the cerebrum was considered to be the locus of high level cognitive processes such as learning that transcended simpler sensory and motor processes. Thus, several conceptual and technical forces were driving physiological psychologists of the time to heavily emphasize research searching for the cerebral correlates of learning. Great changes, however, were occurring about this time, and a number of technical developments appeared that changed the face of this kind of research in profound ways. These developments were so profound that it seems appropriate to draw a line at about the mid-twentieth-century mark between what I have referred to as the early and intermediate stages of research on the neural processes of learning.

5.4.2 The Intermediate Stage

One of the extraordinary new technological developments that demarcate the first and intermediate stages of research on the neural correlates of learning was the invention of the microelectrode. Microelectrodes (Ling & Gerard, 1949) are tiny electrodes that can be inserted for hours or days at a time into single neurons. They thus provide a means of measuring the activity of individual neurons in response to external and internal stimuli. This major technological development led to a series of studies in which the role of individual neurons located at particular places on the brain was examined.

Microelectrodes were particularly useful in exploring the transmission codes used by the sensory and motor systems. They were, however, of less value in exploring high-level, less-well-defined cognitive processes such as learning and attention. The reason for this difference is that there is a major problem with microelectrode studies. Their great advantage has always been the ability to focus attention on a highly localized portion of the brain—indeed, a single cell. However, this extreme focusing on individual cells has its corresponding disadvantages; microelectrodes tend to divert our attention away from the role of all of the other non-impaled neurons that may be involved in the same cognitive process under study. Thus, they can overlook the distributed systems nature of neuronal representation and lead us toward a single-cell interpretation when we should be thinking about the interactive aspects of complex networks. Although all neuroscientists acknowledge the wonderful achievements that this new technology offered, it was for this reason relatively rare for investigators to study the global aspects of learning with microelectrodes once a corresponding single neuron type had been identified. Few microelectrode studies have attempted to explore what other neurons or other parts of the nervous system were doing during the learning process once the investigators found a correlate of a learning process at the tip of their microelectrode.

Thus, there emerged a kind of implicit support for the idea that wherever a microelectrode showed highly localized activity correlated with learning—the antithetical opinion to Lashley's (1950) notion of equipotentiality—that was *the* place at which learning occurred. The hypothesis that learning, or for that matter any other cognitive process, was much more narrowly localized than distributed received a kind of intrinsic support because of the limited perspective of the microelectrode.

Of course, ignoring other possible activated regions was not always the case. One rare and outstanding exception was an experiment carried out by Olds, Disterhoft, Segal, Kornblith, and Hirsch (1972). They studied the responses to a classical conditioning paradigm by placing their microelectrodes in many scattered portions of a rat's brain. Olds and his colleagues discovered that neurons whose responses correlated with conditioning were distributed throughout virtually the entire brain of the rat. Although not all nuclei at all levels contained neurons that were associated with the conditioning process, there was no brain level from the brainstem to the cortex that did not contain at least some neurons that seemed to be so responding. Olds and his colleagues (1972) reported that the activated neurons were most common in the posterior nucleus of the thalamus and a few other thalamic nuclei, the pontine reticular formation, and the ventral tegmentum. These activated neurons were also found in the CA3 but not in the CAI region of the hippocampus as well as in a number of parts of the cerebral cortex. These regions were the ones to which Olds and his colleagues specifically attributed a role in the learning process. The general thrust of these results, however, was to argue that the mechanisms that mediated learning, whatever they were, were to be found in widely distributed regions throughout the entire brain. A corollary was that the engram—the memory itself—was also widely distributed.

As exciting as these results were, the idea that one should examine the neuronal correlates of learning at many places with this method never took hold. Once a correlation was found between a microelectrode response and a learning phenomenon, a study usually ended. There were several reasons for this narrow perspective. First, it was just too ponderous a job to exhaustively carry out the full survey of all brain regions, and, second, distribution of responses just did not fit conceptually within the dominant consensus of the locationist theories that had become so much a part of the contemporary physiological psychology Zeitgeist.

Microelectrode studies of the neural basis of learning became ever more directed at working out the details of how individual neurons and their synapses changed their degree of interconnectivity during the learning process. In this context we learned a lot about the chemistry of synaptic transmitter substances and the growth or potentiation of synaptic junctions. However, this work was all proceeding at the wrong level of analysis if our interest was in cognitive neuroscience; it is aimed at the chemical and functional properties of the individual neuron and not the complex of spatiotemporal interactions among the huge number of these neurons that seems more likely to be involved in even the simplest cognitive process. (See my earlier work [Uttal, 2005] for a more extended discussion of the fragility of modern single-cell theories of mind.)

Some of the most important work on learning at the cellular level has been carried out by Eric Kandel and his colleagues on habituation and classical conditioning. This work was summarized in Kandel (1991) and was the basis for his Nobel Prize in 2000. However exciting these results were, it is not clear that the activity observed in their simple animal model (the nervous systems of the sea hare, *Aplysia californica*) is homologous with comparable processes exhibited behaviorally in vertebrate learning. Much is yet to be learned how these neuronal mechanisms relate to the behavioral analogs observed in higher animals.

The EEG and event-related potential, or ERP, have also been used in many studies, but after many years, these global electrical signals do not seem to have contributed much to our understanding of how we learn. These electrical field-based theories also are problematic for reasons that are different than those based on single neuron, microelectrode recordings. Electrical fields pool the activity of many neurons and, thus, lose the critical information—the details of neuronal interactions as well as the activities of individual neurons. This topic is also discussed in considerable detail in Uttal (2005).

However, there was one technological change that occurred at about this time that was to underlie much of the progress that was accomplished during the intermediate stage of research in this field. It was the enhanced ability to identify and operate on smaller portions of the cerebrum and the brainstem than had hitherto been possible. The ability to keep brain-damaged patients alive after severe trauma or surgery also contributed to new developments in a profound way. In the paragraphs that follow I present a very brief review of the relation between research carried out on the brain and learning during this stage of modern cognitive neuroscientific history that is based primarily on the idea that spatially restricted damage to the brain can inform us about the learning process.

An essential point about this second intermediate stage of research on learning and the brain was that much of its origins lay in fortuitous case studies of humans. Case studies do, unfortunately, have a number of difficulties associated with them, not the least of which is that each seems to be almost idiosyncratic; replication, we find, is the exception rather than the rule. It is, therefore, difficult to draw general conclusions from individual case studies, especially when the anatomy of the injuries is ill-defined and the cognitive deficits ambiguous. Nevertheless, even the most idiosyncratic case can become a powerful heuristic pointing the way to a line of research that might not have otherwise been undertaken.

The predominant modular localization theory that organizes current neuroscientific theories of learning and memory has two parts. The first is essentially Tulving's taxonomy of the different kinds of long-term learning and memory processes described in section 5.3. The second is that each of these cognitive components or modules is assumed to be localized to a major degree in a particular part of the brain. This version of this neuroreductionist

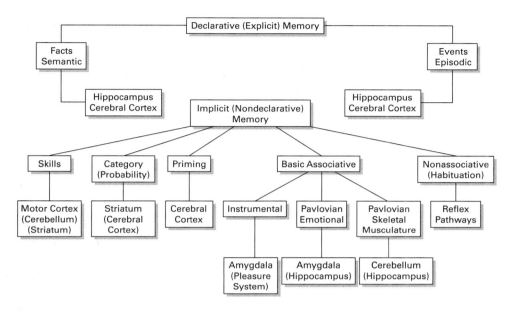

Figure 5.1
A theory of learning and memory types and the brain regions that have been associated with each type. From Thompson (2005), with the permission of Annual Reviews, Inc.

theory of learning and memory has been graphically summarized by Thompson (2005) and is presented in figure 5.1.

However incomplete and regardless of its validity (does any one really believe that declarative memory is represented solely in the medial temporal lobe and the diencephalon?), this is the standard model that characterizes current brain models of memory. Unfortunately, however "standard" and "influential" it may be, it is almost certainly incorrect and misleading. At best, it is a working model of a system whose full complexity is not yet appreciated. At worst, by emphasizing the modularization of learning components and the localization of these functional modules in particular regions of the brain, it may have misled and detoured us from the development of a correct theory—one in which distribution of function rather than localization holds sway. All of this not withstanding, no one can deny its practical value in organizing current research in the biology of learning, and I use it as such in the remainder of this chapter. Without such a framework, psychology would be in even deeper trouble.

A substantial portion of the research dealing with brain mechanisms of learning in the second half of the twentieth century has been directed at the medial temporal cortex. This is a region about half-way between the occipital primary visual receiving areas and the tip of the temporal lobe.

The proposed role of the medial temporal lobe in learning and memory has been brought up to date in a comprehensive review by Squire, Stark, and Clark (2004, p. 279). They describe the anatomy of the system in the following way: "The medial temporal lobe . . . consists of the hippocampal region (CA fields, dendate gyrus, and, subicular process) and the adjacent perirhinal, entorhinal, and parahippocampal cortices."

Slightly anterior to the hippocampus is the amygdala, another region that seems to be involved in the learning process. These temporal regions are also heavily connected to the frontal lobe, which also, as we shall see later, is deeply implicated in the learning and memory process.

Hippocampus

The most widely accepted brain-learning correlation concerns the hippocampus. This association was originally based on the results of a single case study. In 1953 a neurosurgeon—W. B. Scoville—performed a drastic and medically necessary operation on a patient, known as HM, who was suffering from intractable epileptic seizures.[16] The operation and its memory effects were described in complete detail 4 years later in what is now considered to be a classic and iconic report co-authored with a clinical neuropsychologist—Brenda Milner (Scoville & Milner, 1957). This iconic case has achieved almost mythic proportions in the literature on brain injuries and learning and has stimulated a substantial body of research using a variety of investigative techniques. Patient HM suffered postoperatively from severe failure in what we now term short- or intermediate-term memory.[17] Although HM could remember events from his childhood, and those that had occurred a few years ago, he could "recall nothing of the day-to-day events of his hospital life" (Scoville & Milner, 1957, p. 14) beyond what happened in the last few minutes. This now classic and iconic study pointed to the role of the medial temporal lobe and its components as being especially involved in the failure to consolidate short-term memory into long-term memory. We now call these behavioral defects a form of "anterograde declarative memory."

Nevertheless, there remained quite a bit of uncertainty concerning the particular portion of the medial temporal cortex whose damage contributed to HM's memory deficits. The critical region was initially identified as the hippocampus. However, the actual damage done to HM's brain involved much more than just that particular region. Indeed, Scoville and Milner reported that the operation "probably [had] destroyed the anterior two thirds of the hippocampus and hippocampus gyrus bilaterally, as well as the uncus and amygdala" (p. 11). In 1997, an fMRI image was made of HM's brain. It turned out that the damage was much more extensive than they thought. Corkin, Amaral, Gonzalez, Johnson, and Hyman (1997) described the lesions as

. . . bilaterally symmetrical and included the medial temporal polar cortex, most of the amygdaloid complex, most or all of the entorhinal cortex, and approximately half of the rostrocaudal extent of the intraventricular portion of the hippocampal formation (dendate gyrus, hippocampus, and subicular complex). (p. 3964)

Obviously the lesion was very different from a simple hippocampal one. Nevertheless, although his seminal result was not promptly published, Scoville's surgical notes from 1953 quickly stimulated a considerable amount of animal research that sought to clarify the role of the hippocampus in learning by Mishkin (1954) working with monkeys and Mishkin and Pribram (1954) working with baboons, among others. Mishkin and Pribram surgically lesioned two regions in search of the essential one for memory consolidation. The first lesion was restricted to the ventral side of the medial temporal lobe, and the second, carried out in other animals, was restricted to the hippocampus. They found that the ventromedial temporal lesions produced a marked decrement in learning visual discriminations but that the hippocampal and lateral temporal lesions did not impair this kind of learning.

In recent years further research studying this problem has been directed at unraveling the role the hippocampus and other surrounding structures play in the learning and retrieval process. It is not too much of an exaggeration to say that the problem remains largely unresolved despite some creative theories by psychologists such as Squire (1992). He proposed that the hippocampus was specifically associated with consolidating declarative memory and that other nearby regions were responsible for other functions such as classical conditioning or procedural learning of skills. His map of the parts of the brain involved in long-term memory consolidation are shown in figure 5.2

Another theory of the organization of visual memory was offered by Mishkin (1982). Mishkin suggested that the system for visual memory consisted of an array of components that dealt with various stages of the learning process. He suggested that the amygdala and the hippocampus had their own separate roles in visual memory; either one could provide an independent pathway to the thalamus. However, neither these two regions nor any of the other components that he hypothesized were a part of this system, operated independently. Instead, he argued that there seemed to be a complex pattern of feedback between them and other regions such as the thalamus and the complex of components of the temporal lobe.

If there is one thing generally agreed on at present, it is that learning is a function of a distributed system rather than of a singular place on or in the brain. This theme will be played out throughout the rest of this book, with the major residual problem under consideration—what do we mean by a "system"?

In other lesion studies, the role of the hippocampus was defined in terms of specific kinds of fear conditioning—fear being defined as behavior suggesting that a painful stimulus was about to be applied. Distinguishing between cued (in which a specific stimulus was used as the CS) and context-dependent conditioning (in which the situation rather than a specific CS was used), Kim and Fanselow (1992) reported that hippocampal lesions only affected the context conditioning but did not affect cued fear conditioning. Other studies, for example research carried out by Phillips and LeDoux (1992), showed that amygdalar lesions damaged both cued and context-dependent conditioning. Obviously the data are not conclusive and inconsistencies abound.

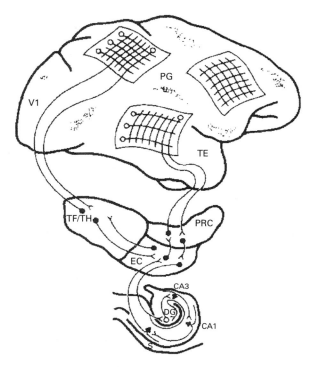

Figure 5.2
A theory of the neural mechanisms of memory consolidation.
From Squire (1992); used with the permission of the American Psychological Association.

There are many problems with this kind of research. Redundant pathways and functions may confuse simple experimental designs.[18] Transfer of function from a lesioned region to an undamaged area could, conceivably, occur between the time of the surgery and the memory test. However well controlled (or not) experiments may be in terms of the surgery performed on or traumatic injuries to human patients, there is a considerable amount of uncertainty introduced into the interpretation of the effects of hippocampal lesions on learning by virtue of the fact that each case is essentially unique.

Furthermore, much of the relevant research has been carried out in a more or less unco-ordinated fashion on the different experimental animals—rats, cats, and monkeys. Jarrard (1995) has pointed out that it is not just the species differences that matter but also the lack of good definitions and incompatible behavioral capacities of the differing species. It is not at all certain what such terms as "spatial," "declarative," "context," and "short-term," among many other descriptors, may mean with respect to other species than our own. Furthermore, Jarrard notes that the psychological constructs represented by terms like this may obscure what are completely different cognitive processes in different species.

In addition, operations on small animals and the fortuitous nature of human injuries and incisions are rarely well enough controlled to assign a specific function to a particular brain center. I recall from my own graduate school days how important it was for my colleagues to carry out postmortem histological studies to determine what the actual damage to brain tissue was during experimental surgery and how it might have differed from the intended lesion. Rarely was the damage to the specific regions as neat as had been hoped. "Hippocampal" damage was often much more widespread than was indicated; in most experiments other surrounding regions had also been damaged. Sometimes, the target region had been missed entirely. Holscher (2003), for example, argued that the uncertainty of the extent of experimental surgery means that many of the memory difficulties attributed to the hippocampus since the time of HM's surgery may actually be due to damage to other regions within or nearby the ventral temporal lobes. In any event, all agree that the data forthcoming from experiments of this class are always "noisy" and unreliable.

Nadel and Moscovitch (1997) have pointed out, furthermore, that the amount of memory loss with hippocampal damage depends on the type of memory task being used. They reviewed a large number of studies to arrive at this conclusion. Their results also reinforced the idea that it was possible that different portions of the hippocampus had different functions, a conclusion that may be less a result of functional specialization then it is a description of the very noisy data from experiments in which the lesioned structure is relatively small and in which the psychological parameters are poorly defined.

In addition to these experimental results, specific to the context of learning, we also know that the hippocampus plays important roles in other cognitive and emotional processes. I have already mentioned its proposed role in the formation of a spatial map of an animal's surroundings. The hippocampus is also considered to be a central part of the limbic system, the collection of centers and nuclei that is especially involved in emotional and aggressive behavior. All of which suggests that it is a part of many systems and that no single behavioral function should be assigned to it.

There are other complications—it is not entirely clear that the hippocampus is really a distinguishable anatomical element in the brain. Thompson and Kim (1996, p. 13443) for example, point out that ". . . a 'structure' like the hippocampus is not really a structure at all; evolution has simply resulted in its appearing so. The hippocampus is not an island unto itself; it is a set of interconnected neurons interconnected with other neurons in the brain. And so it is with all other brain structures."

It must not be overlooked that any expression of a relation between a particular brain region and a cognitive process is more of a theory than an empirical finding. Bitterman (1994) in a review of MacPhail (1993), for example, noted that even the most widely accepted mind-brain association—the role of the hippocampus in learning and memory—is confused by multiple theories and inconsistent interpretations. Bitterman (1994) said:

In the end MacPhail is bound to admit that none of the competing theories of hippocampal function comes off very well. The highly touted mapping theory is clouded by the facts that there are many fewer "place" cells than originally imagined, that their fields are variable, and that hippocampal injury fails to impair performance in some spatial tasks while it does impair performance in some nonspatial tasks. (p. 1637)

Bitterman then proceeds to list several other theories (e.g., selective attention, short- and long-term memory) of the role of the hippocampus and shows how they, too, are challenged by the complexities of this center in a number of other tasks. Nothing we know, he points out, is adequate to assign a narrowly defined cognitive process to such a narrowly defined neural location. Bitterman concludes by pointing out that it is the psychology that is driving these theories not the neurophysiology and by stating (p. 1635) "It certainly is not to work on the hippocampus, for example, that we owe the distinction between place and response learning; nor to work on the cerebellum an appreciation of the limitations of the stimulus-substitution account of classical conditioning . . ."

The point is that it is most often psychology that informs neuroscience and not the reverse. Almost everything we know about the brain as a cognitive machine is guided by what psychologists have uncovered. One has to dig very deeply once one goes beyond the sensory and motor systems to find instances of the neurosciences informing psychology.

The bottom line of this analysis is that the specific link between the hippocampus and the consolidation of short-term to long-term memory remains far more speculative than is usually appreciated.

Amygdala

Another medial temporal region often specifically associated with learning is the amygdala. This is a small olive-shaped region of the cerebrum at the base of the medial temporal lobe anterior to the hippocampus. The amygdala has long been known to have many different functions including polysensory representation, attention, and emotion. It is heavily interconnected with other regions of the brain including the frontal lobes. The amygdala has, in the context of the present discussion, been reported to be involved in many different kinds of learning and memory processes, especially those of highly emotional (especially fear- producing) situations and classical conditioning. Although it had been thought for many years that the amygdala was involved in some way in learning, the first report emphasizing its role in storing emotional memories was made by Goddard (1964) who showed that electrical stimulation of the amygdala could block "fear–motivated learning" but not food-motivated learning.

In addition, the amygdala has been studied in relation to its role in habit formation, in controlling the storage of information, in shuttle box learning, in learned avoidance, and in the evaluation of the quality (i.e., potentially harmful versus potentially pleasurable) of incoming stimuli. According to McGaugh (2004, p. 1) this diversity of function maybe summed up by saying that "The amygdala modulates the consolidation of memories of emotionally arousing experiences." However, the amydala's rich interconnections with other portions of the brain, particularly the limbic system, and the potential for redundant pathways make any definitive statement about a singular role for it in learning, elusive. Obviously, the regulation of emotional learning is only one of many different functions in which the amygdala is involved; it would be incomplete to assert that its sole function is controlling the storage of emotional memories.

A further complication is that the amygdala is also composed of several different regions that appear to have different functions. The constraints on our ability to precisely control surgical lesions always leaves a residuum of doubt concerning exactly what regions have been excised and, therefore, leaves much uncertainty about the amygdala's role not only in learning but also in other cognitive and regulatory processes. Given the new view that most regions of the brain, are parts of distributed neural networks that collectively account for complex behavior and cognitive processes, any assignment of a specific function to the amygdala is probably disputable. The best we can say at the present time is that the amygdala plays some role in many learning processes especially those that deal with emotional learning.

Thalamus

The region of the diencephalon known as the thalamus has been implicated by a number of studies of learning and memory processes. Early studies of human brain injuries had strongly suggested that diencephalic lesions (including the thalamus) were followed by anterograde amnesia—the failure to consolidate new memories. Although most early studies were more or less indiscriminate about the role of other portions of the diencephalon (e.g., the mammillary bodies), Aggleton and Sahgal (1993) were among the first to suggest that the observed amnesia was actually a specific result of damage to the anterior thalamic nuclei. However the small size and ambiguous subdivisions of this structure have made any firm conclusions uncertain. Many other regions of the diencephalon have, furthermore, been shown to have memory effects.

Over the years, research in this field has been complex, and currently attention has been directed at what seem to be the roles of the various parts of the thalamus. There is great uncertainty about the meaning of current experimental results because of the small size and propinquity of the various thalamic regions to nearby structures. It is possible that thalamic lesions, so close to the medial temporal lobe, may actually be a *necessary* part of that system but not have *sufficient* capacity to control memory formation or to serve as a repository of information. It is also possible that the role of the thalamus in the memorization process may be simply explained in terms of the spatial relation of these nuclei to certain critical tracts and pathways. Since parts of the thalamus also conduct sensory signals, the possibility of diminished afferent flow must always be considered before specific high-level cognitive processes are attributed to it. Nevertheless, whatever their specific role as quasi-independent units or parts of a more complex system, there is no question that damage to certain of the thalamic nuclei of the diencephalon can produce learning defects in humans and animals.

Striatum

The striatum is a collection of subcortical nuclei at the top of the brainstem. It is considered by anatomists to be a part of the basal nuclei of the brain and to include two major divisions—the caudate nucleus and the putamen. There is a long history of the striatum's role in what Balleine, Delgado, and Hikosaka (2007) refer to as affective learning—that is, as a modulator of learning depending on the nature of the reward. Montague and Berns (2002) have suggested a more subtle role—namely that the role of the striatum is to set the subjective value of a stimulus in the learning process. Thus, the striatum is proposed to have the very specific function of determining relative costs and potential payoffs during the learning process. They (Montague and Berns) formalized their ideas in a "predictor valuation model." In this model a distinction is made between the actual reinforcement (such as food) and the "value" of that food. Although the former may remain constant, the latter varies depending on the state of the animal, and it is the striatum, they argued, that encodes this distinction.

The striatum is also thought to be involved in instrumental conditioning, a form of procedural learning. As we see later in this chapter, recent work with fMRI has suggested to some investigators that the two parts of the striatum may have separate roles in this process—one part regulating the value of the reward and one part concerned with remembering the appropriate behavior. As with all other aspects of instrumental conditioning, this process may proceed without any conscious awareness, a result consistent with the subcortical nature of the striatum. Damage to the striatum (or a deficiency of dopamine transmitters there) may also be involved in Parkinson disease in humans, a condition that also displays memory loss as well as its better-known motor dysfunctions.

Frontal Lobes

Many other regions of the brain have also been reported to be involved in the learning and memory processes. Of particular interest is the role the frontal lobes play in these processes. There are well-established connections between the medial temporal lobe regions and the frontal lobes that suggest some kind of interaction. However, the empirical literature is vague about such interactions because so many other functions have been attributed to the frontal lobes including short-term episodic memory, emotions, attention and selective attention, imagination, self-awareness, executive control, thinking in general, and even humor. The iconic case of Phineas Gage implicated planning and decision making, and control over the sequences and awareness of the implications of our behavior, but curiously little effect on learning in the classical sense of the word.[19]

Nevertheless, patients with frontal lobe damage are reported to be poor in working memory tasks. However, long-term memory is seemingly not lost after damage to these regions. This suggests, but does not confirm, that because of possible redundancy the frontal lobes are not the site of the stored information we call memory. Instead, it seems that the frontal lobes are involved in the control of information processing that ultimately leads to long-term storage in a way that is comparable to that of the hippocampus. Neither region's role, of course, should be considered to be exclusive of the others.

A recent review (Simons & Spiers, 2003) emphasizes the interaction of the prefrontal, as well as the medial temporal lobes, in learning and memory. The authors conclude that the prefrontal region acts to control the acquisition process by "regulating" the essential region for information storage—the medial temporal lobe. The frontal lobes are also active in controlling the retrieval process, according to these reviewers, by specifying retrieval cues and thus by specifying what will be recalled.

Damage to the frontal lobe may produce widely different results that vary from individual to individual. Deficits in language may imitate differences in other cognitive processes. The inability to interpret or retrieve stored information may be confused with an absence of that stored information. Thus an inability to carry out some task may not be a fault in the storage of the engram or even in the retrieval of that information but ,instead, an inability to make the necessary associations that take a memory from storage to performance. One place that the frontal lobes are clearly involved is in the control of working memory (Fuster, 1985; Goldman-Rakic, 1987). "Working memory," however, is such a generic term, comparable in its ambiguity to "paying attention," "thinking," "thought," and perhaps even "consciousness" itself, that the particular experimental tests may reflect only a small portion of the true complexity of the role of the frontal lobes.[20] Indeed, the higher and more complex the cognitive process, the poorer are our definitions and the empirical results that are obtained.

As a result, the literature on working memory and the frontal lobes is still contentious, and no consensus has yet appeared that offers more than heuristic enthusiasm to mind-brain theorists. Many of the associations between cognitive processes and brain mechanisms are highly speculative and poorly validated. As is so frequently the case, an early iconic finding (in this case, that of Phineas Gage) sets the tone for what currently may be a very uncertain set of explanations.

Cerebellum

An entirely unexpected discovery drastically changed our conception of the role of the cerebellum in learning, specifically with regard to classical conditioning. The cerebellum had traditionally been thought of as an organ associated with the more or less passive coordination of muscular activity. Lesions of the cerebellum were well known to produce tremors, paralysis, and other motor disturbances.[21] There were a few curious results (e.g., Brogden & Gantt, 1937) in which direct stimulation of the cerebellum produced a kind of conditioned reflex that seemed to be indistinguishable from that produced by a UCS shock to the foot. However this effect was clearly antithetical to the strong consensus existing at that time that the cerebellum was merely a sensory-motor coordination center, albeit a very complex[22] one.

During this intermediate period, attention (based on a discovery by McCormick & Thompson, 1984) was directed at another aspect of cerebellar function that had previously been obscure. Richard Thompson (see summaries of his work in such papers as Kim & Thompson, 1997; Thompson, 2005; Thompson & Kim, 1996) has been the leading proponent of its role in mediating classical conditioning of the eyelid and other simple motor responses.[23]

The 1984 paper showed that the cerebellum contains certain regions that appear to be necessary for this type of learning. However, the cerebellum alone appears not to be sufficient to account for the model system under study—the conditioned eyelid response of the rabbit; instead, it is a part of a complex neural system (shown in figure 5.3) all of which must be intact for this kind of learning to take place. Thompson (2005) went even further in attacking one of the great questions of cognitive neuroscience: he argued that this system not only controls the conditioning process but is also the locus of the memory trace itself.

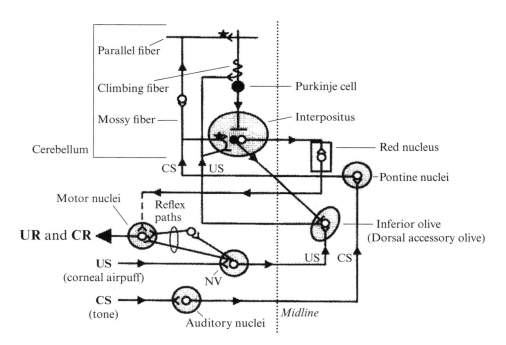

Figure 5.3
A theory of how the nervous system might process cerebellar learning. Stars indicate sites of plasticity.
From Thompson (2005), with the permission of Annual Reviews, Inc.

Figure 5.3 is the hypothetical model proposed by Thompson and Kim (1996; reproduced from Thompson, 2005) to suggest how an air puff, the UCS, can come to be associated with an acoustic tone (the CS) such that the tone will produce a conditioned response (an eye blink).

Despite the compelling argument put forward by Thompson and Kim, they were appropriately cautious in drawing their conclusions. For example, they reminded us that "The message here is not that all learning occurs in the cerebellum; it does not. Certain structures, cerebellum, hippocampal system, and amygdala, play key roles in processes of learning and memory" (Thompson & Kim, 1996, p. 13443).

This neurophysiological theory of a particular kind of learning—classical conditioning—reemphasizes an important general point—no single region of the brain is likely to account for even the simplest kind of learning process. All studies, however much they dote on the *necessary* role of a particular center, must ultimately acknowledge that their findings have to be interpreted in the context of a distributed system of brain components interacting in complex manners that are *sufficient* only in the collective sense.

It must be kept in mind that the psychological taxonomy (or theory) of learning types proposed by Tulving (1972) provides the intellectual foundation of much of this neurophysiological approach. Researchers have not only sought mechanisms for the psychological constructs but have also been guided in the design of their experiments by these hypothetical cognitive processes. It must not be forgotten that any such classification scheme by itself is actually neutral with regard to the physiological mechanisms. There are no physiological premises or assumptions implicit in the Tulving model of learning types. Only when links are made to particular brain sites (as shown in figure 5.1) are neuroreductionist assumptions added. Should the psychological model change, it would be a colossal source of confusion and disorder; ambiguous neurophysiological correlations would probably have to be drastically reinterpreted. All of this would have to happen in the absence of any change in the neuroscientific findings. That a whole science is so susceptible makes it logically possible that there is a much more tenuous link between the psychology of learning and the neuroscience of the brain than is generally appreciated.

Finally, as they are in most other sciences, the empirical data are the final arbiters. In much of this stage of cognitive neuroscience—the intermediate stage—there has been a huge variability in findings with many experiments that were initially supposed to replicate each other demonstrating conflicting results. It is for this reason that so many publications end with the admonition that "these data conflict with those of my colleague Professor X" or admit that "this theory" is a plausible, but not definitive, explanation of what has been observed. This is not at all surprising given the complexity of the task—the disentangling of the functions of the many interconnected regions of the brain—undertaken by what are admittedly fairly crude techniques.

This, then, brings us to the most modern stage of cognitive neuroscience—the one in which brain imaging techniques seem to have taken over most of cognitive neuroscience.

5.4.3 The Current Stage—Brain Imaging

The course of the first stage of neural studies of learning was dictated by fortuitous brain trauma to humans and some preliminary and crudely formulated animal experiments. The second half of the twentieth century was exemplified by more sophisticated brain surgery and, to a lesser degree, by the use of microelectrodes to determine what regions of the brain showed neural activity that might be associated with learning tasks. As we have seen, all of these techniques posed severe interpretive problems when the raw empirical data were converted into robust conclusions about how the brain instantiated the behavioral and cognitive changes that occurred with experience.

However, a remarkable change in technology had been in the making even while the first and second stages were running their courses. In the 1930s developments in the physical study of materials using magnetic resonance imaging (MRI) had been producing exciting new discoveries in quantum theory. The real breakthrough for medical science, however, came almost 40 years later when Damadian (1971) first proposed and then actually constructed a device that used the differential tissue responses to magnetic fields to image the anatomy of the human body.[24] This magnetic resonance imaging (MRI) technique was able to discriminate between different tissues of the body by virtue of the different susceptibilities of protons to recover their original orientation following the application of strong magnetic fields.

The next step in this extraordinary development was the invention of functional magnetic resonance imaging (fMRI) by Ogawa and his colleagues (1990). It was at this point that cognitive neuroscience seized on what has become the main theme of current research. Ogawa's group reported that the magnetic susceptibility of blood varied depending on its oxygen content. It was suggested, therefore, that images could be made not only of the anatomy of the brain but also of its function. The technique depends on the brain's metabolism consuming oxygen during mental activity. As the blood oxygen level dependent (BOLD) magnetic resonance signal varied, active regions could be discriminated from inactive ones. The basic idea was that the regions of depleted oxygen should indicate where neural activity corresponding to mental activity had been located. (See section 1.5.4 for a more complete discussion of the logic behind this process.)

The rest is scientific history! Perhaps no other development in cognitive neuroscience changed the research environment for psychology and cognitive neuroscience as thoroughly and as quickly as did the development of the fMRI.[25] During the 15 years since Ogawa's group's development, everyone who was anyone in cognitive neurology and neurochemistry was collecting fMRI measures of the brain from intact human beings. No longer were we dependent on fortuitous brain injuries in humans, surgical lesions of uncertain extent, or questionable cross-species comparisons; in their place, the conscious, thinking, cooperative, and verbal-reporting normal human being became the subject of choice. In the section that follows I explore a few of the many studies in which fMRI brain imaging was used to study human learning.

At the outset, I must apologize once again for the spotty coverage of this overview. In the last decade and a half, many hundreds of articles on the use of brain imaging as an indicator of learning and memory have been published. There are far too many studies and resultant articles to even consider a comprehensive coverage in a book such as the present one. These studies typically strive to show changes in the distribution or amplitude of the brain image as a result of changes in controlled learning experiences. However, the range of these studies is enormous. Work has been done on visual skill learning (Poldrack, Desmond, Glover, & Gabieli, 1998); comparisons of passive and active motor movements (Lotze, Braun, Birbaumer, Anders, & Cohen, 2002); the effect of rewards on learning (Delgado, Miller, Inati, & Phelps, 2005); motor sequence learning (Toni, Krams, Turner, & Passingham (1998); procedural learning (Kassubek, Schmidtke, Kimming, Lucking, & Greenlee, 2001); and working memory (Olesen, Westerberg, & Klingberg, 2004) to mention only a few examples in this huge corpus of research.

Although it is impossible to review all of this vast body of work in a book such as the present one, I now present a few general examples of how this work fits (or, as is so often the case, how it does not fit) with the findings that had been observed in the intermediate stage in which human case studies and surgical interventions had previously dominated. Once again, I organize this minireview in terms of the anatomical structures that have been associated with Tulving's taxonomy of learning types.

Hippocampus

The hippocampus, as we have seen earlier, has long been considered to be a critical brain component in the storage and retrieval of information. There is virtually no evidence that it is the site of the engram, but there is a substantial body of evidence that suggests that it is involved in some way in the consolidation process—among many other roles. Unfortunately, the role of the hippocampus and that of its subdivisions in this complex network of interacting regions remains poorly understood even under the illumination that was supposed to be thrown on it by the new fMRI studies. One source of this uncertainty is that the hippocampus is heavily interconnected with other parts of the brain that have also been shown to be involved in the consolidation process. Empirical studies, as a result, usually display related activity in many other parts of the brain.

However, there is another conceptual issue that mitigates against a clear-cut answer to the question of what is the role of the various brain regions in learning. That is, as I have noted earlier, virtually all of this work is based on the theoretical model of learning types proposed by Tulving (1972) shown in figure 5.1 or derivatives of that typology. This has led to a substantial diversity of learning tests being used as the independent variable in studies in which the fMRI image is used as the dependent variable. A few of the variations of learning tasks that have been used in fMRI studies of the hippocampus's role in learning include these tasks:

- Context fear conditioning
- Cued fear conditioning
- Classical conditioning
- Instrumental conditioning
- Exemplar novelty
- Perceptual novelty
- Relational memory
- Artificial language acquisition
- Episodic memory
- Semantic memory
- Memory consolidation
- Memory retrieval
- Transitive interference
- Conscious versus unconscious memory
- Motor sequence learning
- Spatial learning

This list of the variety of independent variables and learning tasks suggests that we have either not actually zeroed in on what specific learning function the hippocampus may play or that its role is extremely varied. In retrospect, all we really have is evidence that damage to it or to a number of the other components with which it interacts produces amnesias of one kind or another, especially anterograde amnesias, those involving a failure of consolidation into long-term memory, and, thus, a loss of the contents of short-term memory. It is not at all certain that this extensive list even correctly identifies what it is that the hippocampus does—our inability to define cognitive processes may mean that Tulving's taxonomy, which is in the final analysis a theory of learning, does not yet represent the full complexity of the role of the hippocampus in learning. After all, it not at all clear what the phrase "episodic memory" actually means biologically. It would be nice if our psychological constructs mapped directly onto anatomic structures, but the empirical data for the two domains are so different that there is no a priori reason to assume that they must do so. Psychological faculties and abilities are transient concepts that vary from generation to generation, always to be replaced by other equally ambiguous terms (see Uttal, 2001).

Stark and Squire (2000, p. 7776) similarly pointed out that even the simplest word may cover up a complex of different cognitive processes. For example, they noted that remembering is far more than just passive retrieval. Instead they stated that ". . . activity during retrieval [contrasted] activity with a perceptual baseline (a broad contrast that includes many cognitive functions, including the intention and the effort to retrieve)." Thus, it is not only the variety and uncertain composition of these learning and memory tasks that make it difficult to form a coherent story about the role of the hippocampus or any other region, but it is also the diversity of empirical results. Contradictory or overly inclusive reports, suggesting an enormous degree of variability in the obtained data, inhibit our search for the exact role of this particular center. Indeed, it is not even certain that it has a well-defined and unique role.

Another problem is that the hippocampus is not uniform in its response. Different regions seem to have different functions. The left anterior hippocampus is often associated with "novelty," whereas the posterior hippocampus seems to react more to "familiarity" of repeated stimuli (Strange, Fletcher, Henson, Friston, & Dolan, 1999). Nor for that matter are the duties of the hippocampus restricted to the learning process. The hippocampus is also considered to be a part of the limbic system, which has long been associated with emotional behavior.

One possibility is that, by emphasizing the particular role of the hippocampus in regulating consolidation, we have been ignoring its more general contribution as a part of a much larger and diverse system. Furthermore the hippocampus is heavily interconnected with other portions of the nervous system, and it is only by making arbitrary decisions about the threshold for activation to be used in the imaging process that signals can be limited to this structure.

Since the hippocampus had a preexisting reputation for being involved in learning, fMRI studies of it were initially directed at it in that context. Despite general agreement that at least one major function of the hippocampus is its role in learning, its exact role in this domain (and what other role it may play) remains elusive; much research has been heavily influenced (some would say biased) by the findings obtained in the previous stages of cognitive neuroscience research. However, it now seems clear that the role played by the hippocampus may be far more complex than simply declarative consolidation. Marschner, Kaslisch, Vervliet, Vansteenwegen, and Buchel (2008), for example, were able to show that the hippocampus had a role in conditioned fear similar to that observed with amygdalar lesion studies, but so, too, did a wide range of other cerebral and brainstem regions.

Other studies also show a much diversified role for the hippocampus in such tasks as relational learning. The suggestion in this case is that the hippocampus is important in defining the relations between stimuli as opposed to its more passive and better-known role in consolidation. Whenever studies of this kind (e.g., Opitz, & Friederici, 2003) are carried out, however, the general result is that it is not only the hippocampus (or any part of it) that is activated; instead, a broad brainwide response is more often observed. In such a situation it is difficult to attribute a specific role to any particular cognitive process solely to the hippocampus.

A distinction has also been made between the hippocampus's role in consolidation and retrieval. Where the traditional view was that it was mainly involved in associative consolidation (i.e., the conversion of short-term memories into long-term ones), Stark and Squire (2000) showed, using fMRI imaging techniques, that its role is much broader—the hippocampus is also robustly activated during the retrieval of words and objects.

A further dimension of interest to some researchers has been the role of consciousness on learning. It is generally assumed that the hippocampus is deeply involved in conscious learning but there is considerable dispute according to Greene, Gross, Elsinger, and Rao (2008) whether or not the hippocampus actually has a role in implicit learning situations such as instrumental conditioning. They note that a number of investigators had suggested that task "awareness" (i.e., conscious awareness of the learning task) is necessary for hippocampal activation. Other researchers have argued that the hippocampus is involved in implicit learning without any awareness on the part of the subject. Greene and his colleagues used fMRI images to make the argument that the hippocampus is, in fact, involved in unconscious (implicit or procedural) as well as conscious, declarative learning by comparing brain responses and reaction times to novel and repeated displays.

Another experimental approach using fMRI attacked the problem of specialized regions of the hippocampus in various stages of the learning and retrieval processes. Zeineh, Engel, Thompson, and Bookheimer (2003) studied the association of names and faces, and they discovered that some regions (the CA fields 2 and 3 and the dendate gyrus of the hippocampus) were active only during the encoding process after which their activity gradually declined. On the other hand, the subiculum was active only during retrieval, and then its activity declined. Both were compared to psychophysical data measuring the learning and recall processes.

A universal characteristic of all of their results is the multiple sources of variability in these studies. Not only are many different stimulus conditions used, but the behavioral measures used as dependent variable vary widely. Furthermore, relatively few subjects are typically used in these experiments (it is an expensive business). Since individual variability is high, this makes for low-power experiments. Furthermore, many investigators are becoming aware that different MRI devices and different environments may introduce some uncertainties into the obtained data. (Stark & Squire, 2000, for example, actually repeated their experiments in two different laboratories in acknowledgment of this possibility. This is rarely done these days, but it may become more necessary as meta-studies make the variability of brain images clearer.)

There is a continuing stress between what we can know and what we want to know about the role of the hippocampus in learning. The complexity and variability of the data reported so far make it difficult to draw any firm conclusions about its role either by inclusion or exclusion. The empirical findings are complex and variable, and few generalizations seem to stand for long. The possibility of a gross mismatch between our psychological and neural findings remains. This is both a compliment to the richness of the mind-brain problem and an extreme impediment to the kind of focused research that has dignified so many other sciences. Whether we will be able to go beyond this plethora of confusing results concerning the hippocampus remains to be seen. For the moment the best we can say is that this remarkable brain region plays many roles, not only in learning and memory, but also in our experience of the world around us.

Amygdala

The amygdala, the almond-shaped nucleus just anterior to the hippocampus, has been specifically associated with emotion and affect for many years (see, for example, the work of Weiskrantz, 1956).[26] However, its potential role in learning is an even more recent discovery (LeDoux 1995; Philips & LeDoux, 1992). Specifically, it was suggested by these researchers that the amygdala acts to accelerate the consolidation of long-term memory (otherwise controlled by the hippocampus) by adding emotional content. One popular notion is that because the amygdala accentuates the learning process, our memories of momentous events (such as the Kennedy assassination in 1963) are deeper and more profound than those of ordinary events. We cannot say whether this is an enhancement of either the storage or the retrieval of the experience. Nevertheless it seems clear from even the most superficial behavioral measures that emotional experiences are remembered better than neutral ones.

The amygdala is also notably active in a kind of conditioning in which the CS becomes associated with a pain or the fear of pain. Phelps (2006) has provided a comprehensive review of the role of the amygdala in emotion. It should not be overlooked, however, that emotional enhancement of learning is not its only function; the amygdala is also known to process visual and auditory stimuli and is a part of the extended limbic system.

Striatum

The striatum, a subcortical region consisting of the caudate nucleus and the putamen, also has had specific learning functions attributed to it. These include various kinds of implicit or procedural learning—that is, learning based on a passive process that does not require explicit attention and for which the learner is typically not able to explain how or what he or she has learned. Examples of implicit learning include instrumental conditioning (reward learning), motor-skill learning, some language skills, and improvements in reaction time. The term—implicit learning—was first suggested by Reber (1967) in studies of rule-based behavior without realization on the part of the subjects of the rules in a study of artificial grammars. It is clear, however, that the implicit learning process, known by a number of other names, was of interest to psychologists for many years prior to Reber's seminal experiments.

The association between the striatum and implicit learning had been suggested by a number of early clinical cases, particularly by patients suffering from Huntington or Parkinson disease. These are diseases in which the striatum was determined to be involved and in which a typical behavioral concomitant exhibited by patients was a deficiency in one form or another of implicit learning. With the development of the fMRI imaging techniques, it was hoped that it would be possible not only to measure striatal activity but also to determine the role of the striatum's parts. Unfortunately, like so many other of these associations, the research is controversial and noisy, at least partially because of the very large number of different implicit memory tasks that have been used to study the effects of striatal damage. There is, so to speak, no standard "behavioral fruit fly" that has been uni-versally used to explore the implicit learning-striatal association. The range of utilized behavioral concomitants that has been used is very broad and includes all of the following ones:

- Implicit learning of phobias
- Impact of schizophrenia
- Sequence learning tasks
- Serial reaction time tasks
- Advantage learning
- Transfer of learning
- Concept learning

A further complication in explaining the role of the striatum is that relatively few studies have gone beyond the striatum to evaluate the role of other centers in the implicit learning process. Thus, once the assumption that the striatum was associated with implicit learning was accepted, research attention was directed at this center and that type of learning, and the activity of other regions was rarely considered thereafter.

However, a few workers exploring other parts of the brain of course also found distinctly different brain regions to be involved in implicit learning. For example, Zedkova, Wood-ward, Harding, Tibbo, and Purdon (2006) using brain images found procedural learning responses in the dorsal striatum, anterior cingulate, and the parietal and frontal cortices among other regions.

As this brief comment on the role of the striatum in implicit language learning especially strongly illustrates, there is a strong influence of the prevailing theory or hypothesis on experimental design and protocols and ultimately, it must also be acknowledged, on the obtained results in this new stage of imaging research. Observed psychological phenomena or—even more important—inferred hypothetical constructs are often used to guide the imaging exploration. Although this is without question a scientific necessity, blind adher-ence to one's initial assumptions often can inappropriately emphasize neural mechanisms in a circular manner in which vague and variable images support ill-defined psychological constructs and vice versa. The process, therefore, can become quite misleading. To illustrate how the problem can become conceptually complex, let us consider several articles that deal with the problem of the functional role of the different areas of the striatum, all of which have been measured with comparable fMRI techniques.

I cite first the work of O'Doherty and colleagues (2004). They base their analysis of the separable roles of the ventral and dorsal striatum on a rather tenuous psychological theory of instrumental conditioning that assumes two processes—a predictor of future rewards and a memory component that remembers the outcomes of previous actions. On this basis, they sought and found that activity in the dorsal and ventral striatum, respectively, represented these two psychological constructs. They associated the ventral striatum primarily with the predictor function and the dorsal striatum with the storage of information about previous outcomes.

Unfortunately, other investigators have also found differentiable responses in the dorsal and ventral striatum that do not map directly onto the psychological functions on which O'Doherty and his colleagues based their work. Reiss and colleagues (2005) report that both the dorsal and ventral striatum were activated when implicit learning took place but to a lesser degree in the ventral striatum than when their subjects did not learn. Attempts to reconcile the two approaches led Reiss and his colleagues to propose that the dorsal regions were associated with "motor responses" and the ventral with "more cognitive roles."

Rodriguez, Aron, and Poldrack (2006), on the other hand, found activity in the ventral striatum that was associated with what they referred to as prediction error. They also noted the conflicting results of similar studies. For example, they noted the following:

Some fMRI studies do report decreases in ventral striatum related to the absence of expected reward . . . but other studies do not . . . and some report it *only* in relation to positive outcomes. In brief, the source of discrepancy between neurophysiological findings and neuroimaging findings of striatal activations, as well as different direction of striatal activations for different tasks, remains to be fully understood. (p. 311)

Furthermore, the role of the striatum is clearly not limited to implicit learning. It has been implicated in a variety of other roles including motor control (Grillner, Hellgren, Menard, Saitoh, & Wikstrom, 2005) and concept learning (Seger & Cincotta, 2002) in addition to explicit learning, and even decision making (Balleine, Delgado, & Hikosaka, 2007)—a process usually attributed to the higher levels of the brain.

A detailed model of the role of the striatum as a component of a complex system subserving perceptual classification (as a subset of procedural learning) has been suggested by Ashby, Ennis, and Spiering (2007). Their model, based on an extensive review of the literature, is shown in figure 5.4. The important point, regardless of the correctness or incorrectness of the details of this model, is that the procedural or implicit learning is not mediated solely by the striatum but that whatever regulatory role it might have should only be conceptualized in terms of a broadly distributed system in which multiple centers interact.

It should be obvious that the role of the striatum, like so many other regions of the brain, is far more complicated and far less understood than is currently appreciated. Whether it is appropriate to even attribute a specific function such as implicit learning to it is questionable. Within this general context of uncertainty, it is problematic what its role in cognition actually is.

Rodriguez et al. (2006), furthermore, made another contribution that is of a type that is all too rare. In addition to their study directed at the striatum, they also did a study of the entire brain's responses to comparable stimuli—in this case, classification learning. In a brief paragraph, they noted that other regions of the brain including many parts of the cerebellum, the cuneus, and the pre- and post-central gyrus of the cerebrum were also activated.

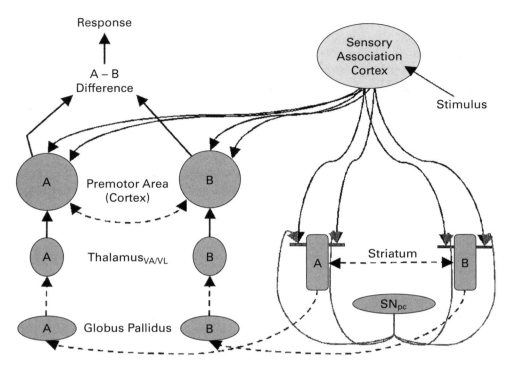

Figure 5.4
A theory of the neural control of perceptual categorization—an implicit learning task. A and B refer to two contrasting categories of learning.
From Ashby, Ennis, & Spiering (2007); used with the permission of the American Psychological Association.

These findings lead to several possible interpretations. First, the stimulus tasks that activated the striatum had some cryptic significance beyond the role played by the striatum. Second, the brain mechanisms for those tasks were not limited to the striatum but were carried out on a more distributed basis by a widely dispersed set of neural centers and nuclei. Third, the cognitive tasks are so poorly defined that they do not reflect the biology of the nervous system. Rather than their being a center for implicit learning, for example, our cognitive taxonomy simply does not map onto the functions that are carried out by this part of the brain.

The variety of research carried out in this field and the indefinite results obtained make it clear both that the striatum has many roles beyond implicit learning and that many different cognitive, sensory, and motor functions produce activations in this region. Indeed, taking this situation as an example, it is possible to add support to the argument that many parts of the brain interact in most cognitive processes. The historic emphasis on specific structure-function associations may represent a major conceptual failure in the past history of cognitive neuroscience.

Cerebellum

Functional magnetic resonance imaging studies of the cerebellum have confirmed that it responds to classical conditioning situations in humans (see review by Gerwig, Kolb, & Timmann, 2007). Based on the results of Thompson (as summarized in Thompson, 2005), this should not be surprising. However, it has been known for over a decade that the cerebellum is also involved in a number of other types of learning tasks. Desmond and Fiez (1998) summarized the results of a number of fMRI imaging experiments that showed that cerebellar responses were associated with a variety of other learning activities including explicit memory retrieval, language, sequence learning, rotor pursuit learning, as well as verbal working memory. Furthermore, Cabeza and Nyberg's (2000) extensive review of 275 imaging studies revealed that the cerebellum was also activated during a wide variety of other kinds of cognitive and learning tasks. They reported cerebellar activations when subjects pay attention, use language, and during working memory processes, episodic memory retrieval, as well as the now well-established responses produced during procedural learning such as classical conditioning.

Cerebellar activity during high-level cognitive processing has been reported in recent fMRI studies by a number of other investigators. Hayter, Langdon, and Ramnani (2007) and Kirschen, Chen, Schraedley-Desmond, and Desmond (2004) have reported that the cerebellum is activated when a person is exercising working memory.

An important point made by both of these groups of investigators (as well as most researchers these days) is that it is not the cerebrum alone that seems to be correlated with these high-level cognitive activities. Instead, all of these studies remind us that the cerebellum is an important part of a complicated network subserving relatively intricate cognitive activities. Indeed both groups reported widely dispersed brain activity during many kinds of mental activity.

Cerebral Cortex

The cerebral cortex—the great hemispheres of the brain onto which we have projected the idea of association areas (among others)—has obviously been the center of attention when it comes to many different kinds of high-level cognitive processes, not the least of which are the processes involved in learning and memory. Once again it must be reiterated that there is still no indication of how or where that information is stored. A second reminder is that despite an enormous amount of research using imaging techniques in the last decade or so, there is only the glimmering of an understanding about how this highly complex organ works to produce cognitive activity.

The current approach has been to provide structured experiences and then to use brain imaging as a means of localizing which portions of the cortex seem to be associated with which particular kind of learning experience. However, here, too, there remains a great reservoir of uncertainty. As we see, the results are typically unreliable and complex, and no overarching theory of the role of the cerebrum has yet emerged to bring order to the last decade of research. There has, however, been a noticeable shift in thinking about the role of the cerebrum during this period. Whereas extreme localization theories were dominant until recently, it is becoming clear that many regions of the cerebrum are involved in most learning processes.

The perennial problem of an abundance of poor or ambiguous definitions of learning and memorial processes continues. Images based on fMRI methods have been correlated with a large number of different cognitive processes, some of which are based on behavioral studies but some of which seem to be ex post facto artifices to explain complex results. For example, Kirwan, Wixted, and Squire (2008) distinguish between "memory strength" and "recollection" and attribute the former to the traditional medial temporal lobe region but the latter to the prefrontal cortex.

In the most recent paper from this laboratory, Smith and Squire (2009) report what has to be considered some of the most provocative and interesting data concerning the engram itself. They used fMRI methods to study the effect of the age of the memory of past news events on the activation of structures in the medial temporal lobe. They reported that activity in the hippocampus, amygdala, and temporopolar regions actually declined when the subject was asked to remember things further in the past. This is a very curious result, but, at first glance, it suggests that a decline in memory recorded behaviorally is associated with reduced activity in these temporal regions. However, quite surprisingly, activation strengths actually increased in most of the rest of the brain including the frontal, parietal, and other portions of the temporal lobe.

We can only speculate what these results mean. Could it be that the engram moves from the medial temporal regions to these other regions over time, much in the way a gas might diffuse from an area of high density to an area of low density? Since the decline occurs mainly over a period of 6 years, after which both the increases and decreases plateau, does this suggest that there are really two different kinds of "long-term memory"—one of which is stored in the medial temporal lobe for the first 6 years and one that is relocated to other regions where the memory-correlated activations increase after that? Or, is it possible that these findings are contaminated by some cryptic, uncontrolled additional factor or statistical error that raises questions about their validity? What is clear is that given the variability of fMRI responses and the potential for misinterpretation, uncritical acceptance of very interesting findings like these should be delayed.

Earlier, Fletcher and Henson (2001) had argued that the lateral frontal cortex was divided into three regions each with its own functional responsibility. The three divisions of the lateral frontal cortex they believed to have their own cognitive responsibility were the anterior, dorsolateral, and ventrolateral regions. These divisions were partially based on anatomical demarcations (e.g., the inferior frontal fissure) and partially on the basis of their

Fletcher and Henson's fMRI findings. Specifically, they argued that the anterior region encoded the "selection of processes/sub-goals"; that the dorsolateral region encoded "selection/manipulation/monitoring"; and the ventrolateral encoded the "updating/maintenance."

Fletcher and Henson's analysis was based on a broad review of the literature as well as their own studies. However, they acknowledged the absence of a "completely consistent picture" attributing this inconsistency to (1) "poorly defined cognitive processes"; (2) "subject specific encoding"; (3) "small subject samples"; (4) "differences in strategies and performance"; (5) "variability in neural anatomy"; (6) "prespecified statistical thresholds"; and, finally, (7) a failure to "emphasize a more global picture of integrated systems in the brain" (Fletcher & Henson, 2001, p. 874). All of these putative sources of inconsistency, so cogently presented by Fletcher and Henson, were largely ignored during the early days of the stampede to brain imaging studies of cognition and are all too often still ignored by researchers who use fMRI methods to "localize" cognitive functions. Most germane to our review at this point was their acknowledgment of the ambiguity of the ways in which cognitive processes were attributed to the frontal lobes of the cerebrum.

It now seems likely that the response of the various frontal regions depends on both the psychological method used to study or encode the information and the cue used to recall a stored memory into working memory. For example, Fletcher, Stephenson, Carpenter, Donovan, and Bullmore (2003) showed that fMRI images varied depending on the task presented to the subject. Very slight differences such as those incorporated within the rubrics of "deep encoding" and "shallow encoding" (variations in episodic memory) led to substantial differences in cerebral responses. Deep encoding referred to stimuli that were processed according to their emotional overtones; this kind of stimulus produced maximum response in the left lateral prefrontal and left medial temporal regions of the cerebrum. On the other hand when spatial cues (such as underlining letters in a word) were used as stimuli, it was the right prefrontal cortex that was most highly activated. Similarly, but on the retrieval side, Otten (2007), showed that when different cues for recollection (a spoken word versus a picture) were used, distinctly different patterns of activity were observed in many regions of the brain including prefrontal, temporal, and parietal cortices.

In point of fact, the very word "learning" may be far too gross a concept for use in these kinds of correlative studies; and efforts to particularize "learning" into subcategories also quickly fall victim to vaguely defined constructs that do not match the actual neural mechanisms of the brain. Different subject matter topics, as well as different methodologies of study or retrieval, seem to invoke activities in different areas of the brain. Delazer and colleagues (2003), for example, studied complicated multiplication arithmetic using fMRI imaging and found that brain regions supposedly encoding these arithmetic tasks were differentially activated by different levels of learning. The regions they suggested that were most deeply involved in this kind of learning were predominantly on the left hemisphere and included frontal and parietal areas where activations seemed to vary as a function of the level of learning. On the other hand when quite a different "learning" task was used, the results turned out to be quite different and inconsistent. For example, Reber, Stark, and Squire (1998) reported bilateral activation patterns that included occipital, frontal, and right anterior frontal cortex when the subject was confronted with a category learning task.

What we see in all of this work is a great diversity of cerebral responses exhibiting an extreme sensitivity to the many variables involved in learning experiments. Aggravating this intrinsic variability is its sensitivity—slight changes in procedure can lead to substantial changes in response.

By far the most instructive argument against the idea that specific localized regions have evolved for "learning" in either a general or a specific sense is to be found in the profoundly important meta-study carried our by Cabeza and Nyberg (2000). Their work still remains the most comprehensive study of its kind up to the present. Although not all parts of the brain are activated by all learning tasks, it is clear from their charts and graphs that the PET and fMRI imaging technique produces extremely variable and inconsistent results (from experiment to experiment) because of technical reasons, because of ill-defined stimuli or tasks, or because of a real biological variability in the way the brain carries out its functions. None of their surveys found narrow localization. The best (i.e., the most concentrated and localized scatter plots) came from semantic memory retrieval experiments. On the other hand, episodic memory responses were scattered over much of the brain for both encoding and retrieval experiments. The salient point is that distinctively different response patterns appeared even when experimenters thought they were evaluating the same learning or memorial task. The most important implication of this meta-study for the present discussion is the lack of consistency and replicability—the keystones of scientific acceptability.

By far the best sampled of memory tasks was Cabeza and Nyberg's depiction of the sites activated by working memory. Although the frontal regions are traditionally most often involved in this cognitive process, almost all of the brain was shown to be activated when the findings from a large number of laboratories were accumulated. (The only exceptions to this generality were the temporal lobes. However, the absence of activity in these areas is better explained by then current technical difficulties with the imaging devices rather than by actual negative evidence.) Table 5.2 shows Cabeza and Nyberg's results for their working memory meta-review.[27] What is obvious from this meta-review is that working memory activates virtually all regions of the brain.

Most of the other kinds of memory functions discussed by Cabeza and Nyberg display this same kind of wide dispersion of cortical activations. It is only when one deals with cognitive processes dominated by motor mechanisms such as language or perceptual processes dominated by sensory mechanisms such as vision that the activations are more clustered. Even then, there is no suggestion of highly circumscribed localizations—widely distributed portions of the brain are still being activated in even the most restricted areas of their meta-study.

Table 5.2

Activation peaks associated with working memory

Table 5: Working Memory		Frontal										Cingulate				Parietal			Temporal								Occip			Subcort		
Study	Contrast	10	9	46	11	47	45	44	6	8	4	32	24	23	31	7	40	39	38	ins	42	22	21	20	mt	37	19	18	17	bg	th	cb
5.1 Verbal/Numeric																																
Paulesu 93	lett: hold English - Korean						●	●									●		●	●	●							○				●
Salmon 96	lett: hold English - Korean						○	○				■					○			○	○							○				●
Smith 96-1	lett: hold - match						○	○				◆				○	○		○										○		●	
Fiez 96b	wd/nonwd: hold 5 for 40 sec	●					○	○	◆																							●
Jonides 98a	nonwd: hold 5 for 40 sec		●				●	○	○								●															●
Awh 96	lett: hold - match						○	○				■				○	○		○										○		●	
Awh 96	lett: 2 back - search						○	●				□				●	○															●
Awh 96	lett: 2 back - rehearse							●								●	○													■		●
Becker 94	wd: 3-wd Rc - rest						○	○			◆					○	●			●	●		○							◆	●	
Petrides 93b	num: gen random - count	●	●					●					□			□	●															
de Zubicar. 98	lett: read random - alphabetic		○	●		●	●	●	●		●	□		■	□	◆	●	●	●			●				●	●	●				●
Schumach. 96	lett (visual): 3back - search			○		○	○	○	●			◆				◆	●											●				
Coull 96	num: update - search	○					○	◆								●	○											●				
Salmon 96	lett: update - Korean	●	●	○													●	●									●	○		■	●	
Cohen 97	lett: load factor (0 to 3 back)		●	●			●	●	■							●	●															
Braver 97	lett: load (0 to 3 back)		●	●		●	●	●	●		○					●	●	○	○											●		
Smith 96-2	lett: 3 back - search	●	●	●			○	○								●	○															
D'Esposito 98	lett: 2 back - search		●					●									●											●			●	
5.2 Object																																
Haxby 95	face: hold 21sec - sm	○					○					□						○				○				○						
Courtney 97	face: hold 8 sec (regressor)	●	●		●	●	●																		●	●	●	●				
Courtney 96	face: hold 3 - sm		●	●	●	●	●	○				◆															●					◆
Smith 95-1	shape: hold - match							○				◆				○								○								
Petrides 93a	shape: SOP - match	○	●					●				◆				●									●							
Belger 98-1	shape: hold - ctrl	●	●													●											●					
Elliot 98b	shape/col conj: hold - sm						○	○				□				◆	○								●		●	●	●	○	○	
Klingberg 97	patt: altern match - simple	●							■							●																
Owen 98	patt: 1 back - sm							●	●										●		●	●		○								
McCarthy 96	shape: det rep - sm	●				○																										
5.3 Spatial																																
Anderson 94	loc: del sacc - fix							●				□	□			○	○					●					●	●	●			●
O'Sullivan 95	loc: del sacc - rest	●						●				◆				●	●					●					●	●	●	●	●	
Sweeney 96	loc: del sacc - guided	●	●				◆	●					○					●										●				
Smith 95-1	loc: hold - match					●		●								●												●				
Courtney 96	loc: hold 3 - sm							●								●												●				
Goldberg 96	loc: hold 4 - match		●	○		○	●									●										○	●	●		●	○	
Owen 96b	loc seq: hold - sm							●								●											●	●				
Lacquaniti 97	loc point: 2 back - 1 back					□						□	□		□	●	●								■	○	○	●		□	◆	
Owen 98	loc: 2 back - sm						●	●				■				●	●									○						
D'Esposito 98	loc: 2 back - search			●				●								●	●			○							●				●	
Smith 96-2	loc: 3 back - search 3	○	●	●				●								●	●										●				●	
Owen 96b	loc: SOP - sm	●	●	●				●			●	■				●	●	●								●	●		●			
Owen 96a	loc: SOP - sm	●	○	○				●			●					●	●								■	■						
Gold 96	del resp altern - sm	○	○	●		○											○							○			●					○
Owen 96a	moves: hold 4/5 - point	●	●	○			○	○				■				●	●				●				●		●					
Belger 98-1	loc: hold - ctrl	○		●	○							■				◆	●	◆					●	○				●	○			
McCarthy 94	loc: det rep - sm		●																													
McCarthy 96	loc: det rep - sm		●																													

After Cabeza & Nyberg (2000).

All of this suggests (as do a large number of other studies that I have not treated in detail here) that there is a widespread activation of many parts of the cerebrum in an irregular and inconsistent manner during learning protocols. These results add credibility to the suggestion that a lack of control of the independent variable in an experiment and normal biological variability are more likely to determine the outcome of an fMRI investigation than any specific learning task, per se.

Furthermore, the frailty of our taxonomies of cognitive processes may also be accounting for the variation in imaging results. It may be that we have to conceptualize this entire enterprise in a new way emphasizing the distributed and generalized nature of the neural processes and the ambiguity of the cognitive tasks presented to the subject. It may be no longer satisfactory to preserve any of the vestiges of the older schema in which cognition is divided up into modular functional components and the brain into selectively functional regions. Much of the data I have surveyed here, however limited in scope it may be, supports the need for a bold revision in our thinking, if not just additional scrutiny. The assumed ability of the brain imaging techniques to tell where something is happening may be blinding us to the actual nature of this extraordinary organ—a nature in which practically all parts are activated in practically all cognitive processes.

5.5   Interim Conclusions

What can we draw from this admittedly incomplete and spotty review of the literature on the neurophysiological basis of learning and memory? To begin, it is clear that a substantial amount of current research effort is still mistakenly concerned with identifying the specific regions where learning and memory are purported to be represented and controlled. With regard to this "where" question, to the contrary, an emerging answer seems to be that the brain responses are observed in many different brain regions for even the simplest learning task. Learning, as this work not unexpectedly confirms, is a process in which many parts of the brain (perhaps all parts) are involved.

There are many unanswered questions in the cognitive neuroscience of learning. Some regions such as the hippocampus and the amygdala appear to be deeply involved in controlling the storage of information but do not appear to be the locus of that stored information—the engram. Where the engram is located remains a great unknown. Even more elusive is the challenge of defining what the engram is. What role the basal ganglia play is especially unclear; it is alternatively possible to think of their activation during learning as a measure of effort or emotion rather than an essential part of the information acquisition process. Thus, we may be confusing processes as effort or attention with learning itself.

Nevertheless, modern cognitive neuroscience persists in searching for the loci of brain activities associated with poorly defined psychological modules. It seems increasingly likely that this is a conceptual misdirection. As we learn how variable the findings are and how many different, dispersed regions of the brain seem to be involved in the many learning paradigms, further doubt is cast on the idea that specific learning processes or capabilities are localized in restricted regions of the brain. It is hard to imagine that each kind of learning studied by psychologists has produced its own regional specialization, but this is a necessary logical precursor of the idea that we might expect to find regional differences in the brain responsible for subtle differences in learning strategies.

Furthermore, there seems to be extreme sensitivity in the observed brain responses to the properties and conditions of the cognitive stimuli used to evoke them. Psychologists have known for years that very slight changes in experimental protocols (e.g., what kind of cue is used in retrieval) can produce dramatic differences in the pattern of brain activations.

A persistent problem with all of the neuroscience research on learning reviewed here is that efforts to measure the magnitude of the recorded brain responses use arbitrary and poorly defined metrics. "Response strength" was often inadequately defined and the metrics of the scales used often hidden away in obscure measures of the brain's response. Some reports used spatial extent of the involved voxels exceeding a threshold value as a dependent variable; however, there is no way to be assured that this metric correlates well with subjective magnitudes or skill levels.[28] Many studies used the mere presence of activation or such soft, quasi-qualitative measures of learning as "greater than" or "decreased" as metrics; the use of these approximations suggests a major difficulty in the quantification of brain images.

Furthermore, not all of the functional relationships were even of the same valence. For example, some studies showed that certain areas increased their activity during one kind of learning; whereas other studies showed decreases. It is not at all clear that a lower activity level at the gross level at which the fMRI operates is actually associated with a smaller subjective experience. Yet, this fallacy pervades much of the current literature.

Another problem with such an idiosyncratic, multi-area response is that it is not certain which parts of the brain can or should be associated with the learning process itself. Many factors can operate simultaneously to modulate the brain response, and it is difficult in any cognitive task to determine the one that contributes most to the variance of a response. This raises monumental problems in deciding on a critical brain image indicator of learning. Indeed, as Hilgetag, O'Neil, and Young (1996) have shown formally, it may be impossible to disentangle the hierarchical structure of a complex network. That is, it is unlikely that we will be able to determine the order of activations in a system with many feedback loops and in which inhibition and disinhibition also both play major roles. Therefore, it is not at all to be unexpected that there may be several different kinds of dynamic changes occurring simultaneously in the brain during learning, only some of which are related to the learning task itself. A further complication is that regions active at one stage of the learning cycle may not be the same as those active later.

Finally, I must reiterate that a lack of change per se in an fMRI brain image is not necessarily indicative of an absence of change in the microscopic synaptic interconnection pattern—a pattern where the crucial and essential neural equivalents of learning are assumed to be taking place. Substantial changes can occur in the detailed coding of the neural network without any change in the cumulative response depicted in an fMRI image. Remember, the brain image is a "blunt" tool; it pools the finer details of the more microscopic neuronal activities that are more likely to be the true psychoneural equivalents of learning into an unanalyzable and possibly irrelevant cumulative score. Enormous amounts of information are lost whenever data are pooled either across subjects or across repeated presentations of the same stimulus! I have expressed this elsewhere in the form of the aphorism "Data pooled are data lost!"

There are also many other technical problems with regard to the cognitive neuroscience research on learning. Like all of the physiological indicators that have been used over the years to compare brain activity and cognitive processes, the responses generated by differences between the experimental and control conditions are often relatively small. Data curves tend to be noisy and irregular and have relatively sparse data points over the continuum of independent variable values. Because of the diversity of responses observed in virtually any brain image, it is always likely that an energetic investigator will be able to find some relationship or some correlate between some physiological indicator and some behavioral response.

In short, although learning is one of the most actively researched areas in cognitive neuroscience, there is still no universally accepted objective brain image measure of any parameter of stored experience. Nor, for that matter, is there any unique relationship between any localized brain region and a particular aspect of learning. Instead, there is a complex interplay of many distributed parts of the brain interacting with a variety of behavioral measures.

In the following statements I try to summarize what I believe this brief review of the relation between learning and brain activity now tells us.

1. A major problem with research in this field is that the psychological constructs we call "learning" and "memory" are composed of so many different processes that there is actually very little replication of findings from one neuroscience experiment to the next. This contributes to a substantial amount of variability and inconsistency among those findings.
2. Both individual differences and the pooled brain activation patterns of a group of subjects in even well-controlled experiments are variable. Meta-studies show even greater variability. Pooling data probably tends to obscure some mind-brain relationships and to artificially enhance illusory conclusions. Where we would have expected convergence, pooling increases diversity of responses.
3. Both behavioral and brain image responses to trauma and surgery are idiosyncratic. Nevertheless, iconic cases set the conceptual tone for further experimentation in ways that may misdirect our research attention.
4. Slight differences in experimental procedures can produce enormous changes in findings. Both brain and behavioral responses are extremely sensitive to the type of learning task for inscrutable reasons.

5. Species differences in both behavior and neuroanatomy often hinder the development of coherent explanations.

6. Microelectrodes often hinder the appreciation of the distributed nature of the neural mechanisms accounting for higher cognitive processes by concentrating attention on highly localized neuronal responses and ignoring what all of the other unimpaled neurons are doing.

7. Currently, the most widely accepted taxonomy of learning processes (Tulving, 1972), although helpful in organizing a scientific study of the cognitive neuroscience of learning, has an inordinate influence on experimental design and the interpretation of the relationships between specific brain regions and particular types of learning.

8. Despite an enormous amount of research in this field, no overarching explanation of how the brain instantiates learning has emerged; nor have the specific roles of individual centers in the learning process been determined. Thus, there is still great uncertainty about how brain activity is associated with the phenomena of learning and memory. The following quotes drawn from some of the literature reviewed here give the flavor of this lack of systematic progress.

• "The medial temporal lobe (MTL) is critical in forming new memories, but how subregions within the MTL carry out encoding and retrieval processes is unknown." (Zeineh et al. 2003, p. 577)

• "The contributions of the separate components of this system [the medial temporal lobe] are not well understood." (Stark & Squire, 2000, p. 7776)

• ". . . the precise functional role of the hippocampus in episodic memory remains elusive." (Strange et al. 1999, p. 4034)

• "Although amygdala activity has been purported to be modulated by affective and nonaffective factors, considerable controversy remains on its precise functional nature." (Costafreda, Brammer, David, & Fu, 2008, p. 57)

• ". . . previous neuroimaging studies on the acquisition of fear conditioning have yielded conflicting results." (Cheng, Knight, Smith, Stein, & Helmstetter, 2003, p. 9)

Obviously much is yet to be understood about the brain mechanisms of learning and memory. We now turn to another topic—attention in which the scientific situation may be even less well understood.

6 Attention

6.1 Introduction

When one studies learning, there are clear-cut operational parameters that help us to design and carry out empirical research studies. These parameters permit us to determine the behavioral transformations that occur with experience and, in some cases, to correlate neurological processes with these changes. The independent variable—experience—can be readily controlled by regulating the number of learning trials or the duration of the training period. The effects of learning are also easily measured by any one of a number of performance tests, including such old standbys as "percentage correct" and "reaction time."

As our focus changes to attention, however, the problem of operationally defining what we mean by this elusive term becomes much more challenging. Attention is clearly a characteristic or property of a covert cognitive or mental state; as such it is subject to all of the vagaries of definition plaguing any mental or cognitive process. The actual dependent variable—the degree of attention—in this case is inaccessible and is very difficult to control. Efforts to control attention, therefore, do not have the force of the manipulation of the number of learning trials. At the most fundamental level attention is both unobservable and inaccessible as well as being practically difficult to specify and control. It is, as are all other mental processes, a private, intrapersonal activity whose properties, at best, must be gleaned from fallible introspection or inferred from behavioral results (both scientific strategies having their own limits and constraints). Profound changes in attention may go on with absolutely no overt behavioral clues.

Attention is, therefore, a much more elusive target for cognitive neuroscience than was learning. The problem is exacerbated because attention varies not only as a result of changes in the external stimulus environment but also as a result of its own dynamics—the inexplicable and uncontrollable sequencing logic that drives one "idea" onto the next. This "wandering of attention" in even the most constant stimulus environment is undoubtedly a result of associative links that may have been established (i.e., learned) between different mental states over an individual's lifetime. "That reminds me of this and this reminds me of that!" The study of the meanderings of the mental activity we call attention, therefore, is severely compromised at the outset because we cannot track these wanderings nor know what are the forces driving our attention from one object to another. In this regard, learning studies are simpler; we usually can define the stimuli and measure the behavioral responses. Artificial situations in which attempts are made to direct attention to a particular target cannot completely overcome this "flight of thoughts." The ravages of this kind of uncontrolled independent variables on research in this field quickly become evident.

A further problem arises out of the inadequate definition of attention as it does with most other cognitive constructs. There are two issues here; first, a number of similar research paradigms (or cognitive processes) may go by the same name, and, second, many names may be applied to what is actually the same phenomenon. Closely related to these ambiguities is that attention (and many other psychological processes) may be incorrectly perceived to be the distinguishable components, properties, or attributes of what are in reality a common process. William James (1890, paraphrased from p. 416), for example, divided attention into a number of distinguishable varieties any one of which could be the focus of an experiment. These include the following examples:

- Sensorial attention in which attention is directed at real environmental objects.
- Intellectual attention in which attention is directed at ideas or represented objects.
- Immediate attention when the object is interesting in itself.
- Derived attention when the object is interesting because of its relation to something else.
- Passive or nonvoluntary attention.
- Active or voluntary attention.

What differences, if any, distinguish each of these varieties of attention from the others remains a major conundrum for psychological science.

A much more modern effort in the same sprit to classify attentional processes was made by Cabeza and Nyberg (2000, p. 7). They offered the following five subcategories of research projects that they cluster together into the supercategory we call attention.

- Sustained attention
- Selective attention
- SR compatibility
- Orientation of attention
- Division of attention

It is interesting to note how little overlap there is between James's and Cabeza and Nyberg's minitypologies. Furthermore, even collectively they represent only a sample of the many different aspects, properties, or subdivisions of what many consider to be a unified process, activity, or procedural construct. The historical trend has been for each new experimental protocol to raise new possibilities that are subsequently reified into real entities and that expand on these two lists. The literature is voluminous and expanding; although the classic problems are still being studied, the variety of attention research has also grown. The even more dramatic tabulation of the components and processes of attention research shown in table 6.1 by various authors illustrates the diversity of topics studied in attention research.

One special problem that emerges from this definitional morass when one tries to characterize attention is the ever-present confusion or conflation of attention with other closely related phenomena. For example, by the substitution of a few words, all of the empirical manipulations carried out in the laboratory directed at the study of "attention" might equally well be considered to be a study of "working memory," "decision making," "span of apperception," or even "consciousness" and "mind" themselves. After all is said and done, attention is a hypothetical construct referring to the results inferred from a group of experiments purported to be evaluating one of the properties of self-awareness—what is it that is

Table 6.1
Components and types of attention

• Working memory	• Effort
• Competitive selection	• Attentional set
• Top-down sensitivity control	• Filtering tasks
• Filtering for stimuli that are likely to be behaviorally important (salience filters) (Knudsen, 2007)	• Voluntary control
	• Shifts of attention
• Serial processing	• Divided attention
• Parallel processing	• Monitoring
• Psychological refractory period	• Automaticity
• Visual search	• Psychophysics of detection (single stimulus tasks) (Pashler, 1998)
• Selective listening	
• Selective looking (Sperling's partial report technique)	To which we might add:
	• Vigilance
• Reaction time to alternative signals	• Orienting
• Divided attention (Wickelgren, 1979)	• Attentional capacity
• Monitoring with attention and without attention	• Integrality
	• Priming
• Limited auditory capacity	• Alerting
• Switching attention	• Stimulus (bottom-up effects)
• Selective attention	• Anticipation
• Arousal and threshold of attention	• Subliminal phenomena
• Conscious or voluntary attending	• Attentional sharing (divided attention)
• Span of apprehension	• Space and object frames of reference
• Attending to multiple inputs (Glass, Holyoak, & Santa, 1979)	• Goal neglect
	• Popout
• Selective attention	• Attentional blindness
• Attentional capacity	• Lapses of attention

momentarily occupying our thoughts? It is, therefore, very difficult to distinguish between attention and thought or thinking in general just as it is to distinguish it from such closely related hypothetical constructs as "working memory."

Just how complex are the interactions between attention and working memory has been highlighted by Awh, Vogel, and Oh (2006, p. 201). Their definitional distinctions between the two processes are at best only emphases on different aspects of a person's momentary cognitive state. Whereas they define working memory as the "temporary maintenance of information in a limited-capacity system," attention is defined as "the efficient encoding of relevant targets in spite of a potentially overwhelming quantity of sensory information." Even a close reading of their two definitions does not provide any operational way to distinguish between the two—if there is any real psychobiological distinction to be drawn. Either one could be encapsulated as that portion of our mental life from among all possible thoughts that is momentarily being processed.

Awh and his colleagues then attempt to disentangle these two processes by describing what they believe are the functions carried out by attention and working memory, respectively. Unfortunately such an effort is carried out at a purely inferential level, based as it is on speculations about the nature of these putative functions. Unfortunately none of the behavioral assay methods Awh et al. (2006) invoke can say anything definitive about internal mechanisms. Thus, we are left where we were—a conflation of two very similar processes whose distinctiveness is arbitrary and uncertain.

A further complication deals with the confusion of attention and consciousness. Although consciousness (or its near synonym—awareness) could easily be used as a synonym for attention, some residual uncertainty arises from the fact that in certain restricted circumstances we are able to appropriately respond to stimuli to which we are not "paying attention" and of which we are, therefore, "unconscious." All of us can recall situations in which we were driving a car and suddenly found ourselves a mile or so down the road with no recollection of having responded successfully (it is hoped) to the roadway stimuli. Nevertheless, the evidence is clear that we are capable of making necessary and appropriate control motions to stimuli that are not a part of our attentive consciousness. Clearly, this kind of "automatic behavior" can be as effective as that constrained by conscious, attentive responses. If behavioral responses can be delinked from stimulus awareness in some cases, what chance is there for a scientific examination of attention based on inferences from behavior?

Despite these difficulties attention has played an increasingly central role in contemporary psychological research. William James (1890) made an important and still valid point— if there would be nothing such as attention—". . . the consciousness of every creature would be a gray chaotic indiscriminativeness, impossible for us even to conceive" (p. 403). Thus, he was influential in establishing the role that attention might play in selecting from among all of the sensory stimuli that which is of interest, relevant, or salient. Whether it is a simple matter of overloading our mental capacities or the result of some kind of a complex filtering process was not dealt with at this point by James, but these ideas were to become the main themes of the kind of attention theory subsequently developed. What he did do was to offer a famous and oft-quoted working definition that, despite its relative antiquity, is as good as anything that we have nowadays.

Everyone knows what attention is. It is the taking possession by the mind, in clear and vivid form, of one out of what seem several simultaneously possible objects or trains of thought. Focalization, concentration, of consciousness are of its essence. It implies withdrawal from some things in order to deal effectively with others and is a condition that has a real opposite in the confused, dazed, scatterbrained state which in French is called *distraction* and in German, *Zerstreutheit.* (pp. 403–404)

Unfortunately, despite James's eloquence, not "everyone knows what attention is" no more than everyone knows what the "mind" is. Although there are hints here of questions that were to be subsequently asked by research psychologists, the links to independent entities or criteria (a property of all good definitions) is inadequate to precisely define attention.

With regard to the possible physiological mechanisms that might control attention, James did not do much better. Of course he did not have the neuroscientific knowledge we enjoy today, but he did speculate about mechanisms that might be involved. Two mechanisms in particular were suggested by him (p. 434):

1. The accommodation or adjustment of the sensory organs.
2. The anticipatory preparation from within of the ideational centers [*sic*] concerned with the object to which attention is directed.

In these two possibilities James laid the foundations for what has become the main controversy in attention research—is attention a selective process carried out early in the neural pathway, or is it a result of late or high-level associative processes? Unfortunately, as we see later in this chapter, this controversy remains unresolved and may possibly be unresolvable. Regardless of how this controversy may play out in the future, both of these suggestions depend on descriptions of a "conceptual nervous system" rather than of a biological one and both represent plausible if extrapolative inferences from common knowledge. Both, however, have within them a more materialistic, if metaphorical idea—the distilling, filtering, or funneling of the totality of our sensory experiences down to that small portion to which we are momentarily attending. Otherwise it would be James's *Zerstreutheit!*

Subsequent scholars have done no better. Indeed, for a longish period ranging from the heyday of Watsonian behaviorism until the second half of the twentieth century, few texts were written and little research was carried out on the subject of attention. Few attempted defining what current cognitive psychologists now accept as a core part of the experimental psychology paradigm. Such distinguished text and reference books as Kling and Riggs (1938) and Stevens (1951a) made only passing reference to attentive processes. This, of course was due in large part to the reluctance on the part of behaviorists to study such covert mental processes as attention and perception.

   Why attention did not play a more important role in the late nineteenth and early twentieth centuries was originally made clear for a very interesting reason by James (1890) himself. James pointed out that the whole idea of voluntarily "paying attention" ran counter to the prevailing empiricism of the nineteenth century. That is, the British empiricists, who had had such an enormous influence on American psychology of that time, taught that the experiences of our minds (including perception and attention) were determined by our life experiences and by knowledge (i.e., stimuli) coming from the external environment. Thus, the idea of having a free-floating and internally controlled process, such as attention, that was not fully determined by experience was contrary to much of their program.

   The second half of the twentieth century brought mentalistic cognitive psychology into prominence and increased psychologists' willingness to consider these very same mental processes as legitimate topics for psychological research. Although many workers finessed the issue of what attention was by simply operationalizing their experiments and avoiding a precise definition, a few efforts were made to make the meaning of the word more precise both in dictionaries and by theoretically oriented psychologists. I now tabulate a few of the offerings. First, we consider some popular definitions:

• Attention: The ability to focus on a selected stimulus, sustaining that focus and shifting it at will: the ability to concentrate. (MedicineNet.com)
• Attention: The concentration of the mental powers upon an object; a close or careful observing or listening. (Answer.com)
• Attention: The process whereby a person concentrates on some features of the environment to the (relative) exclusion of others. (wordnet.princeton.edu)
• Attention: Mental focus or serious consideration. (Dictionary.msn.com)
• Attention: The cognitive process of selectively concentrating on one aspect of the environment while ignoring other things. (en.wikipedia.org)

These definitions are by no means bad, but they get no operational gold ring. So, let us consider some more formal definitions by the scientific community to capture the essence of what we mean by attention.

• Attention is consciousness and something more. (Sir W. Hamilton as quoted in Ward, 1887).
• Two primary themes or aspects characterize the phenomenon people allude to with the term attention: selectivity and capacity limitation (Pashler, 1998, p. 2).
• To pay attention to something is to be consciously aware of it (Farthing, 1992, p. 11).
• Attention is not a single process, but an organized set of procedures. A procedure is a series of physical or mental acts used to perform a specific function (Glass, Holyoak, & Santa, 1979, p. 183).
• Endogenous attention [is] defined as executive and directed by voluntary acts. Exogenous attention [is] defined as automatic and directed by external stimulation (Peretti et al., 2008).

Although these definitions still fail to meet strict criteria of good definitions, most psychological studies of attention have attacked the twin properties of capacity and selectivity in one or another of their manifestations. These topics arise covertly, sometimes in forms such as distribution of attention, divided attention, or attentional switching time. In other experimental designs, processes such as serial or parallel processing can stand as surrogates for attention.

Thus, it seems clear that despite the large amount of research that it has stimulated, the term attention may be far too general and ill-defined (by any of its many definitions) to be a precise assay of psychological activities. What is actually being studied, therefore, are the properties or attributes of something we really can neither precisely define nor directly measure.

This result of the multiple meanings of the word attention was brilliantly developed by Allport (1993). He asked the rhetorical question—"Have we been asking the wrong questions?" Among his other contributions to answering this question, Allport tabulates some additional meanings of "attention" and some closely related terms such as "selection." We can add his list of possible definitions to those already presented.

- An obligatory process versus an available strategy
- Spatial orienting
- Selective facilitation
- Entry to a limited capacity short-term memory
- A cognitive outcome
- A causal mechanism
- A processor
- A response

Allport wisely pointed out that "Unless all of these, astonishingly, denote one and the same underlying operation, there can be no a priori grounds to expect just one 'locus of selection'" (p. 185). By arguing this point, I believe he was both attacking the value of the debate over early, middle, and late models of selective attention (to be discussed more fully later in this chapter) and the naïve idea of localization of such cognitive processes in the brain.

The question is, therefore, raised about the actual biological reality of attention. Can it meaningfully be defined, identified, described, or located in the brain? Or, on the other hand, can attention better be understood as a residual concept left over from earlier mentalist psychologies that currently only serves as a heuristic for certain kinds of behavioral research? Whether it has any reality as a tangible structure or a definable and unique process remains uncertain. The word attention, as I have previously noted, may not stand for anything; instead, it might be nothing other than another word for mind or thought as explored by a particular experimental protocol. Its transformation from an empirical property or experimental result to a "thing" whose physical equivalent must be located in the brain may be an example of what some psychologists refer to as "reification." Pashler (1998) phrased it well when he made this distinction:

The dangers of taking substantive words from ordinary language and assuming a corresponding entity have been noticed for a long time, of course; philosophers as far back as Bacon (1620/1960) have warned against assuming that where there is a word there must be a thing (this is often called reification). Closer at hand, one of the pioneers of modern attention research, the late Donald Broadbent (1982) emphasized the dangers in the uncritical use of the word "attention." However, like all vices, reification is more easily deplored than prevented . . . (p. 4)

When in place of a "word" we reify a "thing," the point being made is that we would be well advised to utilize behaviorally well-defined operations.

At best, attention may be considered to be a hypothetical construct or theory used to coordinate the results of a variety of experiments that tend to cluster together under the much-too-broad rubric of cognitive psychology. Attention in this context is hardly something that we can search for using the array of physiological techniques now available to us. It may be as much an inaccessible phantom as any other cognitive process and less likely than most of achieving anatomical tangibility. The idea of a place in the brain that serves as a biological marker for attention may be one of the biggest conceptual errors perpetrated by cognitive neuroscience. To better understand how such an error in scientific conceptualization might have occurred, let us now turn to some comments on the history of research on attention.

6.2   Psychological Research on Attention

The history of research on attention is nowhere as constant over the years as were experimental studies on learning. As I have noted earlier in this chapter there was a lacuna in this kind of research that lasted for almost 40 years. The original pioneering work in the late nineteenth century lay almost dormant until a resurgence of activity in the second half of the twentieth century. Why should this have been the case? One answer, as I noted earlier, is that this kind of research on otherwise inaccessible mental processes was frowned on during the ascendency of behaviorism. Another was attention's conceptual conflict with empiricism. Whatever the cause, interest in research on attention did not recover until the coming of the cognitive revolution in the 1950s. We can, therefore, think about psychological research on attention to be divided upon into two stages; a classic stage that started and ended in the nineteenth and early twentieth century and a modern stage that began in the 1950s. A dark age during which little research was done on attention existed between the two epochs.

6.2.1   The Classic Stage of Psychological Research on Attention
How we attend to some as opposed to all of the parts of our external environment had been a curiosity to philosophers for many years. Aristotle (384–322 BCE) spoke of such a process

as did Alhazen (965–1040 CE), the great Arab polymath. Some scholars suggest that, as long ago as the Renaissance, scholars such as Juan Luis Vives (1492–1540) had speculated about the role of attention in memory formation. Less cryptic is the work of Gottfried Wilhelm Leibnitz (1646–1716) who linked attention and consciousness and that of Herman von Helmholtz (1821–1894) who noted in his great *Handbuch* (Helmholtz, 1867) that an attended region would be "perceptually enhanced" compared to an unattended one. Helmholtz also was one of the first to suggest that attention and gaze could be separated and that attention could be shifted faster than gaze. Mangun and Fannon (2007, p. R171) recalled Helmholtz' words concerning attention. "These experiments demonstrated, so it seems to me, that by a voluntary kind of intention, even without eye movements, and without changes in accommodation, one can concentrate attention on the sensation from a particular part of our peripheral nervous system and at the same time exclude attention from all other parts."

Another early specific attempt to deal with the nature of attention is to be found in the work of the Scottish philosopher-psychologist Dugald Stewart (1753–1828). In a compendium of his writing (Stewart, 1829) he spoke of attention in the context of visual learning:

It appears from the acquired perceptions of sight, that a process of thought may be carried on by the mind, without leaving any trace in the memory; and many facts prove, that impressions may be made on our organs of sense, and yet be forgotten next moment. In such cases, our want of recollection is ascribed, even in ordinary conversation, to a want of *attention;* so that it seems to be a principle sufficiently ascertained by common experience, that there is a certain act or exertion of the mind, necessary to fix in the memory, the thoughts and the perceptions of which we are conscious. This act is one of the simplest of all our intellectual operations, and yet it has been very little noticed by writers on pneumatology. (p. 389)

After commenting on the ubiquitous, but overlooked, nature of this "exertion of mind," Stewart went on to make a comment that is extremely interesting in the context of the present discussion—namely that attention is a general "principle for the explanation of other phenomena" rather than a entity or thing itself. Specifically, speaking of attention, he presented the following argument:

Having established the certainty of the general fact, by an induction of particulars, we are entitled, by all the rules of sound philosophizing, to employ it as a principle for the explanation of other phenomena. Many very curious ones, which are commonly referred to other causes, are resolvable into this principle, in a manner equally simple and satisfactory. (p. 389)

I read this as his view that attention is a very general mental attribute or property that can be used as an organizing principle for a wide variety of observations; nevertheless, it is only an inferred or derived attribute of those "particulars" and not an isolatable, tangible thing in itself. This is expressed very much in the same sense as MacCorquodale and Meehl's (1948) concept of the hypothetical construct. Here, in one of the earliest statements identifying attention as an object of scientific study, its very existence as a thing unto itself is challenged—a harbinger of things to come.

The main wave of empirical work that can be specifically defined as research on attention, however, seems to have been initiated by Franciscus C. Donders (1818–1889). Donders (1868) is still well known as the inventor of a research technique that has been in continued use since his time–mental chronometry.[1] He applied his method to the study of attention summarizing his view in an oft repeated quotation: "Distraction during the appearance of the stimulus is always punished with prolongation of the process" (primary source unknown).

The next flurry of research on attention seems to have been carried out in Leipzig in what has historically been considered to have been the first laboratory of experimental psychology. Among the most notable early students of "attention" was the laboratory's founder—Wilhelm Wundt (1832–1920). Wundt studied attention using an introspective method. He believed that his "physiological psychology" carried out in the controlled environment of the laboratory was the only way to study consciousness. He considered attention to be another process that modulated consciousness; it was a measure of the degree to which something was in consciousness or not. This great pioneer in the establishment of scientific psychology, therefore, also appreciated that attention may not be so much a thing as a dynamic and ever-changing property of generalized mental functioning. However he also believed that properties such as attention could be measured; a conviction that allowed him to consider what was later to be called the "span of attention" or "apperception" as a target for his empirical studies.

Wundt produced an enormous body of publications and a very large number of students who pursued the psychological science he helped to create. These include such luminaries as Oswald Kulpe (1862–1915), James McKeen Cattell (1860–1944), Hugo Munsterberg (1863–1916), and E. B. Titchener (1867–1927), the last three of whom migrated to the United States where they had enormous influence as leaders in the newly emerging university-based departments of psychology and psychological laboratories. Many of these Leipzig-trained psychologists attacked the problem of attention to a greater or lesser degree in their subsequent research activities.

In addition to the psychology and physiology students, Ludwig Lange (1863–1936), a physicist, also worked for many years in Wundt's laboratory. Lange (1888) made use of Donder's technique to produce what many consider to be the iconic, if not the first, experimental study of attention. In this experiment he showed that the reaction time depended on to what the subject was attending—either the sensory (stimulus) or the motor (response) aspects of the experimental design.

The kinds of research that followed from Lange's were extremely varied with attention becoming a major part of the Leipzig research program. In particular, a dominant theme of Wundt's group was to determine the effect on reaction time of effortful attending to a stimulus compared to an inattentive set; the general effect was exactly what one expects—the more one anticipates a stimulus, the shorter is the reaction time.[2]

Another main question asked during this classical period of attention research was—What is the capacity of attention? Even then, it was obvious that we were able to attend to but a small amount of the enormous inflow of sensory experiences. Questions such as these remain open, and much current research deals with these very same issues.

6.2.2 The Modern Stage of Psychological Research on Attention

Although there were numerous publications from a number of psychological laboratories on the problem of attention in the early twentieth century, as I noted earlier, there remains a lacuna—a dark age—between that period and the middle of the twentieth century. It was not until the end of the World War II when the information-processing model became popular and the cognitive revolution emphasizing mentalistic psychologies occurred that research was directed anew to the problems of attention.

At the risk of offending those who may have preceded them, it seems widely accepted that the renaissance of interest in attention as a psychological research topic began with the publication of several key research articles on selective hearing by Cherry (1953) and by Cherry and Taylor (1954). This research was motivated by such surprising observations as that people are able to selectively attend to a single one of a babble of conversations (the cocktail party effect). Another important discovery was "dichotic listening" a listener's ability to select which of a pair of auditory messages was attended to when the two messages were introduced separately, but simultaneously, into opposite ears.

In what was considered to be a seminal experiment, Cherry and Taylor measured the amount of time to switch attention from one ear to another (0.2–0.3 seconds) when the recorded speech messages were switched from one ear to the other. The second part of their study determined that although two very different messages could be fed into the two ears, only a single speaker was "heard." This confirmed one of the major results of Cherry's earlier paper where he had shown that the perception of the information from one ear could be completely blocked.

The next important development in this renewed interest in dichotic listening was carried out by Moray (1959). He showed that the attentional cutoff in the dichotic listening situation was not complete; instead, it depended on the salience or emotional content of the signals to each ear. For example, if the subject was attending to the right ear message and the subject's name was read into the left ear, the subject would respond to his own name significantly more often and faster than to an unrelated word. The main conclusion drawn by these investigators was that it is neither the raw properties of the stimulus nor our volitional ability to direct attention that completely determines the acquisition of information. The semantic content can also be a powerful influence. Attention can, therefore, be a major confounding variable in many other kinds of psychological experiments.

This is, of course, a complication for psychologists who would like their phenomena to be influenced by as few variables as possible.

These results also led to the modern theoretical debate on selective attention—at what level of the mind–brain does the selection process that filters out some stimuli and enhances others occur? Is it early, in the middle, or late in the cognitive-processing chain? Several names stand out in this debate—Broadbent (1958), Treisman (1960), Deutsch and Deutsch (1963), and Norman (1968) for their theoretical as well as their empirical contributions to this problem.

The debate still depends on a conceptual model of the attention system that is made up of a number of different modules or mechanisms as shown in figure 6.1.

Broadbent's original theoretical explanation was based on the hypothesis that the filtering or blocking of the unattended information occurred very early in this system. According to his model, in a dichotic listening experiment the information from both channels is temporarily stored in a sensory memory or buffer. At the next stage, the information in the "unattended channel" (i.e., the ear to which one is not attending) is blocked by a selection mechanism that prevents it from being passed up to the short-term memory, working memory, or whatever it is that we call the site or process of attention.

Broadbent's (1958) early filtering theory was quickly challenged, however, by some curious results from the early experiments carried out by Cherry and others. It was observed that the filtering or blockage of the unattended information was never complete. There was some leakage of information from the unattended ear, for example, and subjects often reported at least partial mixtures of the two streams of information, especially when the

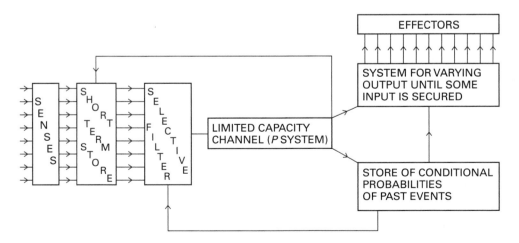

Figure 6.1
A functional theory of low-level attentional filtering.
From Broadbent (1958), with the permission of Pergamon Press/Elsevier Publishers.

incoming information had some personal significance to the subject. This result suggested that high-level cognitive processes might have more influence on attention than had been thought by Broadbent.

Treisman (1960) emphasized the importance of these mixtures or leakages in her proposal of another version of the early filtering idea. In Treisman's model, unlike Broadbent's, it was acknowledged that the filtering was never complete; instead, it permitted intrusions (from the unattended ear to awareness) based on the speaker's gender, the emotional content of the word, or a failure of the filtering action. This partial failure of the filter led Treisman to assume that attention was operating at an early level. On this basis Treisman proposed a model in which the filtering was "attenuated" by high-level or late mechanisms and could break through into attention under some conditions.

A distinction was often made between the perceptual and the response mechanisms in this discussion; perception implying the *availability* of the information up to high levels of the processing mechanism (although it might be unattended) and response being associated with the actual *awareness* (i.e., it was being attended) of the information. Treisman and Geffen (1967) as well as Norman (1968) interpreted the available data to support the perceptual version theory, but it was still mainly an early filtering approach to the explanation of this phenomenon as shown in figure 6.2. That is, the process of filtering out the unattended information occurred at the peripheral level, although it could be affected by

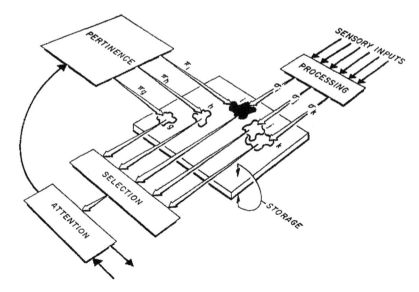

Figure 6.2
A functional theory of high-level attentional filtering.
From Norman (1968), with the permission of the American Psychological Association.

high-level processes.[3] Forgetting was often implicated as a low-level culprit since there was little ability to recall the information presented to the unattended ear (Moray, 1959).

The alternative to the early filtering theories assumed that attention was a high-level or late process that excluded the information from our attention rather than an early one. Deutsch and Deutsch (1963), for example, argued that although we were not aware of the unattended information, it existed at relatively high levels of our cognitive system, and it was not blocked from awareness until it arrived there. It was only at these high levels of the cognitive nervous system that the final determination was made based on the relative "importance" of the high-level information whether or not it would be attended. "Importance" in their model was an actual physical dimension in a manner analogous to choosing the tallest from among a group of boys (their analogy).

Knudsen (2007) has provided anther pictorial model of the cognitive processes that he believed constituted the essence of attention. Shown here in figure 6.3, Knudsen's theory, like Norman's and many of the others, involves a feedback process from the higher levels to the lower that acts as a regulator of what will come to the subject's attention.

As the database became more complex and more often internally inconsistent, intermediate (between early and late) theories of attention proliferated. Examples of this kind of accommodation were the hybrid theories of Johnston and Heinz (1978) and Yantis and Johnston (1990). They argued, as with the feedback model of Norman (1968), that both early and late processes were involved. Early selection occurred, but according to this point of view, the filtering mechanisms were controlled by a high level "semantic" analysis. Hybrid theories such as these are compromises that have developed as the data accumulated and the empirical inconsistencies became apparent. As such these intermediate-level theories may simply have been introducing new degrees of freedom into the discussion that permitted plausible, but still untestable, models to be constructed. The persistent problem in the study of attention or any other high-level cognitive process, for that matter, is the underdetermination of the underlying mechanisms by behavior.

Another kind of argument that the incoming information is available up to a high level of the cognitive system even though it may not be "attended to" is the well-known Stroop test (Stroop, 1935). In this test contradictory cues to the name of a color are given, and the subject is told to respond to one cue and ignore the other. For example the word "red" may be printed in green ink, and the subject told to attend (i.e., read the printed word). The increase in the reaction time when the word red is printed in an incongruent color and the word red printed in the color red has been used as an indication that the irrelevant, unattended cue (color) still has an impact on reading the printed name. Thus, the information must be getting up to a "high level," and the blocking or filtering must be occurring there.[4]

In this contex, the high-level theories began to look a lot like memory theories. A plausible, but untestable, hypothesis is that on close inspection attention is not actually an "attention" phenomenon, but merely a manifestation of a memory failure![5] That is, a

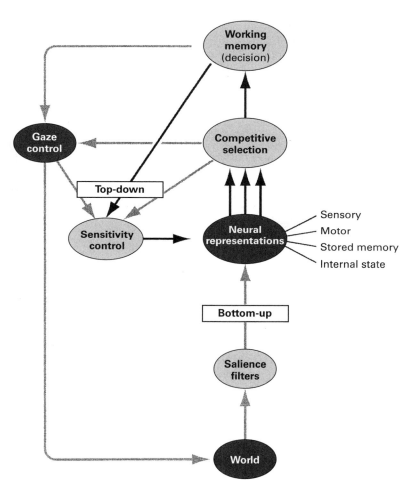

Figure 6.3
An alternative functional theory of high-level attentional filtering.
From Knudsen (2007), with the permission of Annual Reviews, Inc.

high-level theoretical explanation assumes that the information from an unattended channel simply was forgotten more quickly than that from an attended channel, although it had been available sufficiently long to influence our responses. From this perspective, we attend to everything but can remember only a part of it; the part that is encoded into short-term memory and then into long-term memory is that to which we attend. Attention, as a scientific term, would tend, according to this theory, to evaporate into a secondary side show for memory. Of course, this will not happen as long as the modular approach to cognitive processes remains dominant.

The analogy, if not identity, of attention and habituation (a form of learning according to the formal definition presented in the introduction of this chapter) should also not be overlooked. Operationally, the wandering of attention in a vigilance task is hardly distinguishable from the reduction in a person's response to a constant stimulus. For example we quickly cease paying attention (habituating?) to the clothing we wear. Again, the point is that "attention" is very difficult to distinguish from other cognitive processes except as a property of cognitive processing.

Perhaps the most currently influential theory of attention is the one proposed by Treisman and Gelade (1980) and referred to as the "feature integration theory of attention" (FITA). Briefly, FITA is based on the idea that a visual stimulus is composed of isolatable features (e.g., color, orientation, and shape) that are processed "early, automatically, and in parallel" (p. 98). This idea seems to have been stimulated by the rush of discoveries preceding the 1980s that the transmission encoding processes of the peripheral visual nervous system were carried out by parallel, but separate, channels for each feature type. Although information about the individual features is available at an early level of the attention system, Treisman and Gelade argue that the perception of the whole object depends on feature combination at a late or higher level within the focus of attention. If certain features were not attended to, the entire object might never penetrate our perceptual experience.

Treisman and Gelade (1980) then went on to assume that the different features of a visual stimulus object are treated differently by the attention system depending on the degree to which they are necessary (i.e., must be integrated) for perception to occur. In the words of another formulation, this is the degree to which the features are integral or separable for the perception of the object (Garner, 1974; Monahan & Lockhead, 1977; Shepard, 1964a, 1964b). These authors argued that integral dimensions cannot be ignored without loosing the entire percept, but ignoring separable ones does not otherwise diminish the experience. In either case, attention is necessary for the features to be combined into a coherent "correct" perception of the whole object. Not only is attention necessary, but Treisman and Gelade (1980) also argued that it must be applied serially to each of the features to determine what is perceived.

Treisman and Gelade (1980) reported the results of a number of experiments that convinced them not only of the plausibility but the accuracy of FITA. These included studies of the following:

- Visual search
- Texture segregation
- Illusory conjunctions
- Identity and localization
- Interference from unattended stimuli

The specific experimental findings reported in their behavioral studies are probably not contradictable. However, the theoretical formulations seeking to explain the observed phenomena at either a functional or neurophysiological level are far less robust.

In sum, FITA is a much more detailed theory of attention then was found in any of the theories previously mentioned. Whether or not it is a compelling explanation to other researchers is arguable, but there is no question that it has been enormously influential in dictating the course of current research on attention.[6] This does not mean that it has escaped challenge, and a number of researchers have sought to refute it. A recent article by Driver (2001) discusses some of the contradictory evidence that continues to fuel this continuing controversy.

Before continuing with this discussion, I should point out that many of us feel that *in principle* there is no way to distinguish between these early, middle, hybrid, and late theories *on the basis of the behavioral data alone*. The "black box" constraint is concerned with the invisibility of internal mechanisms in a closed system, means that *in principle* there are an infinite number of possible internal mechanisms that could account for the behavior. Thus, the so-called "theories of attention" debated during this time were in actuality arguments from one cognitive or behavioral response to another; analogies, ambiguities, and uncertain data simply drove the discussion from one "plausible" explanation to another. No robust refutation or confirmation of any of them is possible since none of these theories are specific enough to be resolved by the empirical findings. Nor are any of them in any sense quantitative enough to predict specific results. Furthermore, they fall victim to many of the same constraints on reduction discussed throughout chapter 1.

Driver (2001) zeroes in on the implications of these constraints when he notes that "A reader surveying the extensive literature on the early vs. late selection debate . . . . might lose hope of any resolution, since roughly half of the evidence seems to support each opposing camp" (p. 61).

Driver then went on to suggest some possible ameliorating explanations[7] for this discrepancy; however, it may be that the problem raised here is much more fundamental than is generally appreciated.

Yantis and Johnston (1990) alluded to the same problem a few years ago in their efforts to resolve the debate when they noted, "In spite of three decades of intensive investigation with a variety of paradigms (including partial report and search tasks) no consensus has yet emerged on the locus of selective attention" (p. 135).

These insightful comments about the difficulty and uncertainty that characterize the search for the "locus of attention" lead one, once again, to ask whether the task is achievable. After all, as the entire content of this book testifies, there is ample evidence that trying to extrapolate from behavioral results to internal neural or cognitive structures may be an impossible quest.

The continuing controversy, however, did not deter a number of people from developing further descriptive theories as new data continued to reveal the full complexity of whatever it is that we call attention. Indeed, given the highly interactive nature of the neural system that must be responsible for those cognitive processes, it is not at all certain that we would be able to determine the independent effect of a neural unit whose inputs come simultaneously from many levels of the nervous system. This difficulty would be exacerbated if the functional nodes for different activities are not spatially separate but actually intermeshed with the fine neuronal network structure of the brain. Certainly, the simplifying and often simplistic assumptions (as illustrated in the pictorial models proposed by each author) that underlie so much of this research may not be justifiable.

None of the problems or limitations of the purely behaviorally based theories seem to have discouraged subsequent research on attention by psychologists. This topic has continued to play a central role in the evolution of cognitive psychology. It has been approached with an enormous variety of experimental protocols, and both new and old questions are constantly being asked such as these:

- What is the capacity of attention?
- How do we switch attention?
- How do we become aware of unattended inputs?
- Do we switch attention based on a place or an object?
- Can attention shifts be covert (without eye movements or must they be overt?
- Is attention made up of separate processes or mechanisms such as engagement, disengagement, and shifting or a single unified mechanism as proposed by Posner (1988)?
- Are attention shifts automatic or intentional or both?
- What is the relation between attention and monitoring and arousal?
- How long and what is the cognitive penalty for switching attention?

A number of workers stand out in the reinvigoration of attention studies in the latter part of the twentieth century when it was realized that the early versus late theoretical debate was going to be either very difficult or impossible to resolve. This next phase of research saw a shift from the traditional problem to other questions.[8] For example, Kahneman's (1973) book shifted the focus of research from the automatic processes that had been emphasized by the previous theories of attention to the ideas that we could direct our attention about at will.

One new direction was "the frame of reference problem; that is, do we shift our attention based on a general spatial frame of reference or one based on the geometry (unity) of an object's frame of reference? In this context Duncan (1981, 1984) reported that there was an advantage in the time taken when the shifts of attention were confined within the boundaries of an object compared to when the shift was to two different equally distant locations that were not part of an object. This added a whole new dimension to Posner, Snyder, and Davidson's, (1980) studies of "space-based" attention shifts. This line of research has become a major topic in recent years with such researchers as Brown and Denny (2007) providing both new data and an excellent review of this twig of the attention research tree.

A further change in research in recent years was the reduction in the number of studies that were acoustic in design (especially the dichoptic experiments) and the increase in visual studies. Another important distinction between the early work and this second phase had to do with the problem of attentional priming—how do our sets or expectations influence that to which we will attend. Neely's (1977) oft-cited work on priming is considered to be another milestone in the ever-changing panorama of attention research.

Psychophysical studies of attention continued to proliferate in the latter half of the twentieth century. Beyond the work on the early-late debate, a number of other investigators tackled other problems. Shiffrin (1977) studied the automatic nature of attention; Logan (1978) discussed the effect of attention on pattern recognition; Cowan (1995) studied the interactions between attention and working memory; and Egeth and Yantis (1997) offered a general review of visual attention. Of course, we must also include the studies of Posner (1978) and Posner and Petersen (1990) wherein the idea of an attention system separate from the sensory and motor systems first began to germinate. Meyer and Kieras' (1997) work on how one switches attention when confronted with multiple tasks is also an important milestone in modern studies of cognitive capacity and dynamics. The role of attention expressed in the organization of Neisser's (1967) paradigm-shaking textbook should not be overlooked. Nor should we overlook the classic paper by Miller (1956) entitled "The magical number seven plus or minus two," which was clearly a study of attentional capacity.

At this point in this brief historical review the number of reported psychological studies of attention has ballooned out much in the same way that those in learning have. It becomes impossible in practice and wasteful in principle given the goals of this book for me to review all of them. I must apologize to the many productive scientists whose work I have passed over.

Clearly, the concept of attention is heavily intertwined with virtually all other cognitive functions. Attention is influenced by as well as able to influence, effort, practice, memory, in addition to a host of other factors. Attempting to identify it as an independent or quasi-independent entity makes little sense in this context.[9] Furthermore the concepts of attention and willful control are also deeply involved in some of the most fundamental problems of philosophy and theology including the perennial task of understanding the degree of "free will" available to humans.

This then brings us to the next step in this review—is it possible to resolve some of the "black box" constraints on understanding how attention works by looking into the black box itself? In other words is a neuroscientific resolution of the many theoretical problems raised when one attempts to study attention possible?

6.3   The Search for Attention in the Brain

We have seen in earlier discussion how a plethora of different meanings of the word attention have been used as targets of psychological investigations. It does not take long, furthermore, when one reviews past neurophysiological and neuroanatomical research studying
attentional brain mechanisms, to discover how equally large and varied is the resulting body
of cognitive neuroscience findings.

However, sheer abundance is not the first or major problem. First we have to consider
that there is no a priori reason why hypothetical cognitive concepts such as "attention"
should isomorphically map either directly or at all on the neural mechanisms that actually
underlie the observed behavior. Our psychological concepts, modules, faculties, or components are defined by inferential processes that may lead us in very different directions than
those that have evolved in the anatomical structures and physiological processes of the
brain. Thus, there is enormous uncertainty that cognitive constructs will correspond to
neural mechanisms in the ways we might initially have hoped. Of course, the informational
processes do have to correspond to some brain activity as argued in the most basic ontological postulate presented in section 1.1.

Despite the logic of this argument, isomorphism of hypothetical mental modules and
localized brain mechanisms is an implicit assumption built into much of the neuroscientific
research discussed throughout this book. Whether it is by means of surgical interventions
or brain images, the unjustified assumption was that if the functional time course or shape
of a neural correlate of a cognitive process such as attention were the same, the neural event
was the psychoneural equivalent code for the cognitive process.

However the intrinsic uncertainty of the relation between attention and the physiology
of the brain was obvious even during the pre-imaging days. The auras of uncertainty and
perhaps even of unresolvability confused the debates that raged for decades and have not
yet been resolved. Given this uncertainty, it would be very surprising if even the powerful
ability of the most modern techniques to observe and measure brain mechanisms would be
sufficient to answer the great conundrum of how the brain instantiates cognitive processes
such as attention.

At this point in our brief history of research on attention, a major new factor can be
introduced into the discussion. Virtually all of the work I have described so far has been
psychological. That is, the discussed experiments are the results of often ingeniously
designed, but fundamentally uninformative, experiments with regard to underlying neural
mechanisms—experiments in which the external environment was manipulated, and the
behavioral responses were measured. Psychologists operating in this domain, therefore, were
essentially studying a "black box" with all of its attendant difficulties and constraints.
However the mid-twentieth century was the golden age of surgical studies of behavior-brain
activity, and it did not take long before these neuroscientific findings began to be included
in the discussion.

Once again it is possible to separate the discussion into two distinct parts to understand the neurobiological context. The first stage is characterized by the classic tradition of surgery, electrical stimulation, and intracellular recording. The second is typified by the revolution in cognitive neuroscience that occurred with the development of PET and fMRI imaging systems.

6.3.1 The Classic Stage

The Great Conflation
The neuroscientific study of attention does not have as long a history as does the study of learning. Nevertheless, from the earliest explorations attention has often been invoked as an ex post facto explanation of performance successes and failures on various kinds of behavioral tests. A recurrent feature of this older work on attention was the difficulty that investigators had in defining and controlling the cognitive process they thought they were studying. As a result, it was quite common to conflate attention with other equally inaccessible cognitive processes such as learning or even general arousal. Much of the earlier research on what was called visual attention, in retrospect, was actually concerned with the motor control of gaze direction.[10]

A major problem leading to confusion and conflation occurs when one concentrates on any particular region of the brain. This difficulty is exacerbated in studies of the frontal lobe. The frontal lobes have been shown to be involved in a variety of different cognitive processes, many of which are difficult to distinguish behaviorally. Duncan (1995), for example, lists a number of behavioral defects due to frontal lobe damage (see table 6.2). Many other examples of ill defined and variable behavioral dysfunctions arise when the frontal lobes are damaged as discussed throughout this book.

Efforts to find some common theme for all of these normal and abnormal behaviors have not been successful, but many of these behaviors seem to closely parallel what we mean by attention. The result was a continuing problem with conflation and, thus, confusion over what is actually being measured when one attempts to determine the brain mechanisms of attention.

Table 6.2
Behavioral deficits associated with frontal lobe damage

• Attention	• Apathy
• Disinhibition	• Unresponsiveness
• Impulsivity	• Perceptual analysis or classification
• Distractibility	• Memory
• Rigidity	• Response Selection
• Perseveration	• Spatial or verbal problem solving

From Duncan (1995).

An example of such a conflation between what are better considered to be quite distinct cognitive processes is work done on the interpretation of the delayed response test. In this study researchers such as Jacobsen (1936) and Jacobsen and Elder (1936) explored the effect of brain lesions on delayed responses.[11] Although this was originally framed as a memory task, Finan (1939, 1942) subsequently demonstrated that the results could not be attributed to memory (the experimental animal did not forget the location of the food) but, instead, were better conceptualized as an inability of the animal to initially associate the food with the location in which it was placed—i.e., a failure in "attending" during the early exposure in which the location of the food was cued. What Jacobsen argued at that time was that it was frontal-lobe damage that mainly seemed to account for this failure in performance. Similar lesions in the temporal or motor regions did not destroy the monkey's ability to locate the food when there was a substantial delay between the original stimulus exposure and the selection of the food-containing cup. This unique association between frontal lobes and the delayed response is now disputed by more modern findings in which the prestrate region was also shown to be involved—a harbinger of the increasing distribution of responses observed for many cognitive processes in the years that followed.

Another seminal and very influential early study in which attention was conflated with something else was Wurtz and Goldberg's (1972) summary of their extensive research on the role of the superior colliculus in the shift of visual gaze. They stated (p. 448), "When an awake monkey shifts fixations from one point in the visual field to another, we can assume that he is shifting his attention from one point to another."

Although it is now widely accepted that attention may be separated from gaze direction (Helmholtz, 1867; Muller, Philiastides, & Newsome 2005; Ohlendorf, Kimmig, Glauche, & Haller 2007; Posner, 1980), the repeated demonstration of this dissociation had been ignored for many years. Many experiments were apparently conflating "shifting of attention" and "facilitating of movement" during this early phase of research on the brain correlates of attention. The result of this conflation was that Wurtz and Goldberg (1972) mistakenly assumed that the superior colliculus controlled attention when their studies, as well as much of the other work done at that time, can in retrospect be seen to only demonstrate its role in the control of eye movements.

Indeed, Wurtz and Goldberg (1972) went even further astray in concluding that the superior colliculus "is not critical for eye movement guidance" (p. 448) a conclusion that runs counter to more recent views (e.g., Sparks, 1999) of its role in the control of gaze direction. Instead, they proposed that a collicular lesion affected the transfer of information concerning visual attention from some higher center to the occulomotor system and that it was not a defect in that control system itself.

A general difficulty in this kind of research is that a shift in eye position to a different part of the visual scene can change the response of what appears to be an "attention"-related brain region even though there had been little change in the attentive state of the animal. Thus, a change in the physical scene could be misinterpreted as a neural correlate of attention especially if attention was incorrectly associated with gaze direction. In an interesting study that sought to reconcile this conflation, Lee, Williford, and Maunsell (2007) reported that although both contrast and attention affected the magnitude of a neuronal response in Visual Area 4 (V4) of the visual cortex, and a shift in contrast affected latency of the response, a shift in attention only minimally affected the latency. Although this was a major step forward in deconflating attention and contrast, it is hard to even guess at how many times ignoring this aspect of the conflation problem had misdirected the conclusions of previous researchers.

Early Localization Studies of Attention in the Brain

A major (if not the major) goal of research during this early stage of cognitive neuroscience was identifying the regions of the brain that were responsible for the attention process. We now appreciate that attention is associated with a variety of different brain regions. This surfeit of associated locales appeared both in research using experimental brain surgery (once past the earliest studies) or single cell recordings and in the modern stage of brain imaging technology. We now review some of the areas that were implicated in the representation of attention during the early stage of brain imaging.

An important early example of the multiple regions that have historically been connected to attention is to be found in the pioneering work on attention and arousal by Moruzzi and Magoun (1949). These researchers built their experimental protocol on the foundation observation that the EEG had totally different properties when a person or an experimental animal was apparently asleep compared to when that person or animal was behaviorally alert. Their contribution was to show that electrical stimulation of a core region of the brainstem known as the reticular system (subsequently known as the reticular activation system or the RAS) led to widespread cortical EEG changes during which high-voltage slow waves changed to low-voltage fast waves. Moruzzi and Magoun attributed this difference to a generalized "activation" of the brain by the RAS. The RAS responded to signals from any one of the normal sensory modalities. The changes in the brain's EEG responses were very widespread and diffuse as opposed to the more localized activity induced by stimulation of any of the sensory pathways alone. Indeed, direct stimulation of the RAS could produce the changes in the EEG even when none of the usual sensory pathways was activated.

Moruzzi and Magoun's (1949) original and very important contribution was, it should be pointed out, purely electrophysiological—they only measured the EEG response. They did not manipulate or measure any mental or behavioral variables beyond the simple observation that their experimental animals appeared to be either alert or asleep. Nevertheless, if one reads their work, it appears that they made the usual implicit, but incorrect, assumption that a behaviorally alert animal was the same as an attentive animal. It seems quite possible for an animal to be generally alert without attending to any particular aspect of its environment. The general philosophical issue raised here is obvious; how do we determine that an animal has any mental activity from its behavior?

As noted earlier, attention was early on associated with frontal lobe injury by a number of researchers (e.g., Milner, 1963). Studies of the effects of removing different parts of the frontal lobes, however, indicated that different regions might have different effects. The complexity of this system has led to the development of a huge variety of "neuropsychological" tests of questionable validity of what is purported to be frontal lobe function.[12]

Indisputably important, but poorly defined, executive functions such as "strategic planning" and "attention" are without question affected by frontal lesions. (This has been known since 1848 when Phineas Gage was injured in his iconic accident.) This simple conclusion is clouded, however, by the fact that the frontal regions perform so many tasks and are involved in so many neural systems that it is difficult either to assign any particular function to any particular region or to exclude any region from participation in particular intellectual functions.

A continuing problem with efforts to study the effects of frontal lesions is that the high-level cognitive processes (including attention) are so vaguely defined that it is not always clear exactly what cognitive process is actually being studied. For this reason experimental tests are sometimes used that are remote from the complexities of human cognition or are trivial and inadequate models of human mental activity. The situation is exacerbated by the fact that many of the behavioral results of frontal lobe damage in humans are extremely variable.

The potential for confusion is also enhanced by the fact that a large number of different brain regions other than the frontal lobes have been associated over the years with behaviors that seem to reflect deficits in the ability to attend. Although there were many reports of frontal lobe involvement in attention during the early years, it is certainly not the only area of the brain that is so involved. For example, Lynch, Mountcastle, Talbot, and Yin (1977) associated single-neuron responses in Brodmann area 7 of the parietal lobe with attention. These cells became active prior to and during eye movements that had been stimulated by target movement but not when the eye movements were spontaneous. The fact that their experimental animals did not provide any direct evidence of "attention" makes their hypothesis that attention was associated with these cellular responses somewhat less than robust. It would be, furthermore, very surprising if these cells alone controlled such a complex cognitive process as attention given that there are so many other areas with which area 7 is interconnected (Goldman-Rakic, 1988).

Moran and Desimone (1985), furthermore, showed that the neural responses of single neurons in both the inferior temporal and the extrastriate cortex of an animal that was trained to "pay attention to a visual stimulus" were dramatically reduced when the animal's attention shifted to a location outside that neuron's receptive field. Interestingly, there was no reduction in the response of cells in the visual primary receiving area to these shifts in attention. This result supports the idea that the problem of neural localization and representation may be very different for sensory and cognitive processes respectively, a problem to which I return in the next chapter.

A number of other brain regions have been traditionally associated with the cognitive processes designated as attention. Among many others, Goldberg, Colby, and Duhamel (1990) have proposed that the lateral interparietal region of the brain is not only a main center for encoding attention but that it is also made up of a number of different subregions that carry out distinct attentional subfunctions.

Adding to the uncertainty of the role of specific brain regions in attention, the traditional assumption that removal of brain tissue creates specific *deficits* in performance is not always justified. Occasionally, removal of brain tissue paradoxically leads to enhanced performance. It has been suggested for a number of years (e.g., Lynch, 1980) that the posterior parietal or parieto-occipital regions of the brain are also involved in attention. Unilateral surgical or traumatic damage to those parts of the brain resulted in what has been referred to as contralateral neglect—the animal seems not to be able to detect or attend to stimuli coming from the opposite side of the body. One study (Lynch & McLaren, 1989) showed, however, that visual neglect could be overcome by additional surgical destruction of the same brain region on the other side of the brain.[13] No completely satisfactory explanation for this paradoxical result of behavioral improvement is available, but it does illustrate the very complex interactions (such as disinhibition) between various regions of the brain.

To add to the difficulty in interpreting the role of various brain regions in attention, in many instances the putative response of a particular region is modulated by both the stimulus configuration and what are presumed to be higher levels of brain activity. Thus, there is an implicit conflation of both high- and low-level influences on the observed responses. In such a situation, it is very difficult to determine what is the proximal "cause" of an observed response. For example Kniermin and Van Essen (1992) showed that neuronal responses in the primary visual cortex varied in concert with the detectability of a stimulus in a complex background—the more components in the background, the less was the response. In other cases, however, control of these very same responses seemed to be exerted from higher cortical levels onto lower ones.

In recent work using single cell recordings, Womelsdorf, Anton-Erxleben, Pieper, and Treue (2006) and Fries, Womelsdorf, Oostenveld, and Desimone (2008) have confirmed that the visual receptive field of neurons in the medial temporal region, and the "early extrastriate" region of the visual system fluctuated with attention. Once again the complexity of the neural interactions precludes any simplistic assignment of attention to a circumscribed brain region.

The complexity of the brain's interactions and the large number of regions involved in attention do not end there. Mesulam (1981) suggested that attention is controlled or modulated by a system of brain regions that includes, in addition to the posterior parietal lobe, parts of the limbic system in the cingulate lobe, a frontal lobe component now known as the frontal eye fields (and alternatively located in the lateral premotor area), and a brainstem reticular component. Each of these brain regions, according to Mesulam, has a specific function in the control of directed attention. The posterior parietal cortex is involved in sensory representation; the frontal cortex in motor representation; the cingulate cortex in motivation; and the brainstem in arousal. This model has been updated based on fMRI imaging data by Gitelman et al. 1999, without any significant change. In this new version of their model, the brainstem regions were particularized to include the basal ganglia and the thalamus. In addition the new findings from fMRI images suggested that the posterior temporo-occipital cortex (a region of the medial temporal cortex) and the anterior insula were also activated during these attention-based experiments.

That the system of neural areas involved in the processing of the cognitive state we call attention is complex is now well appreciated. For example the network shown in figure 6.4 is another author's (Johnson, 1995) effort to describe the extended neural system involved in attention.

This type of hypothetical system emphasizes the complex and distributed nature of the "network" of brain structures that are involved in the regulation of what we call attention. In particular it is especially important to note that all incorporate "top-down" structures that make the stimulus-driven aspects of attention almost pale into insignificance. They also require us to reconsider the many formal difficulties in unraveling such heavily fed-back systems from brain images or from behavioral inferences.

The variety of experimental designs used to control the cognitive state of an experimental subject leaves much to be desired. Thus, we never can be sure what the animal or human subject is actually doing when asked to perform a task in which attention is manipulated.

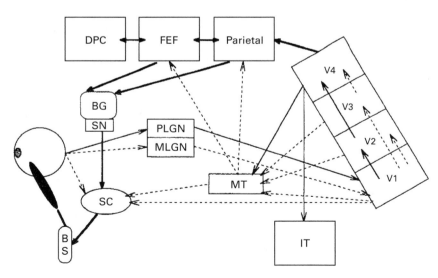

Figure 6.4
A neural model of visual orienting and attention.
From Johnson (1995), with the permission of MIT Press.

There are always several different alternative cognitive strategies that can confuse and distort our interpretations of what may be happening at the cognitive level. Attention may be confused with distance judgments (e.g., Cowey & Irving-Bell, 2006), poor memory, or any one of a number of other factors that are inextricably entangled in even the best-possible controlled experimental design. Not only can people not report their mental strategies in solving problems, but all of the techniques we use to modify behavior during such tests are rarely able to provide the degree of control necessary to unravel the interactions within the exceedingly complex system that includes our brain and its behavioral and conscious consequences.

The major conclusions to be drawn from this early search for the neural bases of attention are twofold:

1. Many different regions of the brain have been associated with variations in attention.
2. Most researchers now believe that attention is encoded as a complex interaction of these many regions rather than being associated with a single area.

An excellent and comprehensive review of the many regions in the brain that have been involved in the early stage of neuroscientific studies of attention can be found in Desimone and Duncan (1995). This is a good jumping off point for discussion of the next stage of research because it was at about this time that brain imaging began to have such a huge impact on cognitive neuroscience.

6.3.2   The Stage of Brain Imaging

The study of attention using brain imaging is new enough that it is possible to identify a clear starting point—the seminal paper of Posner, Petersen, Fox, and Raichle (1988).[14] It was here that some of the earliest findings linking PET images and cognitive processes were first published. Even more important, however, was the clear statement these authors made of what has been the most fundamental and continuing question permeating the entire field. That question was the degree to which the brain mechanisms for cognitive processes such as attention were localized or distributed. Posner et al.'s (1988) answer to this question at that time was a most specific one:

The hypothesis is that elementary operations forming the basis of cognitive analyses of human tasks are strictly localized. Many such local operations are involved in any cognitive task. A set of distributed brain areas must be orchestrated in the performance of even simple cognitive tasks. The task itself is not performed by any single area of the brain, but the operations that underlie the performance are strictly localized. (Posner et al., 1988, p. 1627)[15]

In so stating this theoretical assumption Posner et al. set the conceptual framework for not only attention research but for almost all of the work on cognitive neuroscience using brain imaging techniques. Although a number of our colleagues have ignored the distributed systems aspect of this theory and have continued to offer up single specific regions for one or another kind of cognitive process or subprocess, it is becoming more and more widely accepted that many parts of the brain are involved in even the simplest cognitive activity.

What remains uncertain and is the current crux of dispute is actually twofold. First, there is the question of the range of brain areas that are involved in a cognitive activity such as attention. Recent research seems to suggest more and more brain areas are so associated. This empirical fact leads to the idea that the "system" so elegantly and forcefully invoked by Posner and his colleagues is actually more than a "distributed system." In fact, an increasing body of research suggests that it may be most of the brain. This will become evident as we identify the very large number of brain regions that have been reported to be involved in attention in subsequent paragraphs.

Second, the nature of the neural nodes that are part of this distributed system remains open to question. Posner and his colleagues (1988) assert that these "elementary operations" are "strictly localized." However, there is still considerable uncertainty about what the elementary operations are and, beyond, that, just how localized are they? A plausible question may be asked—does any part of attention actually exist as an independent and "strictly localized" entity? Similarly, we must also inquire into the specificity of these "strictly localized" brain regions. If localized, does it mean that they have no other function with respect to phrenology, or does it means that they also play a role in other cognitive processes as well? Furthermore, what is the extent of their "strict localization?"

These questions, it should be acknowledged, may not have simple answers. Instead, it may be possible only to answer them in terms of a judgment call concerning what constitutes "localization." In other words we may be called on to judge how wide a region of activation can be before we would consider it to be localized. Much of the remainder of this section deals with the evidence that pertains to these questions.

The initial answer of Posner et al. (1988) to these questions is that attention without intention to perform motor acts mainly activates the medial frontal lobe and the anterior cingulate gyrus. They arrived at this conclusion on the basis of PET responses.

More recently, Posner and Rothbart (2007) have invoked a more complex tripartite explanation of attention based on research such as that carried out by Fan, McCandliss, Fosella, Flombaum, and Posner (2005). Using fMRI imaging and appropriate psychophysical tasks that they believed distinguished among "orientation," "alerting," and "executive attention," they argued that different clusters of brain regions were associated with each of these three aspects of attention, respectively. Orientation, according to them, is associated with activations of the superior parietal, temporoparietal junction, and frontal cortices, and the superior colliculus. Alerting, according to their data, is instantiated in activity localized in the thalamus, the locus coeruleus, and the right frontal and parietal cortices. Finally, they suggested that the purest from of cognitive attention—executive attention—is represented by activity in the anterior cingulate, the lateral ventral and prefrontal cortices, and the basal ganglia. This is, on reflection, pretty much the whole brain.

The task at hand nowadays is to spell out sufficiently precise cognitive tasks to distinguish between the three systems. It is not at all certain that this is possible. At the very least, we know that the each of the clusters of brain regions they mention has many other functions. At the very worst, the hypothetical model of three separable or isolable systems with specific functions may be a conceptual convenience to explain a diversity of otherwise incoherent observations rather than a neurobiological reality! At the roots of this difficulty are the poor definitions and distinctions, for example, drawn between "alerting" and "executive attention" as well as the high degree of variability and inconsistency of the empirical findings when one depends on brain imaging devices.

The imaging data provided by Posner and his colleagues is very attractive; however, they leave much too much leeway for scientific interpretation. For example, when one looks at the actual data displayed in Fan et al.'s (2005) figure 2, it is clear that the regions of activation are not quite as clear cut as either the verbal descriptions or the graphic depictions shown in Posner and Rothbart's (2007) figure 2 suggest. The fMRI images indicate that even the responses of the "localized" activations are broadly distributed about the brain. There is considerable overlap in the fields associated with each of the three "aspects" in their model.

Posner and Rothbart (2007) then cite a dozen research articles (see their table 4) that they assert are studies of networks. In fact, none of the cited reports specifically examined the properties of interacting networks; what they actually did was to study the wide distribution of brain regions that are activated to a greater or lesser degree when certain cognitive tasks are carried out. Furthermore, there was little consistency among the 12 papers with regard to the location of the activated regions.

It is interesting to compare Posner and Rothbart's (2007) results with those of other investigators. A review (Behrmann, Geng, & Shomstein, 2004) that was aimed at the role of the parietal lobe in selective attention in both fMRI images and human neuropsychological cases suggests a considerably different pattern of responses than Posner and Rothbart proposed. Where all of these investigators agree that parietal regions are deeply involved in representing selective attention, Behrmann and her colleagues (2004) emphasized a strip of parietal and temporal regions running from the superior parietal region down to the medial temporal lobe. (On the basis of idiosyncratic human neuropsychological data, they also believed that the globus pallidus and the putamen of the basal ganglia were also involved in attention.) Posner and Rothbart (2007), however, paint a different picture of the involved brain regions adding other regions more to the anterior and posterior portions of the brain.

Despite their differences, both of these groups agree in implicating broad swaths of cerebral tissue in the representation of attention. This, however, has not always been the case for others using fMRI as their measure of cortical activation. Wojciulik and Kanwisher (1999), for example, reported very restricted regions associated with several different kinds of attention. They suggested that two relatively small regions—the junction of the

intraparietal and transverse occipital cortex (IPTO) and another region at the anterior intraparietal cortex (AIPS)—are the only regions that are always activated no matter what test of
attention was being used.[16]

To what can discrepant results in associating particular brain regions to attention be
attributed? It seems clear that the type of behavioral test that is used strongly affects which
brain areas will be activated. For example Weissman, Roberts, Visscher, and Woldorff (2006)
used reaction time as a surrogate indicator of attention and found that when there was a
reduction in fMRI recorded activity in the anterior cingulate and right prefrontal regions
prior to the presentation of a stimulus, there was a prolongation of the reaction time to
that stimulus. They hypothesized that this was neurophysiological evidence that these
regions were involved in the subject's not paying attention in preparation for the next trial,
in other words, exhibiting a "lapse in attention."

However, Weissman and his colleagues (2006) went even further and showed that when
the reaction times were long, the amount of activity induced in the visual cortices was
concurrently reduced, thus suggesting that the attention-related mechanisms may be even
more widespread than suggested by the predictive regions—the anterior cingulate and the
right prefrontal regions. This alternative "top-down" view argues that these regions facilitate
or gate information to the visual cortices. Such a theory probably does not give due credit
to any possible "bottom-up" influences from relatively low levels, which have also been
invoked as participants in the attention process by other researchers.

For readers interested in a comprehensive review of the "top-down" versus "bottom-up"
approach to attention, I recommend the review article by Kastner and Ungerleider (2000).[17]
They indicated that fMRI studies indicate that a wide variety of brain areas are activated
when a subject is directed to attend to different attributes of a visual stimulus such as color
or shape. The visual areas that selectively respond in this manner include areas of the extra
striate cortex including the posterior and midanterior portions of the fusiform gyrus and
the medial temporal region. However, they also list other areas implicated by fMRI studies
of attention including a "network of areas outside the visual cortex" including the frontal
and parietal regions as well as the frontal and supplementary eye fields.

Other workers also report widely distributed fMRI activations in response to cognitive
tasks that seem to be associated with variations in attentiveness. In an attempt to unravel
the interactions of the eye movements associated with ocular gaze and what is now generally appreciated to be a separable attention mechanism, Ohlendorff et al. (2007) designed
a complex multifaceted task in which gaze shifting and pursuit were compared with attention shifting and pursuit. The fMRI activations that remained after the subtraction of the
eye movement activity from the attention plus eye movement activity (the residual activations were assumed to be a purer form of attention) was associated with superior and inferior
parietal lobe and postcentral gyrus activations, the latter being a region traditionally associated with somatic sensation.

Attention has been shown to modulate a somewhat different set of brain regions by Vuilleumier, Armony, Driver, and Dolan (2001). When subjects were directed to attend to faces, maximum fMRI activations were reported in the right and left fusiform and temporal-occipital regions. These responses were independent of any emotional effects. Curiously, if the stimuli were houses instead of faces, then a somewhat different set of brain areas was activated. Instead of the mainly fusiform activations, the main regions responding to this kind of stimulus were the parahippocampal, retrosplenial, and lateral occipital regions.

The role of the parietal regions in attention has been reemphasized by Uncapher and Wagner (2008) who were interested in the problem of how attention affects episodic memory. They suggested that two regions in the post parietal cortex–the dorsal and ventral regions—were responsible—independently and respectively—for effortful (i.e., conscious) and automatic (i.e., reflexive) attention shifts. Despite the recentness of this report, it is surprising that they did not indicate the role of any of the many other brain regions that had previously been associated with attention. Perhaps this was intentional since their interest had been restricted to the post-parietal cortex. Nevertheless, by showing that this region had important contributions to make to those that had been primarily associated with either learning or memory, they also illustrated the high degree of functional interconnectedness between both the regions of the brain and the cognitive processes that all too often had been dealt with separately in the past. Their findings support the contention that the post-parietal cortex is a part of a complex and distributed system of intertwined cognitive and neural processes, not the least of which is attention.

The complexity posed by the many interactions among brain regions and the difficulty of defining and controlling cognitive processes are becoming increasingly clear. Depending on the nature of the task—whether one is attending to auditory sentences or visual images—the involvement of areas previously unequivocally associated with attention has now come into question. The anterior cingulate, for example, is one of the regions that many researchers had previously linked to attention (e.g., Bush, Luu, & Posner, 2000; Heilman & Valenstein, 1972). However, newer work (Fellows & Farah, 2005) indicates that that area may not play a critical or even necessary role in the process we call attention. Similarly, Newman, Keller, and Just (2007) showed that activations of the prefrontal region are also regulated by the nature of the stimulus and what the subject is directed to attend to rather than having a dedicated and unchanging association with a particular cognitive process such as attention.

There are many other examples of brain areas whose involvement in attention-related activities depend on the task or test but areas whose exact roles remain variable and uncertain. For example Culham, Cavanagh, and Kanwisher (2001) devised an experiment that distinguished between two different sets of brain regions based on the attentional load. (Load was defined by the difficulty of tracking a computer display of a bouncing ball in a visual psychophysical task.) They found one group of brain regions—the frontal eye fields, superior parietal lobe, parts of the precuneus, and the medial temporal region—that seemed to quickly reach a high level of activation at low attentional loads, but did not further increase parametrically with the load. On the other hand there was another group of brain regions that seemed to track the varying load as regulated by the difficulty of the psychophysical task. These included the superior frontal, precentral, and supplementary regions, the anterior, posterior, and intraparietal regions, and a region where the occipital and parietal lobes adjoined. Within these two sets of regions, however, there was some overlap, and a few voxels that were load dependent were found in regions that were otherwise not thought to be load dependent.

Culham, Cavanagh, and Kanwisher (2001) concluded that those regions that did not vary with attentional load were, therefore, associated with processes other than attention—for example, the control and suppression of eye movements. They proposed that those cerebral regions whose activations varied with attentive load actually mediated the elusive process of attention itself. In my opinion, these post hoc explanations do not take into account the inconsistency of findings in both the earlier and current literature.

There appears to be an emerging consensus that extensive control information is fed back from higher attention-mediating levels of the brain even to the most peripheral sensory areas of the brain. For example Chawla, Rees, and Friston (1999) have shown that if a subject is asked to attend to the color or the motion of a stimulus, the response in the different extrastriate regions supposedly associated with each of those respective stimulus attributes is activated *before* a stimulus is presented. Similarly, a subject who is directed to attend to a particular stimulus position displays heightened fMRI brain activity in the brain regions associated with the retinal position also *before* the stimulus occurs (Kastner, Pinsk, De Weerd, Desimone, & Ungerleider, 1999). How much of the variability of results in sensory experiments is due to inattention or anticipation on the part of an experimental subject remains unknown. Nevertheless, what these experiments do strongly argue, once again, is how difficult it is to control the independent variable called attention; it is a difficulty that may help us to understand the failure of the many studies that tried to answer the superficially simple question—what parts of the brain encode attention?

The list of brain areas that have been shown by fMRI images to be involved in attention continues to grow. Relatively low-level or peripheral areas in the visual system (i.e., the visual cortex and the lateral geniculate nucleus of the thalamus) have been shown to increase their fMRI signals when subjects attend to a specified location (O'Connor, Fukui, Pinsk, & Kastner, 2002). Corbetta, Kincade, and Shulman (2002) and Beauchamp, Petit, Ellmore, Ingelholm, and Haxby (2001) implicate the intraparietal lobe and the frontal and precentral regions in attention. Interesting, although slightly outdated, reviews of this topic may be found in Corbetta, Kincade, and Shulman (2002) and Yantis and Serences (2003). A somewhat newer review of the field can be found in chapters 8 through 17 in Posner (2004b).

There remains no better source for summaries of the brain areas involved in attention by brain imaging techniques nor a more fitting place to conclude this discussion than the heroic meta-review carried out by Cabeza and Nyberg (2000). Although their review of attention-based activations was based on a smaller sample than those they cited in their review of learning and memory studies, it is of interest to examine their results as reproduced in table 6.3. Unsurprisingly, there is a considerable amount of activity observed in the parietal region by the 42 studies that are summarized in this table; there is also considerable activity indicated in a number of other regions. For example there is substantial activity in the occipital and frontal lobes as well as in the basal ganglia and in the cerebellum.

Table 6.3 indicates that at least some investigators have reported activations in virtually all parts of the brain. It is interesting to note that no region of the brain is excluded by these data from participating in attention despite the different tasks that were used to define attention. It must also be remembered that this selection of activation sites is further biased by the fact that the temporal lobes were not being imaged very well with fMRI techniques during the period that preceded Cabeza and Nyberg's important meta-review.

The general impact of these experimental results is to argue strongly for a very broadly distributed system responsible for the process we call attention. Clearly, the answer to the question of what parts of the brain are involved in encoding or representing attention is "nearly all of them!"[18]

This, then, is a sample of the empirical data. In themselves these findings do not mean very much; it is only when we seek to interpret these findings that we make the transition from robust observation to fragile explanation. In the concluding section of this chapter, I seek to build on the observations presented earlier to develop an interim view of the current status of research on this topic.

6.4   Interim Conclusions

It is clear from this review, however spotty and incomplete it may have been, that the distribution of brain regions that have been associated with attention is very large and very variable. Although some of this can be attributed to the lack of control over the independent variable we call attention, some to flawed experimental design or statistical analysis, and some to simple randomness, it seems to be a biological fact that attention should not be considered to be represented by one or a few isolated or specialized brain regions. Instead, it has been shown that almost all of the brain is involved in its representation.

The multiplicity of brain activations involved in attention is supported by the anatomical fact that all of these responsive areas are heavily interconnected. New techniques such as diffusion tensor imaging, known as DTI, provide additional vigor to the traditional anatomic study of brain white matter by showing the many connections that course among virtually all portions of the brain. Neither the traditional surgical approach nor the PET and fMRI procedures that have been used in recent years are capable of disentangling the functionally

Table 6.3

Activation peaks produced in experiments involving attention

Table 1: Attention		Frontal										Cingulate				Parietal			Temporal									Occip			Subcort		
Study	Contrast	10	9	46	11	47	45	44	6	8	4	32	24	23	31	7	40	39	38	ins	42	22	21	20	mt	37	19	18	17	bg	th	cb
1.1 Sustained																																
Pardo 91	lum: det dimming - rest	●							●							●	●											❖				□
Pardo 91	touch left: det pause - rest	●				●	●	●								●						●						❖			□	
Cohen 88	tone: det targ - rest	●	●																													
Cohen 92	tone: det targ - rest	●	●																													
Meyer 91	touch: det change - (touch + calc)															●																
Benedict 98	syll: det targ - nontarg	■	●							■		❖	❖			○	○											❖	●			
Coull 96	num: (RVIP) det seq of 2 - rest	●	○					❖	■	○						❖	○											❖	■			
Coull 96	num: rest - (RVIP) det seq of 2	□	□									□		□	□		❖					●		○								
Lewin 96	lum: det dim - rest	●							●																							
Kinomura 96	*lum: det change - rest*																															□
1.2 Selective																																
Corbetta 90	shape: det shape Δ - det any Δ																					❖		●	❖	○	○	○				
Corbetta 90	patt: det velocity Δ - det any Δ																○															
Corbetta 90	col: det col change - det any Δ																										❖	❖				
Heinze 94	symbols: attend left - pass enc						□					■															●	○				
Heinze 94	symbols: attend right - pass enc																											○			□	
Pugh 96	*wd/tone: dichotomous - binaural*						●									❖	❖															
Woodruff 96	num: det targ aud - det targ vis																				○	○	○									
Clark 97	obj: attention: col - face																										●					
Beauchamp 97	*mot (speed): spat/speed -spat/col*																									❖						
Büchel 98a	vis mot: det change - pass enc	●	●		❖			❖								❖	❖										❖	●		❖		
Vandenb. 97	obj: single feat discr - rep 2wd							●	●							●	●													○		
Rees 97a	obj: col and orient - col or orient									●																						
Allen 97	*shape/col: det targ - pass enc*																															○
1.3 SR Compatibility																																
Pardo 90	Stroop: wd/col - name wd col	□								○		❖					○						●					❖		○		
Bench 93-1	Stroop: wd/col - name fix col						●						■			❖																
Bench 93-1	Stroop: wd/col - name wd col															○	●															
Bench 93-2	Stroop: wd/col - name fix string col	●										■																				
George 94	Stroop: wd/col - name bar col		○			○						□	❖				○						○					○		●	❖	
Taylor 97 - 1,2	Stroop: wd/col - neut wd/false font					○	○																									
1.4 Orientation																																
Corbetta 93	asterisk probe: LVF/RD - cent det								●			■				❖	❖															
Corbetta 93	asterisk probe: RVF/LD - cent det									○		■	□			❖																
Corbetta 95	*col/mot: det targ - pass enc*															❖																
Nobre 97	lett: discr targ - baseline					❖						■					●					●				●				○	□	■
Coull 98	shape: (PET) orient spat/temp-rest		❖	❖			❖		○							❖										○	❖	❖		○		❖
Coull 98	shape: (fMRI) orient spat/temp-rest	❖	❖	❖			❖		○							❖			❖							○	●		❖	❖	❖
Le 98	det targ col - sel shape or col											❖																			❖
Kastner 98	periph stim: attend cent - blank																									○	○	□	□			
1.5 Division of Attention																																
Benedict 98	text/syll:det targ+ text-det targ- text						○	○																								
Vandenbergh 97	obj: dual feat discr-single feat discr		○				○	○				□				○								○		○						

From Cabeza & Nyberg (2000).

interconnected regions of the brain. Clearly we do not yet have a coherent conceptual model of the mind-brain system that is adequate to provide answers to the question of how attention is represented in the brain—all of the modern technology notwithstanding. This deficiency becomes especially evident when one considers that we may be examining attention at the wrong level of analysis of the brain.

It is also important in evaluating the implications of this review of the cognitive neuroscience of attention to remain aware that every one of the areas that has been associated with attention in this chapter has also been associated with other cognitive processes. A comparison of the activation areas mentioned in each of the chapters should remind us that none of the regional associations made in this chapter with attention should necessarily be interpreted as being exclusive of other cognitive processes. It is clear now that not only are many areas involved in each cognitive process but that many cognitive processes are represented by activity in any given area.

Whatever the specific results or associations, one undeniable interpretation is continuously reinforced—the response to any cognitive process is widely distributed on and within the brain. The list of different regions that have been associated with attention seems unending and includes to a greater or lesser degree virtually all areas of the brain. The early emphasis on the parietal lobe may well have been a "culture of science" artifact. Initial discoveries were concentrated there, and some of our most influential scholars have tended to direct the focus of the collegial community to that part of the brain. The preponderance of recent data suggests otherwise—the parietal lobe no longer seems specialized for the processing of the elusive phenomenon we call attention.[19]

However this is not the most difficult problem highlighted by the array of findings discussed here. The most exasperating is the aura of unreliability that surrounds virtually all of the reported experiments. Meta-studies emphasize that the lack of replication is profound. Obviously a number of factors contribute to the inconsistency of findings. These include poorly defined and controlled attentive states and tasks, the large number of possible interacting parameters, and technical and statistical uncertainties in analyzing data.

There are a number of misconceptions permeating the cognitive neuroscience of attention that may possibly be misdirecting us on the path to understanding. Lurking in the background is, for example, the continuing influence of the localization assumption; the phrenological ghost that simply will not go away. Implicit, if not explicit in all of this research, is the idea that there is a locale on or within the brain at which a particular cognitive process (or some part of it) is represented. It is difficult to find an experimental report that is not framed in terms of the query—what macroscopic part (or parts) of the brain accounts for attention? This, of course, is the question that imaging devices are designed to answer. Nevertheless, despite its simplicity and the gross spatial "tuning" of the imaging devices, this may be a misleading (i.e., bad) question since the answer to the "where question" increasingly seems to be "everywhere."

Whatever is the eventual empirical outcome, attention should probably not be conceptualized in the form of an "organ system" as proposed by Posner and Fan (2008). Instead, attention is better conceptualized as a "process," "state," or "property," rather than a "thing" or a "place." The attentional "organs" are nether isolatable functionally or anatomically nor are they yet adequately defined operationally. Nor, for that matter, do they have the tangible nature of anatomic structures that distinguishes the components of other organ systems from each other.

Implicit in Posner and Rothbart's (2007) network idea is that attention is represented by an aggregation of functionally specialized nodes; explicit is that these nodes "can be associated with a particular function or mental operation" (p. 17). Whether or not this idea is correct is still open to question. Much of the logic behind the rigid localization of "mental operations" is also a byproduct of the persisting emphasis on the modularization of mental processes that permeates so much of cognitive neuroscience. An alternative idea is that the "nodes" are just regions of general functionality that can be recruited to participate in a variety of cognitive functions without any special or exclusive functions attributed to them.

A further problem in this context is that the idea of a "network" can be little more than a metaphor for wide-spread brain activity; it is not necessarily a system in a formal mathematical sense that can be analyzed into its independently functioning parts, their interconnections, and their respective roles in representing attention. A different set of assumptions (as well the mathematical proof that the analysis of such heavily interconnected network is impossible) has been offered by Hilgetag, O'Neil, and Young (1996). They argued that the network metaphor may actually be empty of empirical or conceptual content since analysis is impossible.

The review carried out in this chapter can now be summarized by the following list of general conclusions.

1. Attention is a poorly defined cognitive or mental process for which, unlike learning, it is difficult both to control the independent variable and to measure any exclusive effects of it on performance.
2. Attention may be a general property rather than an isolatable module of cognition. It is very difficult to isolate it from other closely related cognitive processes such as working memory or even the more general notion of mind or consciousness. Some theories actually assert that attention (or, better, inattention) is a memory "defect," not a filtering process.
3. Responsiveness to stimuli does not depend solely on attention or awareness. It is, therefore, conceptually difficult to design an empirical experiment based on the assumption that attention and responsiveness are parametrically related in any simple way.
4. Psychological studies of attention rarely provide clear-cut answers to even the simplest questions of mechanism and internal process. Great issues remain unresolved after over a century of research in this field. Where progress has been made, it is terms of the behavioral and information-processing transformations.

5. However, there is no possibility of confirming or rejecting any purely psychological theory of attention with neurophysiological methods. This constraint also holds for theories of all other cognitive processes. Only when a theory contains neuroreductive postulates is it subject to test.

6. The designs of attention experiments are often conflated with or confounded by other closely related cognitive processes. The most obvious example is the confusion of effects due to eye gaze direction with the cognitive state of "paying attention."

7. It may not be possible to neurophysiologically isolate what are actually tightly interacting cognitive processes.

8. Many experiments on attention are known to be heavily dependent on the psychological task demanded of the subject. It is difficult to compare such experiments when each may unavoidably utilize different combinations of cognitive abilities and properties as stimuli.

9. Virtually all parts of the brain have been implicated in the representation of attention. Whether this represents a contamination of the findings by poor concept definition, inadequate control, or task differences or reflects a real psychobiological fact is still unknown. For the moment, it seems prudent to conclude that attention (and perhaps all other cognitive processes) involve broadly distributed portions of the brain. This is the position taken by almost all current researchers although the details of the distribution remain unknown.

10. A major question remaining, even if one accepts the distributed brain region network idea, is the nature of the nodes—are they rigidly, narrowly, and uniquely associated with particular functions? Or, to the contrary, are they simply regions of general capability that are recruited as needed and whose function and extent fluctuate with the nature of the cognitive task? It is also worthwhile to ask, given the variability of these responses—are these nodes just random peaks of activity representing irregularities in the degree of brain activation with no particular psychobiological significance?

11. Each of the many brain areas that have been associated with attention has also been implicated in other cognitive processes. There are no pure "attention" loci; meta-studies show us that most parts of the brain participate in most cognitive process.

It is possible, but by no means certain, that this area of science, like that of the stock market, may represent an unobtainable quest to detect order in a sea of randomness. That we may all be suffering a mass delusion of seeing order when none exists should not be rejected at this early stage of the development of cognitive neuroscience.

7 Consciousness and Other High-Level Cognitive Processes

7.1 Introduction

If there were difficulties and uncertainties regarding the neural nature of attention, learning, or emotion, they are greatly exacerbated when we turn to those elusive phenomena referred to as "higher cognitive processes." As a result of the most extreme kind of inaccessibility (higher cognitive processes can go on in the total absence of any kind of behavior), these phenomena are certainly the most theoretically intractable issues in our search for understanding of what our brains are doing when we cogitate, think, or make decisions. This chapter is aimed at an examination of the progress that has been made in studying these higher cognitive functions.

What are the higher-order cognitive processes? Clearly they are many including these topics:

- Consciousness
- Perception
- Attention
- Awareness
- Thinking
- Reasoning
- Problem solving
- Decision making
- Understanding
- Judging

This list does not exclude many others, however, especially the elusive topic of consciousness itself. We have touched on a number of these topics already in those contexts in which it was possible to link some behavior with them. However, consciousness is quite a different matter when it comes to carrying out meaningful research. Therefore, it is to the psychology of this topic to which I now turn as an introduction to the cognitive neuroscience of the higher cognitive processes.

7.2 Consciousness

There is perhaps no other field of psychology in which so many theories have been proposed, speculative discussions presented, and so little concrete scientific evidence accumulated than with the subject of consciousness. What is consciousness? Can we measure it? How does it affect our behavior? How does consciousness differ from other cognitive processes such as attention, perception, or thinking in general? Or, does it? How does the brain "make" consciousness? All of these queries are manifestations of the basic problem of defining it. Chalmers (1995, p. 200) refers to consciousness as encompassing "the most baffling problem[s] in the science of mind." Indeed, he may have been too modest—it may be the most baffling problem in all of history.

Of one thing we can be sure, unless we are to wander off into some nonscientific dualism, consciousness depends totally on the existence of neural mechanisms that are of unrivaled combinatorial complexity. Out of this complexity, mysteriously arises both the sense of self-awareness that we as individuals have of our own consciousness and the difficulty we have of determining the existence of consciousness in other people.

Despite the probable intractability of measuring, defining, and understanding what consciousness is and how it arises, societies and research centers abound, discussion at meetings continues unabated, and there have been thousands of speculative papers and hundreds of books written on the topic.[1] Yet, the word "consciousness" remains difficult if not impossible to define or operationalize; as a result, many studies, supposedly of this mysterious process, turn out operationally to be studies of more behaviorally manipulable derivatives of it such as perception, attention, or memory. Nevertheless, consciousness (or its absence) lurks in the background, interpreted or inferred by investigators, but not actually assayed by anything but the most indirect means. What empirical "evidence" we have of consciousness usually turns out to consist of suggestive inferences, introspective reports, and plausible but remote neural correlates. All of these forms of evidence could as well be produced in an examination of a competent automaton, someday if not now, without answering the basic question of the presence or consciousness.

Another issue that is often raised in discussions about consciousness concerns the possible effect of consciousness on behavior. Clearly, it is at least possible that an organism could be conscious and yet that consciousness could have no influence on the neural and behavioral processes accompanying it. This possibility is encompassed within the word "epiphenomenon," that is, awareness could emerge from the complex neural processes but not be a part of the causal chain from receptor neuron to motor behavior and, thus, not be able to influence any process in that chain. At this point discussion often wanders off into the matter of "free will," a philosophical issue that goes far beyond the range of the matters covered in this book.

The problem of animal consciousness, in particular, has befuddled philosophers and psychologists for centuries. Romanes (1883), a follower and close friend of Charles Darwin's, saw mental processes evolving from primitive and partial shadowy states of awareness to full blown sentience in much the same way as our bodies structurally evolved from the simple to the more complex. Romanes argued that it was possible to ascribe simple forms of consciousness to animals by assuming behavioral analogies between their covert mental processes and our own reportable ones.

The antagonistic side was taken by scholars such as C. L. Morgan (1894, p. 53), who argued against the analogical method without, according to some historians, denying the possibility of animal consciousness. His pronouncement was that "In no case may we interpret an action as the outcome of the exercise of a higher psychical faculty, if it can be interpreted as the outcome of one which stands lower in the psychological scale." This statement, now known as Lloyd Morgan's canon (a term synonymous in meaning with the fourteenth century "razor" of Ockham), has come down to us over the years as a basic tenet of behaviorism. Skinner (1938) and many other modern behaviorists also subsequently argued against anthropomorphization—the attribution of human properties to animals. William James (1890), with his admonition against ascribing one's own thought processes to others (the "psychologist's fallacy"), should also have been uncomfortable with any attribution of mind to animals; however, his avowed mentalism in other regards suggests that he was not. This is a notable inconsistency in the thoughts of one our most influential psychological theoreticians.

Without question the issue of whether or not it is possible to even study consciousness remains as contentious today as it was in the time of Descartes. In fact, a strong assertion has been made by philosophers (e.g., Nagel, 1974, among many others) that no direct measure of consciousness has ever been made and, in point of basic principle, cannot be made. Others, mainly cognitive psychologists, argue on the contrary that measurement of consciousness is a tractable problem; in fact, they contend that we have successfully been doing it for years.

An excellent way to appreciate the depth of uncertainty surrounding even the most basic issues at all levels of analysis is to read the *Stanford Encyclopedia of Philosophy* (internet version available at <http://plato.stanford.edu>) article on consciousness. The philosophers who authored this article have been joined by a number of psychologists who still adhere to the basic idea of behaviorism with its attendant concepts of inaccessibility and behavioral neutrality. The rise of consciousness research in recent years is largely attributable by many of us to the uncritical reductionism of cognitive mentalism into modular and isolatable functions that holds sway in modern experimental psychology.

The absence of direct accessibility is especially challenging since consciousness may exist in the total absence of any observable behavior. A person may be absently staring off into space but be extremely active mentally, working through the process of solving some problem or reveling in past memories of some enjoyable experience. Obviously, there is no direct or immediate link between publically observable behavior and intrapersonally private consciousness—our minds may be completely active even though our bodies are not. The situation is even further exacerbated because some of the covert mental activity subsumed under the term "conscious" is reportable, whereas some of it plays out in a domain that has been called "subconscious." This suggests that in some cases we may not be aware of the involved logical (or illogical) steps in our thought processes and thus not able to report them at some later time. Neither overt behavior nor introspective reports are, therefore, windows to the essential nature of consciousness; nor do they provide the basis of a clear definition. The extreme difficulties of defining what we mean by consciousness become crystal clear in this context.

Because consciousness and behavior can be dissociated, any study of consciousness is fraught with technical and conceptual difficulties should we wish to pursue it in the laboratory. Many of these difficulties have been discussed by Edelman and Tononi (2000). The situation is so unconstrained that innumerable untestable interpretations and theories of what is going on during conscious mental activity are both possible and prevalent. Each of these alternative interpretations may seem plausible, but none is confirmable. This is not a good setting for the pursuit of objective science, and the results, as we see, of much of the research, both neurophysiological and behavioral, now being carried out is neither empirically robust nor theoretically enlightening. In preview it should be noted that, at the present, determination of the nature or even the existence of consciousness in humans or animals remains one of the great conundrums of modern science. As a result there are many practical problems (such as evaluating the conscious state of a person in a persistent vegetative state) that remain unsolved. Both modern medical practice and cognitive neuroscience theory struggle with this lacuna in our knowledge.

The problem is terrifyingly complex from the outset. We must not underestimate the difficulty of even defining such a high level, relatively behavior-free, cognitive process as consciousness. It does not take a heroic survey of dictionaries, textbooks, and encyclopedias to appreciate that, like all other mental processes, consciousness is defined more on the basis of the intuition of psychologists who have observed experimental outcomes or taken introspective reports more seriously than they should have, than in any precise operational terms. Although not yet widely appreciated, it is, nevertheless, increasingly accepted as being true, that virtually all of the words used to define consciousness are really hypothetical constructs conjured up to categorize the outcomes of experiments; whether they are real psychobiological objects remains uncertain.

The problem of inadequate definition is pervasive throughout cognitive psychology. For example, consider the problem of intelligence: people differ in their abilities to perform on certain tests. The guiding hypothesis is that the capability of the underlying cognitive mechanism (e.g., intelligence) varies from person to person. However, it must be remembered that intelligence or graduations of it are only hypothetical constructs inferred or intuited to explain a certain kind of variability in human behavior. Unfortunately, it may be that this is the best we can do given the inaccessibility of our thoughts or any direct means to measure, much less explain, the mental mechanisms that account for this behavior.

However compelling are the arguments that we follow this strategy, we cannot ignore the fact that a host of other cognitive terms such as "thinking" or "consciousness" are also indirect and nonexclusive inferences from either specific experimental paradigms or other forms of human interaction, including person-to-person conversation. Whether those terms correspond to actual and specific neurobiological mechanisms remains one of the great mysteries of modern psychological thought.

As a result of the inferential nature of our study of consciousness, almost all efforts to define consciousness end up being irretrievably intertwined with other high-level cognitive processes. It is not all certain that we can actually study consciousness independently of any of the others. The list of high-level mental activities comingled with consciousness studies includes virtually all components of the rest of cognitive psychology listed at the beginning of this chapter.

How then do we define consciousness? This elusive term has also escaped precise definition for millennia and continues to do so to the present day. Of interest is a recent issue of the *Journal of Consciousness Studies* devoted to nothing other than the search for a suitable definition. One author (Vimal, 2009) offered a list of 40 different meanings of consciousness and argued that even this list was not exhaustive. All, Vimal contended, were based on the individual investigator's preliminary assumptions or his or her personal theory guiding the research. None could be distinguished operationally from the others. He went on to conclude that "the prospects for reaching any single, agreed, theory independent definition of consciousness thus appears remote" (p. 9).

The problem of definition of consciousness is even further exacerbated since a distinction is sometimes made between the mental process of consciousness and its contents; the first refers to the awareness of knowledge, and the second to the knowledge itself. The problem of definition, as we shall repeatedly see, is further complicated by the fact that it is not easy to discriminate between consciousness and other cognitive processes—attention having a particularly intimate relation with them.

This raises, once again, the important point of separability of a cognitive process such as consciousness from the other that were listed in section 7.1. It seems likely that none of the items in this list are activities that can be experimentally isolated from each other; the severability of cognitive modules (i.e., pure insertion) is a chimera rather than a scientific likelihood. Much more likely is that any artificially isolated cognitive activity is actually a part of a much greater system (both psychological and neural), the other parts of which are at least interacting and at the worst do not exist as independent modular entities. Certainly consciousness is so completely integrated into the other processes that considering it a cognitive module or seeking some sign of it as an independent process seems totally inappropriate.

Various attempts have been made to define consciousness over the years. One example was the very specific statement offered by Thatcher and John (1977) highlighted as the only specific definition in Dennett's (1987) encyclopedia entry for consciousness:

[Consciousness is] a process in which information about multiple individual modalities of sensation and perception is combined into a unified multidimensional representation of the state of the system and its environment and integrated with information about memories and the needs of the organism generating emotional reactions and programs of behavior to adjust the organism to its environment. (p. 294)

Freeman (2007) offered the following definition of consciousness:

Consciousness fully supervenes when the 1.5 kgm mass of protoplasm in the head directs the body into material and social environments and engages in reciprocity. While consciousness is not susceptible to direct measurement, a limited form exercised in animals and pre-lingual children can be measured indirectly with biological assays of arousal, intention and attention. (p. 1021)[2]

Other researchers in the field of consciousness studies tried to tease apart the monolithic idea of consciousness into a set of subcomponents. Revonsuo (2001), for example, distinguished among three different kinds of consciousness:

• Phenomenal consciousness, which is the raw experience itself, the qualia.
• Reflective or access consciousness, which is the subjective experience that can be "conceptualized, categorized, named, reported, and voluntarily acted upon."
• Self-awareness.

Pinker (1997) also distinguished different types of consciousness including the following interpretations (abstracted and paraphrased from Pinker, 1997, pp. 134–135):

• Self-knowledge: The sense of awareness of our own existence.
• Access to information: The introspective response to our self-knowledge.
• Sentience: Subjective experience and the "raw feels" that collectively make up our conscious states.

Some authors prefer not to make any attempt to define consciousness; instead they consider it is a process with certain properties. For example, Edelman and Tononi (2000) listed the following properties (abstracted and paraphrased from Edelman and Tononi, 2000, pp. 146–152):

• *Unity* Consciousness cannot be decomposed into components.
• *Privacy* Consciousness cannot be observed by an external observer.
• *Coherence* A person cannot be conscious of two contradictory thoughts simultaneously.
• *Multiplicity* There are many possible conscious states.
• *Distribution* The neural mechanisms of consciousness are distributed throughout the brain.

- *Limited capacity* The contents of consciousness are limited to a relatively small amount of information; parallelicity is limited.
- *Seriality* One state of consciousness leads to another in serial order.
- *Dynamic* Consciousness is constantly changing from one serial state to another.

In the final analysis, however, even these thoughtful scholars reverted to a simple kind of metaphorical definition and a realization of the limits of scientific examination of its properties. They proposed (reminiscent of William James's famous definition of attention): "Everyone knows what consciousness is: It is what abandons you every evening when you fall asleep and reappears the next morning when you wake up" (p. 3). Of course, all of these definitions overlap considerably, and none of them overcomes the difficulties of applying the kind of empirical method that the physical sciences have found to be so effective.

Others finessed the issue by associating cognitive processes such as consciousness with some metaphor, that is, with a known mechanical or electronic system that seems to exhibit common properties with consciousness. For example Bourne, Dominowski, and Loftus (1979) simply asserted that cognition is a system for processing information; they used the computer as their metaphor to establish a connotative meaning for the word "cognition" and hoped that the model or metaphor would convey enough information to at least limit its meaning. It is possible, of course, that this kind of metaphorical meaning is all that can be done when attempts are made to define consciousness.

The use of the computer metaphor is an example of the enormous influence that newly emerging technologies have had on psychological theory over the years. The superficial similarity between the observed behaviors of these two kinds of information-processing systems led many psychologists to incorrectly assume, in the post-WWII period, that the internal mechanisms of the two must also be the same. Computer programs that produced behavior analogous to that of humans then took on a potent explanatory role. However functional analogy is not tantamount to mechanistic homology, and the explanatory theories so generated may be no better than illusions of understanding. In retrospect it seems that many of these models of cognitive processes were, just that, simple analogies drawn from the known nature of computer circuits and programs rather than deductions from the known neurobiology of the mind–brain.

In one glaring example of this fallacious analogical reasoning, the concept of discrete functional units of the computer was transferred willy-nilly to the brain. The human mind was conceptualized as a system of separable blocks in the manner of a computer. These modules included sensory (input), decision-making (central processing unit), and motor (output) components. A specific analogy was drawn between the CPU and consciousness. It was there that decision making occurred and where it was presumed that consciousness would reside should a brain model become complex enough.

We now know that the brain is a much more integrated system and probably is not well modeled by a system with isolatable chunks. During the heyday of computer metaphors, detailed models were built that attempted to simulate or imitate human behavior. We now appreciate, further, that the same explicit behavior of an organism can be simulated on the computer using a vast number of different programs and algorithms. We therefore have no a priori reason to believe that these computer algorithms are the same as those being used by the organic brain.

The study of consciousness, as discussed in this chapter, is particularly vulnerable to underdetermination (the fact that there is not sufficient information in any associated behavior to determine a unique, or even a most plausible, explanatory mechanism) because the underlying process of awareness is so poorly linked to the stimulus and task parameters. This is quite unlike learning and perception and, to a lesser degree, emotion: uncontrolled cognitive penetration and even the effect of our attempts to measure consciousness can dramatically alter the results of what was thought to be a relevant experiment. It should always be, for example, a matter of concern to investigators of consciousness, as well as any other higher-level cognitive processes, to understand that their instructions may mean something different to the experimental subject than they do to the experimenter. Paradoxical effects, past experience, and differences in the personal meaning of words may often lead to instructions producing quite different results than an experimenter intended.

To sum up, whatever it is that we mean by the term "consciousness" is still uncertain. It is not even clear that it is an impendent psychobiological entity that can be isolated from other cognitive processes. It interacts (possibly inextricably) with a broad range of other mental processes and activities. The network of cognitive processes is often difficult to define and control and, in any case, cannot be directly measured. One thing that all agree on is its intrapersonal privacy or inaccessibility to direct examination. Indeed, it is not at all certain that we can study consciousness as a distinct cognitive process although there is an increasing amount of effort to do so. In previous chapters I have artificially parsed out four areas of cognitive psychology (attention, learning, perception, and emotion); however this has merely been for pedagogic reasons and may not reflect the psychobiological reality of their relationship with other high-level cognitive processes such as consciousness.

Thus, most attempts to define consciousness immediately fall back into trivial circularity such as "consciousness is self-awareness." Similarly, any attempt to distinguish between consciousness and awareness also quickly fails. Like other cognitive processes, our consciousness, sentience, knowing, experiencing, or self-awareness (all essentially synonymous terms) goes on unmeasured and totally inaccessible to the outside observer. Indeed, there is only one irrefutable piece of evidence of consciousness—the awareness we all enjoy as first-person observers and which we all report to be very real, indeed. The neurophysiological source of this personal self-awareness of "I" or "me" remains what many agree is the greatest mystery of modern science. Some philosophers wish to deny its reality; however, the power of the first-person experience makes it a predominant interest of psychologists as well as most humans.

The nature and measurement of consciousness as well as its attribution to others are not new issues; they have perplexed humans since the dawn of our history. Theologies have explicitly dealt with such problems long before psychologists and philosophers appeared on the scene. In the context of religion consciousness was usually considered to be a separate and immortal entity (the soul) that persisted after the death of the body. Nowadays all aspects of the mind including first-person consciousness are considered to be just another process or activity of the brain. Unfortunately, this neuroreductionist postulate has not solved the problem of consciousness, just reframed it in a new arena of discourse. The questions now driving psychology and cognitive neuroscience concerning consciousness are, nevertheless, the perennial ones:

- Can we measure consciousness?
- If yes, how do we measure consciousness?
- If no, why do we continue to try to do so?
- Are there stages or degrees of consciousness?
- Does behavior or introspection provide adequate means of describing or explaining consciousness?
- How does consciousness emerge from the activities of the brain?
- Are other people and other species conscious?
- How do we distinguish conscious from automatic responses?
- Can consciousness exist in machines?
- Is the existing biochemical nature of our brains the only foundation for consciousness?
- When did consciousness first emerge in evolutionary history?
- What are the possible biomarkers of consciousness?

Questions like these are not going to be fully answered in the foreseeable future. However, it is thought by some that progress can be made in at least introducing some insights into how they might be answered. In my opinion the most difficult challenges are those that concern the psychological questions—those that are concerned with the detection, if not the measurement of consciousness. These remain among the most obstinate, recalcitrant, and unanswered issues in science.[3]

Although my main interest is in the cognitive neuroscience that surrounds this topic, it is necessary to briefly review the preneuroscience behavioral research on consciousness to fully understand the neuroscientific findings.

7.2.1 Behavioral Research on Consciousness and its Difficulties

Over a century ago, Romanes (1883) raised the issue of whether behavior can be a key to unlocking access to the mind when he made the discerning statement:

Thus it is that we may have a subjective analysis of mind and an objective analysis of mind—the difference between the two consisting in this, that in our subjective analysis we are restricted to the limits of a single isolated mind which we call our own, and within the territory of which we have immediate cognizance of all the processes that are going on. . . . But in our objective analysis of other or foreign minds we have no such immediate cognizance; all of our knowledge of their operations is derived through the medium of ambassadors—these ambassadors being the activities of the organism. (p. 1)

It could not be said better nor would any modern phraseology further clarify the fundamental nature of the problem. The issue is—how effective are these "activity ambassadors"—now known as behaviors—in providing robust information about the state of consciousness of an individual? This is such a divisive issue that no definitive answer can be given to this query. (It lies, as some of my readers may appreciate, at the heart of the long controversy between behaviorists and mentalists.) However, a current view is that there is no definitive public evidence of whether or not a person is conscious nor can there be. At best, we have some correlated physiological signals but behavioral indicators will always be ambiguous and indeterminate. Conscious awareness (the experience of knowledge), according to this view, is a totally private experience to which each of us is individually privy and for which there is no public accessibility.[4]

Nevertheless, the assumption of "me-ness" or self-awareness exerts a powerful influence on human thought. We each "know" that our own consciousness exists, and, therefore, we draw the conclusion (based on only analogy as suggested by Romanes) that the other people with whom we interact are also conscious in the same way. To not make this leap of analogy would make human existence joyless if not meaningless. Still, the joy must be tempered with the intractability of the problems encountered when one attempts to study such an elusive concept as consciousness.

Clearly, the state of consciousness of a person is very difficult to determine, if it is possible at all. Lack of behavior cannot be taken as evidence of lack of consciousness. The extreme "locked in" syndrome, observed in cases of brain injury, is accepted as a real medical possibility. In this state the human may be fully conscious and even quite aware of the effects of stimuli but be completely incapable of responding. However it is extremely difficult to determine if such a state actually exists in the absence of subsequent reports by the patient—a relatively rare occurrence.[5] The possibility of continued consciousness and sensory experience without motor responses has been documented in experiments (Smith, Brown, Toman, & Goodman, 1947) in which the subject was given a high dose of a curare derivative (D-Tubocurarine). Although curare-like substances can completely paralyze a person to the point of total unresponsiveness, subjects under its influence are still able to subsequently report that they were aware of sensory stimuli.

On the other hand, just as the absence of responsiveness cannot be taken as the absence of consciousness, the presence of adaptive behavior cannot be taken as evidence for the presence of consciousness. Highly proficient electronic automata can ever more frequently and competently simulate human behavior without the necessity of assuming any kind of underlying awareness. Similarly, the question of animal consciousness raised by Romanes has never been resolved; we simply are not able to distinguish between a conscious, sentient organism and a smoothly functioning automaton operating purely on the basis of reflex or programmed action. Indeed, we cannot even make such a distinction for other people.

Because of these profound conceptual and technical difficulties, many psychologists have suggested arbitrary and indirect standards for measuring consciousness. Seth, Dienes, Cleeremans, Overgaard, and Pessoa (2008) categorized some of the behavioral tests that they believed could be used to indicate the presence of conscious experience. These included:

• The ability to choose accurately under forced choice conditions.
• The ability to use or not use knowledge according to instructions.
• Verbal reports of mental states—introspection.

Unfortunately, on close scrutiny, such indicators are inadequate to establish the existence of consciousness. They represent a confusion of the contents of consciousness with consciousness itself. A number of forced choice experiments (e.g., Hernandez & Lefton, 1977; Nisbett & Wilson, 1977) have been carried out in which the subject responds appropriately but without any conscious awareness of the logic behind his or her decision or even of the critical information that was necessary to make the correct decision.

Surprisingly, there is very little behavioral research that *directly* attacks the problem of whether or not a person is conscious. Most such research is indirect and appears to be seeking some kind of marker or indicator of an ethereal consciousness underlying publically observable behavior. (Once again, I refer my readers to the discussion of surgical anesthesia in chapter 8 wherein it is shown how uncertain are even the best clinical indicators of consciousness.) In its place, a substantial corpus of current activity is aimed at finding what are supposed to be neural correlates of consciousness. The goal is well intended; however, the correlations may be one sided, having been drawn between an objective brain measure and what is still an ill-defined and immeasurable cognitive phantom.

The nature of consciousness, thus, continues to challenge scientific psychology. On the one side are those cognitive psychologists such as Seth, Baars, and Edelman (2005) who proposed that there is a constellation of neural and behavioral indices that strongly indicate whether a person or an animal is conscious. They list 17 different criteria of consciousness. These include the following indices (paraphrased from Seth, Baars, and Edelman, 2005, pp. 121–122):

1. Typical EEG signature
2. Thalamocortical activity
3. Distributed brain activity
4. Wide range of conscious content
5. High information content of the stimulus
6. Adaptive and fleeting content
7. Singularity of response to ambiguous or alternative stimuli
8. Limited capacity and seriality of consciousness

9. Sensory binding of distributed events

10. Attribution by the observer of the conscious experience to observer

11. Accuracy of reporting when it is possible to compare introspective reports and expected response to a stimulus

12. Availability of conscious events only to the person

13. Influence on consciousness of "fringe" events, e.g., familiarity

14. Facilitation of learning (or more accurately, the lack of learning) when the person is unconscious

15. Consciousness remains stable over prolonged periods

16. Allocentricity, the property of relating to others as opposed to egocentricity, the property of relating to oneself

17. Conscious knowing and decision making

Setting aside the three initial neural correlates, which I discuss later in this chapter, we now examine Seth, Baars, and Edelman's behavioral indices.

Seth, Baars, and Edelman (2005) provided a useful service by analyzing the limitations of many of the behavioral criteria they enumerated. For scholars who accept the existence of animal consciousness, this is an especially worthwhile effort. Seth and colleagues noted, in particular, that the criteria they proposed "vary considerably in their testability" (p. 134). However, this may be a more general criticism than they appreciated. At this point it becomes a judgment call, virtually a statement of belief, about whether any of their behavioral criteria for the existence of consciousness can unequivocally test its presence or absence.

The basic problem with all 14 of the behavioral criteria proposed by Seth et al. (2005) is that they are not, as described, measurements of consciousness. They are, at best, indirect behavioral indicators or correlations that depend on the fragile assumption that they are sufficiently strongly linked to that which we call consciousness to act as a surrogate measure of the immeasurable stuff itself. However by no means are they convincing and robust measures of consciousness, and in no way do they point with any degree of demonstrable validity to whatever it is that is consciousness. What behavioral observations can do is to serve as heuristics to generate hypotheses about what *might* be happening *within* the organism. Unfortunately they are not either necessary or sufficient proofs of one or another interpretation, nor do they answer even the most basic question—the very existence of consciousness.

In fact, all of these behavioral indicators depend on inferences and sometimes grand logical leaps across vast conceptual and empirical gaps that strain scientific methodology, credulity, and logic. Some are simply tautologies; criteria 12 and 17, for example, on close inspection, simply turn out to be synonyms for consciousness camouflaged by words of equal inscrutability; they offer little additional denotative power. Number 11, accurate reportability, depends on the assumption that it is possible to have a reference against which introspective reports can be compared for accuracy. The perpetual problem faced by number 11 is that such meaningful and independent standards of comparison are not available. What is generally meant by accurate reporting is that different, but equally weak, measures of behavior can be shown to agree when compared with each other. However, such equivalence may result for many different reasons and does not provide any robust proof that such measurements are valid indicators of consciousness.

Others of the criteria proposed by Seth, Baars, and Edelman are actually "answers" to ill-posed or bad questions themselves. For example criterion 9 suggests that "sensory binding" is an indicator of consciousness. However the whole issue of binding may be a poor answer to a meaningless question in the context of the more homogenous and distributed models of mind-brain activity now gaining popularity; a robust distributed neural model does not require binding, merely simultaneity or synchrony. Anatomically, brain regions and activities are now considered to be so heavily interconnected that the concept of a collection of semi-independent processes requiring binding may be irrelevant either to the measurement of consciousness or to any other cognitive process.

Many of the other criteria proposed by Seth, Baars, and Edelman are no more than hypothetical extrapolations from behavior that has not been empirically validated. Behavior and consciousness are, as we have seen, not connected strongly enough to permit us to use the one as the indicator or measure of the other. There are three aspects of this lack of connection: standing between us and any proof of the existence of consciousness (beyond our own first-person experience) are (1) the possibility that a clever automaton (a Zombie system in the words of Chalmers, 1996) of sufficient complexity would be capable of creating all sorts of behavior, yet be totally unaware of itself; (2) humans are capable of thinking without any public behavioral manifestations of those thoughts; and (3) humans are capable of behaving without conscious awareness.

Furthermore, many of the individual criteria in the Seth, Baars, and Edelman's list are logically circular: each is an example of confirming the consequent—that is, each assumes that consciousness exists and then seeks hypothetical correlates or properties that support this assumption. Some of these hypothetical properties only indirectly support our hopes that such a system would operate in a manner that Zombies could not emulate. Others assume a causal relation between consciousness and behavior that is well known to be violated in some instances (e.g., Nisbett & Wilson's 1977 demonstration that certain kinds of problems can be solved by logical processes that do not enter into consciousness).

Unfortunately, all of the rest of the criteria proposed by Seth and his colleagues are similarly flawed, imperfect, and individually inadequate indicators that require us to draw remote inferences or generate untestable hypotheses about what might be going on in the conscious mind, but they are indicators for which no validation is possible. Of course, this constraint is not true for the problem of consciousness alone; all cognitive and other mentalist psychologies are confronted with this same dilemma. The mind being inaccessible and immeasurable puts us in the position that our theories must in the final analysis depend on analogies, metaphors, and inferences from behavior in a way that makes the problem of studying consciousness in both animals and other people extremely difficult.

There are other behavioral criteria that have been used as indicators of consciousness beyond those tabulated by Seth Baars, and Edelman. Mather (2008), for example, suggested traditional indicators of human consciousness including language[6] and meta-cognition.[7] However, these tests cannot be used with animals, and most investigators agree that these criteria are of limited use in the demonstration of animal consciousness because of their inherent anthropocentric prejudice.

The ultimate question is whether totally automatic or Zombie systems of a complexity comparable to that of the human brain must necessarily be conscious. Adaptive and behaviorally competent computer programs are not good evidence of consciousness; complex behaviors can be equally well produced by automata as by sentient organisms. We are no more able to confirm the presence of consciousness in a computer than in a rabbit or a human. The ability to simulate complex and adaptive behaviors using computer programs suggests that there is nothing there that can be used to establish the existence of consciousness.

In principle it seems more likely that consciousness cannot be rigorously measured or even proven to exist, no matter how many individually weak, redundant, or tautological behavioral arguments may be invoked to make the case for Fido or Aunt Jane. Indeed in such a situation it comes down to choosing between two alternative postulates. The first is that consciousness exists and that we must seek out the best possible indirect indicators of it in an effort to support that belief. The second is that the question is unanswerable and any hypotheses we may generate concerning its nature or reality are little more than hand waving.

An instructive way to illustrate the current state of consciousness research would be to comprehensively review the logical foundations of experiments carried out to test the presence or absence of consciousness. This is what I have done in previous chapters. However, there are few formal experiments that I find sufficiently compelling to fill the role of interesting exemplars in my discussion. In fact many of the currently available "proofs of consciousness" turn out to be superficial demonstrations rather than robust experimental findings. For example a number of recent demonstrations of animal consciousness have been based on phenomena known as mirror self-consciousness. The test, originally proposed by Gallup (1970) required that a spot of paint be applied to an anesthetized chimpanzee's forehead. The paint, of course, was hidden by the animal's prominent eye ridges and could not be directly seen by the chimp. When the animal was awakened and allowed to look in a mirror, however, it touched its forehead in a way that suggested that the animal realized that the image in the mirror was of itself. Recent research has extended this phenomenon to other of the great apes such as orangutans (Parker, Mitchell, & Boccia, 1994), questionably to gorillas (Patterson, 1984), but not to animals lower on the phylogenetic tree such as monkeys (Suddendorf & Collier-Baker, 2009) or dolphins (Marten & Psarakos, 1995).

Needless to say, even this simple test has been subject to considerable controversy. (See, for example, the controversy between Anderson & Gallup, 1997, on the one hand, and Hauser, Kralik, Botto-Mahan, Garrett, & Osher, 1995, on the other.) However strongly one wishes to accept mirror self-recognition as a sign of animal consciousness, its expansion to ideas such as a "theory of mind"—the attribution of consciousness to others has all of the aroma of hyperbolic extrapolation.[8]

The problem of animal consciousness has also been discussed by Mather (2008), specifically regarding a behaviorally rich cephalopod—the octopus. Acknowledging that self-recognition is not a property of octopi, she alluded to three other behavioral criteria that led her to conclude that "cephalopod mollusks may have a form of primary consciousness." (p. 37). One of the three is a set of neural similarities between the animal's nervous system and that of higher animals—specifically including lateralization. This is hard to accept as a compelling argument. There are certainly many more dissimilarities, both neurally and behaviorally between octopi and humans, to negate the impact of this superficial neuroanatomical similarity.

Mather's second and third criteria attesting to consciousness in the octopus are both behavioral—the well-confirmed capability for learning by an octopus and this animal's equally well-documented responses indicating a kind of positional awareness. However, these two arguments are also very weak struts on which to build a theory of cephalopod consciousness. Two points need to be reiterated here: first, behavioral similarities might well be encoded by vastly different cognitive or neural mechanisms; thus, any neuroanatomic similarities or differences are inconsequential. Second, as I have repeatedly noted, automata (e.g., computers or Zombies) are conceptually capable of producing complex behaviors that can be influenced by experience. Simple computer programs can learn, and even a device as simple as a gyroscope exhibits it own kind of "positional awareness." Mather's criteria, thus, come up against the same barriers and challenges as do all other proposed behavioral indicators of consciousness.

When we turn to the human being, research at first seems to be much more direct and consciousness more accessible. Humans can and do report the details of their own states of consciousness; they can speak, and they have a much broader repertoire of other potentially significant behaviors. However, fundamentally, the problem remains the same—can we demonstrate consciousness unequivocally, or must we always face the possible option of a powerful automaton in which awareness is at best epiphenomenal and at worst, illusionary. There is ample evidence in human behavior that consciousness is not necessary for either overt behavior or covert problem solving. We are perfectly capable of driving an automobile while unconscious (or at least not attending to the driving task itself), and some of the greatest discoveries of human intellectual and scientific history have reputedly been made while their discoverers were reportedly asleep.

Another phenomenon often used to support the separation of consciousness and behavior is "blindsight" (Poppel, Held, & Frost, 1973). Damage to regions of the visual cortex of patients were reported to produce near total blindness to the shape or even presence of visual objects in the corresponding portions of the visual field. However, as Poppel et al. (1973) first noted, there was a surprising sparing of the ability of patients to direct their gaze toward an object that could not be "seen," that is, perceived. That is they responded appropriately to an object of which they were not aware. Obviously we are entering into a domain of lexicographic uncertainty here that makes much of this discussion less than satisfying.

Later investigators (Perenin & Jeannerod (1978) found that similarly brain-damaged patients were also able to manually point to an otherwise "invisible" object. Furthermore in subsequent experiments using forced choice procedures, these ostensibly blind subjects also showed discriminative behavior that required some knowledge of the position and shape of a stimulus object. In other words objects below the level of conscious awareness could still lead to adaptive motor responses to objects (such as appropriately grasping a hammer) that were introspectively reported to be invisible to the patient.

Initially, this phenomenon was explained by information transmission by a secondary visual pathway that passed through the colliculus of the brainstem. However, a considerable argument (Fendrich, Wessinger, & Gazzaniga, 1992) has erupted over the past couple of decades that blindsight might not be the outcome of a secondary pathway; instead, it might be the result of sparing of small islands of residual neural reactivity passing through the normal geniculate-striate pathway.

Regardless of the exact neurological mechanisms accounting for the blindsight phenomenon, the phenomenon itself is another piece of strong suggestive evidence for the separability of adaptive behavior (i.e., pointing or orienting) from the conscious experience (i.e., the subject's introspective report of what was perceived). Phenomena such as blindsight further complicate the question of how we might distinguish between automatic behavior and conscious experience.

Thus, a major difficulty for the measurement of consciousness is that behavior and even our best efforts to assay consciousness do not necessarily coincide. A priori, according to this point of view, behavioral measures are virtually useless in determining whether or not a responsive human is conscious or aware of a perceptual or cognitive process.

What kind of measures could we then use to bring any possibility of scientific studies of consciousness to respectability? Seth, Dienes, Cleeremans, Overgaard, and Pessoa (2008) have considered this matter in detail. They accept the utility of both behavioral and neurophysiological measures of consciousness. Seth and his colleagues suggest that there are three theories of consciousness that can be used as the foundation for its measurement. The first is designated as "worldly discrimination theory" (WDT). This approach is based on the assumption "that any mental state that can express its content in behavior is conscious" (p. 314). Unfortunately, it is clear that such a point of view in its rawest form begs the question by assuming a link between consciousness and behavior that, as we have already seen, is not otherwise supported.

The second theoretical approach proposed by Seth et al. (2008) on which measures of consciousness might be based on is a set of "integration theories" (IT). This point of view suggests that "According to these theories a mental state is conscious if it provides a sufficiently informative discrimination among a large number of possible states, in which successful discrimination requires both differentiation and integration" (Seth et al., 2008, p. 316). This approach is based on the idea that conscious information is available to many different "cognitive/and or neural processes" (p. 316), and our ability to distinguish between them is a sign of consciousness. The discriminative measure obviously fitting this bill most comfortably is signal detection theory (SDT). The role of SDT in this theoretical approach is to provide a measure of our ability to discriminate between mental states and, thus by implication, of an awareness of the different properties or aspects of a stimulus.

The third theoretical approach is based on what Seth and his colleagues (2008, p. 316) refer to as "higher-order thought" (HOT) theories. In this set ". . . a mental state is conscious when a person is actually aware or disposed toward being aware of being in that state." Consciousness, from this point of view, depends on our perceiving or thinking something about our own mental state, a process we have already encountered under the rubric of "metacognition." This third approach is also obviously logically circular and, therefore, a not very useful criterion. In this case "consciousness" is simply associated with a different but synonymous word, "awareness." What "disposed toward" means in an empirical context would always remain opaque.

Obviously, all three of these approaches differ more in their vocabulary than in their substance. All three are examples of the more or less circular logic embedded in the most basic aspects of their definition. Furthermore, none of them solves the problem of measurement raised when we try to determine whether consciousness is present or not. Instead, they collectively demonstrate the extreme conceptual difficulty of trying to measure this inaccessible mental state.

Another question now arises—is experimental psychology able to do a better job in studying consciousness in humans than with animals given the tremendous advantage provided by human abilities to verbalize and introspect? Achieving an answer to this rhetorical as well as scientific question is clouded by the enormous interest in consciousness and its connection to a huge array of philosophical, spiritual, and religious ideologies. It is clear, furthermore, that there are many other technical and conceptual obstacles beyond inaccessibility that obstruct the study of consciousness. These include the simple, but fundamental, issue of experimental reproducibility; consciousness research produces research that is typically extremely variable and inconsistent. However, there are also a number of other barriers to our applying experimental psychological methods to this most fundamental of psychological problems. The technical difficulties of carrying out research on consciousness have been eloquently described by Jahn and Dunne (1988) in the preamble to their book. In their words:

. . . formidable obstacles oppose such investigations. The physical and psychological relationships between consciousness and the physical world entail subtle effects and processes that in some cases appear to violate the most fundamental scientific premises of space, time, and causality. The parameters bearing on such interactions are numerous and widely interdisciplinary, and various subjective and aesthetic factors not normally accommodated by traditional scientific methodology seem crucially relevant. Even in the most incisive and carefully controlled studies, systematically replicable effects appear only as marginal deviations from the normal statistical behavior of probabilistic systems, predicating extreme sensitivity and stability of detection equipment and acquisition of huge data bases if valid indications are to be unequivocally discriminated from the intrinsic noise of random processes. (p. 204)[9,10]

Another problem with measuring consciousness is a kind of psychological Heisenberg principle. As noted by Koch and Preuschoff (2007), the very act of asking someone about her or his state of consciousness may alter that state. For example, that of which we might not have been aware could be called to consciousness by the probe question itself. At the same time, our awareness might diminish to a stimulus when our attention is directed elsewhere by some aspect of the experimental protocol.

Notwithstanding the technical and conceptual difficulties inherent in consciousness research, there has been a persistent interest in recent years in what was hoped would be a more objective and scientific psychological attack on the problem. Human psychological research on consciousness can be exemplified by investigations that invoke an intermediate or surrogate process such as decision making (e.g., Persaud, McLeod, & Cowey, 2007), control of the response according to instructions (e.g., Jacoby, 1991), or (looking far further back into the history of psychology) expression of the degree of confidence that something had happened (Peirce & Jastrow, 1884). The supposed purpose of these intermediaries, according to Koch and Preuschoff, is not to force something into consciousness, but rather to use "a more implicit, a more indirect way to assess awareness" (p. 141) that does not require introspection. The indirectness of this approach, necessary because of the fundamentally inaccessible nature of consciousness, leaves open the possibility, of course, that what is being measured is not conscious experience but something that might be influenced by it—a secondary effect that actually begs the question of its presence or absence. Here, we once again, confront the definitional difficulty, so prevalent throughout scientific psychology, not only for the central property—consciousness—but also for what we mean by the words "direct" and "indirect." The difficulty of measuring consciousness by behavioral indicators remains as difficult now as it was in 1884.

Another of the pioneering scholars who asked how we might go about determining whether an animal or another person was conscious was Ayer (1936). He reformulated what had been a persistent query about consciousness when he said these words:

The only ground I can have for asserting that an object which appears to be conscious is not really a conscious being, but only a dummy or a machine, is that it fails to satisfy one of the empirical tests by which the presence or absence of consciousness is determined.

Unfortunately, to the best of my knowledge there are no "empirical tests by which the presence or absence of consciousness is determined." Thus the search for consciousness and its attendant cognitive processes such as thought remains an unfulfillable one.

In conclusion, after considering some of the behavioral or psychological research on consciousness, it is becoming increasingly clear that much of the research in this field is based on circular reasoning—specifically the premise that consciousness exists—and the companion assumption that consciousness leaves traces of its presence in behavioral responses. It must be reiterated, however, that there is no way to distinguish between behavior driven by automatic mechanisms and conscious ones. All modern behavioral research on consciousness is subject to this constraint; inferences and theories not withstanding, consciousness remains inaccessible to all of our current experimental tools and protocols as it has been to philosophical speculation in the past.

7.2.2 Brain Imaging Neuroscientific Research on Consciousness and Its Difficulties

Much of the research now being carried out on neural correlates asks questions that promise, even if it has not done so yet, to answer some of the most difficult questions about the nature of consciousness. Although there are many variations on the basic question, in its simplest form it is—what are the neural correlates—the biomarkers—that might be associated with consciousness? This present section attacks that question with the understanding that any hope of actually finding a neural correlate of consciousness is mitigated by the elusiveness of mental states—no matter how objective and precise may be the neural measures.

This area of research is motivated in large part by the importance of the effects of anesthesia in surgical operations. I deal in detail in chapter 8 with the conventional methods of monitoring consciousness in that arena. It is clear from that discussion that none of the traditional biological correlates of consciousness (such as the EEG) is a dependable indicator. Whatever neural recording method is chosen, there is considerable statistical fluctuation in its association with consciousness as indicated behaviorally. By this I mean that whatever signal one chooses to measure the degree of consciousness, neuronal response, EEG, ERP, or brain image, exact replication is elusive. No matter how objective a neural measure may seem to be, it is not definitive simply because we have no access to consciousness itself. Obviously, this constraint has serious consequences for surgery; but, it also has serious consequences for the more theoretical aspects of cognitive neuroscience.

Any review of the literature in which brain imaging has been used to investigate consciousness leads to an immediate frustration—the literature is still fragmented, inconsistent, and controversial. Indeed a substantial portion of the literature has been dedicated to the question of whether or not these methods are capable of answering the questions we most want to answer. The debate has revolved down to the matter of the fundamental plausibility of finding neural correlates of consciousness and what these correlations might mean in terms of a theoretical explanation of it. For example, Revonsuo (2001) points out that each

of the currently available neurophysiological research tools attacks the problem of the organization of the nervous system at a different level; yet, none of them operates at the level—
that of the great neuronal networks of the brain—at which complex cognitive processes
such as consciousness are presumed to originate. He summarized his thoughts on this matter
with the words:

> We have currently no methods for imaging (or otherwise capturing empirically) the levels of electro-
> physiological organization in the brain that would allow the reconstruction of a mechanistic model of
> neuroconsciousness, or the phenomenal level of organization in the brain. Thus, for the time being,
> the imaging of consciousness or discovering consciousness in the brain is not feasible. (p. 20)

Although Revonsuo goes on to assert that this does not mean that some of the cognitive-
neural *correlations* may be of interest or useful (perhaps as diagnostic "biomarkers"), his
argument concerning the limits of "literal discovery" should specifically remind all of us of
the difficulties in the search for this most elusive mental process—consciousness.

A further observation made by Revonsuo (2001) was that the literature on possible brain
mechanisms of consciousness is extremely confused. Virtually every part of the brain has
been associated with consciousness by one or another investigator. We currently have no
consensus concerning either the necessity or sufficiency of any part of the brain to encode
consciousness.

Obviously, one comment by even the most distinguished neuroscientist is not sufficient
to detour an army of cognitive neuroscientists from their search for a neural correlate of
consciousness. Many others, either explicitly (e.g., Lloyd, 2002) or implicitly (any of a multitude of cognitive neuroscientists), have accepted the feasibility of using brain imaging
techniques for the study of consciousness.

As discussed in the preceding commentary, consciousness itself remains inaccessible. As
a result much of the experimental work that has been done on consciousness has been done
in the context of its effects on other cognitive processes such as perception or learning. As
we have noted earlier, the inference is usually made that if discriminative responses can be
observed, then consciousness must have occurred. For example, binocular rivalry (an alter-
nating of perception between two visual stimuli that cannot be fused into a meaningful
composite perception) has been used as a vehicle to assay the neural locus of consciousness
with fMRI imaging. Typical of this line of research was a study by Haynes, Deichmann, and
Rees (2005) in which both V1 and the lateral geniculate body were selectively activated (as
indicated by fMRI images) as the subject's percept shifted from one eye's stimulus to the
other. Unfortunately, other comparable studies detected activations in many other regions
of the brain; this leaves us with great uncertainty concerning not only the idea of a localized source of consciousness but also whether or not these regions are actually the necessary
and sufficient components of the conscious experience.

Another comparison of conscious and unconscious visual perception has been carried
out using contrast-varying letter stimuli that were either clearly visible (supraliminal) or

behaviorally invisible (subliminal) by Heinzel et al. (2008). Subjects were required to choose between two alternative responses in a forced choice paradigm. A control condition in which no letter was presented was also used. Heinzel and his colleagues applied event-related fMRI imaging techniques to the two conditions and found that there were distinct differences between the brain responses to each of the two types of stimuli. Activation differences were found for both the supraliminal and the subliminal stimuli when these were compared with the control condition, however in different regions of BA 37. However, when the supraliminal fMRI responses were compared to the subliminal ones, the results were quite different—significant activations were found in BA 9, 44, 45, and 46. Similarly when the subliminal responses were compared with the supraliminal ones, significant activations were found in BA 19 and 21.

The work of Heinzel and his colleagues (2008) suggested that BA 37 (an extrastriate region near the junction of the temporal and occipital lobes) was deeply involved in the sensory processing of letters but in a way that did not distinguish between consciousness and unconsciousness. On the other hand, conscious perception of letters did seem to depend on BA 9, 44, 45, 46 regions of the frontal lobe.

Other experimenters using visual experience as an entre to consciousness have, to the contrary, associated other regions of the brain than those already mentioned with consciousness. Dehaene et al. (2001) found that masked words produced a much lower level of activation than did unmasked words in prefrontal and parietal areas. The role of the prefrontal area was supported by research published by Lau and Passingham (2006).

A major problem with all of this research that goes beyond even the inconsistency of the associations made by the various investigators is the fact that none of these experiments directly measures any property of consciousness. It seems that the philosophers were more or less correct: consciousness—the process—is inaccessible to the experiment and private to the individual experiencing it. There probably is no way to separate this process from others with which it shares common attributes. This point is made clear when we move on to the next topic in this discussion—thinking.

7.3 Thinking

Although there has been an immense amount of thinking about *thinking* over the centuries by philosophers, theologians, psychologists, and artificial intelligence types, our thinking processes, like all other cognitive processes, remain observable only through the behavior they elicit. Should thinking not lead to overt behavior, there would be no evidence of any thought processes being executed even though our minds might be very active. Thinking, in a behavior-free context, would remain covert and beyond the reach of scientific inquiry.

However, this does not mean that the mind is not active or that a person is not thinking when there is no behavior; it means only that such activity is hidden from the experimenter's inquiries. In such a situation many of the goals of cognitive neuroscience concerning thinking remain unobtainable. Under normal conditions (excluding such states as the locked-in syndrome or vegetative states where there is always some question of residual thought), there is little doubt that we (our brains and our minds) can be and probably are at work mentally (whatever that means physiologically) almost constantly as we adapt, solve problems, muse, worry, and generally deal with environmental problems, probably including at least some of the time we are asleep. However, it must be reemphasized, the link is weak—behavior is not a necessary accompaniment of conscious thinking, and it is possible to conceive of behavior without consciousness (for example a reflex) as easily as consciousness without behavior.

How can we distinguish between consciousness and thinking, should we wish to make that distinction? One way is to remember that consciousness was conceived of as a more or less passive process; thinking can be distinguished from it (barely) as a more active, effortful process that subsumes the presence of consciousness. Necessarily the two (if they are actually distinct psychobiological processes) are deeply intertwined.

Beyond these generalities, however, it is remarkable how difficult it is to define each or to operationally separate the two concepts. Herein is the crux of the difficulty in distinguishing between concepts such as "passive" consciousness and more "active" thinking—the latter presumably involving active and effortful transformation as opposed to simple awareness. Here too, lies another source of difficulty in distinguishing between the two—both are representations, and both are encoded by processes totally invisible to the external observer. Thinking does have one advantage over bare-bones consciousness as an object of study by psychologists. A cognitive task can be phrased in specific terms and the behavioral consequences measured and evaluated. Thus, although we cannot know what the internal processes were that led to a solution, we can control the situation in a way that is not possible with studies of raw consciousness. Whether or not the two can be separated from each other in any useful empirical sense is a question that remains to be resolved in the future.

Other obstacles that make it challenging to distinguish consciousness and thinking also exist. For example, it is obvious that insentient automata are also capable of reasoning, problem solving, and decision making at relatively complex levels. Many of these computational analogs of the equivalent human process can be carried out by even the simplest computer. Unless we are willing to assign consciousness to a computer (or even a device as simple as a mechanical governor), then, it is not a priori necessary to assume that a human problem solver is conscious. Nevertheless, this assumption is often made that tests of thinking are also indicators of consciousness. I make no such assertion in the following discussion.

Nor is the matter clarified by the many alternative definitions of what we mean by thinking including its synonyms—thought, contemplation, or deliberation. At best, thinking has been defined operationally by the kind of task that a subject confronts in an experiment. As a result, much of the research in this field is concerned with some other influences (e.g., music) or cognitive parameters (e.g., intelligence, mental dysfunction, or age) of thinking.

In such a context it has been notoriously difficult to define thinking. The most general definition of thinking I have encountered is that proposed by Holyoak and Morrison (2005, p. 2) when they said "[thinking is] the systematic transformation of mental representations of knowledge to characterize actual or possible states of the world, often in the service of goals." However, this is hardly a satisfactory operational definition for experimental design purposes. As a result it has become fashionable to dissect thinking into components such as reasoning, problem solving, and decision making among many other related mental activities. (I use this trichotomy to organize the following discussions.) Even these subdivisions are not monolithic, however, and each has been further subdivided. Investigators such as Prabhakaran, Smith, Desmond, Glover, and Gabrieli (1997), for example, break down reasoning into even finer categories such as analytic reasoning, figural or visuospatial reasoning, and pattern matching. As we shall see there are many other subdivisions suggested as we pursue this review of brain correlates of the covert behavior we call thinking.

In what is still the most comprehensive meta-study of brain imaging investigations of cognitive processes, Cabeza and Nyberg (2000) cluster problem solving with working memory. Others have gone so far as to extend the basic trichotomy of types of thinking to include the mental activity guiding in motor skills such as dancing (Fink, Graif, & Neubauer, 2009).

However, all of these categories and subcategories of thinking are more or less arbitrary. Their meaning depends more on the design of experiments—the tasks that serve as independent variables—than they do on any psychobiological reality. We can use them as convenient taxonomies to guide our reviews or as experimental operations to help us design our research protocols, but on close examination it is extremely difficult to distinguish between any of these categories. Indeed, there remains an unanswered question—does this plethora of psychological modules, faculties, and components of thinking have any neurophysiological meaning? Are they merely arbitrary and artificial categories into which we jam the huge and endless variety of experimental variables that psychologists manipulate? Can we really separate any of these hypothetical constructs so that they are as pure and pristine as our current postulates of psychological research imply? Even more specifically, can we assign particular brain regions to each of these constructs? Certainly it does not seem to be the case from Cabeza and Nyberg's (2000) review. Their charts suggested that there was no location that was repeatedly activated when the problem-solving research prior to 2000 was reviewed. Instead, the pattern of activations was erratic with even seemingly identical tasks producing different results scattered broadly across the brain.

Because of the special intransigence encountered in the process of defining such a term as thinking, I shall not delve deeply into any further discussion of its psychological meaning. Much of it has already been incorporated into the discussion of consciousness, and there is little additional insight to be gained by a further review of what are intangible and inaccessible processes. Instead, I will concentrate in the rest of this section on the cognitive neuroscience of thinking as it has been defined by researchers who are active in this field.

7.3.1 Traditional Neuroscience Investigations of Thinking

The use of the EEG as a measure of any thought process is an attractive idea that has been pursued virtually from the time that Berger (1929) reported the first successful human recordings. Since then, however, most of the important questions concerning the relation of the EEG to mental activity remain unanswered. For example, it is not yet fully understood which portions of the brain produce the alpha rhythms. It was originally (e.g., Lindsay, 1938) believed that they originated from the occipital and temporal regions of the brain. Nowadays most investigators (e.g., Sabbagh & Taylor, 2000; Shaw & Bodner, 1999) emphasize the role of the frontal and parietal regions in generating EEGs. Within these broad areas different experiments produced different answers to the question of where the various components originate. Furthermore, different regions of the brain may respond by either enhancing or degrading the EEG signal strength as a function of thought.

As Jacobs, Hwang, Curran, and Kahan (2006) noted, EEG measures of thinking are concurrently influenced by a wide variety of experimental conditions and manipulations. It is, therefore, difficult to isolate and control any one of them in even the best-controlled experiment. Among the many conventional properties of psychological function that may be confounded with thinking are "task difficulty, stimulus type, memory load, attention, and recognition of previously viewed stimuli" (p. 978). Furthermore, other EEG frequency bands than the most familiar alpha rhythm may respond differently than does the alpha. All of this leads them to conclude that ". . . recent reviews . . . describe a diverse array of relations between oscillations and behavior, with no single pattern emerging clearly" (p. 978). The absence of a clear pattern of EEG and behavior relations is ubiquitous throughout the entire field in which this type of brain electrical activity is measured. The problem is not restricted to higher cognitive processes, but it is accentuated there by the wide distribution of activations, the complex interactions between the subject and the environment, as well as the high degree of instability of even the simplest qualitative measures of the EEG.

Reasoning

Over the years a number of different tests of reasoning (as distinguished from either problem solving or decision making) using the EEG as the measuring instrument of choice have been reported. Some experimenters have used overall power measures of the various components, whereas others have concentrated on the location of sources of activity of one or another of the components of the frequency spectrum.

An interesting aspect of this research is the effort to link music and mathematical reasoning. Sarnhein et al. (1997) and Shaw and Bodner (1999), for example, reported that listening to Mozart's music enhanced activity in the right frontal and left temporoparietal regions. This increased activity was associated with improved performance on some synchronized spatiotemporal behavioral tasks.

Similar tasks have been used to study mathematical reasoning in an effort to control the vagaries of a completely free-running "stream of consciousness" as it would be measured with a standard EEG. One of the first such studies (Glass, 1964) concluded that the alpha rhythm was markedly reduced during mental arithmetic over the occipital lobe. This confirmed and extended the original observation by Berger of alpha suppression when a person became mentally active. But, as we see shortly, some kinds of mental activity increase, rather than decrease, activity in other frequency bands of the EEG.

Mathematical reasoning has also been reported to activate the frontal and parietal lobes by Sakkalis, Zervakis, and Micheloyannis (2006). However, they also pointed out that the frontal lobes are integral parts of other brain systems, and this may lead to an underestimation of the full range of regions contributing to the encoding of mathematical reasoning. Furthermore, in reviewing the literature they also pointed out that a number of other brain regions have been involved in mathematical thinking including the frontal, central-parietal, parietal, and cingulate lobes (Sakkalis et al., 2006, p. 57). Clearly, the ambiguity of what we mean by reasoning and the variety of experimental conditions make any such localization of this or any other kind of high-level cognitive process extremely tentative. There remains in addition the possibility that any attempt to localize reasoning may be naive. Or, phrased somewhat differently, in the world of distributed brain mechanisms that is increasingly becoming clear, the "where" question may be totally inappropriate in our search for the neural underpinnings of cognition.

Decision Making

When we turn to studies of thinking that seem to be better classified as examples of decision making, we find that the concept of a highly distributed system also recurs in the relatively sparse published research on this topic. Spydell and Sheer (1982), for example, found that a 40-Hz EEG signal was enhanced over both cerebral hemispheres during what they called problem-solving tasks.

Philiastides and Sajda (2007) used a combination of EEG measurements and fMRI images to locate the neural sites for the three components of their theory of perceptual decision making. Their previous EEG experiments (Philiastides & Sajda, 2006) had suggested that the three stages of this kind of cognitive process were (1) early visual perception; (2) a task difficulty component; and (3) postsensory decision events. The decision events were reported to activate the lateral occipital cortex, the right ventrolateral prefrontal cortex, and the fusiform gyrus. Although the exact extent of the activated voxels may not have been fully represented by this trio of regions, it is notable that the involved regions extend from the front (the frontal region) to the back (the occipital lobes) and also included the temporal lobe (the fusiform gyrus). These findings suggest that virtually the entire brain is involved in the kind of decision-making task used by Philiastides and Sajda to evoke these neural events.

However, in contemporaneous EEG-based research, a very different distribution of activity than that reported by Philiastides and Sajda was associated with decision making by Jacobs, Hwang, Curran, and Kahan (2006).[11] Jacobs and his colleagues described how it was not the occipital, frontal, or temporal regions that produced the maximum EEG activity associated with decision making, but rather, it was detected by an electrode that was placed on the centerline on the top of the head.

It is difficult to determine from the published literature why this discrepancy in reported location exists; one possibility is that different frequency bands of the EEG were used to identify different regions of the brain. (Jacobs et al., for example, used a 4- to 8-Hz band, whereas Spydell and Sheer used a 40-Hz band). On the other hand, there is such a variety of ill-defined psychological tasks (what, indeed, does the activity known as "mental arithmetic" mean?) that it is often the case that there is little correspondence between two tasks verbally described as being the same. Considering the number of variables (some controlled and others uncontrolled) that are involved in producing these EEG signals, it becomes understandable, if not explicable, why there is such variability and inconsistency in the published literature. Whatever the reasons, clearly it is not yet established where in the brain such a high-order cognitive process as "problem solving" is instantiated. The likelihood that there is no possible answer to this question should not be overlooked.

Problem Solving

EEG studies of the third component of thinking—problem solving—also produced a pattern of inconsistent results. Jausovec (2000), for example, compared alpha rhythm power levels associated with such tasks for gifted and average subjects. Their results depended on the specific problem-solving task asked of their subjects. Tests that involved logical thinking (which Jausovec referred to as "closed" problems) indicated that the alpha activity was enhanced for the more intelligent students but not so much for the less intelligent ones. On those tests that involved more creative ("opened") problems, however, the more creative subjects were found to produce less alpha power. This latter finding suggested that they did not have to work as hard mentally to solve the problem. Although Jausovec was more interested in the power levels of the EEG, he also provided topographic maps of the EEG signal distribution. These maps show the highest amount of EEG activity was to be found for all subjects in the posterior portion (occipital and parietal regions) of the brain for the conditions of Jausovec's (2000) experiments.

An idea of the inconsistent results in this field can be found by comparing the Jausovec (2000) study with a more recent one by Fink, Grabner, et al. (2009). In a two-part study using EEG and fMRI images respectively, they found that the EEG produced when subjects were carrying out "creative problem-solving tasks" was also highly dependent on the type of task. For some (e.g., an "object characteristic task" associated with behaviorally measured creativity) there was a substantial increase in the alpha activity over the whole brain compared to resting levels. However, when another type of task (e.g., "a name invention task associated with behaviorally measured verbal intelligence) was used, there was a limited area of increased alpha activity in the frontal lobe and a limited area of decrease in the occipital lobe. Most of the brain did not display major changes in the alpha power levels. Further, EEG differences were observed for subjects of different levels of psychological competence (e.g., originality).

The results of the Fink, Grabner et al. study are novel and interesting. Indeed their intrinsic interest may not be in the bare-bone empirical results but, rather, what these findings have to say in terms of the variability of their findings and the sensitivity of the EEG changes to task demands, subject selection, and other uncontrolled variables of which we can only guess. In fact, this is the capstone on this section's discussion—the inconsistency of the pattern of EEG results associated with all of the kinds of thinking considered in this section. There remains, therefore, a real question about whether or not the EEG research is actually capable of answering any of the basic questions about thinking per se. Asking questions of the cortical locations of specific cognitive function certainly has not led to any consensus on what parts of the brain are involved beyond the general conclusion that frontal lobes are involved. Once again it is important to remember that the frontal lobes are implicated in so many different functions, including higher-order cognitive, learning, and emotional processes, (not excluding many other aspects of mental activity) that no consensus about their specific role in thinking is possible.

Furthermore, when EEG power level is the dependent variable, there are also wide differences in reported effects—some laboratories reporting increases and others reporting decreases.[12] The possibility remains that the EEG is simply not measuring the salient codes for cognitive processes but some other neuroelectric activity that, however well correlated, may be nothing more than an irrelevant sign.

In this context of inconsistent results and a general lack of replicability when one uses the EEG methods as the measure of choice, I now turn to the other major measuring device used by current cognitive neuroscientists—the fMRI—to see what other investigators have to say about the brain regions possibly involved in various kinds of thinking.

7.3.2 Functional MRI Investigations of Thinking

We can bridge the discussion from the putative EEG-determined neural correlates of thinking to fMRI measures by considering another part of the report by Fink, Grabner, et al. (2009). As noted in the preceding section, their experiment was a two-part one in which both EEG and fMRI measures were used. This study is of interest not only because it one of the most recent neuroscientific explorations of thinking (in this case problem solving) but also because comparisons can be made between methodologies within the context of the same laboratory using the same behavioral tasks.

It turned out that Fink, Grabner, et al. (2009) reported quite a different pattern of results when the fMRI measures were used to evaluate brain activity than when the brain responses were examined with EEGs. The first outcome of the fMRI part of their study was that any of the four behavioral tasks they used produced the same pattern of widely distributed brain image responses when compared with passive visual fixation. Virtually all regions of the brain (including the cerebellum, the hippocampus, and the thalamus) showed some activation; however, there was a notable difference in the two hemispheres. With the exception of the occipital cortex and the cerebellum, which were bilaterally activated, major neural activity associated with thinking seemed to be on the left side of the brain.

Although some subtle differences in the fMRI activation areas were elicited when the images to the four behavioral tasks were compared, the summary table of Fink, Grabner, et al. (2009) make it clear that there was little agreement between the EEG and the fMRI findings. Specifically, these investigators state that:

However, the hemispheric fMRI activation differences between the AU and OC task [*sic*] are difficult to reconcile with the EEG data with respect to their interpretation as cortical activation or deactivation. . . . Moreover, this finding appears to stand in contrast with [other] findings of simultaneous EEG-fMRI which suggest a negative relationship between alpha band power and brain activation as measured by the hemodynamic BOLD response. (p. 746)

Given this evaluation in one of the most recent studies of the purported relation between brain images and EEG measures, we are led to ask—is there any consistency among the fMRI findings themselves that shows reliable brain activations associated with such nebulous mental processes as reasoning or problem solving?

Cabeza and Nyberg (2000) have already given one answer to this question; there was substantial variability in the regions associated with problem solving (one of the main categories of thinking) in the published literature prior to the turn of the millennium. Their tabulation is shown in table 7.1.

In the three subsections that follow, I update their meta-review by considering the same question for publications occurring after the year 2000. Again, for conceptual convenience rather than any suggestion that they truly represent different categories of thinking, I examine a small sample of findings from those reports that self-identify as example of reasoning, problem solving, and decision making.[13]

Reasoning

First, let us consider a few recent examples of what cognitive neuroscientists have identified as the brain regions involved in what are characterized as reasoning experiments. The most striking development in the field of neural correlates of reasoning has been the relatively recent emphasis on a particular region of the frontal lobe as being a localized center for this kind of cognitive processing. Although the frontal lobes have been known for years to be involved in higher cognitive processes, it was not until the early twenty-first century that

Table 7.1

Table of activation peaks produced in problem-solving tasks

Table 5: Working Memory (continued)		Frontal										Cingulate				Parietal			Temporal								Occip			Subcort		
Study	Contrast	10	9	46	11	47	45	44	6	8	4	32	24	23	31	7	40	39	38	ins	42	22	21	20	mt	37	19	18	17	bg	th	cb
5.4 Problem Solving																																
Rao 97	conceptual reasoning - ctrl	●		✦		●			✦	●		✦				✦		✦								●		●	✦ ✦		● ●		✦
Nagahama 96	card sorting (MCST) - rest							✦		●	○	□		■	■		✦	○										●				✦
Goldberg 98	card sorting (WCST) - ctrl	●	✦	✦			○	✦				■					✦	●										●	✦ □	○ □ ○		
Berman 95	card sorting (WCST) - ctrl	●		✦	✦	○	○	✦		●		✦				○	✦	○				✦	●		○			✦ ✦		✦	
Goel 97	sent: deduction - understand					○	○																					○			
Goel 97	sent: induction - understand	○	□			○				□		□	□											○			○				
Owen 96a	Tower London (hard) - ctrl		○						●	✦						✦	●										●	● ✦	○		
Baker 96	Tower London - ctrl	●	✦				●		●	✦		■	□			✦	●										✦	✦ ✦		■ ○	
Elliot 97	Tower London - guess					✦	●		✦																		✦		●	● ●	
Flitman 97	covered maze - sm ctrl	●							●																		●				
Prabhakar. 97	Raven figural - match		●	●								■				✦	✦									●	●				
Prabhakar. 97	Raven analytical -match	●	✦	✦			✦	✦	✦			✦				✦	✦	✦						✦		✦	✦ ✦				
D'Esposito 95	dual task - single tasks	●	✦	✦																											
Klinberg 98	dual task - ctrl	○	●					○								✦			○	●											✦
Goldberg 98	dual task - single tasks							●		○								●	○	○ ●										✦
Goldberg 98	single tasks - dual task	○	○	○		○			○												○				●	● ✦			✦
5.5 Other																																
Barch 97	delay (8 sec > 1 sec)		○	○			○	○								○	○														
Barch 97	difficulty (interaction w/scan)					●	●	●	■			■															●				
Jonides 98b	lett: hold & inhibit prepot resp - hold					○																									
Bonda 96a	tactual identity - ctrl															✦	●														✦
Zatorre 94	melody: compare notes - listen	✦	✦		●	✦		○	□			✦				✦	✦			✦			●							■	■

From Cabeza & Nyberg (2000).

a particular region—the rosterolateral prefrontal region (a region at the lower edge of the frontal lobe) became associated with a wide variety of thinking processes. Among those who made this association early on were the groups of Christoff et al. (2001) and Kroger et al. (2002).

Based on these earlier suggestive studies, Wendelken, Nakhabenko, Donohue, Carter, and Bunge (2008) concentrated their attention on the rostrolateral prefrontal cortex. They showed that this region was especially strongly activated when a subject was carrying out an analogy type of reasoning task. However, they also reported that this was not the only area being activated during this type of cognitive task. Several other regions were also activated across the brain including sites in the brainstem, the insula, the cerebellum, premotor regions, and the occipital lobe. The initial interest in the rostrolateral prefrontal cortex, therefore, may be an example of selective attention on the part of earlier experimenters rather than a true selectivity on the part of the brain.

Melrose, Poulin, and Stern (2007) based their investigation of frontal brain activity and reasoning on the known connection between the frontal cortex and the caudate nucleus, one of the basal ganglia of the brain. Using fMRI techniques while a subject was carrying out a novel reasoning task in which judgments had to be made by following a sequencing rule, they found that broad regions of the cerebrum, as well as a number of brain stem regions, were more strongly activated than during appropriate control conditions. Specifically, the list of activated regions and nuclei contained many areas of the cerebrum including several regions in the frontal (especially the now familiar rostrolateral prefrontal cortex), parietal, and temporal lobes, and, of special interest to them, the caudate nucleus head, the putamen, and the globus pallidus. The left caudate head was specifically associated with their reasoning task in accord with their original anatomical assumption of a strong connection between that subcortical region and the frontal cortex.

Rodriguez-Moreneo and Hirsch (2009), quite to the contrary, using a syllogistic reasoning task and fMRI techniques implicated a different system of brain regions involved in this type of reasoning process. The components of this system included areas in the prefrontal, the parietal, and the caudate nucleus. The areas activated shifted as a function of what part of a syllogism was being processed (i.e., whether it was processing the first or second premise or drawing the conclusion). The published brain images in this study show, in disagreement with other studies in this section, a more sparsely localized pattern of activations.

There are two implications of this body of work on reasoning. First, there is little agreement among the various studies. Second, the range of activated regions is very broad; it is harder to find brain regions that are not activated during reasoning than those that are.

Problem Solving

One of the most important preliminary roles of the experimenter is to structure a task for the subject that hopefully emphasizes the desired cognitive activity; in this case, problem-solving behavior. A number of standard protocols have been utilized over the years including mathematical problem solving and games such as the Tower of Hanoi or the Tower of London, the latter of which was probably first suggested as a standard tool by Owen, Downes, Sahakian, Polkey, and Robbins (1990).[14] Two similar studies using the Tower of London provide an opportunity to directly compare their respective results for this kind of problem solving with the findings for the reasoning tasks discussed in the previous section on Reasoning as well as with each other.

The first study of problem solving to be considered using the Tower of London was reported by Schall et al. (2003). Their subjects viewed two samples of Tower of London displays on a computer display screen and were asked to mentally solve the problem of determining how many moves it would take to go from the first position to the second as fMRI brain images were constructed. The parts of the brain that were activated in this study included several regions of the frontal and parietal lobes as well as the cerebellum.[15] Because of the importance of comparison I draw here, it is important to be more specific about the location of the fMRI activations. For this experimental protocol Schall and his colleagues (2003, table 1, p. 1158) reported that the responding areas included the following regions:

- Left superior and middle frontal gyri
- Right middle frontal gyrus
- Right inferior frontal gyrus
- Left parietal lobule

- Right postcentral gyrus [parietal]
- Left cerebellum
- Right Cerebellum

The second study of problem solving using the Tower of London task was reported at nearly the same time by Newman, Carpenter, Varma, and Just (2003). Their use of the Tower of London task produced fMRI activations in the following regions (table 1, p. 1673):

- Left dorsolateral prefrontal cortex
- Right dorsolateral prefrontal cortex
- Left superior parietal cortex
- Right superior parietal cortex
- Left inferior frontal gyrus
- Right inferior frontal gyrus
- Left inferior parietal cortex
- Right inferior parietal cortex

Newman and her colleagues (2003) pointed out that since none of the inferior frontal or parietal regions of the brain co-varied with task difficulty, they focused on the bilateral dorsolateral prefrontal and the superior parietal cortices. They also went on to associate these brain regions with highly specific aspects of cognitive functioning. They contended that the right dorsolateral prefrontal cortex was encoding planning activities, whereas the left dorsolateral prefrontal cortex was controlling the execution of the plan (p. 1676). On the other hand, the right superior parietal region was associated by them with attention, and the left served as a "visuo-spatial work space" (p. 1677).

The task now before us, however, is to consider whether these two patterns of activation are consistent or inconsistent when compared. At first glance they share a certain superficial similarity. Both patterns involve the frontal and the parietal lobes of the brain. The main discrepancy is that Schall and his colleagues involve the cerebellum and Newman and her colleagues do not. This kind of discrepancy may be due to the technology and procedures used and by itself would not justify a "no match" conclusion. The major agreements are to be found in the fact that the two studies both emphasize the frontal and parietal regions in their response to what is as close to a "standard" problem solving task as there is in this field.

However, a more detailed examination suggests that the findings from these two studies do not agree as much as they may have initially seemed. Newman et al. report a more diverse group of brain loci than do Schall et al. Furthermore, the activated parietal regions are on opposite sides of the brain in the two studies. The bilateral dorsolateral prefrontal cortices that play such a central role in the Newman et al. (2003) study are not represented in the Schall et al. (2003) study.

Parts of these discrepancies may be accounted for by the rather loose terminology that is used by these investigators (as well as all others) to localize activation areas. Some of it may be explained by discrepant thresholds of activation. Other sources of disagreement may be due to the subtasks involved.[16] However, beyond the fact that the broad swaths of the frontal and parietal regions were activated, the finer identification of subareas within these areas seems highly questionable.

When we shift attention to another problem-solving type of task—mathematical thinking—the situation becomes even more confused. First, the psychological processes involved (e.g., mathematical fact retrieval as opposed to calculation per se) are categorized quite differently than are the reasoning or game-playing tasks previously discussed. Second, the brain regions that are reported to be activated are quite different for each of the mathematical processes of interest. The implication is that this kind of problem solving is different at both the psychological and neurological levels. Mathematical problem solving can also be divided into subprocesses, and there is no a priori reason why any of these need activate the same places in the brain. Thus, for example, Grabner et al. (2009) attack the problem of the cerebral localization of mathematical problem solving and find that the left angular gyrus is the main region when one is either retrieving mathematical facts or solving arithmetic problems requiring retrieval.

Grabner and his colleagues (2009) then went on to report that "application of procedural strategies" activates a much more widely distributed region of the frontal and parietal lobes. These included a number of regions that do not correspond to those reported by Krueger et al. (2008). Krueger and his colleagues were more concerned with integral calculus problem solving. They attributed this kind of "procedural thinking" to a system of brain regions including the inferior parietal sulcus, dorsolateral prefrontal cortex, posterior superior parietal lobe, precuneus, and posterior cingulate (all of which were on the left side of the brain except the precuneus that was bilaterally activated.) They claim, however, that this is the same system involved in basic arithmetic problem solving. Once again the overall conclusion is that these studies of problem-solving behavior produce results that are inconstant with each other. The main agreement shared by all of these studies is the broad distribution of neural responses regardless of the type of thinking task.

Decision Making

The third proposed category of thinking is decision making. If anything, the trail to a clear definition of what we mean by this type of thinking gets even muddier. The range of processes that might be included under the rubric of "decision making" is virtually unlimited. Indeed, just one subdivision of decision making—executive processes—has taken on a following of its own. Executive processes studied by psychologists also come in numerous guises attended by a host of special names such as volition, planning, as well as circularly returning to some of the processes already discussed—such as problem solving or reasoning.[17]

"Executive function" or "decision making"—whatever one calls this process—sounds very much like the more inclusive term "thinking" itself. It is more likely that what we are considering here are a set of names for the design of psychological experiments in which one or another high-level cognitive process was being manipulated. There is far less support for the notion that these hypothetical cognitive processes represent or correspond to specific neurobiological entities at this molar level of analysis. Even so, there have been efforts to further subdivide executive functions into subcategories. For example Wager and Smith (2003, p. 271) fractionate decision making into two subdivisions:

- Manipulation of information in working memory
- Updating and prioritizing information in working memory

These subdivisions obviously are tied to other theoretical constructs from the literature of psychology. The question of interest in the present discussion is whether or not such categorizations are necessarily linked to demarcatable brain regions? A little preliminary thinking suggests that there is no logical reason why the psychological dimensions of behavior and thought need be encoded by different places in the brain. It is equally likely that this is a misconception reflecting the persistence of the phrenological-localization hypothesis that still afflicts cognitive neuroscience.

Nevertheless, interest in locating executive functions in the brain, stimulated by the pioneering psychological studies of Baddeley and Hitch (1974), has dominated this aspect of research on decision making in recent years. Despite a substantial amount of research in this field, it remains extremely difficult to operationally distinguish between decision making and executive processes. Indeed, it is difficult to operationally distinguish between either of these two categories and thinking or such widely accepted processes as working memory. Clearly, for reasons good and bad, a compelling, useful taxonomy of these high-level cognitive processes remains elusive. This has led to a mass of what are often uncoordinated neuroscientific findings that not only do not fit together very well logically but that are in large part empirically inconsistent with regard to the activated brain regions.

Over the years both clinical and experimental evidence (Fuster, 1989; Luria, 1966; Stuss & Benson, 1986; Wagner, Maril, Bjork, & Schacter, 2001) has tended to associate the frontal lobes with executive and decision-making functions. However, as should be clear by now, the frontal lobes seem to be involved in every kind of emotional, learning, or high-level cognitive processes ever described. The very universality of frontal lobe activation in all mental processes may make meaningless any attempts to pin down the specific role of it or any of its subparts in any of the huge variety of mental activities in which it may participate.

Jurado and Rosselli's (2007) meta-review of executive functions and the brain also made it clear that although the frontal lobes are involved in many different kinds of decision making, it is not to the exclusion of many other brain regions. Even within the context of the frontal lobes, there is a great variance in which of this lobe's putative subdivisions are activated during this kind of thinking. A considerable amount of theoretical controversy concerning the role of the poorly demarcated brain regions still pervades the field. Proposed associations between one or another particular kind of decision making and specific regions of the frontal lobe often disappear in the randomness of the results from a variety of experimental procedures.

Just a few of the many recent brain imaging studies that have dealt with some aspect of decision making are considered here. Sylvester et al. (2003) examined the fMRI images produced when subjects were faced with two different kinds of executive function—attention switching and response inhibition tasks—respectively. They found that both tasks enhanced activations in the bilateral parietal cortex, the left dorsolateral prefrontal cortex, the premotor cortex, and the medial frontal cortex; however, other areas became active with the attention-switching tasks including the occipital lobe and a superior parietal area.

Wager and Smith (2003) meta-reviewed 60 neuroimaging studies that aggressively investigated the problem of executive decision making. They reported that various executive subtasks produced activity in regions widely distributed over the entire front half of the brain as well as in the posterior portion of the parietal lobe.

Hampton and O'Doherty (2007) commenting on a variety of brain imaging studies of decision making implicate the anterior cingulate cortex, the medial prefrontal cortex, the dorsolateral prefrontal cortex, the orbitofrontal cortex, the amygdale, and the striatum as being especially strongly activated in situations in which decision making was required.

The major conclusion emerging from this brain imaging literature on decision making was that the broadly distributed portions of the frontal lobes are involved in our thought processes as they are variously defined. This confirms what has been known for years. We can look as far back on the iconic study of Phineas Gage or on the pre-imaging work of Luria (1966) in which the general ability to carry out complex psychological activities (i.e., thinking) could be seriously disrupted while other speech, sensory, and motor skills go unscathed after frontal lobe damage. Similarly, one of the justifications for the rash of frontal lobotomies in the mid-twentieth century was that only (or mainly) pathological thought processes would be affected by frontal lobe surgery. (See Valenstein, 1986, for a full discussion of this sad excursion into a particularly horrific side of cognitive neuroscience.) Also in similar fashion, experimental brain surgery carried out by such workers as Kamback and Fife (1975), among many others, had already associated frontal lobes and what appeared to be behavioral correlates of brain lesions there. How much progress and deeper understanding the brain image movement of the past two decades has added to these generalizations is unclear.

Considering the sample of reports discussed here, the main conclusion is that broadly distributed portions of the brain are activated when we "think." The frontal lobe, in particular, seems to be generally accepted as the part of the brain that is most often activated during high-level cognitive processes. However results vary drastically from subject to subject and from experiment to experiment. Wendelken, Nakhabenko, Donohue, Carter, and Bunge (2008) reminded us that "The precise regional boundaries associated with this functionality remain an open question" (p. 682) and Rodriguez-Moreno and Hirsch (2009) asserted that

". . . there are substantive differences between the findings with respect to the specific regions engaged in reasoning. . ." (p. 949). Furthermore, even within the context of a specific report, the verbal statements and the sample brain images do not always agree. The sources of this variability have been discussed in several places in this book. At this point, I briefly summarize some of the reasons for the observed variability and inconsistency of the brain responses that are characteristic of high-level cognitive processes such as thinking.

1. The anatomy of the brain may vary from person to person, and, therefore, any assignment to a particular region may be uncertain.
2. The tasks presented to the subject, although categorized with different words (e.g., reasoning, decision making, problem solving) may not map onto different brain mechanisms. In other words the psychological terminology may not be congruent with the neural terminology.
3. Since fMRI thresholds are arbitrary, slight differences in criteria may lead to different brain regions being associated with thinking.
4. Different control conditions may have prevailed.

What does this general finding of variability and inconsistency mean? There are two possible answers to this question. It may be that, despite the unfortunately large amount of variability, the results are real; any apparent inconsistency results from the complexity of the quest on which cognitive neuroscience has set out. Less than robust or misleading statistical analysis procedures, poor task control, and other covert influences may all contribute to producing results that are extremely sensitive to the plethora of variables influencing the cognitive task. In such situations, the slightest differences in protocol may produce enormous differences in activated areas. Thus the true nature of the brain may be that it is organized in a modular manner that may correspond in some rough way to psychological constructs. In other words valid and stable "signals" may not yet have risen above the "noise" produced by inadequate experimental control. Following this point of view, our results, although quite noisy, are generally correct; there are, in point of empirical fact, some specialized functions assignable to specific parts of the brain.

There is, however, a much more disconcerting possibility. That is, all of these data are essentially artifactual! It is possible that the fMRI procedure and the complex analysis techniques being used are producing what are essentially phantom activations because of the poor signal-to-noise conditions. Ill-defined psychological modules such as "mathematical problem solving" or "reasoning" simply may not correspond to the way the brain is neurologically organized. There is no logical or a priori reason why the plethora of hypothetical constructs invoked by psychologists should map directly onto brain organization. From this perspective brain imaging findings simply may not be germane to the problem of measuring the true neurobiological level at which the brain encodes thought, reasoning, problem solving, decision making, and all of the other high-level cognitive processes that have intrigued psychologists for centuries. The imaging techniques, in this eventuality, simply may be incapable of unraveling the mind-brain question. This may be a case of the appearance of order emerging from what is essentially a random process.

The general point here is that rather than looking for specific regional functions, we should be considering the frontal lobes as a general purpose information-processing engine. It is likely that it will show some activation to a greater or lesser degree to almost any stimulus task to which it may be confronted. Differences in details may have more to do with the momentary needs for information processing than the nature of the stimulus or task.

Answering the question of which of these two possible answers is the correct one is a task for the future. However, to ignore the possibility of the second answer—it is all artifact and illusion—is foolish. Such a misjudgment could lead to an enormous waste of valuable resources as well as a total lack of confidence in the cognitive neuroscience of the future.

7.4   Intelligence

In the previous section I examined the scientific literature related to the process we call thinking. A closely related but slightly different way to look at thinking is to consider its quality—in other words, how good are the thought processes in solving problems and making decisions. Measures of the quality of our ability to carry out thought processes are subsumed under the rubric of intelligence. In the broadest sense the property we call "intelligence" is simply another synonym for "mind." However, in a more specific sense (and the one I pursue in this section), it is a measure of our ability to carry out high-level cognitive processes.

Surprisingly, although the focus of research efforts in thinking and intelligence may actually be the same (distinguished only by the choice of the task, the measurements being made, or the vagaries of our psychological language), the two fields of inquiry seem to have grown almost independently. Whereas reports of the various aspects of thinking are usually found within the literature of a more arcane experimental psychology, students of intelligence often are associated with personality, educational, and clinical psychology. Unfortunately, the two cultures often do not speak to each other. Needless to say this is an artificial dichotomy, and neither field has come close to its own consensus concerning what intelligence is. It is worthwhile, therefore, to look at intelligence as a separate facet of the general problem of high-level cognitive processes.

Although consciousness and awareness are more or less binary—a person is either conscious or he is not[18]—intelligence is, in principle, much more fundamentally scalable. The reason for the special role of intelligence in this list of high-level cognitive processes is that degrees of intelligence can be quantitatively measured in terms of the relative amount of success in accomplishing some behavioral task (including a wide variety of "intelligence" tests). Thus, a person or a laboratory animal can be challenged with a problem, and the degree to which the individual successfully solves the problem (which may differ from individual to individual and from species to species) can be measured with considerable accuracy and reliability.

In some ways the nature of intelligence is also akin to that of memory and learning since both are tightly linked to behavioral outcomes. Thus, the outcomes of both intelligence testing and learning are measurable properties of often highly standardized stimulus conditions—unlike consciousness or thought that can proceed with no observable stimulus or behavioral correlates. However the underlying mental or neural processes of all of these cognitive processes remain as inaccessible as ever.

A continuing problem in the study of intelligence is the comparison of different species on tests of performance. It is of interest to measure the relative capacities of different species to solve problems in an effort to calibrate what are assumed to be differences in intelligence. Yet interspecies comparisons are fraught with uncertainty for a number of reasons. One of the most perplexing complications concerns the environment in which a species has evolved and the differing skills that each species must develop in order to survive and prosper in its own particular niche. Thus, intelligence, however it is measured, is likely to mean different things to different species. Human tests of intelligence are obviously inappropriate for lower animals, and gradations in their ability to solve problems encountered in their environment may be equally inappropriate for us.

A long-term historical debate concerns whether intelligence is a single parameter or property of cognition or a cluster of separate measurable abilities, each of which can and should be assayed separately. The idea of a unified, general intelligence is usually attributed to Galton (1879). During the early days of twentieth-century psychology most psychologists agreed with Galton and with Spearman (1904) that there was a single general intelligence. In more recent times Thurstone (1938), to the contrary, proposed that intelligence was made of seven primary abilities all of which are assumed to be measurably independent properties of conscious thought:

- Verbal comprehension
- Verbal fluency
- Mathematical ability
- Memory
- Speed of perception
- Reasoning skills
- Spatial visualization

Nowadays, there is a consensus emerging (e.g., Sternberg, 1985) accepting some version of the multiple factors idea and minimizing the importance of a single, generalized, universal intelligence. Specifically, Sternberg suggests that there are three aspects to intelligence: (1) analytic intelligence; (2) creative intelligence; and (3) practical intelligences. There persists, however, a feeling among many researchers that there is a kind of umbrella intelligence, signified as "general intelligence," that consists of "fluid intelligence," which itself may be distinguished from "crystallized intelligence"; the former refers to the ability to solve new problems and the latter to the ability to apply stored knowledge to new problems (Cattell, 1971).

Nevertheless, the task of defining intelligence is as difficult now as it was years ago. The best we can do is to note that people differ in their ability to carry out certain cognitive tasks, and this variation is in some way a property of the mind–brain that we call intelligence. The nature of the tasks used to measure intelligence varies from time to time but the idea of a scale of abilities to comprehend and to solve problems persists at the heart of virtually all of the psychological research concerned with this cognitive property. As a high-level cognitive process, it is assumed that it is a brain process; this has led to the hope that we might be able to find some kind of a neurophysiological marker that could serve as a biomarker or correlate of whatever it is that is intelligence.

Until the development of neurophysiological recording equipment (e.g., the ERP and the EEG in the twentieth century), most research on intelligence was in the domain of psychologists; however, since the 1920s there have been continuing attempts to find biological markers of intelligence. It is to this topic to which I now turn.

7.4.1   Traditional Neuroscience Research on Intelligence

At the present time, the brain properties that account for differences in human intelligence remain unknown. Studies of brain size have, in general, been equivocal. For example, Burrell, (2004) discusses the failed attempts to correlate Einstein's brain structure with his extraordinary intelligence. Haier, Jung, Yeo, Head, and Alkire (2004, p. 425) also allude to the fact that "total brain volume accounts for about 16% of the variance (a very small proportion) in general intelligence scores."

Whenever a new instrument capable of measuring brain activity becomes available, cognitive neuroscientists converge on it in an effort to provide some entrée to the solution of at least a limited part of the mind-brain problem. Given the strong interest over many years in the many aspects of individual differences and abilities among people, the immediate application of the ERP and the EEG at midcentury to the study of intelligence was preordained. It was a perfect match of a higher-level cognitive process whose behavioral correlates could and had been measured by a plethora of different "intelligence" tests. However obvious it may have seemed in the early days, the history of EEG measures of intelligence has been fraught with uncertainty and controversy throughout its later history. As in so many other cases when electrophysiological devices were applied to cognitive neuroscientific topics, the persistent uncertainty and inconsistency of the ensuing results did nothing to dissuade the faithful.

Electroencephalograms were used in the search for a brain correlate of intelligence from virtually the beginning. Among the first researchers to attempt to find correlations between the standard EEG and intelligence was Berger (1933) himself. In an EEG study that may have literally been the first application of EEG-based cognitive neuroscience, he applied the new technique to study the intelligence of low-intelligence subjects. A series of similar articles followed from the laboratory of George Kreezer (e.g., Kreezer, 1937; Kreezer & Smith, 1936) exploiting what was then perceived to be a positive correlation between the EEG and these large individual differences in intelligence.

The a priori attractiveness of applying the EEG to study intelligence led to a subsequent burst of activity throughout the 1930s and 1940s. However the literature emerging from those times was wildly inconsistent; many investigators reported positive relations, and others did not observe any correlation. In subsequent decades, several reviews (Ellingson, 1965, 1966; Lindsley, 1944; Ostow, 1950) came to the conclusion that there was no empirical justification for assuming the EEG was strongly enough correlated with intelligence to be used as a practical biomarker. Whatever correlations did exist, these critics argued, were due to third factors (e.g., retardation, brain damage, etc.) rather than to a real relation between intelligence and EEGs.

Not to be outdone, a vigorous group of supporters continued to report correlations in the massive amounts of data that were so easily accumulated with the EEG device. Reviewers such as Vogel and Broverman (1964) came to the antithetical conclusion that positive correlations between intelligence and these brain signals existed at least during childhood. On the other hand, even these enthusiasts acknowledged that experiments on adults were equivocal. Vogel and Broverman attributed the earlier inconsistent findings with adults to methodological issues, especially to which band of the EEG spectrum (among the many possible frequency bands) had been used in the evaluation. The debate between Vogel and Broverman and Ellingson continued with a rebuttal by Vogel and Broverman (1966). Indeed, the debate continues to this day, however in the new context of brain imaging.

Despite the explosive impact of brain imaging on cognitive neuroscience, there is continued interest in using the EEG as a measure of intelligence. Nevertheless, after many decades the evidence remains mixed and the conclusions controversial. Positive results were reported by modern researchers such as Mundy-Castle (1958) and Anokhin and Vogel (1996), whereas researchers such as Oswald and Roth (1974) claimed there were no such correlations. A phrase common to many investigators working in this field is ". . . the question of whether basic EEG characteristics are associated with intelligence in normal adults remained controversial." (In this particular instance the quote is from Anokhin & Vogel, 1996, p. 1.)

Despite the controversy and uncertainty surrounding the use of the EEG as a biomarker of intelligence, it continues to be used by some investigators who believe that they have found some frequency component or processed measure of it that can reliably be associated with intelligence. Currently, popular measures include the total power[19] of the entire EEG spectrum of frequencies, the power of the alpha rhythm alone, and the coherence or phase delays among the various frequency components, as well as nonlinear systems analyses.

Among the most committed appliers of the EEG power measure to the study of intelligence have been workers in Klimesch's (1999) laboratory. His approach was based on the observation that the alpha (~10 Hz) and theta (~5 Hz) frequency bands of the EEG behaved quite differently when each was compared to intelligence scores. The reason, he argued, that simple EEG measures did not always correlate with intelligence test scores was that it was a nonlinear combination of the activity in the different frequency bands. He argued further that much of the problem resulted from the fact that the alpha and theta frequency bands actually responded in complex and often opposite directions that depended on a flexible and arbitrary assignment of what was assumed to be the meaningful constituent range of frequencies. Klimesch also has claimed that different frequencies of the alpha band correlated differently with different intelligence tests (Doppelmayr, Klimesch, Stadler, Pollhuber, & Heine, 2002).[20]

A parallel program of research utilizing power measures of the EEG frequency components has been carried out by Fink and Neubauer (2006). Unfortunately much of the possible impact of their results was reduced by the fact that many of their correlations between tasks and alpha power were qualified by the phrase "just failing to reach statistical significance" (pp. 50 and 52).

More complex nonlinear analysis methods[21] have been utilized by a number of current workers. However the results using this approach are also typically controversial. For example Anokin, Lutzenberger, and Birbaumer (1999) reported a negative correlation between nonlinear measures of the EEG and intelligence, but other investigators such as Lutzenberger, Elbert, Birbaumer, Ray, and Schupp (1992), seemingly from the same group of co-workers, reported a positive correlation.

Obviously efforts to use the EEG as a measure of the various kinds of mental activity we subsume under the rubric of intelligence have not been successful. There is an extraordinary ambiguity and inconsistency of the findings reported over the last 80 years. No matter how elaborate the analytic techniques, experimenters (sometimes coming from the same laboratory) report that their findings do not agree with other similar studies and/or that the significance levels barely meet the criteria for reliability.

In the face of this uncertainty, one is compelled to ask—why do some workers persist in their search for what is at best a weak predictor of mental capabilities? In large part the answer to this rhetorical question is the intuitive attractiveness of a tangible, neurophysiological biomarker of what is an elusive indicator of otherwise inaccessible properties of our minds such as intelligence. To put it simply, EEGs, as measurable signals from the brain, have a compelling attractiveness and face validity; so much so that these characteristics overpower the actual evidence measured by modest correlations, insignificant, unreplicable, inconsistent, and, typically, small differences. A positive aspect of the current situation is that there is reduced interest in the EEG's ability to fulfill this role as newer techniques have come along. Two in particular have redirected the interest of students of intelligence and the brain—the ERP and brain imaging. It is to the topics of the ERP to which I now turn.

If the EEG has been controversial, but persistent, so too have been attempts to use the ERP as biomarker for intelligence. One of the first studies using the ERP was reported by Chalke and Ertl (1965). They measured the averaged ERPs to visual flash stimuli and showed that the latency of the response was inversely related to the intelligence test scores measured for their subjects. This was supported by earlier psychophysical studies that showed a similar inverse relationship with reaction times—a correspondence that suggested to them that more intelligent subjects were responding neurologically more efficiently than less intelligent ones. The idea of intelligence being expressed in the form of faster or more efficient neural information processing, however, was not supported by subsequent research. For example Davis (1971) carried out an extensive study with over 1,000 subjects and could not replicate Chalke and Ertl's original observation.

A more comprehensive review of the ERP literature (as well as the work using standard EEGs) has been published by Robinson (1993). He listed many of the problems in interpreting this kind of experimental finding, especially with the neural significance of the ERP waveform itself. His main contribution, however, was to highlight some of the conceptual and methodological problems involved in associating the ERP with intelligence. These problems involved individual differences in both the ERP waveform and the intelligence scores, unreplicated findings, spurious high correlation from some laboratories, incorrect data analyses, and inadequate presentation of data and sample waveforms. Of particular importance, Robinson pointed out that alternative explanations of whatever correlations were observed were not adequately considered. For example, arousal and attention could also produce similar effects on the EEG and ERP (e.g., reduced reaction-time latencies) that had nothing to do with intelligence per se. Robinson's review was an early but particularly compelling and robust criticism that might well be read in the modern context of the brain imaging approach.

Despite the well-noted deficiencies in both the empirical and conceptual arenas, the effort to find such a relation has continued over the decades. The original inverse correlation between intelligence and ERP latency has been occasionally replicated even in the most recent research, for example, by Liu, Shi, Zhang, Zhao, and Yang (2007).

Currently the study of intelligence with ERPs and EEGs is a highly suspect enterprise. Despite the fact that there have been a long series of articles and reviews challenging the validity of the basic idea—that scalp-recorded signals can serve as a biomarker of such subtle cognitive processes as intelligence—there, nevertheless, continues to be a considerable amount of effort being expended to find support for this hypothesis. At the very least we have not yet found the proper link between these brain signals and intelligence tests. One possible reason is that the interactions are so complex and the involved variables so numerous that we have not yet been able to establish the actual connection or even the degree to which the brain signal and the intelligence test result do correlate. However, as with the search for biomarkers for thinking in general, another possibility is that the reported correlations are actually spurious or artifactual and do not represent solid and replicable evidence. If this second alternative is correct, it can be argued that any continued effort to establish this relation using these techniques is not likely to produce any breakthroughs in theory or practice.

In short, the presumption that any EEG or ERP brain signal is a meaningful indicator or sign of intelligence, then, may be driving any residual attention to these poorly understood measures rather than a succession of mutually supportable empirical findings. The neural mechanisms underlying behaviorally measured intelligence are almost certain to be considerably more complex than the simple assertion that smart people's brains work faster or are more efficient than those of their less fortunate brethren. One dismal conclusion is the neuronal networks underlying such a subtle high-level cognitive process as intelligence are so complex that they will be forever inaccessible and unanalyzable.

7.4.2 Brain Imaging Research on Intelligence

In this environment of invalid presumptions, inconsistent results, and inexplicable complexity, it was a given that any new and promising measuring tool would be quickly applied to the study of intelligence. The next technological development—brain imaging—was not long in coming. Unfortunately one main theme—the hypothesized efficiency of the brain exhibited as shorter reaction times and less activation for the bright compared to the less bright—remained unchanged. The neural efficiency hypothesis originally suggested by the EEG methods (originally pioneered by the work of Chalke & Ertl, 1965, and Kreezer, 1937) became the foundation of the modern brain imaging work on intelligence.

The first experiment to specifically study the relation between PET brain images and intelligence was reported by Haier et al. (1988). Their main finding that was that the brain of more intelligent subjects utilized less glucose to solve problems than did those of less intelligent subjects—and, thus, should be considered to be more "efficient." However, in their recent and comprehensive review of this "neural efficiency" theory, Neubauer and Fink (2009) pointed out that modern data are far less convincing than the earlier results. In fact indicators pointing to differences in neural efficiency are modulated by a number of interacting factors including gender, task type, complexity, and, unsurprisingly, the degree of learning experience a subject may have with the experimental task. Based on their review of the "neural efficiency literature, Neubauer and Fink (2009) concluded that, "From integrating this evidence, we concluded that the neural efficiency phenomenon is observable mostly when individuals are confronted with tasks of (subjectively) low to moderate task difficulty and is most frequently observed for frontal brain areas" (p. 1021). In other words, there are so many subjective and neural variables that one can probably find brain image correlations with intelligence someplace, under some conditions, at some time. Although Neubauer and Fink go on to suggest that the neural efficiency hypothesis is not totally lost, some major changes are obviously necessary in its formulation before any sense can be made of it.

Other workers seeking a brain imaging biomarker for intelligence have aimed in different directions. Instead of seeking a generalized neural efficiency, many investigators have concentrated on finding which regions of the brain seem to respond in ways that appear to be significant for intelligence. This renewed emphasis on localized function is guided, of course, by the capabilities of the imaging devices. It is their presumed ability to highlight locations (answers to the "where" questions) that influenced this change in direction.

For example Duncan et al. (2000) using PET techniques reported what they believed to be the site of a neural mechanism underlying general intelligence in the lateral frontal cortex. Their results were offered in contradiction to the idea that more challenging tasks would recruit more extended regions of the brain. They observed no such distributed recruitment for the more challenging tasks.

An important improvement in the quality of much of this research was the standardization of the behavioral measures of intelligence provided by the test known as Raven Progressive Matrices (Raven, 1936).[22] The convergence on this method has provided a considerable amount of order to what was a chaotic and ill-formed cluster of intelligence tests. Nevertheless, Raven's matrices are not perfect, and there is no a priori assurance that what is being measured by this test is what we otherwise mean by the term intelligence. Despite these caveats the use of this test has been a major improvement over the vague definitions of intelligence typical of so many of the other tests. If only the forthcoming data had emerged equally well standardized, some progress might have been made. As we now see, using the best of modern equipment, such standardization was not to be. We now have no more confidence that a biomarker of intelligence has finally been discovered than we did before the use of this test.

The next step, the introduction of the fMRI system, promised to regenerate some of this lost confidence. Unfortunately, here, too, different investigators found different regions of the brain corresponding to what were supposed to be different degrees of intelligence. Gray, Chabris, and Braver (2003), using fMRI images for example, reported that in addition to the frontal regions, activations in such other regions as the dorsal anterior cingulate, the cerebellum, and other regions scattered within the parietal and temporal cortices correlated with intelligence. No localization here, but, instead, these findings suggested a distributed network of many different regions that correlated with general fluid intelligence.

Quite to the contrary and depending on the specific behavioral tasks, workers such as Waiter et al. (2009) reported broadly separated regions in which activations varied with the particular cognitive task. Unfortunately, as they reported, "We did not, however, find any correlation between BOLD activity and intelligence" (p. 205), although there were correspondences to processing speed and working memory.

Finally, in this brief survey of brain imaging studies of intelligence, a meta-review of the scientific literature by Jung and Haier (2007) incorporating the findings of 37 different studies came to the conclusion that distributed activity in virtually all of the brain was involved in intelligence. Specifically, Jung and Haier invoked roles in intelligence for regions in the frontal, parietal, temporal, and occipital lobes. Although not all of these studies reported activations in all areas, almost all of them indicated multiple regions across the brain that did so correlate. Unfortunately the behavioral tasks were so varied as to prohibit any firm conclusions concerning possible brain mechanisms.

In sum, there is not yet any robust neurophysiological biomarker of intelligence. The consensus is that, as for all other high-level cognitive processes, widely distributed systems of functionally generalized regions of the brain are involved in encoding whatever it is that is meant by the factor we call intelligence. Unfortunately, beyond that generalization both the traditional and the modern data are so inconsistent and unreliable as to preclude any neurobiological explanation of intelligence at the present time.

7.5 Interim Conclusions

Determining the neurophysiological nature of consciousness and other high-level cognitive processes represents the ultimate goal of psychology's long search for a solution to the mind-brain problem. Yet, these intrapersonal experiences are among the least amenable to any kind of reductive scientific analysis. They exist at the most personal and inaccessible level of mental processes; as such they represent the most formidable challenge to any plan for neuroscientific study. Indeed, we still do not know whether our self-awareness is a cause or an inconsequential side effect (an epiphenomenon) of behavior. The two (behavior and consciousness) seem not to be inextricably interconnected; behavior can occur without consciousness as well as consciousness without behavior.

A factor that further exacerbates the problem of a scientific study of consciousness or thought of any kind is that we do not have a well-ordered taxonomy of the relations among the various components or the meanings of the mentalist terminology. Can we think without being conscious? Or, on the contrary, are these words just synonyms for exactly the same thing? Questions like these have perplexed those intrepid investigators who seek to apply the techniques of both traditional psychological and modern neurophysiological research to mind-brain studies. It seems likely that both the mental processes we call conscious thought and the brain mechanisms that instantiate them are aggregates of many components. A major question arises, therefore: can we separate out any of the components? Or, are these features of cognition so thoroughly entangled that they must be treated collectively? Will consciousness evaporate as a result the very effort to dissect it?

It seems clear now that the existence of consciousness is more an inference than a solidly proven fact. There are no neurophysiological measures that can be used to either accept or reject the existence of consciousness in a person or a machine. There is neither a "Turing test" nor a constellation of behavioral indicators that can distinguish between an automaton and a sentient entity. Our ideas of consciousness depend solely on the single datum of own personal self-awareness and the analogies drawn between ourselves and other minds. Many of the questions asked about consciousness are bad questions that cannot be answered. Animal research does not ameliorate this problem; it accentuates it.

The following list summarizes some of the empirical evidence from investigations that have purported to have studied such high-level cognitive processes as thought and consciousness.

1. So far, there are no reliable single neurophysiological indicators of consciousness.

2. Consciousness is inferred, probably incorrectly, from indirect behavioral measures such as discriminability or by using indirect logical connections involving such imprecise constructs as subliminality.

3. Whatever else can be said of the literature on brain imaging of consciousness, one firm conclusion is that it is characterized by a lack of consistency and a high degree of variability among the reported results. It is difficult to find studies that agree on what brain regions are activated even when the experimental design appears to be relatively similar. The higher the level of the cognitive process under investigation, the more profound is the inconsistency. The most consistent report is the involvement of the frontal lobes in high-level cognitive processes. However, as we have noted, the frontal lobes seem to be involved in all cognitive activity, and, therefore, activity there has little to say specifically.

4. Electroencephalographic and brain imaging studies typically differ in their reports of which brain regions are activated.

5. Like most other brain imaging studies carried out on any of the other topics in this book, the inescapable conclusion is that broad swaths of the brain are involved in virtually any cognitive process including the current topics of consciousness and thought. Narrow localization is a misunderstanding of the past. Not only do the most recent studies suggest this to be true, but meta-studies make the conclusion more robust.

6. Thinking, a term sharing many common features with consciousness, is also an inference based on indirect behavioral responses. Indeed, it may not be possible to distinguish between the two; they may be either the same process being evaluated by slightly different experimental methods or slightly different aggregations of a set of overlapping functional components. The main connotative distinction is that consciousness is assumed by many researchers to be more passive than is the act of thinking.

7. Problem-solving ability, decision making, or reasoning—one tripartite model of the components of thinking—are also more alike than recent experimental designs suggest. This is another result of the failure of precision in our definitions.

8. There is rarely any exact replication of experimental reports; investigators seem to have their own individual definitions of what are the essential features of each kind of cognitive process. This leads to a lack of standardization of experimental designs and is probably a major factor in the widespread inconsistency reported in the scientific literature.

9. Intelligence remains an elusive phenomenon neurophysiologically. Although there are a number of behavioral tests that can reasonably well quantify intelligence, there are no

known biomarkers that can be used to measure it. Indeed, it has not yet been determined whether intelligence is a single attribute or property or if it is a composite of many different abilities or factors.

10. There is a continuing controversy over the use of EEGs or ERPs as a measure of intelligence. Despite decades of research there still is no convincing evidence that the EEG (or any processed version of it) or the ERP is functionally related to intelligence.

11. Brain imaging techniques, of course, were immediately applied to the search for an electrophysiological correlate or marker of intelligence. None has been successful. Whether a generalized metabolic indicator of brain efficiency or differences in the regions of the brain activated for people of different intelligence was used, the results have always been controversial and erratic.

12. It is still unclear whether brain images and EEGs are real psychobiological measures of cognitive activity or merely irrelevant artifacts. The worst-case possibility—that brain images are neither correlated (signs) nor measures of the true psychoneural equivalences (codes) but are artifacts driven by other unknown factors—cannot be entirely rejected at the present time.

8 Applications

8.1 Introduction

Cognitive neuroscience, as discussed throughout this book, is one of the most exciting and fastest-growing fields of scientific biology. Impressive developments have been made in the study of the anatomy and physiology of the nervous system. For obvious reasons, philosophical as well as technical, the possible application of such powerful modern technologies as the fMRI to the study of the brain has generated an enormous amount of interest. Because the brain is the organ of the mind, the link between the two seems self-evident. As a result the association of the brain mechanisms associated with cognitive processes promises to be what many consider the major development ever in this burgeoning new science. Certainly the amount of effort and resources currently being expended in using such technologies as fMRI to study cognitive activity has been exceptional. The ultimate goal in such a quest would be to discover some kind of a "biomarker" or neurophysiological signal that was sufficiently reliable and quantitative to be used as a practical indicator of a cognitive process in a variety of applications.

Unfortunately, however much we may desire it to be otherwise, we have already seen that cognitive neuroscience is still in a relatively underdeveloped stage with a huge bag of empirical results crying out for interpretation, understanding, synthesis, and comprehensive theory. For many reasons a profound misunderstanding of many of the accomplishments of cognitive neuroscience has led to optimistic hope taking the place of critical evaluation. In point of fact we really know less about the brain-mind relationship than is generally appreciated.

Despite the promise, at this relatively early stage of development it is difficult to determine what the successful applications are going to be. Although some are likely to be of great value, it is equally certain that many explorations will be dead ends at least in the foreseeable future. The main reason for this uncertainty of application is that even at this date, the empirical data are inconsistent, and the explanations and interpretations of those data still depend more on speculation than empirical proof.

We have at this point encountered some of the difficulties and challenges and begun to appreciate that the ultimate goal of cognitive neuroscience—to understand how mental activity arises in neural tissue—is far more remote than virtually everyone at every stage of its history had thought. With so much promise and yet so much uncertainty, it would be irresponsible at least not to ask a few preliminary questions concerning plausible applications that might make use of these findings and understandings that are currently available. If nothing else, it would be useful to appreciate some of the already known limits of this science.

It is likely that some suggested applications can already be deemed to be impossible and others to be so improbable that discarding some of the existing behavioral techniques they might have promised to replace would be injudicious. Because hyperbole runs amok in this field to a degree that is unprecedented in modern times, this is a worthwhile exercise. The purpose of this chapter, therefore, is to distinguish between probable and impossible or unlikely applications of cognitive neuroscience.

The major barrier to the application of brain imaging techniques to some fields is the clash of levels at which they operate and the level at which most high-level cognitive processes operate. This has been a main theme of much of our earlier discussion: that is, subtle personality and other cognitive and behavioral properties of people (indeed, all mental activity) are most likely manifestations of the intricate neuronal connections among the huge number of neurons in our brains. Unfortunately the imaging techniques lose all of the details of these interactions as they cumulate, pool, and average them into an irresolvable sum. Thus, properties such as intelligence are not likely to be explained at the molar level available from brain images.

Before we continue this discussion, there are some caveats that have to be raised in light of the current stage of development in brain imaging. First, it is quite clear that we still are nowhere near an answer to the general and very hard mind-brain question—how does the brain make the mind? Indeed, many scholars believe that we still know virtually nothing about how this magical transformation occurs. Others raise the possibility that it is an unanswerable question.

Second, despite the hype, much of the progress that has been made is not going to be transferable to any practical application. There is a strong tendency to take some kind of a preliminary, suggestive, but unreliable finding and to draw from it a premature conclusion that "just a little more effort," "a little more funding," or "a slightly more powerful machine" will bring us to the brink of something that would truly revolutionize both science and human life.

Third is the probabilistic nature of even the best research. Although we may someday be able to say something about group averages, it is unlikely that at any time in the future we will be able to use these probabilistic distributions to diagnose or measure individual human capabilities, proclivities, or dysfunctions.

Fourth, like so many of the other approaches to cognitive psychology, many cognitive neuroscience findings exist in the form of isolated, fragmented, and surprisingly unreplicated observations. As much as we hate to admit it, hope and the powerful human drive to understand this most difficult of scientific enterprises drive more of the expectations and hopes than do solid, reliable, empirical facts. Hyperbole and exaggeration dominate both scientific and lay communications, most evident when the two meet in the popular media. Unfortunately, in such a situation much of these hopes for the future are not likely to be fulfilled.

Please understand that in no way am I denigrating the powerful uses of brain imaging (or any of the other earlier neuroelectric techniques that preceded it) in solving problems of anatomy and physiology—that is, of structure and function. The criticism that is expressed throughout this book is with the application of neuroscientific techniques and findings specifically to our high-level mental or cognitive processes—exactly the kind of processes for which we have the most critical clinical and other applied needs. It is in this domain that much of the misdirection, hyperbole, and unwarranted expectation have most often been encountered.

A current example of the exaggeration and unwarranted expectations that characterize the application of cognitive neuroscience to a practical field can be found in a recent report by a committee of the NRC (2009) entitled *Opportunities for Neuroscience for Future Army Applications*.[1] This report deals mainly with the selection and training of military personnel. Throughout the report, there was a continuous overestimation of the successes achieved so far by neuroscience research. It seemed that hopes and needs were often conflated with plausible possibilities. "What would be wonderful," if achievable in some distant future, was uncritically reified into "what can be done—later!" Often "what can be done—now" had to take the place of "what would be nice." The undeniable operational needs of the Army stimulated fanciful extrapolations from very preliminary and statistically uncertain results. For example, it was asserted at the very outset (p. 2) of this NRC report:

. . . neuroscience offers new ways to assess how well current training programs and accepted assumptions about learning achieve their objectives.

On page 6, the comment was made:

Neuroscience has identified the risk factors associated with the development of PTSD and related stress disorders.

On page 30 we read:

. . . noninvasive tracing of major fiber pathways provide an opportunity to learn how we can use these novel methodologies to enhance training and personalize it to meet the needs of the soldier . . .

On page 53:

Neuroscience techniques . . . can be used to measure the training status of individual soldiers.

On page 58:

Imaging techniques could be used to detect individuals who are at high risk for experiencing deterioration of performance . . .

On page 149:

. . . psychologists are able to test cognitive models of the human mind against functional data.

This last is actually a hotly debated issue in cognitive science. Many argue that cognitive models cannot be tested by fMRI because the cognitive models have no neural postulates. In point of empirical fact, there is virtually nothing in the scientific literature that supports any of these wild leaps of fancy. These remarks and others like them are not supported by even flimsy empirical data. At best there are very preliminary and surprisingly infrequently replicated observations that suggest that it might be possible, however improbable, that at some remote future time such an application of neuroscientific techniques might substitute for the kind of behavioral measures that have been so successful in treating or teaching human beings. On the other hand there is increasing evidence that some of these goals may be chimeras whose capture will never happen.

Finally, on page 179:

. . . individual differences in behavior, cognition, and performance of skilled tasks are deeply rooted in the neural structures of individuals. . . . This common theme offers great opportunity to the future army.

This last statement sums up the flawed logic that underlies the incredible overoptimism and hyperbole that pervades this entire report. Of course all mental and behavioral processes are dependent on the nervous system. We have known this for centuries. This is a basic postulate of modern cognitive neuroscience as discussed in chapter 1. However true this may be as an ontological tenet, it does not logically support the conclusion that it is likely or even possible to link these cumulative and early brain measurements to mental processes specifically enough for us to begin to think of substituting a brain image or some other electrophysiological biomarker for a behavioral measure of some cognitive process. The search for such biomarkers will go on for centuries, probably well beyond even the most optimistic time lines expressed in this NRC (2009) report.

The remainder of this chapter deals with the preliminary nature of such claims and the evidence that suggests that our hopes, in many cases, may be running far ahead of scientific credibility, or, for that matter, that they have already been tested and found lacking.

8.2 Anesthesia

The idea of a controlled and reversible decent into unconsciousness to minimize pain and discomfort was one of the most important developments in medical history. The control of surgical pain by drugs or gases (e.g., ether, chloroform, nitrous oxide) dates from the middle of the nineteenth century. However, natural narcotics (e.g., cocaine and opium) and alcohol must have had a much longer history. What is considered to be the first use of nitrous oxide as a surgical anesthesia was by a dentist—Horace Wells—in 1844, as discussed by Jacobsohn (1995).

How efficient such agents were, however, could only be guessed at by surgeons. The task of monitoring the depths of anesthesia remained a major challenge. At first purely behavioral indicators were used. Was the patient responsive? Was there any reflex action such as increase in the heart rate when an incision was made? Were there any movements, or in the most extreme case, complaints made by the patient? Later on as modern surgical technique improved, more direct physiological measures such as blood oxygen levels, breathing rates, blood pressure, and even measurement of the residual amount of anesthetic in the exhaled breath of the patient, were added to the measures that it was hoped would be good indicators of the depth of unconsciousness and, thus, insensitivity to pain.

There is no question, of course, anesthetic unconsciousness and insensitivity to sensory stimuli is primarily a brain state; these other physiological measures, regardless of how well they work, are indirect and not directly related to the absence of consciousness. Although we have only limited knowledge of how anesthetics work to reduce consciousness (as reviewed by Urban, 2002), there has been a prolonged search for correlated "biomarkers" that are sufficiently closely associated with consciousness to provide indicators of the depth of anesthesia. One of the applications of modern neuroscientific technology that has been a long time coming was monitoring the brain state of a patient undergoing surgery. The ultimate goal is to develop an electrophysiological measure of brain activity that is sufficiently well correlated with consciousness to be used as a measure of the depth of anesthesia.

One early promising indicator was the EEG. Although the neural origins of the irregular cyclic waves that are recorded when a high-gain amplifier is connected to contact electrodes on the surface of the skull are still not unequivocally known, the EEG has been an object of considerable research as a potential tool for monitoring the depth of anesthesia.

The EEG is cyclic electrical activity recorded from the surface of the skull. The first indication that there was such a signal recorded from animal brains was reported by Caton (1875) and from the human skull by Berger (1929). The first application of the EEG to monitoring anesthesia was reported by Gibbs, Gibbs, and Lennox (1937)—a surprisingly recent date. Initially, simple visualization of the mixed array of frequency components of the raw EEG was applied to measuring anesthetic depth. However, it is now generally agreed that the raw signal is not a satisfactory measure; it is too irregular to simply act as a measure of consciousness and is useful only as the grossest of measurements. For example, changes in the raw EEG may indicate that not enough oxygen is getting to the brain or that some other major discontinuity in the anesthetic process has occurred.

Although a considerable amount of research still goes into the use of the raw EEG signal as an indicator of anesthetic unconsciousness, a number of new analytic techniques have been developed that process the signal to extract or emphasize certain features of it. (See Rampil, 1998, for a good introduction to the kinds of signal processing that have been and are currently being used.) Foremost among them is a simple Fourier or frequency analysis in which the various frequencies of the EEG are separated from each other so that each can be used as a specialized indicator. Frequency analysis can also be used to measure the power or energy in the individual components of the frequency spectrum of the EEG. However, this "power spectrum" is only part of a frequency analysis; a second part, the phase spectrum in which the temporal relations of the various frequency components are examined, has also been considered to be potentially useful in measuring the degree of consciousness.

Higher-order statistical analyses (the bispectrum and the trispectrum procedures, respectively) of the EEG have also been studied. Specialized techniques such as the bispectral (BIS) system (Mashour, 2006) that process the raw EEG data are now being offered by commercial organizations. Yet even the most vigorous proponents of the use of such techniques report that they have many limitations (see, for example, Jeleazcov & Schwilden, 2003). For all practical purposes, and despite a vigorous and extensive amount of research, the utility of these higher-order statistical measures remains controversial. They have not been unequivocally shown to have any added value beyond simple measures such as the mean and variability of the raw EEG signal. Indeed, despite a major effort to link the EEG components or high-order statistical measures to consciousness, some investigators would argue that we have still not gone very much further than the original observation by Berger that the resting signal (mainly characterized by the alpha wave—a 10-Hz frequency component) is suppressed when the subjects looked at or thought about something.

A problem with the EEG as an indicator of mental processes during anesthesia is that this signal is sensitive to a number of other factors than the state of consciousness of the patient. For example electrical signals are often recorded that are related to electromyographic artifacts. In addition, the EEG varies in different ways depending on the particular anesthetic substance being used. Thus, it may be only indirectly related to the actual conscious state of the surgical patient. As with any study of cognition or consciousness, the difficulty of directly linking an indicator variable with the degree or state of consciousness remains formidable.

At the current time there is a substantial amount of disagreement and controversy concerning just how effective the EEG is in supplementing the traditional physiological and behavioral measures of anesthetically produced unconsciousness. One particular problem (beyond the desire to keep a patient immobile and within normal hemodynamic limits) concerns the risk of residual awareness (i.e., insufficient loss of consciousness) to the degree that the patient might experience pain or discomfort during surgery or remember the pain or discomfort following surgery. Although relatively rare, as many as 26,000 cases of awareness during or after surgery are expected in the United States each year (Sebel et al., 2004).

The *Swedish Council on Technology Assessment in Health Care* issues evaluative reports on the value of new medical techniques. In a recent report (SBU, 2008) based on an extensive review of the relevant literature, it was considered whether there was any advantage of EEG monitoring compared to the traditional methods for avoiding unexpectedly high levels of consciousness during surgery or for improving recovery from anesthesia. The conclusions were that there was insufficient evidence to answer these questions.

In general anesthesia, the scientific evidence is inadequate to support routine use of EEG-based monitoring of anesthetic depth aimed at reducing the incidence of awareness or improving patient recovery. The council stated that there seemed to be little advantage of any kind for using EEG monitoring. In general the report concluded that If EEG-based monitoring is used, it should only complement traditional anesthesia monitoring and should not be accorded greater importance than traditional monitoring. The risk for misinterpretation, and the resulting consequences (too deep or too shallow anesthesia), must be considered carefully in each individual case." (SBU, 2008, Unpaginated)

Earlier research in the United States had also raised questions about the value of some of the more elaborate EEG processing devices such as the BIS. For example, Sebel et al. (2004) pointed out that such machines may actually increase the occurrence of awareness due to low levels of anesthesia by providing a false measure of conscious state of the subject.

In general the literature describing the use of such analytic methods is filled with ambiguous and contradictory results that are at best merely suggestive and at worst counterindicative of the routine use of the EEG in either the raw form or in any of its processed versions to monitor surgical unconsciousness.

Therefore, the one conclusion for which the surgical community (see, for example, Jameson & Sloan, 2006) has achieved closure, it seems, is that the EEG at best can only be a supplement to the traditional physiological measures of anesthetic unconsciousness and should only be used alone in the most unusual circumstances.[2] Although I have not been able to find any statistics, it does appear that the uncertainty surrounding the utility of the EEG is reflected in the relatively small proportion of times that it is actually used by anesthesiologists in the surgical arena.

Given the limits of the EEG, other electrophysiological signals have been suggested as alternative means of monitoring anesthetic depth. Another example of such a measure is the evoked brain potential (EVBP) or, as it is more familiarly known nowadays, the event-related potential (ERP). Following up on some wartime RADAR developments in small-signal detection, Dawson (1950) developed an averaging technique for the detection of very small brain responses to impulsive sensory stimuli. The averaging was required because the amplitude of these tiny evoked potentials (about 10 μV) was an order of magnitude less than those recorded from the standard EEG (about 100 μV). Because of the randomness of the EEG and the time-locked nature of the EVBP, repetitive stimulation and averaging resulted in the extraction of the evoked potential as the random "background noise" of the EEG averaged to zero.

Evoked brain potentials or ERPs can be recorded to many sensory stimuli, and many of them show some relation to the conscious state of a patient; drastic differences are shown between the somatosensory evoked potential when the subject is asleep compared to the wakeful state. The key is having sufficient control over the repetitive sequence of stimuli so that the averaging process will begin at the same point each time a stimulus is presented.

For this reason auditory clicks and light flashes as well as electrical pulsed stimuli to the somatosensory system have proven to be superior to stimulus modalities for which the timing of the stimulus is not so easily controlled such as gustation or olfaction.

The averaging technique has many flaws, but it has been suggested that it too might be a better indicator of the state of anesthesia than the EEG. In particular, the auditory evoked potential (AEP) or auditory brain response (ABR), a particular kind of ERP, has been thought to hold special promise for this application (Thornton & Sharpe, 1998). The advantage of the AEP is that it is a compound signal responding not only to the early acoustic nerve responses and late cortical responses but also to brainstem responses in intermediate parts of its cycle. (See fig. 2.7 for a complete analysis of this sequence of signals.)

There are, however, a number of problems inhibiting progress in any attempt to use the AEP as an indicator of anesthetic depth. The amplitude of acoustic signal may be modified by other anatomic and physiological states of the patient; the response may habituate after the repeated averaging necessary to detect the signal; even how well the body temperature of the patient is maintained can influence the AEP. Nevertheless, there are a number of arguments in its favor. The middle-range components are thought to reflect brainstem activity, and components of the brainstem have long been associated with consciousness and wakefulness. The later components also vary in amplitude with some components dramatically disappearing, doubling or tripling, or changing in their latency as a function of the depth of anesthesia. Remarkably, some of the components of the AEP may disappear completely at various stages of anesthesia, thus also limiting their value as quantitative indicators. A full discussion of the technique for producing AEP responses as well as a review of how the various components co-vary with anesthetic depth can be found in Thornton and Sharpe (1998).

As promising as the method may seem, the problems with the ERP technique are not inconsequential. There are numerous technical difficulties involved in acquiring and averaging the signals. Electrode placement and the prolonged time that it takes for a sufficient number of signals to be averaged may preclude use of the ERP.[3] Also, as with the EEG, it is known that different anesthetic materials may produce different kinds of changes in the ERPs.

In this environment of uncertainty, as well as the great need for a way to determine anesthetic depth, it is not surprising that any new technological development will be targeted as a means of measuring consciousness. So it was that the development of brain imaging techniques, especially the fMRI, stimulated a new round in the search for a brain indicator or biomarker of anesthetic depth. From, the outset, however, such an application of a system that requires the presence of a very large magnet is likely to be problematical. Instruments, other measuring equipment, jewelry, and even stray pieces of metal in the patient's body (e.g., rods, plates, and pins from orthopedic surgery; bullets) are going to present hazards that were not of consequence until this new system was proposed for intrasurgical use. Indeed any suitable instruments would have to be specially designed for this application as described by Karlik et al. (1988) and Peden, Menon, Hall, Sargentoni, and Whitwam (1992). Even space considerations are important in evaluating this application given the small size of the bore of a typical MRI magnet. It is also possible that combinations of chemical anesthesias and fMRI imaging system may introduce other unanticipated technical and environmental incompatibilities that may interfere with the successful use of either technique.

Although it remains very difficult, intraoperative use of the fMRI as a monitor of surgical progress is now being carried out in a few surgical theaters. This requires that all of the magnetic materials be removed from the surgical environment with many of the instruments made of titanium or even ceramics. Even more important is the design of special MRI magnets (e.g., the Signa SP manufactured by GE Medical Systems) that permit the surgeon to have access to the patient, itself a formidable design requirement described by Mittal and Black (2006).

There are other ways in which anesthesia and brain imaging may productively interact. One is the use of anesthesia to reduce activity in patients who must undergo the difficult psychological experience of being thrust into the confined quarters of an MRI system. Here, the anesthesia is secondary, the real problem is—how do you sedate a patient so that he or she is minimally disturbed or disruptive during the fMRI test? The questions of why, how, who, and when to monitor a patient who has to be sedated for an MRI test have been discussed by Kanal and Shellock (1992). In such an environment it is especially important that the added value of an fMRI image as a biomarker of anesthetic depth be established in a way that significantly adds to both economic as well as medical considerations.

The second useful contribution of the fMRI technique in surgery has to do with the preparation of a patient prior to surgery or for evaluation of a patient after surgery. Here, there have been considerable research carried out and many contributions made. The position of tumors, improved precision of definition of brain structure and anatomic details, and selection of the best surgical trajectory to a deep portion of the brain can all be evaluated both preoperatively and postoperatively using an MRI. These are clear examples of how the MRI system can be used in productive and useful manners. Remember, however, that these applications are primarily anatomic and physiological and do not speak directly to cognitive issues.

My interest in the present context, however, is with a third kind of application, one in which the MRI system is used as an indicator of the depth of anesthesia to maintain clinical unconsciousness. It is here that the conceptual, logical, and empirical trail becomes confused and is ultimately lost. To the best of my knowledge, the practical details of large machines and powerful magnetic fields make any routine use of an imaging system in monitoring anesthesia extraordinarily rare at the present time. In a few cases (for example, in ultrasound treatment of tumors [Jolesz, 2009] or in brain surgery [Mittal & Black, 2006]), fMRI systems have occasionally been used intraoperatively, rather than pre- or postoperatively. However I can find no mention of such a system used to monitor anesthetic depth.

There has been some progress in developing small fMRI machines (for example, the PoleStar N-10 developed by Odin Medical Technologies of Israel) that may fill this lacuna in the future, but at the present, it seems to be a promise unfulfilled.

8.3   Vigilance, Alertness, Wakefulness, and Fatigue

Another possible field of cognitive application of neuroscientific techniques that has become of considerable interest is the use of such devices as the EEG, the ERP, and the fMRI to monitor what is generically called vigilance.[4] It is well known in the behavioral literature that performance on many kinds of tests declines with time. That is, as a result of work overload, prolonged periods of sleep deprivation, the cognitively complex process we call boredom, and any number of other factors, people show diminishment in their ability to detect, identify, and appropriately respond to stimulus objects in their environment. Although much of the work in this field has been done using behavioral methods in which the decline in vigilance (defined behaviorally) is directly measured, it has been frequently proposed that indicators of brain function may offer a neurophysiological means of monitoring performance of this kind.

Work on the EEG correlates of wakefulness, a closely related problem, can be dated back to the pioneering work of Loomis, Harvey, and Hobart (1935) in which they followed up on the earlier work of Berger (1929), the investigator who first detected the EEG in humans. Loomis, Harvey, and Hobart attached a primitive EEG machine consisting of a single channel of amplification connected to only one electrode on the skull of a subject and examined the resulting signals when the person was asleep or awake. On the basis of their measurements, they concluded that they were recording a true brain electrical response ("potential rhythms") that was in some unknown way correlated with the states of wakefulness. Although they did not call it an "EEG," it obviously was the same kind of measure described by Berger. They also reported that the recorded electrical response varied depending on the depth of sleep of the subject—at low levels of sleep, acoustic stimuli could produce a burst of response; at deeper levels there was no response to such a sound.

Their next contribution (Loomis, Harvey, & Hobart, 1937) was to show that there were systematic changes in their potential rhythms associated with different levels of sleep. Indeed, Loomis and his colleagues suggested that measurable differences in the brain potentials characterized five different stages of sleep.

The next major breakthrough concerning the EEG and sleep, however, came in a research article authored by Aserinsky and Kleitman (1953). These investigators found that there were two distinct classes of sleep EEGs. The first was the set of three or four different frequencies of slow waves that had been identified by Loomis, Harvey and Hobart, now known collectively as nonrapid eye movement sleep (NREM). The second was a higher frequency pattern of activity associated with rapid eye movements (later to be made famous as REM). If the subjects in their experiment were awakened during REM sleep, most reported that

Table 8.1
Frequency of EEG waves in stages of sleep

Stage	Frequency in Hz
1	4–8 (no spindle activity)
2	3–15 (with spindle activity)
3	2–4
4	0.5–2
REM	20–28

After Dement and Kleitman (1957)

they had been having some kind of a dream. Thus was an association made between the EEG and the mental state of the subject.[5]

At the present time, the first three or four stages of NREM sleep are characterized by a progressive decline in frequency from the typical awake frequency of the 8-Hz to 10-Hz alpha wave[6] as a person passes through what are assumed to be deeper states of sleep, followed by a final stage—REM sleep, as indicated in table 8.1. In addition to the changes in alpha frequency, the progression of other fluctuations in the EEG was also used to characterize these changes by Dement and Kleitman (1957).

There are, unfortunately, several problems facing anyone who desires to use the EEG as a measure of the depth of sleep, that is, of stages of consciousness, just as there are those that limited its use in the measurement of anesthetic depth. One is that the frequency ranges associated with each of these stages overlap those measured at other stages. There are no clear demarcations between stages; any such system will always lead to diagnostic calls that are, to a substantial degree, arbitrary.

Furthermore the variability of the signals at any sleep stage makes any tight correlation between the depth of sleep and the frequency spectrum of the EEG problematical. Far more disconcerting is that we really have no validating data from the cognitive side of this correlation to indicate what even the best conceivable frequency analysis really means in terms of the stages of consciousness associated with sleep. Thus, the sleep researcher (or any one who chooses to use this measure as an indicator of sleep or wakefulness) is using a very blunt tool to estimate how a particular EEG pattern is connected to sleep stages. Even the most advanced analytical processing techniques suffer from this handicap; no matter how precise and regular the measurements of the EEG may be, they have never been and can never be linked directly to a subject's conscious experiential state! What we can do, on the other hand, is to associate these neuroelectrical signals with other physiological or behavioral measures, but this does not overcome the lack of validation introduced by the inaccessibility of the mental state. Another difficulty arises from the fact that sleep is not a monotonic descent through the various sleep stages. Instead, people cycle back and forth between different stages in what may appear to be an almost random order.

In addition and hardly surprising there remains the perpetual problem of individual differences. The brain is so complicated and the precision of our definitions of psychological processes so vague that no single EEG classification system seems to work for all experimental conditions and subjects. It is in this context that we see the relatively large effects of word meaning and semantics or ecological significance that can completely obscure small changes in any kind of electrophysiological signal. (For example, see the work of Carretie, Mercado, Hinojosa, Martin-Loeches, & Sotillo, 2004.)

Despite these enormous experimental challenges, there is continued interest in the possibility of using the EEG to monitor that state of alertness or vigilance of an awake person. Although the work of Loomis and his colleagues, of Dement, Kleitman, and others provided an initial insight into the changes in the EEG as the subject made the transition from a state of wakefulness to one of sleep, most recent work has essentially ignored the changes that might occur within the wakeful state. As a result, using EEGs as a measure of the state of behaviorally defined alertness of a subject in a vigilance task offers quite a different challenge for research. The challenge in this case is to use behavioral responses to calibrate the EEG measures for awake subjects in various, controlled states of alertness. To do so, of course, requires that the signals are not so noisy and that individual differences are not so great as to negate the possible advantage accrued to the objective nature of the EEG.

Roth (1961) was one of the first to seize on this opportunity and to appreciate the advantages that might be available to an investigator working with awake subjects, a situation in which behavioral observations and introspective reports are more easily obtained. He classified the EEG signals during wakefulness as shown in table 8.2.

Because of the erratic nature of the relation between alertness and the EEG, over the years a number of other schemes for the stages of wakefulness have been put forth. A modern example has been proposed by Olbrich et al. (2009). Their system, based on the previous 50 years of research in this field, includes the following four stages from an eye-closed resting stage to the onset of sleep (abstracted from Olbrich et al., 2009, p. 319)[7]:

Table 8.2
Frequency of EEG waves during declining vigilance

Stage	Characteristics
1	Disintegration of ~10-Hz alpha activity
2a	Flattening (zero activity)
2b	5–6 Hz
2c*	3–4 Hz

*Followed by stages 3, 4, and REM, which are sleep stages. Onset of sleep is also characterized by the appearance of high-frequency bursts called spindles.
After Roth (1961).

1. Posterior alpha is mostly seen after eye closing with a frequency of 8–12 Hz and an occipital focus. This oscillation has been referred to as "idling rhythm because it marks a state of relaxed wakefulness corresponding to vigilance stage A1 . . .

2. Alpha power anteriorisation [*sic*] occurs increasingly after several minutes of relaxed wakefulness. Alpha peak frequency shows a slight decrease. This phenomenon is reported to occur during transition to drowsiness . . . and corresponds to vigilance stage A2 and A3 . . .

3. Low voltage EEG is observed during low vigilance stages. The alpha rhythm disappears . . . This EEG pattern corresponds to vigilance stage B1 . . . The low EEG-amplitude in this state is similar to that during intense mental activity and eye open condition.

4. Increase[d] delta (1–4 Hz) and theta activity is observed in parallel with increasing subjective drowsiness . . . corresponding to vigilance stages B2 and B3. The appearance of sleep spindles and K-complexes characterizes sleep onset.

Olbrich his colleagues summed up these verbal descriptions with the chart presented in figure 8.1.

One of the most important aspects of this classification system is its explicit appreciation of the fact that the use of such a system will always be confounded by other variables than solely the alertness state of the subject. For example a major confound exists between the onset of drowsiness and attentive effort. That is, similar EEG response changes will occur to both the state of wakefulness or alertness and the degree of attention paid by the subject

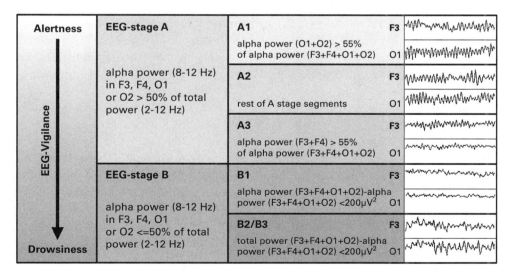

Figure 8.1
EEG stages associated with various stages of alertness.
From Olbrich et al. (2009), with the permission of Elsevier Science and Technology Journals.

to the task; whatever effects of fatigue might have been measured, they may be at least partially counterbalanced by an increase in attention dictated by the onset of a probing stimulus. A further complication is the presence of circadian or even more finally tuned intraday rhythms over the course of an experimental cycle. The situation is further complicated by the fact that the mere presentation of a stimulus has the capability of producing massive changes in alertness when a stimulus is presented during the period in which sleep is restricted and vigilance is low.

Clearly, any physiological measure purported to be a correlate of alertness is going to be extremely noisy, variable, and unstable. It is not at all clear that any further processing will be able to pick out salient and stable measures that can be associated with performance sufficiently well to justify their use in applied settings. Heaped on the general noisiness of the EEG signal, the hopes for a purely electrophysiological indicator of wakefulness, alertness, or vigilance such as the EEG are yet to be fulfilled.

Another possible signal that has been considered as an objective electrophysiological indicator of alertness and vigilance is the event-related potential or ERP. Two early demonstrations that the RAS also affected the ERP in humans were published in 1964. Uttal and Cook (1964) initially showed that there was a distinct difference in the ERP when subjects were asleep compared to when they were awake. In the sleep state, when electrical stimuli were applied percutaneously to the wrist, the ERP consisted solely of two early, brief positive waves occurring less than 20 msec after the stimulus. These responses were localized over the somatosensory region of the brain. When subjects were awake, however, there was an additional very large and more prolonged negative wave occurring about 100 msec after the stimulus. Haider, Spong, and Lindsley (1964), in a comparable experiment, showed that not only were detection scores correlated with similar ERP changes (early plus late components) but so too was a generalized visual vigilance. The next question is whether or not this change can be calibrated in a way that will permit it to be used as an indicator of vigilance or alertness.

Although a number of investigators have attempted to use a late positive component (variously identified as the P300 or P3) as an indicator of vigilance or alertness, many of the studies reporting positive results showed only modest changes in the ERP and barely significant statistical test scores even when there were massive changes in behavioral measures of vigilance. For example, Schmidt, Kineses, Schrauf, Haufe, Schubert, and Curio (2007) carried out a driving test in which the subject was fatigued by 3 hours behind the wheel. Both the EEG and ERP measures were taken every 40 minutes. The results were modest at best. The ERP declined in the first 40 minute period and then barely changed as the driver presumably became more and more fatigued and bored. Thus, there was a dissociation between the ERP and the state of wakefulness of the drivers that casts cold water on the use of this signal as a quantitative measure of wakefulness or alertness. The EEG was taken from both the frontal and parietal areas; however, neither region showed major and consistent changes over the course of the experiment.[8]

In the final analysis, all other arguments should be put aside and the empirical data determine the answer to the question—can the ERP be a useful indicator of fatigue, alertness, or vigilance? The answer to this question seems obvious at the present time—it is not yet ready to serve this function. Typically the ERP responses to different conditions differ by only a relatively small amount (with the exception of major changes from full wakefulness to sleep). Yet, it is on these small differences that many of the conclusions about the practical promise of this work have been based. Furthermore the issue of the practical applicability of the ERP is clouded by the considerable controversy that arises from the inconsistent results. Despite continued assertions that the P300 amplitude varies as a function of prolonged sleep deprivation or fatigue (e.g., Humphrey, Kramer, & Stanny, 1994; Kato, Endo, & Kizuka, 2009), there is considerable contrary evidence that this positive excursion is not associated with fatigue or a decline in alertness over a prolonged period of time (Falkenstein, Hoormann, & Hohnsbein, 2002).

Finally, we can consider the possibilities of the newest candidate—the fMRI—to serve as a biological marker of fatigue or as an indicator of a reduction in alertness over time. Clearly it is going to be difficult to design an experiment that permits both the recording of brain images and measuring behavioral indications of a fatiguing task simultaneously simply because of the practical mechanical problems brought on by the sheer size of the magnet as well as the prolonged temporal dimensions of the decline in alertness.

A continuing problem with this new technology is that it is difficult to know what stage of alertness or vigilance a subject may be in at the time the fMRI image is recorded; behavioral measures are all affected by the stimuli, the environment, and the attention demanding aspects of an experiment. Despite these initial practical problems, a number of investigators have sought to carry out studies that seem to embody this challenging paradigm. One such report documents the work of Olbrich et al. (2009). They attempted to solve the problem of determining the state of arousal by simultaneously recording fMRI activations and using the five-point scale described in figure 8.1 to suggest when a subject was in a particular stage between full wakefulness and the onset of sleep. The results of this comparison were surprising; there was an increase in the strength of the fMRI signal in many parts (e.g., occipital, some frontal regions, frontal, and temporal cortices) with decreasing vigilance and a somewhat lesser increase in others (e.g., the thalamus and some other regions of the frontal lobes).

Olbrich and his colleagues have made a major contribution in this report; however, there are many doubts and uncertainties raised by it. The spatial images they published represent a complex multidimensional vector with each voxel providing some information. Elaborate information-processing algorithms are, therefore, necessary to extract a stable metric that could be routinely used to calibrate vigilance levels. Furthermore there are empirical inconsistencies between the two measures—EEG and fMRI—that must be resolved before they can be incorporated into a single analytic method. The broad conclusion that one draws from EEG data is the *progressive reduction* in the alpha rhythm as the subject moves toward the onset of sleep. The broad conclusion from the fMRI data, however, is of *substantial increases* in activity in the occipital, frontal, parietal, and temporal cortices as well as the anterior cingulate cortices over the same time course. At the same time as activity increased in these brain regions, activity was reduced in the brainstem as well as a few restricted portions of the frontal lobe.

This discrepancy—high alpha activity and low blood oxygenation level dependent (BOLD) activity in the wakeful state—leads to the suggestion that it is *the absence of coordinated activity* that produces the changes in the alpha rhythm. On the contrary, it is *the presence of coordinated brain activity* that produces the activations and deactivations observed in the fMRI. This issue is further complicated by some observers (e.g., Fransson, 2006) arguing that the fMRI is enhanced during early stages of wakefulness and others (e.g., Olbrich and his colleagues) suggesting that the fMRI activity is reduced during these same early stages. Obviously the situation is much more complicated than is generally appreciated. As recently as 2009 Olbrich and his colleagues quite properly concluded that "[n]o generally accepted knowledge about the functional meaning of these BOLD signal fluctuations exists" (p. 320).

Ideally, if we were to calibrate the fMRI system as a means of measuring alertness or vigilance on the part of an observer, we would have to simultaneously run a different kind of experiment—one in which performance on a conventional test of vigilance, for example, was combined with an fMRI survey. Correlations would then be sought with the behavioral scores. Although complex and certain to produce very variable results, it is conceivable that such a study could be carried out with coherent results, possibly in conjunction with an EEG study.

To sum up, the uncertainties in all of these protocols that attempt to measure neurophysiological correlates of wakefulness, sleep, alertness, and vigilance suggest that the routine use of the fMRI as a substitute for a behavioral measure of alertness or vigilance would be a relatively high-risk project. At the present time I can find no research that speaks to this issue and feel that, for both theoretical and practical reasons, it would be an extremely difficult and risky experiment to carry out. The case for the use of the EEG, however, is not so dismal. There are extenuating circumstances that distinguish between electrophysiological measures of alertness and other higher-order cognitive processes. One such factor is that alertness may be a global arousal function of the brain as a whole rather than a cognitive process in which detailed encoding at the network level is required. To analogize, alertness may be more like the power than the information-processing aspects of computer operation.

8.4   Native Ability, Training, and Skill Level

Next we come to a group of applied behavioral topics of great interest to many components of society including our military and business worlds. The basic question is how do we select people who have the necessary native ability for particular jobs, train them to perform at optimum skill levels, and then evaluate their competence in executing the trained tasks? The basic idea is to determine if some of the less tangible aspects of human cognition such as native ability and skill-level activity can be monitored, measured, and correlated with neurobiological activity of one kind or another. I broadly discussed the topics of intelligence in chapter 6 and learning in chapter 5. Here, I consider a more restricted view of abilities and training, not just in the abstract and esoteric realm of psychological or neuroscientific theory, but in terms of the practical aspects of selection and specific motor-skill training.

Learning, has been a mainstay of psychological research and theory building since the origins of psychology as an independent science. It was shown in chapter 5 how the well-defined stimulus attributes and response measures made it possible to make progress in studying the stimulus-response transformations we call learning in a way that had not been possible for most high-level cognitive processes. There is considerable practical interest, furthermore, in understanding how best to learn to execute and then to measure the execution of some important skills. The range of skills is very broad and varies from a task as complex as playing the piano to what seem to be such simple tasks as rhythmic finger tapping. In general we refer to this kind of research as being concerned with motor-skill learning.

The major approach during the early period of interest in motor-skill training was behavioral; that is, parameters of the protocol were varied in order to find the best training strategy or to improve those that were current. Dependent variables were relatively straightforward; behavioral performance scores were measured by evaluating changes in such familiar variables as reaction time, time on target, or error rate. Understanding how these processes worked in terms of their neural underpinnings, on the other hand, was severely limited since these input–output measures did not and could not implicate any specific neurophysiological mechanisms.[9] Therefore, theoretical speculation was unconstrained and all too rife. Theories of motor-skill learning were suggested by many psychologists among whom the most notable were Hull (1943), Fitts (1954), Bernstein (1967), Adams (1971), Pew (1974), Schmidt (1975), and Willingham (1998). Although most of these theories did a fair job of *describing* empirical results, they were confronted with the usual problems encountered when one tried to infer internal structures and mechanisms from behavior—underdetermination.

As a result, rather then converging on a consensus theory, much of the twentieth century was spent either in controversy and argument over the postulates of each of the theories or in the demonstration of practical training strategies. For example questions of behavior-behavior relations were asked such as—Does covert mental rehearsal improve motor-skill learning?—that tell us almost nothing about internal mechanisms. Feltz and Landers (1983) carried out a comprehensive meta-review of the literature concerned with this question and concluded that the field was so rift by controversy due to contradictory findings that it was not possible to conclude that there was anything more than a modest effect of implicit rehearsal, if that. Others asked about the transfer of skills between hands, how best to distribute or clump training trials, or studied many of the other standard questions that had been used in earlier work on simpler forms of learning such as classical conditioning.

During this epoch, motor learning was attributed to various portions of the brain on the basis of neuroanatomy. Florens, the great nineteenth century debunker of phrenology, was the first to discover the association between the cerebellum and motor skills.[10] However, the details of the cerebellar theory were not spelled out until well into the twentieth century when histological techniques were more fully developed. (See the review by Houk, Buckingham, & Barto, 1996 for a summary of the various cerebellar theories of motor-skill learning that were prevalent at the end of the twentieth century.)

The primary motor cortex has now been shown to be heavily involved in motor-skill learning. Kleim, Barbay, and Nudo (1998), for example, demonstrated this association by showing that the areas for the limbs in this region were functionally reorganized following training. Their tool of choice was the microelectrode. Sanes and Donoghue (2000) review the role of the primary motor cortex in this kind of learning. The striatum has also been implicated in motor-skill learning. However, it is clear that many other regions of the brain are also involved in motor-skill learning.

The earliest attempts to use neurophysiological techniques to study motor-skill learning were complicated because the system was obviously influenced by many other regions of the brain than those traditionally associated with motor-skill learning per se. Just how complicated the interactive roles of the various brain areas could be was illustrated by the considerable amount of work over the years resulting in paradoxical outcomes. Ades and Raab (1946), for example, had shown that two-stage extirpation of portions of the motor cortex resulted in such a paradoxical effect. The first stage produced a contralateral paralysis—the second stage, surprisingly, produced some recovery of function.

Furthermore there is the well-known and typically observed contralateral recovery of function (e.g., most recently demonstrated by Frost, Barbay, Friel, Plautz, & Nudo, 2003). This type of finding adds to the difficulty of rigidly attributing any motor-learning process to any limited brain region because widely separated regions on both sides of the brain may eventually represent the same behavior. This is an important point because it also makes plausible the suggestion that nearby regions on the same hemisphere might also be capable of representing similar behaviors. If one follows this logic to its conclusion, it also makes plausible the idea that whatever localization there may be can be extremely variable from one person to another as well as from one time to another time.

The prevailing current view, therefore, is that a system of brain regions is involved in this process. One proposed system is shown in figure 8.2.

The use of the EEG as a measure of motor-skill proficiency has persisted over the years with what has to be considered to be only moderate, if any, success. One problem is that, once again, any measure of ongoing learning per se is confounded with that of attention

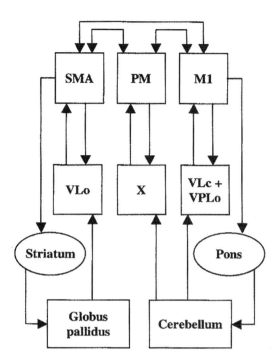

Figure 8.2
A theory of the neural mechanisms involved in motor-skill learning.
From Ungerleider, Doyon, &Karni (2002), with the permission of Elsevier Science and Technology Journals.

and effort as well as the achieved level of expertise. The classic result, mentioned so frequently in this context, is that the alpha rhythm typically changes with virtually any measure of mental activity. Thus, as learning progresses, there is no a priori reason to make this nominally 10-Hz signal (or any other EEG frequency band) the single salient measure of skill acquisition—too many other processes are concurrently active. In any such situation the effects of learning would have to be balanced against the effect of the need for lessened effort. Indeed, as one was balanced against the other, the net effect on the EEG could be negligible or even null; what seems plausible could actually turn out to be paradoxical. Hatfield, Haufler, Hung, and Spalding (2004, p. 144) express it well when they say, "Simply stated, skilled athletes perform tasks in their sport with minimal effort or accomplish their intended work or muscular performance with minimal effort as constrained by the task demands."

The important point here is that the multiple forces driving changes in the EEG may make such measures neutral with regard to underlying mechanisms and make it very difficult to extrapolate results from one situation to another. In this multidetermined situation, effects would be expected to be counterintuitive, subtle, relatively small, erratic, and not particularly diagnostic of the state of motor-skill learning per se even in those situations in which modest correlations may be observed between performance and the EEG. This, indeed, is what the scientific literature in this field suggests is the usual outcome. For example, Cross (2002) in an exceptionally well thought out senior thesis found very small EEG effects as skill increased when subjects were playing a computer game. The work of Etnier, Whitwer, Landers, Petruzzello, and Salazar (1996) also illustrates this same point—significant but modest increases were observed in the alpha rhythm with increased expertise in mirror tracing.

To further illustrate this point, the review by Hatfield et al. (2004) is especially instructive. These authors summarized the results of 17 reports that used EEGs to determine if there were any stable indicators of motor-skill learning. The impression one gets from this table is that, although there were some gross effects (typically an increase in the alpha rhythm and a small increase in the symmetry of the responses of the two sides of the brain with practice), these results were different for different athletic skills and even for different electrode placements on the skull.

Furthermore the observed changes in the EEG with increased proficiency in a motor skill have not always been monotonic. For example whereas Sterman and Mann (1995) showed that there was a progressive suppression of the alpha rhythm during the progress of an aviator's flight training, others have been equally emphatic that the alpha rhythm recovers to original levels with increasing training. This latter finding generally agrees with the classic Berger result that the alpha rhythm is suppressed with mental effort or viewing a visual stimulus. Its recovery may be due to the lessened mental effort required by the expert to carry out the task.

Hatfield et al. (2004) went on to review and tabulate the work that has been done using various components of the ERP to study motor-skill training. The cited work using slow potentials is rather limited; the corpus of literature is mainly from a single laboratory (that of N. Konttinen of Finland), and the slow components of these recordings dealt primarily with the different body posture of novice and expert riflepersons. The main reported effect was that the slow potential varied with body stability, a measure that improved with training. Increased negativity of the slow potential was associated with "increased readiness to respond," whereas an increased positivity correlated with "an inhibition of neuromuscular activity."

The work on other components of the ERP reviewed by Hatfield and his colleagues was limited to two studies; the main result of one (Radio, Janelle, Barba, & Frehlich, 2001) was an increase in the P300 latencies and smaller amplitudes with increased expertise. It is interesting to note that whereas the P300 latency was shorter for the novices, their reaction times were longer—a temporal inconsistency that also suggests that neural and behavioral latencies are not always congruent. One possible explanation of all of this inconsistency may be that it is the amount of "mental effort" or task load or some equivalent third variable that may actually be accounting for much of the variance in this line of research.

Few other studies using ERPs as a measure of motor-skill learning have appeared. One rare one was published by Ranganathan, Siemionow, Liu, Sahgal, and Yue (2004). The main goal of their experiment was to consider if mental training could enhance motor-skill learning; they also included an ERP measure of the increased performance attributable to "mental exercise." Although there was a substantial behavioral improvement in the force applied by the fingers with this mental exercise (although less than with actual motor training), the ERP changes were modest over the course of the experiment.

To conclude, so far no one has shown a simple, reliable metric of motor-skill training using any of the EEG or ERP techniques. It is, therefore, somewhat surprising that in this arena of modest and idiosyncratic results interest in the EEG and ERP should be continuing. It is almost as if a cult of enthusiasts has grown up around the use of these "objective" measures of brain activity. Despite the fact that they tell us little about the basis of the mind-brain relation and that their findings, although significant in a statistical sense, are not often significant in a theoretical sense and have yet to be proven to be significant in application, they remain a part of the current scientific environment.

As a partial result of this general dissatisfaction with EEG-type techniques, interest in finding neurophysiological correlates of motor-skill training has shifted mainly to the use of brain imaging. Before I consider some of the current research in this field, I should reiterate a point made several times in this book. That is, there are advantages to dealing with both sensory (such as vision) and motor topics (such as skill learning). Although it is by no means certain that our efforts to deal with motor and sensory topics with neurophysiological methods will not ultimately turn out to be as recalcitrant as those embodying our "higher-level" cognitive processes, at least motor and sensory functions have two substantial advantages: (1) they are tightly anchored both to the stimulus and to measurable aspects of behavior; and (2) they are mainly concerned with monodirectional transmission codes, at least with regard to the initial and final pathways. In this regard they are conceptually much simpler than such elusive mental processes as consciousness or thinking.

The advent of the new brain imaging technology changed the way in which cognitive neuroscience approached the problem of finding biomarkers for motor-skill training. Compared to the EEG, brain images were much more detailed, their spatial resolution was vastly better, and they seemed at first to offer a much more direct means of measuring brain states during the varying stages of motor-skill training. Early studies, however, were inconsistent even concerning which brain areas were involved and whether or not neural responses increased or decreased with training. To add to the confusion, some early imaging studies suggested that a number of brain areas decreased in the extent of their activity over the course of training (Jenkins, Brooks, Nixon, Frackowiak, & Passingham, 1994). On the other hand other investigators such as Grafton, Hazeltine, and Ivry (1995) reported that there was an increase in the extent of regional activations. It did not clarify matters when researchers such as Karni et al. (1995) reported that both trends occurred—but in serial order. As a subject became more proficient in a finger-tapping task, BOLD signals from the primary motor cortex first increased and then decreased. The results were not huge; at best there was only a 10% increase in the number of activated pixels as a result of the extended training. However, to confuse the issue further, there was a diminishment of the BOLD signal during the first day of the training.

Toni, Krams, Turner, and Passingham (1998) later reported a similar pattern of fMRI responses; however, the brain response findings were distributed over broader regions of the brain than just the motor cortex. A further inconsistency was that the valence of the responses varied from area to area. Indeed, some areas showed only a gradual reduction in the BOLD signal. Areas involved in motor-skill learning, according to Toni et al. included frontal, cingulate, premotor and motor, somatosensory, and parietal cortex as well as the subcortical basal ganglia, thalamus, and the cerebellum.

It has been proposed that there are two phases and possibly two distinct mechanisms at work when a person learns a motor skill. Doyon, Penhume, and Ungerleider (2003) (as summarized by Doyon & Benali, 2005) proposed a theory of motor-skill learning based on this interpretation. According to their model, during they early phase portions of the cortico-striatal (CS) and cortico-cerebellar (CC) systems, working in conjunction with the hippocampus, are activated. In later stages of learning only one of the two systems is involved; which one this is depends on the nature of the motor skill being trained. Kincses et al. (2008) also accepted the idea that there were two systems at work during the early training periods. The first was a fronto-parieto-cerebellar system that decreased during the early training, and the other was a collection of posterior parietal and premotor relations that were activated during the early training.

In the last decade several active groups of researchers have worked on the problem of the neural representation of motor-skill learning using the fMRI as the research tool of choice. Despite this activity, however, there remains little agreement on which areas are involved in the process or how the activation changes as a function of the degree of training. Poldrack et al. (2005, p. 5356), for example, suggested that during the training period "a wide network of frontal and striatal regions, as well as the parietal lobe" was activated during motor-skill learning. When the subjects were well trained, decreases in activity were observed in "bilateral ventral premotor regions, right middle frontal gyrus, and right caudal body; activity in other prefrontal and striate regions" also decreased.

An alternative, if overlapping, allocation of brain resources during motor-skill learning was reported by Orban et al. (2010). During the training period activity in the putamen and the contralateral lobule VI of the cerebellum correlated with their behavioral learning task. However, there was a serious confound in this work, As Orban and his colleagues (2010) pointed out, both learning per se and performance are intertwined so thoroughly that it is difficult to distinguish between the learning and the motor control representation at any given point in the experiment. They summed up the problem in the following manner:

However, much controversy exists as to which components of these anatomical loops actually code for learning per se, notably because performance changes inherently occur as a function of learning, and thus may contribute imaging results in human studies. . . . The potential confound arises from the fact that brain activity can be parametrically modulated outside a learning process. (pp. 694–695)

When Orban and his colleagues (2010) isolated these performance measures, they described a very different set of brain regions that were involved in encoding what they hoped were the separable aspects of performance as opposed to learning. These included a second cerebellar lobule as well as motor and premotor cerebral loci. They believed that these areas were the ones in which the attained skill level guiding performance was "represented," implying that these were the regions in which the engram for the motor skill was stored.

It is clear despite the relative conceptual simplicity of the motor system and its solid anchoring to physical performance measures (compared to the much more elusive higher-cognitive processes) that our knowledge of the neurodynamics of even as simple a task as finger tapping is quite limited. At best, the current research is still constrained to identifying the regions that may be involved in this kind of learning. However, there is still no region or system that has been shown to uniquely instantiate the learning process and certainly no neurophysiological quantitative measure of how well a person is performing. Perhaps in the future such an fMRI-based scale of motor-skill competence might be available; as far as a current or near-future application of brain imaging to monitor task performance is concerned, there are still too many unknowns to justify the use of such a measure to evaluate training level or task competence. Some of the most basic issues remain controversial. There are a wide variety of different brain areas that have been implicated in this conceptually simple learning process ranging from the frontal cortex to the depths of the cerebellum. Some of the obvious confounds have been identified by workers such as Orban and colleagues (2010), but it is virtually certain that others lurk just beyond our ken.

8.5   Personnel Selection

In this chapter I deal with a group of practical applications for which all agree it would be wonderful if we had any objective biomarkers. Unfortunately, at the present time such indicators do not exist. Although I have generally considered the concept of intelligence in the previous chapter, there remains considerable doubt whether or not such an ephemeral property of the human mind as native ability for a particular job can be found in a brain image. Despite the paucity of scientific findings for such an association, the idea that we could use brain imaging or EEGs as a means of selecting individuals with particular abilities has gained widespread popular acceptance. Indeed, however unjustified and premature, commercial enterprises have been set up to exploit the idea that imaging can be used as a means of selecting personnel for jobs.

Unfortunately, with human nature being what it is, intelligence or native ability being among the most elusive of human mental components to identify and to measure, and brain activity being so variable, it remains extremely difficult to find acceptably high correlations between any brain measure and ability. Not only are the psychological concepts so elusive, but it seems likely that ability actually represents a conglomerate of interacting components that may not be separable, interchangeable, or interpredictive. At the present time, in which we have very limited ideas of where specific skills are located in the brain (if indeed they are localized), it seems even less likely that we would be able to find a bio-marker in an EEG or fMRI recording that would correlate with such subtle proclivities. Indeed, an extensive search on my part for research supportive of such an idea turned up nothing that currently exists that would suggest that brain signals of any kind could be used for personnel selection. Despite a popular commitment to this concept, injudiciously extended to the idea that behavioral-based aptitude tests (as inadequate as the best of them are) could be replaced by any known brain activity measure, it must be concluded that such a possibility at present falls in the realm of science fiction rather than science.

8.6 Deception Detection

Since it is not possible to peer directly into the mind of a potential prevaricator, there has been a historic search for biological indicators of one kind or another that could reveal when a person was not telling the truth. Trovillo (1939a, 1939b) and Adler (2007) provide insightful histories about the behavioral and obvious physiological markers that have been used over the centuries. These include such behavioral indicators as "downcast eyes," "shivering," "stooped posture," and other forms of "body language." Biological markers associated with autonomic responses including such phenomena as "flushing" and a "dry mouth" have also been used probably since prehistoric times.

The fact that some early methods incorporated the use of what we now appreciate were autonomic nervous system responses reached fruition in the later nineteenth century when Lombroso (1895) suggested that the newly developed instruments for measuring blood pressure, pulse rate, and respiration rate could individually be used as a lie detector. The general theory in this case was that lying led to emotional distress that would be reflected in the physiological reactions of the autonomic nervous system. This "theory" culminated in the simultaneous use of all of these measures as well as the galvanic skin reflex (GSR) in a single modern lie-detection instrument—the polygraph—an invention usually attributed to Larson (1921).

Although the polygraph remains an integral part of our legal and investigative systems, well-designed experimental studies have never shown it to be reliable, and its validity has been continually challenged. Government reports (Anonymous, 1983; NAS, 2003) have concluded over the years that the device does not adequately correlate with lying to the level that would justify its use in our courts, in any criminal investigation, in personnel selection, or, for that matter, any serious commitment to further research. Their conclusion is made clear by the following summary of the NAS (2003, pp. 212–213) deliberations.

• Almost a century of research in scientific psychology and physiology provides little basis for the expectation that a polygraph test could have extremely high accuracy.
• The theoretical rationale for the polygraph is quite weak, especially in terms of differential fear, arousal, or other emotional states that are triggered in response to relevant or comparison questions.
• Research on the polygraph has not progressed over time in the manner of a typical scientific field. It has not accumulated knowledge or strengthened its scientific underpinnings in any significant manner.
• The inherent ambiguity of the physiological measures used in the polygraph suggest that further investments in improving polygraph technique and interpretation will bring only modest improvements in accuracy.

That the polygraph has persisted as an investigative tool as long as it has in this context of such scientific criticism reflects the compelling power of the popular but increasingly suspect idea that mental states can be measured by physiological means. Thus, it was not surprising with the advent of the brain imaging techniques that the PET and fMRI devices would also be applied to deception detection. The superficial directness and face validity of a brain signal was sufficiently seductive to produce a substantial amount of serious research into what we now appreciate to be only the remotest possibility that we may eventually find a biomarker of lying.

Although it is true that several authors report correlations between lying and brain images, it is unfortunate to observe that none of these studies agrees with any of the others. Although we cannot be sure at this point if the studies in this field are so variable because the methods used were so varied or if they represent a true biological variability, it is clear that there is no support at the present time for their use as an alternative to the equally ineffective polygraph.

I was able to locate 16 research articles[11] that had been published up to 2006 that dealt with what regions of the brain were activated when a subject attempted to deceive. Each of them attributed a relatively small number (1–10) of brain regions as being selectively activated under the deception condition. However, as figure 8.3 shows, the regions were spread over the entire brain with little if any clustering indicating a region or group of regions selective for lying. Most important of all was the observed fact that the 16 reports did not agree with each other concerning the location or dynamics of the areas they believed to be associated with deception.

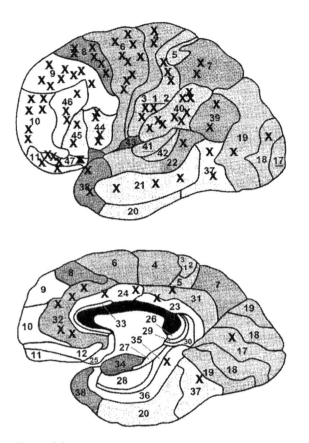

Figure 8.3
Distribution of activations during deception from 16 relevant lie detection experiments.
Data from Uttal (2009b); background brain image through the courtesy of Mark Dubin of the University of Colorado.

    The implication of this graphic is that there is nothing special within the context of this group of experiments about any brain region or any group of brain regions that could help us to signify deception. In other words there is no localized brain region or group of regions selectively associated with lying. Indeed, the counterargument is being made—if these activations are really correlated with lying, they are broadly distributed across the brain. Furthermore, in conjunction with the corpus of experimental results that we have discussed throughout this book, there is a strong implication that much of the brain is involved in virtually any cognitive process. These 16 studies collectively make the supplementary point that brain imaging systems are unlikely in the future to provide answers to the question of the relation between brain activity and such cognitive processes as deception.

8.7   Mental illness and Cognitive Dysfunction

Probably transcending in social importance all of the other applications of brain imaging is the need for some objective biomarker of various kinds of cognitive dysfunction. Included among the most demanding applications are such topics as

- Schizophrenia and other mental illnesses
- Hyperactivity and attention deficit disorder (ADHD)
- Posttraumatic stress disorder (PTSD)
- Autism

Although there are well-established behavioral symptoms of each of these mental dysfunctions, as a preliminary generalization there are at the present time no well-established biomarkers for any of them. There is a very long history of searches for some biochemical or neurological indicator of mental illnesses, most notably schizophrenia, and a shorter but equally unsuccessful search for something to help us predict susceptibility or measure the progress of autism, PTSD, or ADHD.

8.7.1   Schizophrenia and Other Metal illnesses

When fMRI systems first became available, there was a major and immediate effort to see if this new approach could provide biomarkers for mental illness. The results have been unpromising in virtually all cases. A recent review (Shenton, Dickey, Frumin, & McCarley, 2001) of the attempts to use MRI systems to explore the possibility that particular brain regions might be useful correlates or biomarkers of schizophrenia resulted in no consistent answer. As Shenton and his colleagues concluded, "After more than a hundred years of research the neuropathology of schizophrenia remains unknown" (p. 1).

Speaking more generally of the use of brain imaging in the study of mental illness, Callicott and Weinberger (1999, p. 95) stated that ". . . functional neuroimaging has not generated any pathognomic findings in mental illness, has not established a clear link between neurophysiology and observable behavior, and has not resolved the potential confounds of medication." These judgments do not, of course, mean that research using fMRI systems to search for a biomarker of any mental illness has stopped; indeed there continues to be an active program of research in this field. However, the results are still inconsistent and erratic, and no robust biomarker has yet been found. The presence or absence of effects in particular regions of the brain differentiating between normal and schizophrenic subjects remains both unreplicated and controversial in virtually all cases. Where there were correlations, their valences were unpredictable. For example the prefrontal cortex has been shown to both decrease and increase its fMRI activations by current researchers. Perlstein, Carter, Noll, and Cohen (2001) argued, on one side of this controversy, that schizophrenic patients exhibited reduced activity in this region, whereas Manoach, Greve, Lindgren, and Dale (2003) presented data that they felt supported exactly the opposite conclusion—increases in frontal cortex activations. Both, it should be noted, used a working memory paradigm as their probe test of this kind of mental illness.

Disagreements like this abound in the field with even the most basic facts still a matter of contention, and few experiments have been validated by adequate and appropriate confirming replications. There has been, recently an increasingly conservative tone expressed by researchers concerned with mental illness. A number of currently active researchers in this field of inquiry have raised caution flags about the ease with which data like these can be misinterpreted. Their warnings are based on the small size of differential neurophysiological effects when normal and schizophrenic subjects are compared, some totally contradictory results, and the possibility that slight procedural changes may be biasing the outcomes of experiments that seek to find a biomarker of schizophrenia. For example in a technical report of their search for differential fMRI responses in normal subjects and schizophrenic patients, Weiss et al. (2007) pointed out the following potential biases in their own work as well as that of others.

- Differences in task performance
- Small sample size
- Mixture of different types of schizophrenic patients
- Differences in baseline activity

Perhaps the most recent comprehensive review of the application of fMRI techniques to diagnose schizophrenia was reported by Demirci et al. (2008). They describe the continuing challenges to interpretation of brain images in this application including bias in classification due to the small samples of schizophrenic patients used in various experiments. That is, there may be too few subjects in the control group to establish a robust experimental comparison. Hence there is a desire to combine patient data from different sites—a procedure that will further confuse the final analyses since even in the most similar labs there will be differences in operators, equipment, and patient samples.

Despite some reported progress in distinguishing between schizophrenic patients and normal controls, according to these authors current progress seems to be characterized as possibilities, potential accomplishments, and promises rather than solid evidence, much less a usable diagnostic tool. The words of Demirci and his colleagues (2008) on this subject are informative ones: "the results are usually not generalizable to larger data sets and require careful definition of the techniques used both in designing algorithms and reporting prediction accuracies" (p.207). And, in further discussing the potential for bias in this kind of research, they say, "We believe that there are important issues to consider both in analyzing fMRI data for classification and in presentation of the results" (p. 224).

They continue, "In summary, with the use of proper validation techniques we believe that fMRI has great potential for use in clinical decision making, but there is still much work to be done" (p. 224).

Clearly, the use of brain images for diagnosing mental illness is still not a practical reality.

Why should this confusion be the current situation? The answer to this question is undoubtedly associated with the inappropriate level of analysis at which brain imaging systems operate. The origins of the behavioral symptoms of mental illness, like all other mental activity, are more likely to be found at the level of the detailed interactions among the myriad of neurons in the brain rather than at the level examined by the macroscopic measuring devices such as the fMRI. The complexity and numerousness of these patterns of interconnections preclude our examining them at the detailed level required. However useful EEGs and fMRI devices may be in other applications, it is not likely that they will ever be able to discern the neurophysiological origins of subtle cognitive dysfunctions such as schizophrenia or bipolar disorder. It has not happened in the past century and, in my judgment, it is not likely to happen in the future.

Given this level of empirical uncertainty, the social needs for a cure, and the ethical complications of diagnoses or misdiagnoses of severe mental diseases, it behooves us to be especially conservative about applying brain imaging methods to categorizing patients with mental dysfunctions. There is perhaps no greater opportunity for dangerous errors than in the field of mental illness.

8.7.2 Posttraumatic Stress Disorder

I now turn to the problem of three other current topics of deep concern to modern society—PTSD, ADHD, and autism—each of which has been the target of searches for brain biomarkers, most recently with fMRI imaging techniques. Each of these debilitating conditions is characterized by changes in behavior, personality, mood, and affect. Because of the societal needs, all three of these dysfunctional behavior patterns have become embroiled in high levels of political as well as scientific controversy. However, it is controversy of a different kind than the technical and arcane matters that have already been discussed. Because of the importance and increasing occurrence of autism, ADHD, and PTSD, there has been enormous pressure to find some kind of brain signal that would be diagnostic of either a proclivity toward, or a full-blown presentation of, these three dysfunctions. The problem is that at the present time none of them has been reliably associated with any brain state, functional, anatomic, or neurochemical.[12] As just noted, it is far more likely that they represent a dysfunction in the details of interactions of the neural network that guide and control normal mental activity in a manner that is virtually indistinguishable at the molar level of a brain image. Indeed, there is a considerable argument that all three of these dysfunctions actually do not represent mental illness as much as being extremes of what we consider normal behavior. Therefore, there may be no special biomarker, and the search for such a neurophysiological biomarker is a profound waste of time and resources. What drives this medicalization of these syndromes may partially be accounted for by social and family issues rather than suggestive neurobiological clues. A supporting argument that this is the case is that at the present time there is no widely accepted medical treatment for PTSD (or for that matter autism)—only behavior-based therapies seem to have any therapeutic value.

Despite a considerable amount of research activity, the search for a brain correlate of PTSD seems to have been unsuccessful. A recent meta-study by Etkin and Wager (2007) explored brain imaging similarities among PTSD, social anxiety disorders, and phobias—a cluster of mental disorders that share many common features. They pointed out that studies of brain correlates of PTSD "vary greatly in their findings" (p.1476). These differences included decreases, increases, and no differences between patients and normal controls in the activation areas occasionally illuminated by fMRI imaging techniques. The only common brain activations for these different but behaviorally related anxiety disorders have typically been found in the amygdala and the insula. This is not unanticipated because these are regions we know to be deeply involved in emotional activity; thus, it seems unsurprising that anxiety disorders such as PTSD might be affected by (or affect) activity in these brain regions. Patients suffering with PTSD were characterized by diminishment of activations in a number of other brain regions including the prefrontal and cingulate cortices and the thalamus. The answer to the question of whether or not such activation patterns are specific enough to diagnose something as ephemeral as PTSD remains elusive.

8.7.3   Attention Deficit Hyperactivity Disorder

In children ADHD is diagnosed on the basis of behavioral disorders that exceed those of normal young children. It is possible that these dysfunctions are not qualitatively different—only exaggerations of those observed during the normal development stages of children. ADHD is characterized by a persistent inability to maintain attention, hyperactivity, and a diminished self-control over impulsive activity. Other behavior characteristics include procrastination and a general reluctance to respond to directions.

The situation is more complicated for ADHD than for PTSD; since Bradley's (1937) introduction of Benzedrine (a stimulant) to treat hyperactivity, a number of other drugs of various therapeutic values have been introduced over the years. Some of them are, also paradoxically, stimulants that seem for mysterious reasons to lessen rather than excite further hyperactivity. However, a few newer drugs such as Strattera and Pamelor are nonstimulants. The problem with all of these drugs is that no one has any idea of how they work, and yet many of them have been shown to work to a certain degree in various kinds of ADHD patients.

Additionally, ADHD has also been the target of extensive research using brain imaging techniques but, once again, with inconsistent results. In their review of the field Bush, Valera, and Seidman (2005) provide a remarkably intelligent and conservative approach to studying these subtle mental dysfunctions with imaging devices. In doing so they highlight a number of problems faced when one attempts to find a biomarker for a psychological dysfunction such as ADHD.

Bush, Valera, and Seidman reviewed 12 SPECT, 12 PET, and 9 fMRI studies of ADHD. Speaking of the nine fMRI studies, they noted that although there were suggestions that there was "less consistency" among these studies with respect to the role of the lateral frontal cortex, there seemed to be preliminary support for the idea that the cingulate cortex was especially dysfunctional in those suffering from this malady. Furthermore, the list of regions supposedly activated in ADHD students was quite extensive. Bush et al. (2005) reported activations in all of the following regions when ADHD was studied using the fMRI technique.

- Frontal lobe
  Ventral lateral prefrontal
  Medial prefrontal
  Bilateral frontopolar
- Striatal lobe
- Fronto-insular network
- Ventral lateral prefrontal cortex
- Putamen
- Cerebellum
- Dorsal anterior cingulate cortex
- Caudate
- Hippocampus
- Inferior temporal
- Left temporal

among others! The distribution and variability of these responses in such a small sample of experiments suggest an alternative explanation—these data cannot be depended on to provide a reliable biomarker of ADHD.

   Bush et al. (2005) concluded that although there were some early suggestions that the frontal, cingulate, and striatal regions of the brain may be "possibly playing roles" in controlling this behavioral dysfunction, findings were insufficient to support brain imaging as a means of clinical diagnosis. Specifically, they stated:

. . . there is currently no accepted role for functional imaging in guiding clinical diagnosis or therapeutic decision making. Simply put, no matter how exciting the preliminary advances might be, none of the imaging modalities has been accepted in the peer-reviewed literature as a proven method for reliably distinguishing ADHD subjects from normal control subjects, distinguishing ADHD subjects from other subjects with other psychiatric or neurological comorbidities, identifying subtypes of ADHD, or predicting treatment at the level of the individual subject. (p. 1281)

8.7.4 Autism

Another area of mental dysfunction of intense current interest is the possible "epidemic" of autism. In recent years there has been an explosion of diagnoses of autism that has been variously attributed to subtle environmental effects or to increased attention by therapists to what had previously been an unnoticed, but equally prevalent, syndrome. Autism is characterized by social withdrawal, repetitive behavior, and poor use of language skills. Currently, whatever progress has been made in treating this illness has also been with behavioral techniques. Thompson (2007, 2008), a leader in autism treatment, pointed out that not only are there no drugs or any other kind of biological intervention that have been shown to alleviate autism, but almost any behavioral strategy seems to work with no advantage of any one over another. What the common factor is in behavioral treatments that work remains mysterious.

Unfortunately for those attempting to design a clear-cut experimental program, the psychopathology of the disorders included under the rubric of what is called autism is not simple. Many different, but closely related, patterns of behavior are currently included in this dysfunction. This has led to considerable confusion in the search for potential biomarkers and collective incorporation of the various syndromes under the term autism spectrum disorder (ASD).

Despite the difficulty in defining and classifying the different kinds of autism (if there really are different kinds at a biological level—not just behavioral differences in expression), autistic dysfunctions have also been the target of an extensive search for neurophysiological and neuroanatomic correlates or biomarkers that might add some material objectivity to the mysterious substrate of the clinical behavioral symptoms. As with PTSD and ADHD, modern attempts have been made to find such correlates of autism using brain imaging techniques. This research has progressed in two different directions. The first is a series of studies that show differences between normal and autistic people in terms of the *function* of various brain areas. The second line is a series of studies that purport to show anatomic differences in various brain areas.

If there is any generalization that all investigators agree on, it is that the findings of this extensive body of research have not yet converged on either a consensus of either a useful physiological or anatomic biomarker of autism. The phrase "evidence from different studies has been inconsistent" is either explicit or implicit in virtually every study from either line of research up to the most recent reports. The possible reasons for this lack of consistency and replicability are several, but they include the following possibilities:

- Poor classification of the variety of behavioral symptoms included within ASDs.
- Difficulty in matching experimental and control groups.
- Differences in experimental tasks.
- Inadequate statistical power of experiments.
- Confounds from:
    Age
    Gender
    Individual differences
    Medication
    Degree of autistic disorder
- Most of all, there may be no macroscopic signal, sign, or marker of this behavioral disorder. Even if there were one, it might not tell us anything about how the system works.

Notwithstanding these potential obstacles to progress, a number of studies have attempted to find some biomarker of autism using both functional and anatomic brain imaging techniques. An early example of a functional study was reported by Baron-Cohen et al. (1999). These investigators were interested in distinguishing between regions of functional activation in normal control and autistic subjects. They were seeking a neural foundation for the elusive, behaviorally defined, concept of social intelligence—a generalized process that they expected would be diminished in those suffering from autism. In their experiments subjects were asked to judge the affect expressed by the eyes of a photograph. How well the subjects did in interpreting their pictures was supposed to assay their social intelligence. Baron-Cohen and his colleagues reported that the normal subjects showed increased activity in the superior temporal gyrus, the amygdala, and some areas of the prefrontal cortex when making these judgments. Although autistic subjects showed the same activation in the frontal regions as the normal controls, they displayed no increased activation in the amygdala.[13] Thus, Baron-Cohen et al. (1999) concluded that a major cause of autism was defective amygdalar function.

However, subsequent reports (albeit with different cognitive tasks) often told a quite different story. For example, Castelli, Frith, Happe, and Frith (2002) reported that normal subjects showed hyperactivity in the medial prefrontal cortex, regions near the temporal parietal junction, and at the poles of the temporal lobe when observing animated sequences. Their autistic patients responded significantly less in all of these regions in contrast to the Baron-Cohen et al. (1999) findings. Furthermore, extrastriate cortex was comparably activated in both groups. However, the images obtained from the autistic patients suggested to Castelli and his colleagues that poor connections (i.e., low correlated interactions) among the various regions that had been activated accounted for autism. They concluded that autism resulted from inadequate communication between regions they believed were associated with "higher order and lower order perceptual processes" (p. 1839), respectively.

A more complex pattern of results purporting to distinguish between normal and autistic children was found by Gilbert, Bird, Brindley, Frith, and Burgess (2008) and also varied with the task. They compared their normal control and autistic subjects on two behavioral tests—a random finger tapping task and a shape recognition task with alphabetic characters, both of which presumably required executive decisions to determine the nature of the response. Somewhat surprisingly, Gilbert et al. (2008) reported that both groups did equally well on the behavioral tests.[14] For the first behavioral test—production of random tapping—the fMRI brain images differed in the cerebellum but not in the frontal lobes. The second alphabetic character perception test, on the other hand, indicated that the autistic subjects produced higher levels of activation in portions of the prefrontal cortex than did the normal controls as well as different locations. Gilbert and his colleagues concluded on this somewhat tenuous basis that the source of autism lay in the hyperactivity of the frontal lobes, but possibly also of the temporal poles and the amygdala. Specifically, they reported increased activity in the frontal cortex for the autistic subjects compared to the normals—but only in the alphabet task.

Just how inconsistent the results can be in this search for neural correlates of such subtle behavioral disorders as autism is highlighted by another report (Luna et al., 2002) published just a few years earlier. Luna et al. (p. 834) reported that "[a]utistic subjects demonstrated significantly less task-related activation in dorsolateral prefrontal cortex (Brodmann area [BA] 9/46) and posterior cingulate cortex (BA 23) in comparison with healthy subjects during a working memory task."

Thus, we see both increased and decreased activation being reported for the frontal lobe of autistic patients. The possible explanations of this discrepancy could be attributed to patient diagnoses, the psychological tasks that were used, local differences in brain structure and/or function, or other procedural differences between different laboratories. Another possibility is that these small and inconsistent differences actually are reflecting a situation in which there are no real differences—only random and irregular responses of such great complexity that anyone can read anything into them at any time. In other words, there is a real possibility that there are no gross activation differences between normal subjects and autistic patients that can be observed with this technology.

Until this basic uncertainty and inconsistency can be resolved, there seems to be little promise that brain imaging could be used as an aid to the clinical diagnosis of autism. It is more prudent to assume that the observed differences in the brain images have little to do with the nature of autistic dysfunction. Instead a more reasonable theory is that they reflect extremely subtle differences in the neuronal network, differences that necessarily go undetected in brain images. Then, of course, there is a further disconcerting possibility. Autism, although behaviorally "abnormal," like ADHD, PTSD, and mental illnesses, may merely represent an extreme of normal human behavior for which brain activations and deactivations measured at the molar level play no role.

The second thread of brain imaging research for the study of autism is directed at anatomic differences that may account for this dysfunctional behavior. The detail possible with brain imaging technology seductively offers us the possibility that even relatively small differences in anatomy might be discernible when normal control subjects are compared with those suffering from autism. However in this literature there is also an enormous problem with consistency that suggests that this problem also may be being carried out at the wrong level of analysis at which to seek a biological basis for autism. As I now show, anatomic inconsistency associated with this kind of research is as bad as that found in the functional data. The inconsistency and lack of replicability are strong enough to add substance to the argument that this new kind of high-tech phrenology is as misdirected as was the older kind. I now briefly review this structural line of autism research in roughly chronological order.

We are fortunate that there have been several meta-reviews of research that attempt to provide a broad view of possible anatomic correlates of autism. The results of all of them are similar—weak replicability from experiment to experiment. For example, Brambilla et al. (2003) carried out a meta-review of structural brain imaging studies published between 1996 and 2003. They reported that although there were some early associations between autism and the size of a number of brain regions, "[n]evertheless, available MRI studies were often conflicting and could have been limited by methodological issues" (p. 537).

Brambilla and colleagues (2003) summed up their findings in a table (see table 8.3) showing the various brain regions whose sizes correlated with autistic behavior. There are a number of interesting aspects of this table. First, changes in the size of virtually all regions of the brain (cerebral, cerebellar, and brainstem) have, at one time or another, been implicated in autism. Second, no attribution of autism to a particular brain region has gone unchallenged. Competing studies have shown both enlargement and reduction in overall size. Others have been contradicted by negative results. Third, the number of negative results is comparable to those reporting some positive effect of size or volume.

This is hardly the kind of support that one would want to depend on for a diagnosis of this serious behavior problem. One can only wonder why as unpromising a line of research as this one should have continued to attract investigators and funding.

Other more recent meta-reviewers have made a variety of attempts to link particular brain-region size abnormalities with autism. Stanfield et al. (2008) concluded from a review of 46 reports that autistic patients had relative enlargement of some brain regions (cerebral hemispheres, cerebellum, and caudate nucleus) but reductions in other portions of the cerebellum, the midbrain, and, most interestingly, the corpus callosum. The corpus callosum was of particular interest because it supported the contention that the problems associated with autism might be a result of poor communication between different parts of the brain due to the relatively small size of this major band of connecting tracts. This hypothesis ("underconnectivity") was also supported by research carried out by Just, Cherkassky, Keller, Kana, and Minshew (2007). They all argued that it was a failure of adequate interaction between and among different lobes of the brain that was the source of autistic dysfunction. Along with the other studies, it contradicts any argument that regional brain sizes or shapes may serve as a biomarker for autism. Their work, therefore, provided little support for any subsequent functional activation differences between autistic and normal subjects.

Despite these uncertainties the search for an autism biomarker has continued. With the foundation provided by the Bambrilla et al. (2003) data suggesting that it was not possible to assign autism to a particular place on or in the brain, other possible correlates were sought. Later, Redcay and Courchesne (2005) summarized research that suggested that it was not a specific place or places on the brain but rather the overall size of the brain that correlated with autistic behavior. Also noting how inconsistent research on this topic had been ("Multiple studies have reported increased brain size in autism, while others have found no difference from normal," p. 1), they argued that the earlier findings were confounded by relative brain size at different ages. Younger autistic children (3–5 years) were reported to display statistically different brain sizes than those of normal controls; however,

Table 8.3

Summary of MRI findings in autism

Structures	Decreased size, N studies (measurements)	Increased size, N studies (measurements)	Negative findings, N studies (measurements)
Cerebellar vermis			
Total vermis			3 (areas and volumes)
Lobules I-V	1 (areas)		10 (areas)
Lobules VI-VII	5 (areas) (same group)	2 (areas) (same group)	11 (areas)
Lobules VIII-X	2 (areas)	1 (gray matter density)	7 (areas)
Cerebellar hemispheres	2 (areas)	3 (volumes)	3 (1 areas, 2 volumes)
Total brainstem	2 (areas)		1 (areas and columes)
Pons	3 (areas)		8 (areas)
Midbrain	4 (areas) (same group)		4 (areas)
Medulla	4 (areas) (same group)		2 (areas)
Total brain		7 (areas and volumes)	5 (areas and volumes)
Cortical lobes			
Frontal		1 (volumes)	2 (volumes)
Temporal		3 (volumes)	
Parietal		2 (volumes)	1 (qualitative signs)
Occipital	1 (volumes)	1 (volumes)	
Planum temporale	1 (volumes)		
Ventricular system			
Lateral ventricles		2 (areas and volumes)	2 (volumes)
Third ventricles		1 (volumes)	
Fourth ventricles		2 (areas) (same group)	7 (areas and volumes)
Hippocampus	2 (areas and volumes)		5 (areas and volumes)
Amygdala	1 (volumes)	3 (volumes)	1 (volumes)
Basel ganglia			
Caudate		1 (volumes)	2 (areas and volumes)
Putamen	1 (areas)		1 (volumes)
Globus pallidus			1 (volumes)
Thalamus	1 (volumes)		1 (areas)
Corpus callosum			
Total	2 (areas)		3 (areas)
Anterior sub-regions	2 (areas)		2 (areas)
Middle body	2 (areas)		2 (areas)
Posterior sub-regions	3 (areas)		1 (areas)

N, number.

From Brambilla, Hardan, Ucelli di Nemi, Perez, Soares, & Brale (2003), with the permission of Elsevier Science and Technology Journals.

the difference disappeared for all older children and adults (6–70 years). This finding was further supported by Amaral, Schumann, and Nordahl (2008). However, the differences in brain sizes of autistic and control groups respectively between age groups were relatively small, and the differences within each group were large. Here, too, one would be hard pressed to justify these results as the basis for either a diagnostic biomarker, an explanatory theory of autism, or a plausible therapy.

The situation regarding the search for anatomic differences that may be associated with autism, thus, remains murky. In recent years other anatomic structures have been singled out as being of importance. To sum up this work on possible brain regional correlates of autism, it is of interest to look at another recent meta-review of the field by Amaral et al. (2008). Based on a number of studies from a number of different fields (some relevant and some not quite so relevant), they proposed that the types of behavioral dysfunction—social impairment, communication deficits, and repetitive behaviors—that had been used to diagnose autism can speculatively be associated with particular brain region activities. These areas include such diverse portions of the brain as the frontal cortex and brainstem structures such as the thalamus. Even they note, however, that these associations are based on small samples, few studies, and low correlations.

Amaral et al. (2008) suggested that the key to understanding autism is the relative volume of the whole brain, gray matter, and white matter, respectively, as a function of the age of the participant. Still elsewhere in their article, they attribute autism to developmental differences in the neuronal organization at the microscopic cellular level following the lead of Casanova, Buxhoeveden, Switala, and Roy (2002).

Thus, at present, there is no conclusive and very little suggestive evidence that robustly supports any of the structural, functional, or cellular theories of autism. It is possible that this is another one of those situations in which the doors are forever closed to understanding by the inaccessibility of mental activity and the complexity of the brain's neuronal network.

In sum, all of the imaging research regarding these behavioral dysfunctions is inconsistent, varying both from lab to lab and with the assigned cognitive task. Comparable experiments produce diametrically opposed results, and all are subject to the caveat expressed by Bush, Valera, and Seidman mentioned at the end of the previous section on ADHD. This inconsistency can be attributed to many factors including small subject sample sizes and a lack of standardized testing methods. Even more likely is that we are looking in the wrong place, the wrong level, and using the wrong instrument to answer to the profound question of the origins of autistic behavior.

There are, however, other possibilities. One is based on the absence of a good taxonomy of the involved psychological processes. It is widely acknowledged by cognitive neuroscientists that it is mainly psychology that informs neuroscience rather than concepts flowing in the opposite direction. If so, any inadequacies in the definitions of the cognitive processes under investigation would undermine any putative associations between those processes and specific brain regions. If the cognitive processes are not congruent with the neurobio-logical mechanisms, the entire enterprise of searching for nonexistent or questionable biomarkers of these ill-defined psychological dysfunctions such as PTSD, ADHD, or autism may be futile. Given the "fuzziness" of our psychological vocabulary, such a possibility cannot be entirely ignored. Although there is no question that these behavioral dysfunctions exist, there is far less certainty that these symptoms can lead us to specific neurobiological causal factors.

There is another disconcerting possibility. Notwithstanding all of the technological, methodological, and statistical elegance, it may be that the question being asked is being asked at entirely the wrong level. If these psychological dysfunctions are actually attribut-able to subtle differences in the states of the neuronal network at the microscopic level, then the macroscopic imaging devices will never see anything other than what in the final analysis must be considered to be indirect random or quasi-random activity. If this is the case, then whatever positive results we do get may be spurious—illusions of order rather than order itself. Whether this uncertainty will be resolved in the future is yet to be deter-mined, but clearly no application to clinical diagnosis of these very preliminary results is yet justified. It just may be that the fMRI is not the right instrument to search for a bio-marker of autism—or, for that matter, any other mental dysfunctions that are defined solely by behavioral symptoms. There is, therefore, the continuing possibility that whatever data are provided by brain images are just noncausal *signs* (that have little to do with the cogni-tive processes in which we are interested) rather than *codes*—the actual psychoneural equiva-lents of cognitive processes. To apply such inferences to clinical applications seems hardly justified.

Finally, a general caveat: our desperate need to find solutions to some of the dysfunctional behavioral problems I have discussed here is only a part of the many mind-brain problems that confront society. There are in addition other applications in which mental states need to be evaluated. Examples of this need range from legal exculpation due to neurological lesions to determination of consciousness when a patient is in a coma, the latter being the topic of the next section.

8.8 Brain Death and Coma

The apparent, but possible illusory, directness of the new brain imaging techniques seduces us to think that we have a direct line into both the brain and the mind even in conditions in which behavior or introspective reports, for one reason or another, are not available. One such condition is the "vegetative state," a coma-like condition in which no behavioral responses indicative of consciousness can be evoked from a brain-injured patient. A defini-tion of what is clinically meant by "vegetative state" and a review of the neurobiological research including brain imaging to study the vegetative state can be found in Riganello and Sannita (2009). Their definition describes the vegetative state:

The vegetative state (VS) is a clinical condition characterized by the absence of awareness (of both self and environment), voluntary or purposeful behavioral responses to external stimuli, and communication in the severely damaged. Subjects in a VS are otherwise awake, often with wakefulness-sleep cycles ... (p. 18)[15]

In general Riganello and Sannita found that of the numerous studies that have been carried out, mainly since 2002, many reported that some residual neurophysiological function seemed to be preserved in some subjects at some places, sometimes, in the brain. However, there were great differences in these responsive locales depending on the source of the brain damage as well as the ultimate prognosis of the patient (80% of patients diagnosed as being in a vegetative state in this study sooner or later recovered consciousness). Thus, the population of patients included within the diagnosis of VS differs greatly. It remains extremely difficult to determine what degree of cognitive activity remains and, much more so, to predict what the specific prognoses of all these patients will be. As a result, controversies over how to deal with individual cases of VS are often subject to exceptional amounts of intrusion for other than medical reasons. The most notable example of this kind of controversy is the well-known Florida case of Terri Schiavo, a fiasco that culminated in federal congressional intrusion into the most private of family matters.

No matter how complex the issues are in studies of VS, a few intrepid investigators have studied and reported about this condition. Among the most interesting cases are vegetative state patients who show discriminative responses in the brain image. These anomalous responses led some neuroscientists to infer that not only was some brain function preserved in the absence of behavioral responses, but so too was consciousness. For example, in one of the most notable cases, it was reported (Owen, Coleman, Boly, Davis, Laureys, & Pickard, 2006) that a patient in what was presumed to be a persistent VS produced distinctively different fMRI brain images when asked to think about one of two different physical activities—tennis playing or navigating about a house. The fMRI brain images obtained from the patient were comparable to those obtained from a group of 12 control subjects who were tasked to produce the same mental images. The implication was that the patient, supposedly in a profound VS, was able to carry out different willful cognitive tasks, which showed up as different patterns of activations in the fMRI records.

This, of course, is an extraordinary and virtually unique report that raises questions about the behavioral and brain image indicators of VS as much as it does of the awareness on the part of the patient.[16] Unfortunately, as is so often true of these extraordinary cases, there are many possible alternative explanations. For example, to the degree that there was actually a differential response to the two tasks, it cannot be excluded that the stimuli (the instructions to the patient by the experimenter to "think about playing tennis" or to "think about walking through your house") could, in some way, themselves excite different neural mechanisms independent of the conscious state of the patient. Furthermore, given that this type of study has not been independently replicated and is so dependent on interpretations on the part of the investigators, it would be desirable to carry out better-controlled experiments (particularly those using double-blind protocols) to fully authenticate this singular report.

The problematic nature of any attempt that purports to associate brain images with consciousness is well illustrated by a recent review of the current literature by Di, Boly, Wang, Ledoux, and Laureys (2008). They carried out a meta-review of 15 articles that discussed studies that used both PET and fMRI imaging techniques to determine if there were any predictors of recovery from this terrible condition observable in the brain images. Ancillary to their main interests in this context (recovery was improved if subjects showed activity spreading to high "association levels of the brain"), they also considered the matter of residual consciousness. They concluded that simply demonstrating passive brain responses to auditory and visual stimuli could not discriminate between conscious and unconscious patients. Only studies such as those carried out by Owen and his colleagues (2006) and Monti et al. (2010) in which active participation on the part of the patient (if that is what was being displayed in this experiment) determined that the results could answer such a question. Unfortunately those reports remain unique and subject to many uncertainties.

Nevertheless, the satisfaction of our scientific interest in this problem is dwarfed by the clinical implications of what may be a clear example of VS. An even more extreme scenario is the "locked-in" syndrome in which a patient does have consciousness but is totally unable to respond to outside stimuli.

At this point the difficulties and uncertainties surrounding VS, the locked-in syndrome, and coma remain serious challenges for future cognitive neuroscience researchers. As we discussed in chapter 7, the conceptual problems of measuring or even finding some sign of consciousness with any kind of neurophysiological measuring method are profound. Given the inconsistencies discussed here and the importance of the social and medical issues involved, it is obvious that much additional research is required. This does not mean that whatever knowledge is available will not be used to treat these massive dysfunctions of cognitive processes. However, much of it will have to be at an ad hoc level without the benefit of a good theory of how the mind may become inactive and the body continue to function—or vice versa.

A closely related problem is that of determining when a person can be declared dead.[17] Traditional signs of death were primarily cardiopulmonary; that is, older medical and religious traditions declared a person to be dead when breathing and the pulse stopped. We now know that death is not an exact point in time but rather is a process that may go on for protracted periods of time. During this period, a number of different metabolic and neurological signs may also continue to be present just as others drop out. Furthermore, it is possible to maintain a patient in some kind of neurological existence by artificial means, for example, with the use of a respirator.

In recent years, therefore, physicians have turned to various neurological signs as criteria for declaring someone to be dead. In addition to reflexes of various kinds, EEGs and fMRI investigations have been applied to this problem. Considerable medical attention has been directed to what many laypersons considered to be a straight-forward decision. The problem is further compounded by the need for organ donations; just when is a person dead enough so that his or her organs can be "harvested" for use in another person. Declaring a person dead, therefore, is certainly no longer as simple as it once was; it was only as recently as the 1950s that brain death was first suggested as a substitute for the cardiopulmonary criteria by French researchers such as Wertheimer, Jouvet, and Descites (1959) and Mollaret and Goulon (1959) and a decade later by a Harvard committee (Beecher, Adams, & Banger, 1968). As shockingly recent as these dates are, there has been considerable progress in making death declarations more specific. There is now a standard and quite extensive protocol for declaring someone dead (Van Norman, 1999), which, although probably rarely fully used, does involve the optional use of an EEG in situations where the behavioral and clinical signs may be ambiguous. The fMRI is also occasionally used in those situations where there is great doubt; but as we have seen there is great ambiguity about what residual brain signals may mean.

8.9 The "Neuro" Neologisms

The excitement surrounding the development of the brain imaging techniques joined with the increasing acceptance of the postulate that all of our thoughts are produced by neural activity of the brain has led to an explosion of interest in a diverse group of new applications of cognitive neuroscience. Most of these involve an enormous leap from measures of the hemodynamics of the cerebrum to phenomena carried out at the most molar levels of the social sciences, even to the level of theology and ethics. The variety of these new "sciences" can be estimated from the following list.

- Neuromarketing
- Neuroeconomics
- Neuroethics
- Neurotheology
- Neuroergonomics[18]

In general the scientific foundations for all of these efforts are sparse. For example neuromarketing is being peddled to a gullible advertising community on the basis of speculations presented at a conference by Smidts (2002) without any semblance of scientific support. Although there have been a number of subsequent attempts to find discriminative judgments on the part of people drinking different soft drink brands (McClure, Li, Tomlin, Cypert, Montague, & Montague, 2004) or their preferences for automobiles (Erk, Spitzer, Wunderlich, Galley, & Walter, 2002), all such studies are heavily confounded by experimental design flaws and what can better be described as emotional activity.

A critical evaluation of neuromarketing, which appeared as an editorial in the journal *Nature Neuroscience* (Anonymous, 2004), put the whole endeavor into perspective:

A more skeptical view of neuromarketing is that cognitive scientists, many of whom watched from the sidelines as their molecular colleagues got rich, are now jumping on the commercial bandwagon. According to this view, neuromarketing is little more than a new fad, exploited by scientists and marketing consultants to blind corporate clients with science. (p. 683)

Since then, the peer-reviewed literature in neuromarketing applications of brain imaging continues to be sparse, to say the least. For example, in a review of the field by Senior, Smyth, Cooke, Shaw, and Peel (2007), positive proponents of the applications of brain imaging in the neuromarketing field, there were no references to specific research concerning the applicability of these techniques beyond the two just mentioned. All other references were either speculations about potential, if unlikely, future applications or citations of solid experimental reports drawn from other fields of inquiry.

Neuroeconomics is a newly defined field dedicated to understanding the biochemical, physiological, psychological, social, and macroeconomic aspects of reward, value, choice, risk, utility, decision making, preferences, and other variables across many levels of scientific discourse. At present it is a mixture of various scientific methods that do not necessarily have anything to say to each other beyond the ambiguous meanings of some of the key terminology. (Reward, risk, value, and other such terms mean different things to the different sciences.) Much of the effort to build bridges between levels is based on flimsy analogies, neutral theories, and misleading definitions. Debate about its future is continuous with many opponents saying that lower levels have nothing to offer to higher levels and vice versa. How all of the more or less conventional cognitive neuroscience could link to macroeconomics remains obscure. Indeed there remains considerable doubt that we can cross the much shorter conceptual bridge between the behavioral and neurophysiological domains. With specific regard to individual human learning, beyond a few interesting heuristics, nothing has been added to the conventional cognitive neuroscience of learning or learned from neuroeconomics. The applicability of this material to practical problems of human behavior, therefore, remains uncertain. There remains considerable doubt, then, that behavioral learning can be realistically monitored by neurophysiological measures. This does not mean that it may not be possible in the future, only that at the present time any attempt to do so would be a very risky enterprise.

Neuroeconomics operates at a somewhat higher level of theoretical abstraction than does neuromarketing, but any hope of bridging the gap between brain images and macroeconomic theory remains equally unsupported by reliable evidence. Although a substantial effort is being made to codify the field (see for example, Glimcher, Camerer, Fehr, & Poldrack, 2009), efforts to link neurochemical, neurophysiological, and brain imaging data to economic behavior are currently limited to similarities in the terminology including such ambiguous terms as "reward," "risk," "value." Whether each of these terms refers to the same underlying process at the macro and neuronal levels seems unlikely. The conceptual bridges between higher levels of macroeconomic and neurophysiological behavior are still elusive. In its place Glimcher and his colleagues attempt to model various kinds of individual behavior in a more classic psychological sense. The great giants of macroeconomics are not mentioned after a few preliminary salutes at the beginning. Much more attention is paid to psychological theories such as those describing reinforcement learning. The hope is that we will be able to make a leap from the individual level to the macro one by using the heuristics and concepts of the former to illuminate the latter.

There appear to be two very different goals of neuroeconomics: the first is mostly conventional cognitive neuroscience attempting to link ideas from behavior to neurophysiology. The second is the effort to link human behavior to macroeconomics. Although activities in both of these areas can be charitably designated as works in progress, any effort to link neurophysiological measures to macroeconomics seems wildly off the mark for reasons that I have repeatedly pointed out in the course of this book.

In the main, neuroeconomics seems to be a game played out under the rules of analogical thinking in which the most superficial relationships are misunderstood to have causal significance.

Specific debates concerning the applicability of neurophysiological methods such as brain imaging to macroeconomics characterize the current literature. For example there was a recent debate between Harrison (2008a, 2008b), a critic of the progress that has been made so far, and Camerer (2008), a strong proponent of the possibilities, if not the realities, of neuroeconomics. The interesting part of this debate was that there was also little if any referral to any robust scientific findings supporting the premise that brain imaging could have any direct impact on economic theory. The discussion was, instead, carried out at an insubstantial level eschewing any mention of data or correlations. As Harrison (2008a) expressed it:

Understanding more about the how the brain functions *should* help us to understand economic behavior. But some would have us believe that it has done this already, and that insights from neuroscience have already provided insights into economics that we would not otherwise have. Much of this is just academic hype, and to get down to substantive issues we need to identify the fluff for what it is. (p. 303)

Harrison (2008a) went on to identify some of the fallacies (he called them "bloopers") that have appeared in the neuroeconomics literature. One of these is the idea that neuroeconomics offers fundamentally new concepts about how the brain works. Neuroscientists might argue this point, however, given much of what I have already discussed in this book. Neuroeconomic concepts are mainly unsupported extrapolations from an especially fragile empirical database. An example is the idea that money directly influences human behavior because of its role as a surrogate for pleasures of other kinds. This may or may not be true, but, as Harrison pointed out, it is hard to understand how neuroscience has contributed (or might contribute in the future) to this conclusion.

Other neuroeconomic ideas deal with the psychological properties of human nature that are supposed to control human behavior. In particular Harrison (2008b) argued that much of neuroeconomics is based on ideas of brain localization and the efficacy of reverse inference—a logically treacherous process according to Poldrack (2006). Currently both cognitive neuroscience ideas are under attack; there is as yet little evidence of any brain region or regions that can be assigned to economic decision making or of any neurophysiological measures that will inform us of these social interactions. It is especially difficult to make such an assignment when the laws of economic behavior are themselves not well understood. To look for correlates of a well-defined behavior in a brain image is one thing; to look for a vague phantom is another.

A new trend in neuromarketing, as in many other of these "neuro" neologisms, has been to ignore the issue of the actual scientific credibility of the problem (i.e., does it work at all?) and raise questions about the ethics of using what may be an nonexistent measure. Murphy, Illes, and Reiner (2008), for example, asked how we can go about protecting people from the pernicious influence of neuromarketing, mainly ignoring the possibility that the whole idea may be a nonsensical nonstarter. Although this may be a prudent thing to do—to anticipate a potential misuse of a possible system—it does seem that it would be a better use of resources to worry about extant dangers that are closer to the horizon than to worry about what may only be a rush of pseudoscientific hyperbole.

Not unexpectedly in this environment of high-technology brain studies, ethical considerations have also led to the invention of their own subfield—neuroethics. The idea of studying the ethics of neuroscience is a reasonable concept even if a neuroscience of ethics is far in the future of even the most hopeful neuroscientists (see for example, Gazzaniga, 2005).

A few studies have attempted to pursue the possibility of finding neurophysiological correlates or foundations of ethical behavior. Greene, Sommerville, Nystrom, Darley, and Cohen (2001), for example, measured the differential effects on fMRI signals elicited by two stories, one loaded with moral considerations and the other devoid of any such implications. Although different regions of the brain were reported to be activated by each tale, the results may easily be explained by the indirect emotional overtones of the two scenarios rather than the direct presence or absence of any "moral" issues—assuming, of course, that these rare results are real and can be replicated. Since the Greene et al. study, the scientific literature has been curiously deficient in empirical studies of how our brain may control our ethical and moral behavior. What seems to have taken the place of this technical topic are philosophical discourses on how we should adjust to the "impending dangers" of mind reading by means of brain images. This would be all to the good if there were any imminent danger that brain imaging devices could actually measure our ethical thought processes. However, we can be assured that this danger does not yet exist—no hard evidence establishes that either morality or ethics has yet become visible in a PET or fMRI image. It is unlikely from the point of view of the current literature that it will ever be.

And if the elusiveness of a bridge between the economic and ethical concepts and terminology, on the one hand, and measures of brain activity, on the other, is not extreme enough, imagine how difficult it is to nail down something as insubstantial as a supernatural entity. Early on in the history of another new "science"—neurotheology, attempts were made to measure brain activity during transcendental experiences associated with religious thinking. Much of this work showed a great diversity of brain responses with responses distributed widely across the brain. Azari, Missimer, and Seitz (2005) reported high levels of activity in the frontal and parietal regions correlated with religious experience; Newberg, Pourdehand, Alavi, and d'Aquili (2003) added the thalamus and limbic system to these regions; and Beauregard and Paquetter (2006) presented data that supported the idea that virtually all of the brain was active during religious experiences.

One recent (and still relatively rare) neurotheological study has been reported by Kapogiannis et al. (2009). The protocol in their experiment consisted of two parts. The first was a purely behavioral experiment that classified their subject's responses (by means of a multidimensional scaling procedure) into three "psychological dimensions of religious belief":

- God's perceived level of involvement
- God's perceived emotion
- Religious knowledge source

The second part of the Kapogiannis et al. (2009) study involved the use of fMRI imaging. A series of three kinds of statements (based on the behavioral tests) was presented to subjects who were simultaneously having their brain images evaluated. The subjects were asked whether they agreed or disagreed with samples of the three classes of statements. A second experimental condition in this part of their study in which the subjects were to make a visual discrimination between different character fonts was also used as a control for the religiously oriented questions.

The results of this complex experiment indicated that the three dimensions of religiosity obtained from the first behavioral experiment activated different regions of the brain. The first dimension, reflecting "God's perceived level of involvement" activated a cluster of regions including various subparts of the occipital, frontal, and temporal cortices. The second dimension, "God's perceived emotion," activated a narrower set of frontal and temporal regions. The third dimension, "religious knowledge source" activated a broad swath of brain regions including the temporal, supramarginal, cingulate, calcarine, fusiform, precuneus, and precentral gyri.

What can we make of this study? First of all, there was no suggestion by the authors that it was in any way intended to present an empirical proof of supernatural entities. It was, they emphasized, only an examination of the brain correlates of the beliefs and perceptions of the subjects in this experiment. Therefore, it is clear that what Kapogiannis et al. were asking in this unusual experiment was the question—where are the brain localizations associated with a particular set of cognitive processes? These cognitive processes may be congruent or closely related to other more familiar cognitive activities such as emotion, thinking, and even learning to deal with other people. This point was strongly made by

Kapogiannis and his colleagues (2009) when they suggested that religiosity ". . . is integrated in cognitive processes and brain networks used in social cognition." As such, they continued, "the evolution of these networks was likely driven by their primary roles in social cognition, language and logical reasoning" (p. 4879). What they were not talking about was the existence of anything or any entity supernatural. Nevertheless, if there is any new study that is most likely to be misinterpreted by the popular press, this one is it. The real issue in unique (i.e., unreplicated) experiments of this kind is their validity. The potential for confounds and artifacts, especially those discussed in chapter 1, requires that we take any such brain imaging study with a substantial-sized "grain of salt." The potential for misunderstanding this kind of finding is great.

We can expect many other neosciences to emerge in the future. Some of them build on the strong needs of our society to provide plausible, if not definitive, solutions to some important problems of humanity. In addition to those already mentioned, neuroergonomics[19] ("the application of neurobiological data to man-machine systems"), neurolaw ("the application of neurobiological knowledge to adjudicating guilt or innocence in our legal system"), and neuropolitics ("the application of neurobiological information to the assessment of political beliefs") are already on the scene. Others are certain to follow.

To what can we attribute this enthusiasm for the insertion of brain imaging into the social dialogue? The answer to this question is subtle but understandable in the context of a complex society with desperate needs to find solutions to crippling social problems. We quite understandably reach out to whatever objective measure of human nature becomes available, regardless of the robustness of the scientific literature on which it is based. There are economies of thought that make it easy to link the psychological and neurophysiological even when the critical evidence is sparse or absent. This is the psychological equivalent of the "minimum energy" concept in physics that explains the way in which a bridge cable hangs. We may refer to that idea as the "least cognitive effort" principle. However, there are more subtle influences that propel us toward an uncritical acceptance of these highly suspect "neuro" neosciences including the underestimation of the weakness of correlational or analogical thinking.

One of these influences is the perfectly valid and widely accepted postulate discussed in chapter 1 that mental activity of all kinds is a function of the material brain. As a philosophical, ontological belief this is cornerstone of much of cognitive neuroscience. However, this postulate, this assumption, this axiomatic principle, undeniable though it may be, is still in its infancy in terms of the scientific foundations required to establish its validity. The problem is that the mind-brain relationship is so complex, both in terms of our behavioral and neurophysiological analyses and the variety of different kinds of neural responses so great, that the plausible possibilities greatly outnumber the rigorous proofs of necessity and sufficiency that should characterize strong scientific inference and explanation.

The point is that because of this great complexity, cognitive neuroscientists—the acknowledged experts in this field—actually know far less about the mind-brain relation than is generally appreciated. In such a context there is a compelling tendency to seize upon even the flimsiest neuroscientific finding as a possible surrogate of what we could previously only observe as molar behavior. Much of the enthusiasm for these new sciences, particularly those that seem to provide some possibility of a solution to a critical social need, is based on a misunderstanding of how little we actually know and how inconsistent are so many of the early experiments. It is all too easy to speculate about a potential application of brain imaging because, in some ultimate analysis, the physicalist assumption that all mental and behavioral processes are products of brain physiology must be true. All too often, however, the empirical foundations for these speculations are still unavailable.

8.10 Mind Reading

Finally in this discussion of applications, it is appropriate to say a few words about the most dramatic application of all—mind reading. To futurists, mind reading is defined as the ability to use a brain imaging system to uncover (detect, reconstruct) what a person is thinking. This would be an extraordinary development if it could be achieved. Although currently there is no unequivocal support for mind reading of this kind (any more than there is by fortune tellers) beyond a few limited findings based on the retino- or tonotopic layout of the primary sensory areas (e.g., Miyawaki et al., 2008),[20] such an accomplishment would certainly be considered to be the holy grail of brain imaging applications. I refer my readers to chapter 3 of this book for a discussion of some of the recent and very preliminary experiments that have used subtle multidimensional pattern analyses to select from among a limited number of alternatives. It must be emphasized that this is not "mind reading" in the popular sense. Rather, it is based on the fact that some brain responses at the macroscopic level may contain some information that distinguishes between what are primarily sensory states. It is not surprising that the overall state of brain activity should differ from task to task, but these measures are almost certainly limited to the grossest of discriminations.

The answer to why brain image-based mind reading should be so difficult, if not impossible, in a general sense has been repeatedly discussed in this book. The basic fact is that brain imaging almost certainly is operating at the wrong level; brain images obscure the fine detail of the neuronal network at which mental processes are most likely represented and encoded. We have no practical or proposed method of examining these microdetails at the level required to read minds.

8.11 Interim Conclusions

Clearly a long-term goal of much of the basic research on mind-brain relations is that these arcane findings and theories be applied to the solution of practical applied problems. At present, however, virtually all of the proposed applications remain promises and expectations rather than accomplishments. Despite continuous exaggeration of what we know about mind-brain relationships, there remain many mysteries, uncertainties, and inconsistencies about the empirical facts as they are reported in our journals.

Coupled with this lack of credible scientific support for many of the proposed applications is the universally observed fact throughout cognitive neuroscience that there is always a substantial amount of inconsistent variability encountered among studies that purport to speak to practical problems. Results from individuals, from groups of individuals, and from meta-reviews all describe limited correlations and partial associations of the various psychological and neurophysiological states. Therefore, the ultimate goal of using brain activity as a selection or diagnostic tool or as a means of "reading the mind" is fraught with uncertainty at the present time. Application requires that we have both a basic understanding of the systems under study and a robust corpus of empirical results linking the neurophysiological measures with behavior. Description and correlation, even if we do not have good explanations, are necessary for any successful application. A strong argument can be made that neither compelling descriptions nor adequate correlations yet exist to permit us to apply any physiological measure of brain activity to the prediction of behavior.

The empirical database supporting any of these proposed applications is sparse, and that which is available is confused and inconsistent. It is especially instructive to examine the scientific literature concerning behavioral dysfunctions and to discover the lack of any progress toward a strong association with any independent neurophysiological or neuroanatomic variable. The optimism that brain imaging will be able to find dysfunctional places in the brain that might underlay dysfunctional behavior is quickly falling victim to the undeniable fact that not only are many areas of the brain activated (rather than only one or a few) but that the pattern of activated regions varies considerably from one person to another.

Any hopes that we can shortly substitute neurophysiological indicators for direct measures of behavior are currently far fetched and fanciful. Some day it may be true, but currently the scientific foundations for such exaggerated hopes do not exist. Some important problems, such as the etiology of schizophrenia, have been pursued for a century or more without success and are not likely to be resolved even with the best of modern technology. This century-old failure should be instructive to any one looking for shortcuts to diagnosing or treating subtle behavioral problems such as PTSD, autism, or ADHD.

The following list presents some of the general conclusions that emerge from the discussion in this chapter.

1. The ultimate goal of the application of neuroscience to cognitive process is the discovery of a robust biomarker or correlate of a behavioral process. The current state of our science has not yet provided such an indicator for any practical application.
2. Promoters of applications often refer to highly exaggerated but nonexistent research to justify risky and expensive excursions into what now exist only in science fiction novels.

3. At best most research results exist as strongly probabilistic statements exhibiting a substantial amount of variance. The application of this kind of cumulative data to individuals is both ethically and practically suspect.

4. Even in situations as important as the effects of anesthesia, the evaluation of the depth of unconsciousness depends on a multifactor evaluation by the anesthesiologist. There is no stable, single measure of anesthetic depth. Specifically, devices such as the EEG, the ERP, and AEP are not now considered to be to be useful adjuncts to monitoring the level of anesthesia.

5. There remains the great imponderable of determining when a person is dead. Because consciousness is not directly accessible, and death is not an event but a process, there is great uncertainty about the moment that a person can be certified as being dead (or dead enough) to harvest organs for transplant.

6. Because consciousness is a general state of the nervous system (as opposed to a cognitively specific task such as learning), it may be possible to find some global measure of alertness or vigilance that varies with rest or sleep deprivation. Such measures, including EEG measures of brain activity during sleep, however, are very irregular and idiosyncratic. The one advantage that such a proposed application has is that it is not a priori implausible.

7. It may also be possible to make some estimates of motor-skill level with neurophysiological measures, but for a very different reason. The motor system, like the sensory system, is closely anchored to the physical world through an efferent system that is mainly monodirectional. Some rough measure of effort is also plausible, but effort and motor-skill level competence may be heavily confounded and counterbalance each other. Unfortunately, the literature in this area, as well, is extremely inconsistent.

8. On the other hand, the idea that we can find a physiological indicator of cognitive processes such as an individual's native ability or talent is a priori implausible. There is, at present, not even suggestive evidence that such a thing is possible.

9. Deception or lie detection, though long sought for and difficult to extract from popular culture, also is devoid of empirical support. What studies have been done produce extremely inconsistent results. What the causes of this chaos are is not known; whatever they are, the use of any EEG or brain imaging device to detect lies has not been shown to work.

10. Subtle cognitive dysfunctions resulting in mental illness or behavioral problems have not yet been successfully correlated with any neurophysiological or neuroanatomic measure.

11. Despite the early stage of development of cognitive neuroscience, entrepreneurs have begun to invent companies exploiting new fields of "neuro-this" or "neuro-that." Ignoring for the moment, the blatant efforts to profit from a premature or fraudulent application of brain imaging, even the more serious scholarly work falls victim to the glaring gap between the way the level at which neuroscience findings and social and economic forces are conceptualized.

9 Conclusions and a New Brain Metaphor

9.1 Introduction

Throughout this book, I discuss a number of individual experiments and describe their findings and results. None of these experiments, no matter how elegantly conceived or precisely executed, however, is of any particular importance. If any one of them, including the classic iconic studies, had never been conducted, another example of the same phenomenon would surely have taken its place and eventually made the same point. Collectively, on the other hand, experiments carry us forward to an ever-changing conception of the mind-brain relationship and to a constant reformulation of the current nature of cognitive neuroscience.

In this final chapter I strive to draw from this collection of observations and my comments about them the general principles that should be guiding our science as it undergoes its continual evolution. Certainly, the modern view of cognitive neuroscience is not the same as the popular view of mind-brain relations millenia, a century, or even a couple of decades ago. As the science accumulates empirical knowledge, the Zeitgeist is in continuous flux. That is as it should be; otherwise there would be no point to the collection of what is now becoming an extraordinary amount of detailed and variable findings concerning the brain, the mind, and our publicly observable behavior.

Brain imaging, as the newest tool in our attempts to solve the mind-brain problem, has garnered most of the attention in this field in recent years. Unfortunately, much of the newly forthcoming body of knowledge highlights our inability to resolve certain of the most fundamental scientific controversies. The problem is that imaging techniques such as the fMRI are gradually demonstrating that however useful they are in studying neuroanatomy and neurophysiology, they are not as useful as was originally hoped in the search for brain correlates of cognitive activity. Indeed, it may not be an exaggeration to assert that the most robust conclusion to be drawn from this work is that *specifically with regard to its application to the study of cognitive processes* brain imaging has demonstrated that it is not doing what it is supposed to do—that is, localize modular cognitive processes in a particular place or a number of particular places on or in the brain. Furthermore, every day we learn more about potential artifacts, statistical misdirections, and other confounds that raise fundamental questions about this approach to solving the mind-brain problem.

Two fundamental assumptions are likely to remain constant as the enterprise goes forward. The first is the basic idea of materialism—that the world is real; that there is only one kind of reality, and that everything else emerges from operations in that domain. The second is that all mental processes (and the behavior that may or may not attend them) are functions of that material reality. Specifically, everything that is mental or behavioral is, in principle, a result of physical (more specifically, neural) processes operating at the level of the great networks of neurons in the brain. This instantiation of the mind incorporates no additional scientific principles other than those that guide biology and physics. Indeed, any phenomenon (e.g., psychic precognition) that violates physical laws must be considered to be on its face –fraudulent.[1] Without at least an implicit acceptance of these assumptions, it would be meaningless to pursue work in the field of cognitive neuroscience; we would have to accept the existence of a set of supernatural and uncontrolled variables that would make any experimental results meaningless.

Where cognitive neuroscience and other sciences part company is with regard to their complexity. It is likely that the brain—with its billions of components and idiosyncratic interconnections—represents the most complex entity in the universe. This irregular three-dimensional array is far harder to study than the one-dimensional (DNA coding) problem faced by geneticists. Even the cosmos, with many more components, is relatively simplified by the uniform nature of its interconnecting forces—a simplification not enjoyed by cognitive neuroscience. It is this enormous complexity, rather than violation of any physical principles, that both overwhelms our analyses and opens the door to illogical speculation.

I carry out three tasks in this summary chapter. First, I list what I believe are the major *general* empirical observations that have been identified in the main body of this book. In this list I integrate across modalities, cognitive topics, and the host of individual experiments, to suggest what they collectively say from an empirical point of view. Second, I list what I believe are the implications of these empirical findings; that is, I step beyond the ever-expanding body of data to draw inferences, some very speculative and some less so, about what the observations mean in general. This second list, then, becomes the source of a revised point of view on which I base my third task, the expression of a new outlook or metaphor of the organization of the brain in terms of its cognitive operations. In my opinion the current view of the macroscopic brain is obsolete and must be replaced with a perspective that is more in step with modern findings. Unfortunately, it will be difficult to surrender some of our most treasured assumptions. Nevertheless, some may have to be replaced, and some of our most revered experiments may turn out to have implications other than the ones originally suggested when viewed from this new perspective.

It is now clear that cognitive neuroscience has not begun to answer all of the questions posed in the preface of this volume. Nor is it likely to do so in the near future. Indeed, some of those questions may be unanswerable for reasons of either principle or practice. What has happened, however, is that to an increasing degree and without many of us realizing it, the brain imaging data reviewed here have actually pushed us in a different general direction—toward the idea that brain mechanisms and regions are much more general purpose and broadly distributed than was previously thought. If this is the case, I believe such a change will lead to new assumptions and hypotheses about the brain and the mind, a new basic paradigm for research, and a new metaphor of brain organization. To flesh out the foundation of this argument, I now distill the scientific findings discussed in the previous chapters of this book into a series of summary statements.

9.2   The Empirical Observations

1. The main empirical finding of contemporary cognitive neuroscience is that many investigators are now reporting widespread and variable responses in the brain for virtually any stimulus event or task. This poses problems that are not only computationally challenging but also make it increasingly difficult both to understand the data and to develop theories and models.

2. In particular, brain imaging meta-studies show that when the results of a number of experiments are pooled, the typical result is to show activations over most of the brain rather than convergence on a single location.

3. As the number of research papers in cognitive neuroscience has proliferated, even the results of what are supposed to be comparable experiments display considerable inconsistency and unreliability in their findings. There is an enormous amount of variability between brain images, between individuals, and between cumulated data from single experiments, not to mention the increased variability and broader distribution of responses suggested by meta-studies.

4. Considerable portions of modern cognitive neuroscience's empirical research support the idea that every cognitive process is a product of the action of a highly integrated system in which many parts of the brain interact rather than function independently as isolated regions. Whether this is a signal of a network of isolatable and specialized nodes or something quite different has yet to be determined. This holds true for both neural and functional systems.

5. Correlative studies produce ambiguous results. Even in relatively simple systems it cannot be certain what the nature of the interactions is among the parts. Excitation, inhibition, and disinhibition can all mimic each other. Furthermore, new techniques such as diffusion tensor imaging make it clear that there are widespread neural interactions along a massive system of tracts interconnecting all parts of the brain. Given these multiple pathways, it is hard to imagine how any portion of the brain could operate independently.

6. In point of empirical fact, there has been little replication of most findings.[2] It is very difficult in an environment that is both underdetermined and very variable to draw general

and robust conclusions about putative relations between mental and neurophysiological parameters. Empirically, based on the typical diversity of responses obtained, even the most extensive meta-study seems to lack the kind of convergence we desire.

7. Many parts of the brain, purported to be functionally and anatomically separate from other parts, are not demarcated by any sharp boundaries. Many of the so-called anatomical regions are defined by arbitrary and accidental criteria such as the paths of the sulci or by imprecise systems such as the Brodmann map. Such boundaries are now beginning to be appreciated as being inadequate means of defining areas of cognitive interest. Further exacerbating the problem of comparing brain areas is the imprecision of the language used to locate regions typified by the use of such vague terms as "the dorsolateral region of the medial frontal cortex."

8. Without exception, every part of every system of the brain so far studied has been shown to participate in a number of cognitive processes. No part of the brain has only a single, unique function. No part of the brain operates in isolation. Modern research is increasingly making it likely that most parts of the brain are active in most cognitive processes.

9. There is a strong bias in the reports that achieve publication. Negative results—no correlation between the brain image and psychophysical results—either do not get accepted for publication or do not get written in the first place. Obviously, the strong biases at work in this field include the vested commitment on the part of investigators to their implicit or explicit assumptions.

10. Traditional experimental brain lesioning and stimulation techniques also exhibit a high degree of variability from study to study because of the uncertain nature of the surgery, the ambiguity of the stimulus conditions, individual variability in brain structure, and different criteria for accepting what was a positive result. Even the best-controlled surgeries leave a residue of uncertainty about exactly what centers have been stimulated or damaged. In general, the challenging problems of cognitive neuroscience are never solved, just passed by as new technologies replace earlier ones.

11. Clinical data, especially with traumatic injuries, do not display high degrees of correlation between particular brain lesions and cognitive states. Even the most widely cited "iconic" clinical studies show relatively low levels of correlation and high variability on close inspection. This is due both to the idiosyncratic nature of the lesions and the complex nature of the brain.

12. An implicit, but generally incorrect, assumption in brain imaging is that the largest activation is the most salient one. This leads to the mistaken idea that when all lesser peaks are reduced to invisibility by arbitrary scaling, the largest remaining peak represents the sole locale of a particular cognitive process.

13. Many statistical problems infect the field of cognitive neuroscience leading to artifacts and misinterpreted data in a surprising number of experiments. Among the most familiar is double-dipping—using the same data both to select and then to establish relationships.

14. Complex pattern recognition algorithms used to extract relationships often obscure the fact that different patterns of neural activation can be associated with the same discriminative outcome. Thus, the results of an imaging experiment may depend on the analytic method used rather than the psychobiological parameters of the experiment. The criteria for choosing the best method are not always clear; simplistic notions of parsimony or best fit may not correspond to the redundant complexity of the brain.

15. Grouping subjects on the basis of such parameters as gender can often produce effects that are similar to but different from those resulting from random grouping of the same subjects. The empirical fact that a distinctive pattern of brain activations occurs does not mean that that pattern is a valid measure of group differences. Indeed, substantial differences between groups can sometimes appear even when the groups are supposed to be equal with regard to the attributes under study. Permutation studies are desperately needed to filter out false differences from real ones.

16. The relation between the BOLD signal and the neural responses remains problematic. Although touted as being a direct measure of brain metabolism, the BOLD measure is very indirect and is mediated by a number of intervening steps that pose many opportunities for misunderstanding and misinterpretation. In a few cases it has already been determined that the BOLD response does not correlate with the neural response it was supposed to reflect.

Here, then, is a distillation of the major empirical developments that characterize the current research literature. Findings such as these are important; however, it is even more important to extract what they mean. That is the purpose of the next section.

9.3   The Implications

1. Above all else, the wealth of empirical research carried out by cognitive neuroscientists in the last century has made it clear that we are dealing with an enormously complicated structure—the brain—that repeatedly throws major conceptual and technical obstacles in our quest to understand its functions. The inferred meaning of the findings from any given experiment is driven by a multitude of factors, some psychological, some lexicographic, some technical, some associated with poorly defined stimuli, some dependent on the complex neural mechanisms themselves, some resulting from covert confounds due to uncontrolled factors, and some from deep conceptual and logical errors in the current Zeitgeist. The net result is to raise questions about the significance of any particular experiment's findings.

2. The current empirical situation emphasizes distribution of responses, the evocation of "systems," and the lack of replication among comparative studies. All of these outcomes argue against any stable and unique localization of cognitive functions in the brain.

3. A major problem with cognitive neuroscientific research of all kinds is how poorly cognitive processes are defined. The referents of such terms as learning, emotion, perception, and

so on are not precisely defined by either these words or the experimental context in which they arise. There is a major disconnect between our understanding of what cognitive processes are and the brain measures we try to connect to them. A penalty is also paid in stimulus control by poor definitions. In particular, asking a person "to think" or "not to think" about one thing or another often produces paradoxical responses.

4. A major conceptual problem with the application of cognitive neuroscience is that the gross anatomical level of analysis (EEGs, brain images, extirpation) open to investigators is not the one at which the neural processes germane to cognition are most likely carried out. Stimulus, lesion, and imaging experiments are carried out at a macroscopic level that ignores the details of the microscopic neuronal networks at which cognitive information and sentience presumably reside. Unfortunately, these microscopic networks are so complex that we have no means of studying them at the level at which mind is probably instantiated. Mind is much more likely to be a manifestation of Hebbian microscopic neuronal interactions that are completely obscured by all of these modern research tools. *It is most likely the detailed pattern, not the sum of the minute neuronal connections, that determines the cognitive outcome.* The pooling of the data from neurons or from subjects tends to obscure the true nature of the underlying processes.

5. For reasons such as complexity at the microscopic neuronal net level, it is impossible to use microelectrodes to establish how mental processes emerge from the network interactions. The basic problem is that the information needed to understand this amazing phenomenon is not available in the activity of a single or a few neurons—it is instantiated in the network activity of countless neurons. *In other words bottom-up explanations of cognition are not feasible because the critical information is not available—there is too much of it.*

6. For a completely different reason, all of the macroscopic measuring instruments such as fMRIs and EEGs also will not be able to unravel the basic mind-brain conundrum. The reason in this case is that all of these measures pool the details of the myriad of neuronal interactions into a cumulative value in which all of the critical information is lost. *In other words top-down explanations of cognition are not feasible because the critical information is not available—it has been pooled out of existence.*

7. Despite years of research searching for correlative biomarkers for such diseases as schizophrenia or bipolar disorder, there are no widely accepted neural measures—brain image, EEG, chemical, or otherwise—for these afflictions; nor are there any for the more normal aspects of human mentation such as leadership, sociability, or intelligence. Indeed, the literature on neural correlates of dysfunctional cognition is so chaotic that it is rare to find agreement between the results reported by any two laboratories.[3]

8. There is another matter that transcends whatever success there may be in correlating brain images and cognitive states. Because of the modest correlations and variability of these brain measurements, there will always be the problem of false positives as illustrated by the overlapping distributions of a signal detection theory analysis. Since there is no practical way to completely avoid false positives or missed detections in any noisy (i.e., realistic)

environment, any brain image indicator of an individual's cognitive process will be inherently wrong at least some of the time. The bottom line of this limitation is that there is at present no satisfactory use of brain imaging in any of the many applied cognitive fields that are in such desperate need for solutions.

9. The subtraction method, which is still at the heart of most brain imaging studies, remains a major source of misunderstanding and misinterpretation. There are many problems with this method; the most important is that an absence of change measured at the macroscopic "activation" level does not mean that there has been no change at the microscopic neuronal network level. It is now becoming widely appreciated that changes in the activation in an fMRI brain image tells us nothing about the degree to which a region may have changed its function or pattern of activity. This is due to the pooling of neuronal responses. The age-old admonition must not be forgotten—*data pooled are data lost!*

10. Mathematical models can be powerful descriptions of neural and cognitive mechanisms. However, since most such models are underdetermined by the available data, they are, like thoughts, behavior, and narrative descriptive theories, neutral with regard to a multitude of equally plausible neural mechanisms. The best they can do is to eliminate possibilities that are in violation of mathematics, logic, and physical laws; otherwise there always remain innumerable plausible alternatives that cannot be distinguished by any method.

11. Any studies using brain images that report single areas of activation exclusively associated with any particular cognitive process should a priori be considered to be artifacts of the arbitrary thresholds set by investigators and seriously questioned. Especially stringent criteria for publication approval should be required because of this obvious artifact.

12. Any studies using brain images to report some extraordinary new relation between a macroscopic cognitive process (e.g., altruism) or societal issue (e.g., economic policy) and a neural response should also be considered a priori to be beyond the limits of scientific plausibility.

13. Finally, as a general summary of the preceding statements, a substantial portion of cognitive neuroscience research is currently being carried out at the wrong (macroscopic) level of analysis rather than the correct (microscopic) level at which cognitive processes are most likely instantiated. Unfortunately, analysis at the microscopic level is intractable because of the complexity and the numerousness of the involved neuronal networks. This results in low-power experimental designs, misdirected attention and effort, and the surprisingly poor quality of the resulting data. *In effect, we are doing what we can do when we cannot do what we should do.*

9.4 A New Brain Metaphor

Cognitive neuroscience is, for all of the reasons that I have spoken of so far, a science driven by what might best be called metaphors rather than theories. By this I mean that at each point in its history there exists a consensual point of view that described how we believe the brain functions and how it is related to cognitive processes. The prevailing metaphor at any time has been composed of words that are neither precise nor literal but reflect a generalized conceptual model of mind-brain organization. Often the current metaphor is not supported by empirical data but rather by preexisting and antique assumptions as well as by the Zeitgeist that emerged from whatever technology was currently available..

The concept of a metaphor, as I use it here, is too loose and too vague to be relegated to the level of a theory since it is not so much a formal set of axioms, derivations, theorems, and conclusions or an integrated expression of empirical findings as it is an overall way of looking at the brain without fleshing out the details. In the absence of relevant proofs or robust data, a metaphor sets the tone for thinking in the field; as such, it can be amazingly potent in guiding research. Whatever its degree of popularity, however, it is important to remember that we have metaphors because we do not yet have a solid scientific foundation on which to establish a full-blown theory of mind-brain relations.

The current guiding metaphor for cognitive neuroscience is the idea that the brain is made of regions or locations that map in some direct way onto the divisible modules of the mind. Although the details are obviously different, this is very much in the spirit of classical phrenology and the locationist theories of the centuries that followed. As we have seen throughout this book, however, there is a new trend developing, one of variable function and broad distribution rather than rigid function and constrained localization. The important fact is that this is a data-driven development. The new metaphor is driven not by philosophical speculation or by a wistful hope for simplification but, rather, by observation.

Unfortunately, metaphors change much more slowly than do empirical observations: sometimes this is for good reasons; sometimes for reasons that involve the conservative sociological nature of science. As a result, the current metaphor is not changing as fast as it should given the corpus of knowledge we now have available.

It is the purpose of this section of this final chapter to propose a new view, perspective, metaphor, or Zeitgeist for understanding the brain that is more in accord with the current mass of empirical observations than is the one currently guiding our science. Such a periodic reformulation not only is desirable but is also a necessary part of any science if it is not to stagnate and simply repeat the faulty paradigms of the past. It is particularly necessary at this moment in the history of cognitive neuroscience because of the availability of new imaging technologies on which we tried to impose the metaphors of the past. Many of the new findings contradict the conventional, currently accepted, metaphor; some are especially frustrating just because they are so internally contradictory and inconsistent, but others speak strongly to the suggestion that our current metaphor is out of date.

The task of coordinating all of these findings—old and new—has not been adequately attended to; the attention of most cognitive scientists has mainly been directed to the collection of new observations. In such a situation it is only subtly and slowly that the changes in our perspective trickle through to change our overall perspective of the foundation concepts of a modern cognitive neuroscience.

Over the long history of interest in the mind-brain problem, a number of controlling metaphors have run their course. Although the various metaphors have contended with each other and coexisted at many points in scientific history, it is possible to disentangle them and appreciate how significant are the differences between them. The dominant metaphors for brain action during the history of our attempts to explain mental processes with brain mechanisms can be separated into two levels of analysis.

The first-level metaphor is the now familiar and widely accepted microscopic one.[4] It asserts that the neural equivalent of the mind is instantiated, encoded, or represented in the incredibly complicated network of interacting neurons—the cells that make up the various portions of our brain. These neurons are assumed to be interconnected by synaptic connections that modulate the behavior of the individual neurons as well as the overall state of the network and, thus, all cognitive processes. The fullest and still most widely accepted expression of this level of metaphor is Donald Hebb's (1949) brilliant intuitive leap to such hypothetical networks as the cell assembly and the phase sequence, arrays of responding neurons that change in accord with the changing state of the many interconnecting synapses. Although we know a lot about the behavior and chemistry of individual neurons, as I have noted earlier, there is actually no empirical evidence to support the Hebbian metaphor in general or in detail. Nevertheless, since there is no plausible and scientifically sound alternative, neuronal networks and synapses are generally accepted as the ways in which the brain works at this microscopic level to produce mind and evoke behavior.

The reason that this first-level metaphor remains unproven and unsubstantiated by empirical results is that the complexity of this vast neuronal network is so great and offers so few means of regularization or simplification. Many of us agree that neuronal networks represent an analytic problem that is both computationally and experimentally intractable. There is no way that we can either model or systematically study the interactions of a system that incorporates 10^{13} neurons each of which is interconnected in an irregular or idiosyncratic (i.e., no repeating or "crystalline") manner and most of which may possibly be involved in the simplest cognitive act.

Thus, almost by default, Hebb's metaphor remains the best possible guess and the one to which almost all cognitive neuroscientists (myself included) adhere these days. However, there is the other level of metaphorical analysis, a second-level, macroscopic one that guides most of our thinking about the operation of the brain just because it fits so well with currently available measuring instruments. I now present a short history of the evolution of this macroscopic level of metaphorical thinking.

9.4.1 A Short History of Brain Metaphors

Primitive Holism

The earliest metaphors that involved the brain were probably holistic. That is, the anatomy of the brain was so poorly understood that it was considered to be homogeneous, and a hit to the head created mental and behavioral problems regardless of where it was struck. Prior to the earliest speculations it was not even certain what role the brain played in cognition and behavior, and what we call "the mind" was attributed to other whole organs such as the heart.

Primitive Specialization

Early Greek philosophers spoke often about the humors or pneuma, or fluids that resided in the ventricles of the brain. This idea lasted for almost 1,500 years, at least from the time of Galen (129–203) to the Renaissance, where it included such luminaries as Leonardo da Vinci (1452–1519). Although the humor-based theory was incorrect in pointing out which part of the brain was important, it was seminal in establishing the idea that different parts of the brain might have different functions.

The Cerebrum

Next came the idea that the solid matter of the cerebrum played a key role in the representation of our mental faculties. Emanuel Swedenborg (1688–1722) is often given credit for this step forward, but it is almost certain that any number of other seventeenth-century anatomists understood this to be the case earlier. However, so little was known about the structure of the brain, and it appeared to be so anatomically uniform, that the brain was generally considered to be a homogeneous organ.

Functional Specialization

Primarily as a result of the growth of anatomical knowledge (including that obtained from observation and analysis of traumatic injuries) especially during the eighteenth and nineteenth centuries, the idea that different brain locations were associated with different cognitive functions emerged from the predominantly holistic ideas of the past. As usual there was an overshoot from the basic idea of localized function to what are now generally agreed to be the outrageous "bumps on the skull" theories of the phrenologists (Gall & Spurzheim, 1808). During the nineteenth century more acceptable versions of functional specialization were professed by any number of workers including Gustave Fritsch (1838–1927), Eduard Hitzig (1838–1907), Charles Bell (1774–1842), François Magendie (1783–1855), Herman Munk (1839–1912), and David Ferrier (1843–1928). Much of this pioneering work, it should be noted, was carried out on the sensory and motor pathways and the primary brain receiving areas for them. Not all were, of course; both Paul Broca (1824–1880) and Carl Wernicke (1848–1904) reported the presence of functionally specialized areas that they thought were involved in the processing of speech at much more central regions of the brain.

A major corollary of the localization idea was that the specialized brain regions are stable and more fixed than not from person to person. On this basis findings from one person to another were expected to be similar; the only corrections to be made would depend on the random meanderings of the brain's gyri and sulci. Thus, for example, if one found a brain region for reading in one person, a basic premise of the localization metaphor is that it would be likely to be found in a similar place in the next person.

The conviction that specific cognitive processes were encoded by specific and stable brain regions grew into what became the dominant current metaphor of cognitive neuroscience. For many of the technical reasons discussed in this book and elsewhere, the metaphorical concepts of specialized brain locales and separable cognitive modules became the driving forces for most of the work in brain and neurocognitive research until the turn of the twenty-first century. (Of course, this metaphorical module was not always without question. For example, Lashley, on the basis of his learning experiments with rats, believed both that the brain operated as a whole and that behavioral changes were only effected by how much of the tissue was excised.)

Most surgical extirpation investigations of the nineteenth, twentieth, and even well into the twenty-first centuries were carried out on the basis of the modularity-localization metaphor. This translated into a specific surgical protocol motivated by the question—what changes in behavior would occur when a particular place in the brain is damaged? When the brain imaging techniques first became available in the 1990s, the guiding question was essentially the same—what part of the brain was activated in particular cognitive contexts?

Distributed Systems of Localized and Function-Specific Nodes

Although the initial imaging experiments (guided by the prevailing metaphor) suggested narrow and specialized localization of cognitive components, further research quickly made it obvious that no such pristine localization actually characterized brain function. Instead, widely distributed regions of the brain seemed to be activated during any cognitive process. This conclusion was robustly supported by every reported meta-study.

Therefore, the metaphor began to change from one of localized functions to one in which "activations" of a "distributed system of nodal components" became widely accepted. It was the collective action of these nodes that instantiated cognition. However, the nodal components of this new metaphorical system retained the old idea of localization—they were supposed to be stable, with several as opposed to a few (or even one) localized components encoding specific cognitive processes. The compelling power of the old phrenological idea that there were functionally specialized regions of the brain was, therefore, retained. The prevailing metaphor was simply being repackaged in a new form asserting that there were several functionally interconnected and specialized locales scattered throughout the brain!

The Holographic Metaphor

Other distributed metaphors for the organization of the brain have come and gone over the years. They arose as a result of the availability of new technologies or a renewed interest in even older mathematical ideas. Certainly, single-cell and field theories had their origins in the development of microelectrode and EEG technologies, respectively. The compulsion is especially strong when there is a preexisting complementary mathematical model on which to build the new metaphor. Thus, when the hologram was first mathematically described by Gabor (1948, 1949), its basic concepts fell on the fertile ground of earlier brain interference theories (Goldscheider, 1906) and equipotentiality (Lashley, 1950) that had been circulating in physiological psychology thinking for many years.

In one notable and very different intuitive leap, Pribram (1969) and Pribram, Nuwer, and Baron (1974) proposed that memory and perception are simultaneously encoded in all portions of the brain. The analogy to the hologram was direct. The brain, according to this metaphor, worked in the same way as did a Fourier analysis—by transforming the stimulus pattern from a Cartesian space into the frequency and phase domains. In this model information was represented everywhere. Although this was one of the earliest suggestions that there was no specialized functional localization, the relation to the data was strained. No experiment showed simultaneous responses throughout the entire brain; nor were the frequency domain transformations ever directly observed. Thus, although Pribram's metaphor was a distributed one, it differs from the one to be described now in that the distributed regions of the brain can and probably do have different rather than identical functions.[5]

9.4.2   A New Metaphor

The force of newly available empirical data suggests that it is time for another evolutionary step in what should be the prevailing conceptual metaphor. As noted earlier the new metaphor that I propose for the organization of the mind-brain has two components operating at two levels of organization. The first, microscopic, level is the still-cogent Hebbian idea of complexly interacting microscopic neuronal networks that change in accord with the efficacy of synaptic connectivity. Nothing further need be said about that now.

The second level, the novel part of this new metaphor, deals with the macroscopic portions of the brain—the hypothetical regions of the brain that are assayed by brain imaging systems. The persisting problem in this case is that it is not at all clear that all measured macroscopic activity is code (i.e., the psychoneural equivalent) for cognition. That is, whatever differential patterns of activity observed at this level may not be directly related to cognition. At the very least these measures are accumulations of the activity from the underlying first-level neuronal network in which most of the salient information has been lost by the pooling process. Thus, while these global, second-level responses may contain some residual information about what is going on at the microscopic level, they do *not* offer a possible road to reductively decode cognition and *cannot*, in principle, lead to a general solution of the mind-brain conundrum. However, these global, second-level responses do point the way to rethinking some aspects of brain organization. The most important empirical findings of recent years suggest that variable and multifunctional brain regions are widely distributed across the brain in a way that belies the traditional idea of stable localized brain regions representing particular modular cognitive functions.

The new metaphor for the macroscopic organization of the brain that emerges from recent work using fMRI and PET systems is substantially different from the previous locationist metaphor even though it may use some of the same terminology; it is based on the following general principles:

- Distribution
- Interconnectedness
- Polyfunctionality
- Weakly bounded nodes
- Methodological sensitivity
- Variable data
- Functional recovery

Distribution

There has been a substantial change in the published literature from older reports that concentrate on single areas of the brain to modern reports that indicate broad distribution of the activated areas by even the simplest cognitive stimuli and tasks. In point of empirical fact it now seems increasingly likely that virtually all of the brain is involved in almost any cognitive process.[6] This is the near-universal conclusion to be drawn whenever research findings are studied by the pooling of data from many comparable experiments, that is, when they are meta-reviewed or meta-analyzed.

Distribution also explains why so many investigators have attributed cognitive processes to localized activations in so many different places. In a world of many candidates it is seductive to assume that any region found to be correlated with a cognitive process is *the* critical region. In retrospect, we appreciate that this may at least be confusing necessity with sufficiency.

Interconnectedness

Modern diffusion tensor imaging techniques elegantly demonstrate the multiple interconnections that run between and among most of the regions of the brain. These connections make it hard to imagine that signals are not repeatedly and recursively transmitted back and forth among widely dispersed parts of the brain during neural processing. Therefore, it seems unlikely on the basis of this anatomical information, as well as on the accumulation of functional findings, that any area of the brain operates in isolation, independently of the rest.

Polyfunctionality

Most brain areas are now known to participate in multiple cognitive processes. No area seems to have a unique function. Regions such as the frontal or parietal lobes, as well as smaller regions such as the hippocampus, are involved in many high-level cognitive functions. Nor are most regions totally silent during cognitive processing during rest. The implication is that any idea of unique localization of function in the brain is a poor approximation to neurological reality.

Weakly Bounded Nodes

The idea of a neural processing node with well-defined boundaries and a unique cognitive function appears to be incorrect. Brain regions are not sharply demarcated from each other anatomically; their boundaries are arbitrary and ill defined. "Nodes" may actually be relatively broad regions of the brain with considerable overlap and no clear boundaries. Anatomical boundaries may be artifacts of our desire to preserve the outmoded concept of localization. Although not quite "equipotential," nodes may be very large chunks of the brain belying the concept of a demarcatable place where a particular function is instantiated.

Methodological Sensitivity

Different analytical techniques produce different patterns of brain activation for what are supposed to be comparable experimental procedures. If our findings are different depending on the method, then any of the answers obtained with different methods are questionable concerning the rigid assignment of any region to any particular cognitive process.

Variable Data

Experimental results, supposedly from similar if not identical experiments, show wide diversity of the activated brain regions even when the methodology is kept as constant as possible. Meta-studies in which results from many studies are compared show a lack of replicability among individual studies as well as exhibiting widespread distribution of the responses. (We do not know whether this is a result of poor stimulus control or a real psychobiological fact, but both probably contribute to this variability.) The net result, however, is that all meta-studies show that virtually all of the brain is involved in virtually all cognitive processes. This point cannot be emphasized strongly enough. The more data we collect, the more diverse are the brain regions we find that seem to be involved in any particular cognitive process. The strongest implication of this empirical fact is that older ideas of localization are substantially incorrect. The more data we collect, the further we are from any specific functional localization. This is unlike conventional statistical studies in which an ever-more precise estimate of a "central tendency" is achieved by adding data.

Functional Recovery

For many years the idea that the brain can restore functions after injury by activating new regions has been shouting out to us that the assignment of cognitive functions to particular brain regions is not fixed but, rather, can be quite changeable. Unfortunately, the implications of this finding have not yet percolated down into the current Zeitgeist. Recovery of function following injury suggests further that the assignment of function (including the initial assignment) may be much more arbitrary than we had thought. Thus, rather than a genetically driven specific functional role for various parts of the brain, the assignment may be at least in part ad hoc and driven by experience and other developmental factors. Certainly, this is reflected in the wide variability of brain activations shown among individual studies and emphasized by meta-studies. It is also reflected in what is often near-normal behavior in persons with severe anatomical brain defects.

The scope of the new second-level metaphor that should guide our attitude toward the macroscopic level is now becoming clearer. It exhibits several features. First, it must dote on broad distribution rather than localized function. Thus, it is a far cry from the classic phrenological-based metaphor. It even deviates from the current one that associates a network of functionally specific cognitive modules with cognitive processes. Specifically, where the phrenological model lived on in the form of cognitive modularity and specific functional localization, the new metaphor, based in large part on recent empirical findings, suggests that the brain mechanisms underlying high-level cognitive processes are to be found in the form of widely distributed and functionally generalized regions.

Second, the idea of static fixed systems (in which either fixed localized areas or fixed systems of localized areas describe brain organization) has to be replaced with the concept of a system that is dynamic and adaptive and that may recruit activity in different places in the brain depending on the needs of the task at hand. A corollary of this idea is that the recruited regions of the brain may not be the same every time or for every cognitive process. Instead, it is possible that identical tasks and stimuli may recruit quite different brain systems as needed.

An implication of this adaptive principle is that the application of brain imaging to determine "where" something is happening can never be productive because wherever that something is, it may not be located in the same place at the next moment or in the next person. Thus, it seems likely that the same brain region may have different functions in different stimulus or task situations and that different situations may recruit different brain regions to accomplish a given task.

Third, the next step in reformulating a new second-level brain metaphor deals with the nature of the nodes in the system. Many researchers have now turned to distributed networks as the prototypical metaphor for macroscopic brain organization. This "distributed network" hypothesis still assumes, however, that the network is composed of fixed nodes with specific "hardwired" functions in the old-fashioned sense. This is just a slight movement from the usual locationist postulate. Rather than invoking functionally specific nodes of limited spatial extent, this current metaphor simply broadens the idea to include many such specific functional locales scattered about the brain. It is these classic (neophrenological) ideas of specificity and fixed functionality that seem obsolescent and need to be replaced.

Fourth, coupled with these neural properties of the new metaphor is a psychological one. We must acknowledge that the current batch of cognitive modules, faculties, and constructs of psychology are inadequate to be used as a guide for probing brain function. They are much too arbitrary, nebulous, and idiosyncratic to have any necessary direct association with brain structure or function. Ill-defined psychological constructs are major factors in explaining why the cognitive neuroscientific data are so variable and inconsistent. In short there is no a priori reason why our currently inadequate psychological terminology should map in any simple way onto brain anatomy. We are badly in need of a more systematic approach to psychology—a more rigorous and robust taxonomy—before we can even think about seeking the neural equivalents of what are currently often only cognitive processes.

To sum up, the new metaphor proposed here asserts that it seems more likely in the light of current research that there are no demarcatable regions nor any regions of predetermined and fixed cognitive functionality in the brain; there are, rather, just "softly" bounded areas that may shrink, enlarge, or be recruited as the current task demands. Furthermore, none of these weakly bounded regions has any specific, preassigned, or fixed function. They all serve as general-purpose processing entities as required by whatever cognitive task is being processed. The whole notion of a place on the brain having a specific identifiable purpose has to be abandoned as an unreliable and outmoded metaphor.

9.5   A Final Note

Finally, there is an important comment to be made about the implications of the new metaphor presented in this book. Modern cognitive neuroscience makes it clear that we still know very little about the way the brain makes the mind. The problem is so complex at the true level of analysis (the microscopic details of the neuronal network) that none of the current research strategies enlightens us on this most important and most challenging aspect of human psychobiological nature. In the domain of cognitive neuroscience inferences have been drawn about the relation between the mind and the brain that are simply not justified by either traditional or modern empirical results. The situation has been greatly exacerbated by the arrival on the scene of brain imaging devices. These techniques are deeply flawed for the study of cognitive processes for a host of statistical, technical, neurobiological, and conceptual reasons.

In this regard cognitive neuroscience differs very much from the physical sciences—we are not building pyramids of knowledge concentrating a broad swath of empirical observations into general laws. Cognitive neuroscience, like its parent psychology, remains an accumulative science with no great syntheses such as those embodied in the great unifying theories such as evolution or in periodic tables that make biology or chemistry coherent.

As I close this book, it is interesting to reiterate one alarming possibility: whereas brain imaging methods are designed to answer the "where" question, it is becoming increasingly clear that data collected with these methods are propelling us toward the conclusion that the brain is not organized in such a specific spatial manner. It would be ironic, indeed, if the methods for telling us "where?" were actually telling us that this is a bad or irrelevant question and that any future effort to push our search for brain locations of particular cognitive processes would be futile. We may have to conclude that brain imaging, however successful it may be in anatomical and physiological studies, is the wrong tool for the study of *cognitive* neuroscience.

What, then, do the activation patterns that are observed with fMRI systems these days mean in terms of cognition? It is not entirely clear, but it seems that the simplistic idea that they represent localized regions of the brain in which specific cognitions are processed has to be rejected. It is not totally implausible to at least consider the possibility that they are not codes for anything but, instead, are quasi-random patterns of activity that have little to do with our thoughts per se. The possibility that the putative associations between brain images and cognition are illusory, therefore, cannot be completely discarded. The variability of brain imaging data raises a serious question—are we reading significance into noise? No one wants to deal with such a possibility, but in the complex world of brain imaging, this possibility cannot be totally ignored.

Afterword

It has long been accepted that the brain performs an integral function in all facets of human behavior, and understanding the mind-brain connection has been a key focus in all of the human sciences, from philosophy to psychology to biology. Recent advances in neuroscience, especially in neuroimaging, have fueled a resurgence of interest and a flurry of research activity in this topic area. There are now a wide range of disciplines that have added a "neuro" focus, ranging from computational neuroscience to neural engineering to neuroeconomics. Just about every area of psychology now seems to have a "neuro" branch of some sort. Even physiological psychology has been renamed cognitive neuroscience.

Along with the rapid growth of neuroscience research, there have also been some sweeping claims about the state of the art. The ideas that the solution to the mind-brain problem is at hand and that it can be seen with neuroimaging are very appealing if not seductive. Many civilian and military leaders as well as academicians believe that cognitive neuroscience can reduce complex cognitive structures and psychological processes to brain images that can be readily interpreted, understood, and used to replace more "traditional" behaviorally based assessments for selection, assignment, and training methods. As scientists, we found it difficult to separate fact from speculation and, until recently, there has been little scientific critical assessment of the assertions made based on neuroscience research.

In the course of seeking a balanced view of the potential of cognitive neuroscience to provide both new theory and practical solutions, we read Bill Uttal's books, *The New Phrenology* and *Distributed Neural Systems: Beyond the New Phrenology*. Bill's well-reasoned assessments of brain imaging and the attempt to localize cognitive functions in the brain based on that imaging were impressive. We contacted Bill in the spring of 2008 and asked him to help us assess the cognitive neuroscience literature and the claims that were being made for its suitability as a replacement for "traditional" cognitive and behavioral research. During the course of helping us to review the pertinent neuroscience literature, especially neuroimaging research, we realized that a book was needed to organize and summarize the findings.

Mind and Brain: A Critical Appraisal of Cognitive Neuroscience offers important perspectives on neuroscience vis-à-vis cognitive and behavioral psychological science, taking to task some of the claims made by neuroscience that have been based either on techniques that need refinement or results that are either not generalizable or do not account for individual differences. Perhaps most important of all, in the last chapter, the book offers some helpful suggestions for the way ahead in thinking about and researching mind-brain issues.

We will use this book to help us more realistically appraise cognitive neuroscience research and, we hope, to help our civilian and military colleagues to make more critical and realistic assessments of the ever-growing cognitive neuroscience literature. Also, we will use Bill's book to help us constructively devise new approaches for developing what we believe to be a more scientifically sound knowledge base for cognitive neuroscience. As an example, we are taking advantage of the large number of extant neuroimaging studies by funding meta-analyses in various domains of interest to the Army, such as the emotional regulation of behavior, to help us make sense of these studies and to resolve differences among neuroimaging techniques of the same cognitive behavior. In his closing chapter, Bill describes the characteristics of a new macroscopic metaphor for the mind-brain connection. We will use these seven general principles, as he calls them, to guide our research and meta-analyses.

We are also following Bill's lead in promulgating the development of new metaphors for connecting the human mind to brain. We agree with Bill and others, like Lisa Feldman Barrett, that lacking a good formal theory of the mind-brain connection, we need good metaphors to help us approximate theory and guide our research. This is particularly true because the brain creates the mind in complex biological ways, and the mind, in turn, generates complex cognition. The structure and function of brain biology, while definitely related to our psychological concepts, are by no means isomorphic with them.

The desire to understand individual and social behavior has a rich history, from its early roots in philosophical discourse, to the rigors of psychological and sociological experiments, and more recently to a flurry of neuroscience research. Each new paradigm claims to have the key to unlock the mysteries of the human mind and tends to discount (or at best redis-cover) what had already been learned in the past. We continue to encourage a full under-standing and appreciation of all of the human sciences as we pursue a multidisciplinary approach based on solid empirical evidence. We hope that others will find Bill's book helpful in fostering a clearer understanding of the cognitive neuroscience literature and will encour-age well-formulated research and conceptual thinking about the mind-brain connection.

Michelle Sams, PhD
Director, U.S. Army Research Institute for the Behavioral and Social Sciences,
and Chief Psychologist of the U.S. Army

Notes

Preface

1. Students are flocking away from traditional psychology graduate programs to work in neuroscientific and artificial intelligence fields that sometimes have little association to psychological problems per se. Part of this exodus is due to the excitement of new technologies, and some of it is due to the intransigence of traditional psychological problems. However important such work is, it is not at all clear that such methods and findings are directly applicable to those of either psychology or cognitive neuroscience. Psychological science needs to regain its birthright by emphasizing a behavioral approach to the study of humankind.

    A further problem for psychological science is that the very expensive brain imaging projects are draining funds away from behavioral studies, studies that are still the gold standard of measurement should one be interested in observing and measuring behavior. This very significant financial investment basically forces faculty to do more and more brain imaging research. Since large research grants are available for this sort of research, a virtual circle is created—universities make huge investments in a particular kind of research program, and the faculty is duty bound to pursue large grants that support that research program. Thus, the technology tail tends to wag the research dog.

    All in all the availability of brain imaging devices, whatever their advantages, come with some built-in baggage for university teaching and research programs.

Chapter 1

1. This is not entirely true. Recently at a meeting of philosophers I found myself contending with a group of dualists who believed that dualism and cognitive neuroscience were not incompatible. It seems to me that accepting this position would make cognitive neuroscience research nonsensical by admitting the possibility of uncontrolled and uncontrollable variables interfering with our experiments. From my point of view, monism and cognitive neuroscience are inseparable, the latter being a practical, scientific expression of the former.

2. I use the word "neuronal" here and elsewhere in this book to refer to nervous cell responses, i.e., the detailed microscopic responses of individual neurons that are typically recorded individually through microelectrodes. This level is opposed to the more holistic response recorded collectively by

means of fMRIs, EEGs, and similar devices. The more general term is "neural," which refers to any response at any level of the nervous system.

3. It is not just the cephalic region of the nervous system that can produce behavior. There are such things as spinal reflexes. However, there is little reason to believe that our mental activities are represented within the spinal cord or autonomic nervous system. Those who would move the mind outside the brain to other organ systems of the body are confusing influence with instantiation.

4. Briefly, arguments that suggest that the mind–body problem may never be solved include: (a) the complexity of the computation problem posed; (b) the variability in human physiology and behavior; (c) unstable psychological laws unlike those found in physics; (d) poor definitions and taxonomies of psychological constructs; (e) defects in all of the theories of mind-brain equivalence including single-cell, field, and localized-function theories; and, finally, (f) simple numerousness and the resulting intractability of the computational problems any relevant theory would face.

5. It is interesting to note that this was a classic example of psychology "informing" neurophysiology——a process that has been repeated many times over the years. It is rare for an idea to flow in the opposite direction, that is, when neurophysiology informs psychology.

6. More complete and specific discussions of their two positions on the nature of consciousness can be found in Crick and Koch (2003), wherein they propose a strategy for identifying the neural correlates of consciousness, and in Greenfield and Collins (2005).

7. Williams and Herrup (1988), pointing out that the number is far from precise, state that estimates of the number of neurons in a typical human brain "range between 10 billion and 1 trillion" (p. 424). Much of the uncertainty lies in the lack of good counts for the cerebellum, which may include as many neurons as there are in the cerebral cortex. If we assume, just for the sake of discussion, that there are as many as 100 brain regions distinguishable with fMRI techniques, the number of neurons included within each of these localized activation regions is still very large—a hundred million neurons or so.

8. For that matter it is not even clear how one would be able to rigorously demonstrate the presence of sentience. There is no test, not even Turing's venerable one, that can distinguish between a clever automaton and some kind of "consciousness."

9. My emphasis in this context is on cognitive processes with one major group of exceptions—the responses to sensory transmission mechanisms. As we see in later chapters, the retinotopic isomorphism of the stimulus and the neural responses may be specific enough to at least reconstruct simple stimulus patterns from fMRI responses.

10. I want to make clear that I am not denying the utility of these devices to make important contributions to science and medicine. However, because they are aimed at the wrong level of analysis vis-à-vis the mind-brain problem, they are unlikely to provide either detailed knowledge of how this almost magical transformation happens, nor are they likely to provide an entrée into the kind of "mind reading" that is being uncritically called for nowadays.

11. Efforts to combine monism and dualism (e.g., the idea of supervenience) usually lead to ambiguities and ultimately back to a position that cannot be distinguished from dualism itself.

12. More complete discussions of these forms of dualism and specific references can be found in Uttal (2004).

13. Counterarguments can be made that the usual laws of macroscopic physics do not hold at the ultramicroscopic levels where quantum probability factors dominate. However, even there, some kinds of lawful relations hold.

14. As so often happens, a particularly sympathetic and eloquent discussion of a topic dear to our heart initially eludes us only to be discovered late in the game. Thus it was with the book review by Fuster (2000), who expressed many of the same concerns expressed here and in my book, *The New Phrenology* (Uttal, 2001). I was not to discover his comments until the summer of 2009. Unfortunately both of our admonitions seem yet to be accepted by the scientific community.

15. A brilliant and detailed history of the battles that raged between the proponents of localization and distribution can be found in the work of Swazy (1970). Swazy argues that there has always been a continuing pendular swing between holistic and locationist interpretations of the data. Obviously the pendulum has for the last half century been strongly locationist. I believe the pendulum is swinging back in a way that suggests broadly distributed and more holistic (but not equipotential) responses and multiple functions for each brain area rather than specialization.

16. A more complete discussion of these issues can be found in my earlier work (Uttal, 2005).

17. One only has to do a Google search for "seductiveness" and "fMRI" to appreciate how widespread is the concern about the extraordinarily compelling but possibly misleading effects of brain images on cognitive neuroscience.

18. The universe of possible uncontrolled variables in both psychological and brain imaging experiments is well populated. For example, although experimenters rarely ask questions about smoking of their subjects, it is now well established that smoking can have significant effects not only on the anatomical and biochemical properties of the brain but also on the activation regions highlighted with fMRI methods (Domino, 2008).

19. Nonlinearities abound in ill-defined cognitive states. It is difficult enough to associate the subjective magnitude of a sensory experience with the amplitude of a stimulus, although the latter is anchored to precise physical measures. Determining the "strength" of an emotion or a memory is far more difficult.

20. This dissociation is different from the well-known "hemodynamic lag"—the prolonged time it takes for oxygenated blood to replace deoxygenated blood compared to the time it takes for the neural responses themselves.

21. Just how wildly "off base" subtle statistical tests can lead investigators was made crystal clear by Bennett, Baird, Miller, and Wolford (2007) in their intriguing study of reading emotions from pictures. The "subjects" in this "experiment" produced positive results in a cluster of brain pixels for different emotional pictures. This kind of report is widespread these days, but, in this case, the surprise was that the "subject" was a dead Atlantic salmon! The positive results in this "experiment" according to Bennett and his colleagues were due to random effects among a relatively small number of the voxels examined

in the experiment and the absence of any correction for multiple comparisons. The important message of this report is that it all too easy to be fooled by spurious results. Bennett and colleagues deserve much credit for this demonstration. (I understand from personal discussions that these investigators are now using this spurious result as a means of educating others how to avoid such artifacts; more power to them.)

22. The vocabulary of meta-studies is sometime confusing. I use three terms here: a meta-study is any study that examines the results of multiple experiments; a meta-review is a meta-study in which the data are simply merged or pooled to determine central tendencies; a meta-analysis, however, is a study in which appropriate mathematical and statistical manipulations are carried out on the findings of the set of reviewed experiments.

23. It must be noted that even the most severe critics of the possible artifacts in the statistical analyses of fMRI data did not reject all of the findings and conclusions. Many of the commentators agreed that although these statistical artifacts are possible sources of erroneous conclusions, they are not a basis for total rejection of the findings. They do raise important questions that have to be resolved, however.

24. Readers are referred to the author's earlier book (Uttal, 2005) for a more complete discussion of this kind of "sampling" error, an artifact that jeopardizes the interpretation of single-cell theories of cognitive processes.

25. The citations for these 77 questionable papers were not made available in the original article by Kreigeskorte and his colleagues.

26. R. D. Luce, in a personal communication, points out that these charges against cognitive neuroscience are equally valid for a wide range of behavioral experimental reports. Few psychological journals show individual results, only averaged data. All too often, the variability is attributed to random errors, not to the very large individual differences that are known to exist. Furthermore, some of the cumulative averages produce spurious fits with well-known "laws" (e.g., the power law) that in many cases turn out to be artifacts of the pooling process. For a further discussion of such "artifactual laws" see Uttal (2008, 131).

Chapter 2

1. However, coding studies can distinguish between competing neural theories that are not resolvable on the basis of psychophysical data alone. The most famous example is the resolution of the debate between opponent and trichromatic theories of color vision—each is correct, but at different levels of the visual pathway.

2. A more complete discussion of the kinds of neural responses that are used to transfer information about the nature of a stimulus to the central nervous system can be found in my earlier work (Uttal, 1973). In the following sections I have liberally drawn from that work discussions on issues of general philosophy with the acknowledgment that many of the specific technical details are now obsolete or have evolved and have been replaced by more modern techniques.

3. Both techniques depend on the repulsive force of two charged objects—a nerve and a charged string or column of mercury. Although slow, the two devices were capable of responding to minute bioelectric

responses. Photographic techniques were then used to measure the displacement of the charged string or mercury column produced by the nervous activity. These techniques were cumbersome, but prior to the invention of electronic recording and display equipment, they were the best available, and some extraordinary progress was made with them.

4. According to Adrian (1926) the problem preventing the earlier use of the oscilloscope was that its trace was too dim to be photographed—a limitation imposed both by the insensitivity of the then available photographic film and the limited light output of the phosphors used to illuminate the cathode beam's trace.

5. An interesting recent report suggests that the concept of tonotopic representation of frequency and intensity suggested by Tunturi may be only partially true. Bandyopadhyay, Shamma, and Kanold (2010) report that while there may be some tonotopic representation at a coarse level of measurement, nearly adjacent auditory neurons may have widely different frequency and intensity sensitivities. In other words neurons in the auditory region of the brain may be much more random in their organization than previously thought. This finding also argues against the idea that locales in the brain that encode specific processes are orderly arranged as suggested by the older work on tonotopic representation.

6. Konorski has been somewhat unfairly tarred with the most extreme version of gnostic neurons. In point of historical fact, he did not believe that a single neuron represented a complex idea. Instead he actually argued that it had to be the result of many neurons working together.

7. Obviously, sensory psychophysicists were aware of this for many years. The joint effects of wavelength, intensity, and purity on the experience of hue, lightness, and saturation have been appreciated for many years. How they interacted at the neuronal level, however, is only now beginning to be understood.

8. An example of the application of autocorrelation functions may be found in Uttal (1975), in which spatial patterns were autocorrelated to produce a representation that predicted the detectability of spatially organized dot patterns embedded in random (dotted) visual noise.

9. See Plaut and McClelland's (2010) counterargument (based on distributed networks) to Bower's single-cell approach.

10. For example, it is now obvious in the information theory world that a simple teletype code is not the most efficient in such a situation. Optimization should depend on the relative frequency of letters in the alphabet. Frequent letters like "e" should have a shorter code than less frequent ones such as "z." By adjusting the size of the code to reflect this kind of frequency effect, much more efficient coding schemes can be achieved. One very efficient means for representing alphabetic letter transmission is the variable length Huffman (1952) code. This system provides the smallest average number of symbols to transmit the alphabet based on the frequency of use of each character. The teletype code is very inefficient because it assigns the same number of symbols to each character regardless of the frequency of use. An analogous "optimum" code is assumed to have evolved in the neurophysiology of the brain. The goal is to find out what it is.

11. This was certainly the case in perhaps the most famous "optimal" coding experiment of all—Hubel and Wiesel's discovery of the extreme sensitivity of the cat's cortical neurons to moving, shaped spots

of light as opposed to the diffuse lighting conditions they had been using. Their discovery was totally fortuitous, at least according to the apocrypha surrounding their Nobel Prize–winning accomplishment.

12. Brindley (1960) has been even more restrictive in specifying what is a good question in psychophysics. He included only such questions as—are these two stimuli the same or different?—in his rubric of "Class A" queries. All others, especially those in which a judgment of some sort (such as the magnitude of a response) must be estimated are probably contaminated or impacted by high-order cognitive factors (e.g., relative strength) and cannot be trusted to be acceptable measures of sensory properties. Brindley calls these "Class B" queries.

13. The simultaneous contrast phenomenon also works with hue as well as with lightness.

14. Meta-contrast is a special kind of backward masking in which a later stimulus inhibits the perception of an earlier one. It has long been modeled by simple neural networks. The problem with all of them is that recognition of the shape of the stimulus is required for the illusion to work. This relegates the problem to a much higher level of perceptual processing than the simple explanations suggest.

15. I will always be grateful to the help provided by Dr. Burton S. Rosner, then of Yale University, in guiding me to the neural recoding techniques and to Professor Leonard Matin of Columbia University, who designed the electrical stimulator used in this work. I had been doing research on electrical stimulation of the skin previously, but the ability both to stimulate and to record percutaneously from nerves in the arm made it possible for me to carry out these early studies.

16. Desmedt and Cheron (1980) also recorded evoked brain potentials in this experiment.

17. One reason that comparable psychophysical experiments could not be carried out in all cases on this preparation was that in order to dissect out individual fibers or small bundles of fibers from the whole radial nerve, it was necessary to cut it "proximally" thus isolating the central nervous system from the stimuli impinging on the distal portions of the neurons. There was, therefore, no information to be evaluated subjectively being conveyed to the central nervous system from the surgically exposed regions in most of their experiments.

18. The idea that there are four basic tastes has a long history and is so deeply ingrained in our language and science that it is often ignored that there is no scientific proof supporting this hypothesis. Erikson (2008) pointed out that the alternative theory—a large number of overlapping taste sensitivities encoded by "across-fiber patterns"—is actually more in line with the empirical data.

19. Although we know (Anderson & Tweney, 1997) that the power function may be a fiction produced by pooling range-limited data (such as the response from the chorda tympani), even this rough approximation suggests that it is the integrated action of many fibers that determines the magnitude of the subjective experience in taste. This result fits well with what we learned from comparable studies in somatosensation.

20. For example, if an ABR does not occur in the intact subject, but one can be stimulated by electrical signals, than such a patient would be an excellent candidate for a cochlear implant. Obviously if there is no ABR with either natural sounds or electrical stimuli, a prosthetic cochlea would be of questionable value.

21. Only rarely have single-cell recordings been taken from the human brain. Most of these rare studies were performed on people with severe brain illnesses or trauma, two conditions that militate against well-controlled experimentation.

Chapter 3

1. By "isomorphic," I am referring to a kind of similarity between a neural response and a psychophysical response either in the time course or form of the respective functions. Identifying the one as the correlate or equivalent of the other due to their functional similarities is often misguided. The classic example is attributing complex cognitive processes to the responses of single neurons.

2. By "stimulus," of course, I am referring to either a physical event or a cognitive task asked of the subject.

3. However, see the discussion in section 3.22 concerning our ability to interpret what is being "seen" from fMRI images.

4. The dorsal-ventral stream dichotomy has appeared in a number of different theories of the organization of the visual system. Goodale and Milner (1992) and Goodale and Westwood (2004) proposed such a scheme in which the two pathways emerging from the V1 went, as mentioned earlier, to the parietal and temporal regions, respectively. However the dorsal stream also had inputs from the superior colliculus. The net result was that the dorsal stream was postulated by them to be responsible for "visual control of action" and the ventral stream for "perception" in this formulation. The difficulty is in the psychological language involved in this cognitive neuroscientific enterprise. Are "action control" and "movement" detection simply different words for the same neural process, or do they refer to what are functionally different phenomena and thus possibly different brain structures?

5. This study was also of interest because it used a novel statistical technique to determine that the frontal (FEF) and interparietal regions were actually responsible for the observed changes in the lower-level visual regions. The Granger Causality test (Granger, 1969) tests for a limited kind of causal relation between two variables by lagging one of the signals behind the other and then determining if the first can be used to predict the other. The Granger test is highly limited in that it does not work for more than two variables; indeed, it can produce highly spurious results if a third variable "causes" or predicts the other two. However, it is one of the few tests of causal relations available.

6. I must admit that I never would have predicted a decade or so ago that such a thing was possible. I consider the work that I am now about to discuss to be some of the most interesting and challenging studies yet encountered. One possibility, should this work not turn out to be some kind of an artifact, is that these signals that correlate with perceptual experience are signs (see section 1.4.5) that do not carry any explanatory impact. Only the future will tell how this will work out.

7. This is much the same scenario that Searle (1980) invoked in his famous Chinese room metaphor in which he showed that an automaton could transmit information without understanding anything that was being transmitted. In other words an unconscious or Zombie entity could simulate consciousness.

8. The three pattern recognizers used by Cox and Savoy included an LDA classifier, a linear support vector machine, and a cubic polynomial support vector machine. However, O'Toole et al. (2007) list a number of others that share common features (although different names) including neural network analyzers, connectionist networks, correlation-based classifiers, back propagation methods, as well as other more familiar statistical analysis techniques. All such methods depend on the analysis of multiple regions or voxels of the brain rather than on the search for a single criterion region.

9. These finding, as well as those of Thirion et al., now to be discussed, differ from the work of Bartels et al. (2008) discussed earlier concerning the nature of the oriented elements being studied. Bartels and his colleagues were concerned with the fMRI determination of the orientation of individual *neurons*. The other two experiments were concerned with orientation of *picture elements*.

10. Similar results were obtained in which the fMRI signal was shown to be related to orientated stimuli by Boynton (2005) and by Haynes and Rees (2005) using different classification procedures. All seem to agree that this effect diminishes once one has moved beyond the most peripheral of the brain's visual areas.

11. For example, respiration and skin conductance may be correlated signs of emotional activity, but few would argue that they are the actual neural (or otherwise) substrate of the *experience* of fear or lust (see chapter 4 on Emotion and Affect). The psychoneural equivalent of any experiential phenomena must be attributed, according to everything that modern cognitive neuroscience believes, to the intricacies of brain activity. Unfortunately every recorded brain activity must be carefully examined to determine if it is a code or just a correlated sign.

12. My hesitant expression of support for this study reflects my general attitude concerning the plethora of startling research results that fill the current literature of cognitive neuroscience. There is such variability and so many opportunities for artifacts, statistical and otherwise, to distort the meaning of these and related experiments that replication is desperately needed to be sure we are not deceiving ourselves. In many cases, no such replication is at hand.

13. The embedded question in this context is where in the nervous system does the psychoneural equivalent of phenomenological experience reside? Clearly it is not in the retina and some authorities (e.g., Crick & Koch, 1995) have gone further to suggest that it is not in the primary visual cortex, either. Thus, there is at least the possibility that fMRI signs of sensory information transmission could be confused with the neural foundations of perceptual experience.

14. It is important to point out that these frequency domain representations are merely a simplified and thus conveniently analyzable means of encoding a picture. If we had an equally good means of encoding in the picture or x-y domain, that would also work. The use of the Fourier frequency space does not mean that brain operates in the frequency domain.

15. Interestingly, Ruben and his colleagues also found that the simultaneous stimulation of the two fingers produced a smaller activation response than the sum of the responses produced by stimulation of the two fingers separately. This confirmed a psychophysical effect of mutual inhibitory somatosensory interaction I reported many years ago (Uttal, 1960).

16. A more complete discussion of the agnosias can be found in Uttal (2008).

17. Indeed there is a contest for the best new illusion. See its results at http://illusioncontest .neuralcorrelate.com/

18. This result was for the relative effect. The absolute magnitude of the adaptation effect diminished as one ascended the visual pathway.

19. This raises the general question—can neuroscience resolve controversies between psychological theories? I argue that it cannot unless the psychological theories contain specific neurophysiological postulates and axioms.

20. "Action understanding" is the essence of the theoretical use of mirror neurons in the view of the members of what has become the Rizzolatti school of thought. It is defined rather loosely (according to Hickok, 2008) as the activation of neurons that encode actions observed or executed for future use. "Understanding" in the neural context is defined as a neural process that accompanies (a weak interpretation) or is the psychoneural equivalent (a strong interpretation) of subsequent behavioral responses. This is closely related to the debate concerning whether complex concepts are "embodied" or only "symbolically" associated with cognitive activity (Mahon & Caramazza, 2008). It is obvious that many of the ideas involved in the leap from monkey multimodal cells to human social behavior are far from precisely defined.

21. Indeed, it may have been the superficial functional analogy between mirror neuron neurophysiology and psychological theory that drew such prompt attention to them. Such functional (often isomorphic) analogies, however, are a potent source of misunderstanding and unsupportable theories in cognitive neuroscience.

22. An unpublished report mentioned by Iacoboni (2009) asserts that mirror neurons have been observed in the human with depth electrodes during surgery on epileptic patients.

23. I have no doubts, however, that some analog of the mirror neuron would be found if we set about invasive recording with microelectrodes in the human brain. At the present time, however, little evidence for their existence is available from brain imaging studies (cf. note 22 above).

24. I must not mislead my readers. Dinstein and his colleagues believe that the mirror neuron is an important topic for future research, especially when it is directly compared to animal behavior studies and when we develop methods to more selectively activate human brain regions with more fully developed adaption techniques.

25. The numbered sections are verbatim quotes from Hickok's article. The comments in brackets are mine. All page numbers are from Hickok (2008).

Chapter 4

1. Agitation may also be interpreted as the antonym of calm, suggesting that any deviation from untroubled "feelings" or any display of abnormal behavior is "emotional." This certainly is an incomplete meaning of the term; behavior does not necessarily follow the underlying emotional state.

2. This traditional view was pioneered by none other than Aristotle. His list included 14 basic emotions such as envy and indignation as well as the more familiar fear and love from which all others were compounded.

3. Two excellent historical reviews of thinking about emotion can be found in Kagan (2007) and Gross (2006). Both consider the role of classic philosophy as well as that of modern cognitive neuroscience in our attempts to understand it. The histories of philosophical and psychological inquiries into the nature of emotions are also well presented in two introductory articles (Solomon, 2000; Stearns, 2000) in the *Handbook of Emotions*.

4. There is considerable criticism, however, concerning the role that such an evolutionary approach can play in understanding human emotions. See, for example, Buller's (2009) critique in which the use of evolutionary theory as a means of understanding human psychology is challenged.

5. Another factor must have been the realization from Papez's work that the system governing emotions was far more complicated than had previously been thought.

6. James, obviously concerned about the priority of the James-Lange theory, cites Lange's 1885 "pamphlet" as containing the germ of the theory but then claims that it was an idea that ". . . I had already broached the previous year in an article in *Mind*" (James, 1890, vol. 2, p. 449).

7. This is not the only set of regions that have been suggested as components of an emotional system. Newman (1999) argued for a system that overlapped only in minor ways with the Papez circuit. This is another piece of evidence that is becoming clearer as we progress through the discussion presented in this book; namely, that an ever increasing number of brain regions seem to be involved in every cognitive process.

8. Papez's original formulation of his circuit included only the following structures: the hippocampus, the hypothalamus, the anterior thalamus, the cingulate gyrus, and the mammillary body.

9. Kruk et al. (1998).

10. The dangers of anthropomorization are clearly evident here.

11. Recent studies have shown that the "pleasure centers" are much more widely distributed in the brain than Olds and Milner (1954) and Old and Olds (1963) had suggested.

12. Phan, Wager, Taylor, and Liberzon (2002) did note that the most commonly activated brain area was the medial prefrontal region of the cortex, which seemed to respond to all emotional stimuli, but other regions also responded almost as frequently for specific emotions.

13. Given that there were three kinds of induction methods (visual, auditory, and recall) and five different kinds of emotional stimuli (happy, fear, anger, sad, and disgust), it is not even clear if there were any repetitions among any of the 55 experiments summarized in this meta-study. The idea that the sample of experiments reviewed can lead us to any general conclusions remains problematical.

14. It must be remembered that this is not an absolute. The amygdala is activated *more* by aversive than by positive stimuli, but both kinds of stimuli tend to activate it. This must be contrasted with the

idea that the amygdala is turned on by aversive stimuli and inhibited by positive ones. We may speculate about the utility of such a process; however, it is clear that no definitive conclusion can yet be drawn about the role of the amygdala beyond its differential sensitivity to what we call emotional stimuli.

15. The arbitrariness of this three-dimensional scheme is becoming increasingly clear. Some authors (e.g., Posner et al., 2009) used a two-dimensional scheme in which only valence and arousal level described emotions. They, too, find correlations between fMRI images and the subjective reports in which subjects rated the emotional impact of word stimuli along these dimensions. Other two-dimensional models of emotion have been used to describe the psychological responses. For example, Britton et al. (2006) proposed that a social and nonsocial dichotomy should be used to describe emotion. Using fMRI imaging techniques, they were also able to find differences in the brain responses to this "dimension." It is likely that there are innumerable other dimensions that would show such differences. Indeed, it is likely that any difference in experimental conditions will produce distinguishable neural responses.

16. Grimm and her colleagues used a different set of emotion-provoking pictures than those used by Johnstone and his colleagues. Grimm's were chosen from the International Affective Picture System (IAPS, 1999).

17. It is becoming increasingly clear that the models and theories of psychology that are necessary to guide the neural studies are quite inadequate in accomplishing this function. Factor analyses or intuitive models suggesting what are some of the properties or components in psychological space probably have little value in reflecting or informing us about the organization of the components of the brain at either the gross or microscopic neural levels. Speculative modularizations of psychological processes, indeed, may have led us seriously astray in our search for brain mechanisms by forcing us to answer bad questions like "where does emotion (or its dimensions) reside in the brain?"

18. This difference was only for the condition in which male activations were subtracted from the female activations. When the male and female activations were examined separately, a wider, but different, range of brain regions was implicated. This curious result should be considered in the context of Ihnen, Church, Petersen, and Schlagger's (2009) experiment described in chapter 1 Both of these studies highlight the substantial potential for artifactual results with brain imaging techniques.

19. This discrepancy between the behavioral and the neural data is another strong illustration of the fact that the behavioral responses are neutral with regard to underlying brain activity and that the perils of any attempt to reduce psychological findings to neural mechanisms persist.

20. The possibility that all of these results are artifacts remains. My readers are reminded of the results of the permutation experiment carried out by Ihnen et al. (2009) and discussed in chapter 1.

21. "Projective tests" are particularly fragile measuring instruments as described by Hunsley, Lee, and Wood (2003).

22. See my earlier work (Uttal, 2009b) in which I discuss the extensive attempts to categorize aggressive behavior and the failure to satisfactorily do so.

Chapter 5

1. In recent years, a considerable amount of research attention has been directed at long-term potentiation (LTP) of synaptic conductivity as the basis of the engram. However, Charles Gallistel, in a personal communication, reminds us of Koch's (1999) summary of the state of research on this kind of synaptic plasticity in the following statement:.

LTP research is very popular: Between 1990 and 1997, over 2,000 papers on LTP research were published. The excitement stems in large part from the hope that LTP is a model for learning and memory, offering the most direct link from the molecular to the computational and behavioral levels of analysis. The field of LTP is also very controversial, so there is a surprising[ly] small number of completely accepted findings. (p. 317)

Even if confirmed, LTP would still not be the answer to the great question of how the brain stores information. LTP would be an answer at the "technology" level, not at the "system" level at which cognitive changes are more likely to be instantiated.

2. The word eidolon (singular) also referred to a phantom or ghost or copy. The eidola of Plato were supposed to be dim and perhaps imperfect copies of real experiences.

3. Although Bacon and the other Europeans have been given credit for the development of the experimental method, other cultures in other times had produced their own "scientists." Among the most often overlooked was the Iraqi genius ibn al-Haytham or Alhacen (965–1039), whose various contributions spanned the full range of science. A new biography of him (Steffens, 2006) is now available that goes a way to filling this lacuna in our scientific history.

4. It must be pointed out, however closely identified with rationalist philosophies, Descartes was also one of the main figures in supporting the mechanical approach to the study of human nature. His work on the nervous system certainly contained the germ of the idea of a law-driven humanity. His strategy (rationalism) may have differed from Hobbes's proto-empiricism, but he certainly shared the idea that some parts of the body, especially the pineal gland, accounted for the processes of the mind.

5. Previously, I pointed out (Uttal, 2008) that psychological time, space, and number are quite different from the comparable parameters of physics. This adds a constraint on the kind of psychological science that can be carried out but does not negate the fact that psychology can be pursued with all of the consequence, if not the precision, of the physical sciences.

6. Although the emphasis in this short history is on the history of thinking about learning, it is important to remember that all of these philosophers and protopsychologists were concerned with other topics as well. The epistemological ideas of rationalism, innate ideas, the human role in nature and society, and the advantages of deduction and induction were all implicit if not dominant in the current discussion. This is quite different from the highly constrained way in which I have presented this material here.

7. Marx and Hillix also include psychoanalysis as one of their "systems of psychology." Although Freud may have something peripheral to say about learning, I don't believe that it is in the same domain as these other schools that specifically deal with the more microscopic mechanisms and processes of how we learn. As an aside, I should point out that this confusion between the therapeutic and scientific

aspects of psychology, in my opinion, is one of the great difficulties that psychology faces in establishing its scientific bona fides.

8. The innate-learned controversy continues, of course, in the domain of developmental and evolutionary psychology. The choice of the subject matter of learning as one's topic of interest more or less removes one from this classic debate as most of the attention is directed to the study of the changes in behavior that result from experience. Innate, instinctive, or developmental activities are dealt with as potential confounds; however, they are actually outside the bounds of much of what we call learning theory. Of course, the genetic heritage and the stage of development of each individual influence and constrain what can be learned, but the current emphasis is on the processes of learning itself.

9. It should be noted that although this is the standard model, it is not universally accepted. For example, Craik and Lockhart (1972) proposed that information coming in through the senses is processed in all of these memory stages (if they exist) simultaneously and that the observed differences in behavior are due to the amount of attentional effort applied to the information. Thus, if one attends strongly to something, it will be stored in long-term memory; and if one does not pay too much attention to it, it will disappear without being consolidated from what appears to be a short-term memory. This alternative theory has been referred to as the levels of processing (LOP) approach.

10. I have added some other terms to their proposal to flesh out their widely accepted minitaxonomy. Keep in mind that all of these processes are inferred from behavioral data and do not neatly correspond to observations of brain activity and function.

11. Cabeza and Nyberg (2000) also included in their study other "nonlearning" areas of research such as attention, perception, imagery, and language. I am concerned in this chapter mainly with the research dealing with learning. It is interesting to note, however, that over half of the studies they cited came from the learning subfield of cognitive research—a reflection of the broad importance and prevalence of learning studies in modern psychology.

12. Whatever its failings and absurdities, it is would be unfair to ignore the contribution of the theory of phrenology. First enunciated by Franz Joseph Gall (1758–1828) and Johann Spurzheim (1776–1832), phrenology was one of the first theories to express the idea of modular cognitive processes located on particular parts of the brain.

13. The sham operation was the same surgical procedure carried on the experimental animal with the exception of the brain lesion itself. It was required because the anesthesia and the surgery themselves could be confounding factors and have their own effects on the animal's learning. It was, therefore, necessary to maintain a control condition to establish that it was specifically the brain lesion and not the operation that accounted for the changes in behavior.

14. This is a continuing problem in modern clinical neuropsychology. Diagnoses of aphasia and agnosia are often conflated by the respective contributions of sensory and high-level cognitive processes.

15. Jacobsen was also the scientist who carried out an experiment on chimpanzees that became the basis of the disastrous frontal lobotomy episode in psychiatry. Jacobsen's equivocal results were leapt on by others such as Egas Moniz (1874–1955) and Walter J. Freeman (1895–1972) to initiate one of the

most unfortunate periods in the history of neurosurgery. The reader is directed to the book by Valenstein (1986) for a comprehensive discussion of this dark epoch.

16. It is not clear from the original report what led Scoville to target the medial temporal region of the brain for his surgery. Scoville and Milner (1957) describe it as "a frankly experimental procedure" based on slim evidence of the epileptogenic qualities of the hippocampus. It is not well known that in addition to HM, nine other patients (all suffering from psychoses) were also subject to roughly ("rough" is a euphemism for what was really done) the same surgery and discussed in Scoville and Milner's paper. Two had no comparable persistent memory defect; five had moderate severe memory defects; and three had severe memory defects.

17. HM died on December 4, 2008. He was identified after his death as Henry Molaison and had lived for 55 years after his operation. Contrary to popular opinion, the operation intended to cure his seizures did not entirely succeed, He was on antiseizure medication until his death. We now await a detailed postmortem analysis of the specific damage that actually had been done by the operation to Mr. Molaison's brain.

18. For example, although the hippocampus has been closely associated with learning in some experiments, other investigators (e.g., O'Keefe & Dostrovsky, 1971) have shown that it also acts to implement a spatial map of an animal's surroundings. O'Keefe and Nadel's (1978) book spells out the details of this theory. The relation, if any, between this spatial mapping process and learning, however, has never been fully explained. But there is the possibility that they represent two manifestations of what is the same more general and equally poorly defined cognitive process. In any event, what it certainly does mean is that a well-defined anatomic region can have two very different behavioral functions. Is it a matter of a lack of anatomical precision such that there are smaller subdivisions with differing functions than we had appreciated? Or, to the contrary, does it mean that our behavioral classifications are not meaningful in this kind of reductive speculation?

19. Phineas Gage was a railroad worker who had very serious damage done to his frontal lobes when a crowbar was explosively thrust through his eye and out the top of his head. The report of his personality changes became the iconic case for frontal lobe damage. I discuss his case more fully in section 4.4.1.

20. Stuss and Levine (2002) have extensively reviewed the role of the frontal lobe in learning and other functions. The reader is directed there for a much more complete discussion from the point of view of clinical neuropsychology than is possible here.

21. It has been known, but largely ignored for many years (see Schmahmamm, 1997 for a historical review of the fact) that damage to the cerebellum produces cognitive deficits. Schmahmamm and Sherman (1997) suggested that cerebellar-regulated cognitive deficits included faulty executive decision making, spatial memory, as well as personality changes.

22. See the discussion by Williams and Herrup (1988), wherein they consider the problem posed by the uncertain number of cerebellar neurons.

23. Much of Thompson's physiological work was done with microelectrodes, but in recent years he has increasingly been applying biochemicals as modulators of the conditioning process.

24. A more complete history and explanation of the technology can be found in my earlier work (Uttal, 2001).

25. Other devices such as positron emission tomography (PET) also were used the 1990s, but they have largely been replaced by the fMRI by cognitive psychologists for many technical and patient-oriented reasons. The story I tell about this third "imaging" period of brain research is mainly about fMRI results.

26. Although Weiskrantz had been the first to specifically link the amygdala with emotion, Kluver and Bucy (1939) had earlier shown that medial temporal lobe damage produces a highly reactive monkey. That generalized damage is now associated with the amygdala in particular.

27. It is important for me to note that Cabeza and Nyberg (2000, p. 35) draw different conclusions form their meta-study than I do. They say quite plainly, "Admittedly, in keeping with the goal of this review, we have emphasized consistencies, rather than focusing on discrepancies from the general patterns." I, on the other hand, have focused on the inconsistencies. Although our conclusions may differ, there is no better source of comparative data than this meta-study by these two important scholars.

28. There is a massive diverging and multiplicative factor of neuronal activity evidenced as a signal goes from a threshold level to the level of perceptual experience. Such recruitment might well swamp out any quantitative differences in brain responses associated with different degrees of learning.

Chapter 6

1. Mental chronometry (a term apparently brought into modern prominence by Posner, 1978) is the method that Donders proposed to explore the temporal properties of otherwise unobservable mental processes. His idea depended on the construction of tasks that involved different combinations of what he believed were modular and separable cognitive components. Differences in the reaction time with and without one or more of the components were supposed to indicate the length of time it takes to carry out the missing function. This resulted from the fact, according to Jastrow (1890), that different neural paths taking different amounts of time would be associated with different mental activities. Mental chronometry thus depends on what a number of workers have called "pure insertion"—the assumption that removing one "modular" process from a multicomponent system would have no effect on any other parts of the system. Pure insertion is a highly problematic concept, and without it the mental chronometric method becomes highly suspect. The classic discussion of the use of reaction times in this way can be found in Luce (1986). It is here that he expresses his "reasons to be skeptical of the [chronometric] enterprise" and concludes that "So, as psychologists, we can hope at best to learn something [from chronometry] about overall organization and very little if anything about the details" (p. 1).

2. Still the most complete history of the Leipzig school is Boring's (1929/1950) *A History of Experimental Psychology*. This monumental history goes into the details of the influence of the Leipzig school in far greater detail than is possible here.

3. In Norman's case, it was an early filtering based on feedback from higher levels. Thus, the sensory signals were analyzed by information at high cognitive (cerebral?) levels and then fed back to the

peripheral sensory regions. Norman (1968) also implies the hopelessness of analyzing such a system when he notes "The simple analysis of each input signal is not sufficient to resolve ambiguities and establish a complete interpretation" (p. 535).

4. A reduction in the strength of the Stroop effect has been associated with damage to the dorsolateral prefrontal cortical regions (Perret, 1974). It is likely that this is but a partial view of a much more complex system.

5. Conversely, as noted in the previous chapter, it has been suggested that the stages of memory in the standard theory of memory are actually manifestations of attentional effort (Craik & Lockhart, 1972).

6. By 2009, Treisman and Gelade (1980) had been cited well over 3,000 times.

7. One possible resolution of this dilemma was suggested by Lavie (2000), who argued that "results apparently favouring [sic] late selection had typically been obtained in situations of low perceptual load, whereas those favoring early selection involved high perceptual load." Thus, both theories may be correct as far as they can be, each in the context of its own experimental design. Whether or not this is merely a Band-Aid on the fundamental impossibility of inferring underlying cognitive structure from behavioral experiments is yet to be determined.

8. This shift of research focus from one topic to another in psychology without resolution is regularly repeated. A question is asked; insurmountable obstacles are found to stand in the way of answering it; and then psychologists move on to new questions leaving the preceding issues unresolved. As I have shown, the problem of attention has been studied in several different stages, not all of which are clear products of the earlier stages. Although many would argue the following point, there seems to be little of the kind of pyramiding of new knowledge on the results of previous research that characterizes the physical sciences. Psychology remains a fragmentary science of controversial data and incompletely resolved theoretical issues.

9. The concept of attention as a target of research has had its ups and downs. The distinguished twin volumes of the *Handbook of Perception and Human Performance* (Boff, Kaufman, & Thomas, 1986) did not have a chapter or section heading dedicated to this topic but briefly embeds a short discussion on attention in a chapter on "Visual Information Processing." In other circles, however, attention is very much alive. As I write these pages it has been announced that the journal *Perception and Psychophysics* has just been renamed *Attention, Perception, and Psychophysics* because 45% of articles in the 2007 volume deal with attention.

10. Exactly what the relation is between eye movements and the cognitive process of attention has been of concern for many years. One view was expressed by Hoffman and Subramaniam (1995) when they suggested that attention guides eye movements but is not irretrievably locked to them.

11. A delayed response procedure is one in which a delay is introduced between initial training and the opportunity to respond. In the Jacobsen paradigm, the food was hidden under one of three cups in full view of the animal, but the animal was prevented from responding (reaching for the food) by an opaque barrier.

12. It should be obvious by now to readers of this book that I am convinced that no psychological test by itself can definitively determine the underlying neural mechanisms. All such associations between

behavior and neural mechanisms depend on correlative studies whose inferred interpretations are sometimes more imaginative than valid. The generalization that behavior is neutral with regard to neural instantiation still holds.

13. Paradoxes of this kind are not all that unusual in cognitive neuroscience. Marsden and Obeso (1994), among others, have noted that surgical lesions of the motor portions of the thalamus tend to *improve* the symptoms of Parkinson's disease.

14. Their pioneering early work (mainly with PET devices) was originally presented in an influential book (Posner & Raichle, 1994) and then in an equally influential article (Posner & Raichle, 1995). In recent years, Posner has developed and expanded his ideas in a number of important and widely read papers including Posner (2004), Posner and Rothbart (2007), and Posner and Fan (2008), among others.

15. Posner and Rothbart (2007) have renewed this assertion: "Results of neuroimaging research also provide an answer to the old question of whether thought processes are localized. Although the network that carries out cognitive tasks is distributed, the mental operations that constitute the elements of the task are localized" (p. 18).

16. It is important to point out a significant generalization; early reports generally reported more localized responses than did later ones. This shift in empirical results is an important development. Whatever the reason for this change—technological, experimental design, or statistical—there has been a major move away from theories invoking extreme localization and toward distribution. These empirical results are being (or should be) followed by a drastic shift toward a more holistic approach to brain encoding of all psychological processes.

17. However, one should be careful of the conflation of reciprocal inhibitory interaction (i.e., sensory suppression demonstrated mainly with microelectrode and behavioral experiments) with potential "bottom-up" effects on attention. These generalized reductions in sensory amplitude produced by lateral interactions do not necessarily produce a diminishment of the attended parts of a stimulus—they actually can enhance some parts of it. This is a distinction that was, somewhat surprisingly, appreciated by Kastner, De Weerd, Desimone, and Ungerleider (1998) in an earlier report wherein they did distinguish between the mutual suppressive effects due to neuronal interaction and the selective reduction of nonattended stimuli.

18. Also, see the discussion of the work of Bush, Valera, and Seidman (2005) on attention-deficit hyperactivity disorder (ADHD) in chapter 7.

19. Culham and Kanwisher (2001) had done us a significant service by listing the many functions other than attention that have been associated with the parietal lobe.

- Motion processing
- Stereo vision
- Spatial working memory
- Nonspatial working memory
- Mental imagery
- Mental rotation
- Response inhibition

- Task switching
- Alertness
- Calculation
- Pain processing
- Swallowing
- Meditation

Adapted from Culham and Kanwisher, 2001, p. 159.

Although some of these cognitive processes may be inadvertent cryptic synonyms for "attention," it seems more likely that this region, like most others, is multifunctional, and any attempt to assign a specific role to it (or any other brain region beyond the most peripheral portions of the sensory and motor systems) "would be absurd" (p. 159) in the words of Culham and Kanwisher.

Chapter 7

1. An illustration of the mass of intellectual activity directed at understanding and explaining consciousness can be found in the Internet site *http://consc.net/online* which lists 5205 items. Countless others may not have made their way to the Internet. Not even a very large book totally dedicated to the study of consciousness could interpret the many views expressed by thousands of authors. Unfortunately, virtually none of this vast corpus of knowledge clarifies the elusive nature of consciousness.

2. "Supervenes" is a term from the philosophy of mind studies that may not be familiar to many of my readers. In brief it means that changes in mind cannot occur without some equivalent changes in physical (i.e., neural) activity. However, there are many degrees of supervenience, and not all of them reflect the bare-bones physical materialism that is currently popular among cognitive neuroscientists. Some, indeed, come perilously close to suggesting a weak from of dualism.

3. Later in this chapter I discuss the biomarkers and neuroscientific correlates of consciousness. In a surprising twist, unlike most other areas of cognitive psychology, and although not underestimating the difficulty of the challenges, more progress has been made because of the medical implications than in the psychological domain emphasized in this section.

4. I deal with the medical problem of controlling consciousness during anesthesia in the next chapter. Although anesthesiologists have a much greater responsibility than do psychologists, it is not clear that the former do any better at either defining or explaining the nature of consciousness than do the latter.

5. Repeated instances of a patient being in a "locked in" state, but conscious, are reported in the scientific and popular literature. Recently a Belgian man was reported to have been conscious, but fully paralyzed, for 23 years. Contact was supposedly recently made between the patient's consciousness and the outside world through a "facilitating communicator" who was able to sense minor muscle twitches in a finger and translate them to a keyboard. Unfortunately this kind of facilitated communication has been shown to reflect the thoughts of the facilitator and not those of this particular patient. For an example of the breathless reporting of this scientific curiosity, access the following site. http://www.gather.com/viewArticle.action?articleId=281474977917571

It should be mentioned that this method of "communication" has been repudiated by the investigator who first reported it. A scientifically more interesting possibility is the use of fMRI signals to communicate with a person who may be in a "locked in" or persistent "vegetative state." However, this too is highly questionable since the different brain activations could be driven by the verbal instructions rather than any volitional act on the part of the patient.

6. The fact that we can self-report our thoughts suggests but does not confirm the presence of consciousness. One difficulty is that communication media such as language are necessarily incomplete replicas of our minds akin to maps or models of the physical world. The flow of language symbols, which can never be as complex as the thought itself, therefore does not fully represent the thought. The essence of consciousness, if it is there, is thus lost by a kind of psychological uncertainty principle in which our very efforts to measure it change it.

7. Meta-cognition is a psychological term that can be defined as "knowing about knowing." In other words it suggests that we can think about what we are thinking about. It has much of the flavor as that of the homunculus or, rather, a nest of homunculi, embedded one within the other, in which the lesser one provides a questionable explanation of the behavior of the greater one.

8. This tendency to exaggerate empirical results of neuronal experiments is widespread throughout cognitive neuroscience. The most egregious current example of it is the extrapolation of a relatively simple neurophysiological observation—the polymodality of certain neurons in the monkey brain called "mirror neurons"—to the highest levels of social interaction.

9. This quotation from Jahn and Dunn's book is from an excerpt of it published in the journal *Explore* (2007), vol. 3. no. 3, 203–204.

10. I refer my readers to my earlier book, *Time, Space, and Number in Physics and Psychology* (Uttal, 2008), for a further development of some of these ideas.

11. It is interesting to note that neither of these two laboratories cross-referenced the work of the other.

12. It is not even clear what an increase or a decrease in the power level of the EEG or any of its components means. An increase in power levels may mean that the idling brain has suddenly gone to work, resulting in an increase in overall neural activity leading to higher power levels. However, an increase in power levels may also be interpreted to mean that the brain has turned to an idling state in which every neuron is doing the same thing, a result that could also result in higher measured power levels.

13. Once again, I must warn my readers that I make no claim that this review is comprehensive. Reports relating brain images and one or another aspect of thinking have ballooned in the last 5 years; my sample cannot do full justice to this vast literature.

14. The Tower of Hanoi is a game in which a set of disks mounted on three pegs must be moved between two prescribed positions in a limited number of trials. The Tower of London is similar to the Tower of Hanoi in which colored balls are used. They may be moved between three pegs or three slots.

15. Additionally, PET images were also constructed. In addition to the parietal, frontal, and cerebellar activations, PET imaging showed activations in the globus pallidus, the cingulate, and limbic regions.

It is important to note that the frontal regions activated in the two procedures were not the same for the two brain imaging procedures.

16. For example, in a follow-up study Newman, Greco, and Lee (2009) found significant differences (compared to fixation) in activation in a number of brain regions that varied with the portion of the task emphasized in the instructions to the subjects. "Goal hierarchy," "number of solution paths," and "processing phase" produced different patterns of activation from the frontal to the parietal regions.

17. For a tabulation of the various mental processes that have been included under the umbrella term of executive functions, I direct my readers to Jurado and Rosselli's (2007) recent review.

18. The term "semi-conscious" is a popular, not a scientific, term. There is no objective scale of consciousness beyond those defined by various levels of behavioral competence. The usual scale for calibrating coma, the Glasgow Coma Scale developed by Teasdale and Jennett (1974), depends solely on behavioral correlations. However, as we have already seen, the links from behavior to consciousness are tenuous at best.

19. Power is defined as the rate of energy being transmitted per unit of time. In this context it is a cumulative measure of all of the power being transmitted by all EEG frequency bands.

20. With so many possible measures and so many plausible interactions, it is clear that there are a sufficiently large number of degrees of freedom to provide support for almost any argument. Adding up different proportions of EEG frequencies, some of which are positive and some of which are negative, provides few constraints on what one might conjure up as a plausible correlate of intelligence.

21. A very readable and informative discussion of nonlinear methods that can be applied to EEG has been written by Stam (2005).

22. The metric of the intelligence provided by Raven's Progressive Matrices is based on a method proposed by Raven (1936). The method is supposed to be relatively culture-free, as it depends more on logical thinking than vocabulary or life experiences. The subject is required to complete 2×2 or 3×3 element matrices by filling in the one element logically suggested by the other three or eight elements. Performance on this test is considered to be an example of generalized fluid intelligence.

Chapter 8

1. The page numbers and exact wording quoted here come from a prepublication copy of this document and may not agree with the final format.

2. The special circumstances in which the use of the EEG is clearly indicated include surgery on the brain itself, especially when a focus of epileptic activity is being sought or cases in which there is an especial danger of oxygen deprivation—carotid artery surgery being the most obvious example.

3. The stimuli used to produce the ARP, as well as all ERPs, must be sufficiently separated from each other so that refractory periods and adaptive responses can dissipate, and each stimulus, therefore, can be considered to be an independent event. Also, enough repetitions are required to average out the ongoing EEG background noise.

4. Vigilance per se has taken on a specific meaning in this field. It refers to the ability to detect small (usually) signals over prolonged periods of time in situations in which the occurrence of the stimulus is relatively rare.

5. In fact it may have been that the EEG was merely artifactually responding to the movement of the eyes and was actually not directly measuring the cortical activity. The important empirical observation, however, was that whatever the EEG is, it was differentially varying in a systematic way between sleep and awakening as well as between different stages of sleep.

6. The exact range of the alpha rhythm—the nominal resting EEG frequency of the human brain—is not agreed to by all investigators. Klimesch (1999), for example, lists 28 reports that differ in their estimate with frequencies ranging from 7.4 to 14 Hz. There are large individual differences that depend on a variety of different attributes of the subject. The important thing is that the alpha rhythm is a relatively slow wave that generally declines in power as vigilance and alertness decline. That it also declines with attention to a stimulus remains one of the paradoxical curiosities that characterize the entire field of EEG measures of behavior. It is, many argue, a very noisy, variable, and inconsistent measure of brain activity. The possibility that it is only an epiphenomenal sign of mental states cannot be rejected.

7. The stages of vigilance referred to in this classification system are those proposed by Roth (1961).

8. It is interesting to note how the effects are often graphically exaggerated in this kind of work. It is very typical for ERPs to be plotted on expanded graphs (i.e., those plotting a lesser portion of the full 100% range) thus exaggerating the raw size of the effect. For those interested in potential distortions of data and how they can influence our theories, the classic work of Tufte (2001) is highly recommended.

9. I am referring here, of course, to the "Black Box Problem" so dear to engineers and so little appreciated by psychologists. In other words, input–output relations cannot *in principle* discriminate between any of the innumerable possible mechanisms that could account for the data. The critical theoretical statement of this principle was written by Moore (1956).

10. Some historians of cognitive neuroscience also attribute to Flourens the general idea that brain locations were specific for particular cognitive processes. However, this seems more likely to be the persistent contribution of Gall and Spurzheim, his antagonists in the great eighteenth and nineteenth century debates on phrenology.

11. The sixteen studies that I located are described and cited in detail in an earlier work (Uttal, 2009b).

12. This sweeping conclusion is likely to be disputed by many investigators. I believe, however, it is justified by the inconsistency of the studies that report such correlations. Of course future research may some day contradict this conclusion, but for the moment there is no agreed-upon biomarker of autism, PTSD, or ADHD.

13. It is interesting to note that although these particular regions of increased activation were emphasized by Baron-Cohen and his collaborators in their text discussion, their tables show widespread activation of many other regions of the brain, indeed, virtually all of the major lobes. This nearly total activation of the brain (to greater or lesser degrees) is now typical of many other experimental brain

imaging reports. Any semblance of narrow localization is increasingly disappearing from the scientific literature.

14. In such a situation, it becomes somewhat problematical what cognitive neuroscience comparison was intended in this experiment. One would naturally have expected that similarities would be observed between changes in the neurophysiological responses that could be correlated with behavioral differences. In this case differences were observed neurologically that had no counterpart in behavior. Thus, the comparison here was between a task and a brain image, a task that did not produce different behavior in the normal and autistic subjects.

15. Although the absence of any behavior alluded to in this definition is indisputable, a considerable controversy revolves around the presence or absence of awareness in such a state. How can we know if a personality exists within an unresponsive body? This is the crux of the discussion in this section.

16. In a recent follow-up article, Monti et al. (2010) reported a more comprehensive survey of 54 VS patients. Of the 54, 5 patients seemed to exhibit some willful control of their brain images. The complexities of this kind of experiment and the possible artifacts suggest that great care is required in interpreting these results as awareness on the part of the sample of patients, not only for those who did seem to respond but also for those who did not.

17. This topic is considered in greater detail in my earlier works (Uttal, 2009a, 2009b).

18. The latest additions to this list include "Neurowar" (a word introduced in a debate reported by the *New York Times* on March 28, 2010) and "Neuroliterature." I gather the former means using brain images to prosecute a war and the latter to evaluate the emotional and literary quality of books. Who knows what lies ahead?

19. An interesting discussion of some of the problems encountered when humans and systems with both artificial intelligence and human-like appearance interact in the future can be found in an article by Roese and Amir (2009). Their central point was that although progress has been made on many of the technical issues, humans still operate functionally at a much higher level than do the best of these artificial systems, and many of the proposed applications are not likely to be implemented for many years.

20. As discussed in chapter 5, other attempts to reconstruct perceived complex images into categories or into images contained in Bayesian priors do not really reconstruct–they merely recognize familiar objects.

Chapter 9

1. This does not mean that psychological processes (as opposed to the material understructure that accounts for them) do not *seem* to violate physical principles. Indeed, I have already discussed (Uttal, 2008) that many cognitive processes appear to violate the laws of physics. Psychological time is flexible, perceptual space can be distorted, and our mental abilities to deal with numbers are vastly different than the laws of arithmetic. However, the apparent discrepancies are not supernatural; they represent misinterpretations and illusions. These interpretive distortions are the source of the discrepancies between the stimulus and the perceptual experiences.

2. This is in contrast to meta-studies in which the results of many comparable studies have been accumulated but always with the same outcome—the more studies involved in the meta-study, the more distributed are brain activations. Apparently, for many reasons, replications do not lead to more precise answers to the questions we are asking, and true replication is less frequent than it seems. The situation where replication is most needed is when some very unusual claim is made.

3. From time to time, various biomarkers are reported for these cognitive dysfunctions. To this date, however, none has been shown to be reliable, much less valid, through carefully designed replications.

4. However widely accepted is the second part of the ontological postulate these days (i.e., that the mind is instantiated in the interactions of huge numbers of neurons), it should be remembered that this postulate is a very modern development. Neurons, synapses, and networks are entities of the twentieth century.

5. Other examples of field theories were discussed in my earlier book (Uttal, 2005). None has stood the test of time.

6. This strongly supports the idea that the microscopic neural nets that actually encode cognition are also broadly distributed during cognitive processing since the distributed macroscopic responses are summation, albeit "informationally deprived" representations, of the microscopic activity.

References

Adams, D. B. (2006). Brain mechanisms of aggressive behavior: An updated review. *Neuroscience and Biobehavioral Reviews, 30,* 304–318.

Adams, J. A. (1971). A closed-loop theory of motor learning. *Journal of Motor Behavior, 3,* 111–150.

Ades, H. W., & Raab, D. H. (1946). Recovery of motor functions after two-stage extirpation of area 4 in monkeys. *Journal of Neurophysiology, 9,* 55–60.

Adler, K. (2002). A social history of untruth: Lie detection and trust in twentieth century America. *Representations (Berkeley, Calif.), 80,* 1–33.

Adler, K. (2007). *The lie detectors: A history of an American deception.* New York: Free Press.

Adolphs, R., Trannel, D., Damasio, H., & Damasio, A. (1994). Impaired recognition of facial expressions following bilateral damage to the human amygdala. *Nature, 372,* 669–672.

Adrian, E. D. (1926). The impulses produced by sensory nerve endings. *Journal of Physiology, 61,* 49–72.

Adrian, E. D., & Bronk, D. W. (1929). The discharge of impulses in motor nerve fibers. *Journal of Physiology, 69,* 119.

Adrian, E. D., & Matthews, R. (1927). The action of light on the eye. The discharge of impulses in the optic nerve and its relation to electric changes in the retina. *Journal of Physiology, 64,* 279.

Aggleton, J. P., & Sahgal, A. (1993). The contribution of the anterior thalamic nuclei to anterograde amnesia. *Neuropsychologia, 31,* 1001–1019.

Aguirre, G. K., & D'Esposito, M. (1997). Environmental knowledge is subserved by separable dorsal/ventral neural areas. *Journal of Neuroscience, 17,* 2512–2518.

Allison, T., McCarthy, G., Wood, C. C., Darcey, T. M., Spencer, D. D., & Williamson, P. D. (1989a). Human cortical potentials evoked by stimulation of the median nerve. I. Cytoarchitectonic areas generating short-latency activity. *Journal of Neurophysiology, 62,* 694–710.

Allison, T., McCarthy, G., Wood, C. C., Williamson, P. D., & Spencer, D. D. (1989b). Human cortical potentials evoked by stimulation of the median nerve. II. Cytoarchitectonic areas generating long-latency activity. *Journal of Neurophysiology, 62,* 711–772.

Allport, D. A. (1993). Attention and control: Have we been asking the wrong questions? A critical review of 25 years. In D. E. Meyer & S. Kornblum (Eds.), *Attention and performance XIV: Synergies in eExperimental psychology, artificial intelligence, and cognitive neuroscience* (pp. 183–218). Cambridge, MA: MIT Press.

Altmann, C. F., Bledowski, C., Wibral, M., & Kaiser, J. (2007). Processing of location and pattern changes of natural sounds in the human auditory cortex. *NeuroImage, 35,* 1192–1200.

Amaral, D. G. (1992). Anatomical organization of the primate amygdaloid complex. In J. P. Aggleton (Ed.), *The amygdala: Neurobiological aspects of emotion, memory, and mental dysfunction* (pp. 1–66). New York: Wiley.

Amaral, D. G., Schumann, C. M., & Nordahl, C. W. (2008). Neuroanatomy of autism. *Trends in Neurosciences, 31,* 137–145.

Anderson, J. R., & Gallup, C. G., Jr. (1997). Self-recognition in *Saguinus*? A critical essay. *Animal Behaviour, 54,* 1563–1567.

Anderson, R. B., & Tweney, R. (1997). Artifactual power curves in forgetting. *Memory & Cognition, 25,* 724–730.

Anokhin, A., Lutzenberger, N., & Birbaumer, N. (1999). Spatiotemporal organization of brain dynamics and intelligence: An EEG study in adolescents. *International Journal of Psychophysiology, 33,* 259–273.

Anokhin, A., & Vogel, F. (1996). EEG alpha rhythm frequency and intelligence in normal adults. *Intelligence, 23,* 1–14.

Anonymous. (1983). *Scientific validity of polygraph testing: A research review and evaluation.* Washington DC: Office of Technology Assessment (OTA-TM-H-15).

Anonymous. (2004). Brain scam. *Nature Neuroscience, 7,* 683.

Armington, J. C. (1974). *The electroretinogram.* New York: Academic Press.

Aron, A., Fisher, H., & Mashek, D. J. (2005). Reward, motivation, and emotional systems associated with early-stage intense romantic love. *Journal of Neurophysiology, 94,* 327–337.

Aserinsky, E., & Kleitman, N. (1953). Regularly occurring periods of eye motility, and concomitant phenomena, during sleep. *Science, 118,* 273–274.

Ashby, F. G., Ennis, J. M., & Spiering, B. J. (2007). A neurobiological theory of automaticity in perceptual categorization. *Psychological Review, 114,* 632–656.

Atkinson, R. C., & Shiffrin, R. M. (1968). Human memory: A proposed system and its control processes. In K. W. Spence (Ed.), *The psychology of learning and motivation: Advances in research and theory* (Vol. 2, pp. 90–191). New York: Academic Press.

Avidan, G., Hasson, U., Malach, R., & Behrmann, M. (2005). Detailed exploration of face related processing in congenital prosopagnosia: 2. Functional neuroimaging findings. *Journal of Cognitive Neuroscience, 17,* 1150–1167.

Awh, E., Vogel, E., & Oh, S.-H. (2006). Interactions between attention and working memory. *Neuroscience, 139,* 201–208.

Ayer, A. J. (1936). *Language, truth, and lLogic.* London: Gollancz.

Azari, N. P., Missimer, J., & Seitz, R. J. (2005). Religious experience and emotion: Evidence for distinctive cognitive neural patterns. *International Journal for the Psychology of Religion, 15,* 263–281.

Baddeley, A. D., & Hitch, G. (1974). Working memory. In G. H. Bower (Ed.), *The psychology of learning and motivation: Advances in research and theory* (Vol. 8, pp. 47–89). New York: Academic Press.

Bahrick, H. P. (1983). The cognitive map of a city; 50 years of learning and memory. In G. Bower (Ed.), *The psychology of learning and motivation: Advances in research and theory* (Vol. 17, pp. 125–163). New York: Academic Press.

Ball, T., Rahm, B., Eickhoff, S. B., Schulze-Bonhage, A., Speck, O., & Mutschler, I. (2007). Response properties of human amygdala subregions: Evidence based on functional MRI combined with probabilistic anatomical maps. *PLoS ONE, 3,* 1–9.

Balleine, B. W., Delgado, M. R., & Hikosaka, O. (2007). The role of the dorsal striatum in reward and decision making. *Journal of Neuroscience, 27,* 8161–8165.

Bandyopadhyay, S., Shamma, S. A., & Kanold, P. O. (2010). Dichotomy of functional organization in the mouse auditory cortex. *Nature Neuroscience, 13,* 361–368.

Bard, P. A. (1928). Diencephalic mechanisms for the expression of rage with special reference to the sympathetic nervous system. *American Journal of Physiology, 84,* 490–515.

Bard, P. A., & Mountcastle, V. B. (1947). Some forebrain mechanisms involved in expression of rage with special reference to the suppression of angry behavior. In *The frontal lobes: Research publication of the Association for Research in Nervous and Mental Diseases* (Vol. 27, pp. 362–404). New York: ARNMD.

Bargh, J. A. (1997). The automaticity of everyday life. In R. S. Wyer, Jr. (Ed.), *Advances in social cognition* (pp. 1–61). Mahwah, NJ: Erlbaum.

Barlow, H. B. (1972). Single units and sensation: A neuron doctrine for perceptual psychology. *Perception, 1,* 371–394.

Barnes, J., Howard, R. J., Senior, C., Brammer, M. J., Bullmore, E. T., Simmons, A., et al. (1999). The functional anatomy of the McCollough contingent colour after effect. *Neuroreport, 10,* 195–199.

Baron-Cohen, S., Ring, H. A., Wheelwright, S., Bullmore, E. T., Brammer, M. J., Simmons, A., et al. (1999). Social intelligence in the normal and autistic brain: an fMRI study. *European Journal of Neuroscience, 11,* 1891–1898.

Bartels, A., Logothetis, N. K., & Moutoussis, K. (2008). fMRI and its interpretations: An illustration on directional sensitivity in area V5/MT. *Trends in Neurosciences, 31,* 444–453.

Bartels, A., & Zeki, S. (2000). The neural basis of romantic love. *Neuroreport, 11,* 3829–3834.

Bartels, A., & Zeki, S. (2004). The neural correlates of maternal and romantic love. *NeuroImage, 21,* 1155–1166.

Baumgartner, G. (1960). Indirekte Größenbestimmung der rezeptiven Felder der Retina beim Menschen mittels der Hermannschen Gittertäuschung. *Pflügers Archiv, 272,* 21–22.

Beauchamp, M. S., Petit, L., Ellmore, T. M., Ingelholm, J., & Haxby, J. V. (2001). A parametric fMRI study of overt and covert shifts of visuospatial attention. *NeuroImage, 14,* 310–321.

Beauregard, M., & Paquetter, V. (2006). Neural correlates of a mystical experience in Carmelite nuns. *Neuroscience Newsletters, 405,* 186–190.

Beck, C., & Rosner, B. S. (1968). Magnitude scales and somatic evoked potentials to percutaneous electrical stimulation. *Physiology & Behavior, 3,* 947–953.

Beck, D. M., Rees, G., Frith, C. D., & Lavie, N. (2001). Neural correlates of change detection and blindness. *Nature Neuroscience, 4,* 645–650.

Beecher, H. K., Adams, R. D., & Banger, A. C. (1968). A definition of irreversible coma. Report of the ad hoc committee of the Harvard Medical School to examine the definition of brain death. *Journal of the American Medical Association, 205,* 337–340.

Behrmann, M., Geng, J. J., & Shomstein, S. (2004). Parietal cortex and attention. *Current Opinion in Neurobiology, 14,* 212–217.

Bekesy, G. von. (1960). *Experiments in hearing.* New York: McGraw-Hill.

Bekinschtein, T. A., Shalom, D. E., Forcato, C., Herrera, M., Coleman, M. R., Manes, F. F., et al. (2009). Classical conditioning in the vegetative and minimally conscious state. *Nature Neuroscience, 12,* 1343–1351.

Bell, C. (1824). *Essay on the anatomy and philosophy of expression.* London: Longman, Reese, Hurst, and Orme.

Bennett, C. M., Baird, A. A., Miller, M. B., & Wolford, G. L. (2007). *Neural correlates of interspecies perspective taking in the post-mortem Atlantic salmon: An argument for multiple comparisons correction.* Paper presented at the 15th Annual Meeting of The Organization for Human Brain Mapping, San Francisco.

Bentin, S., DeGutis, J. M., D'Esposito, M., & Robertson, L. C. (2007). Too many trees to see the forest: Performance, event-related potentials, and functional magnetic resonance imaging manifestations of integrative congenital prosopagnosia. *Journal of Cognitive Neuroscience, 19,* 132–146.

Berger, H. (1929). Uber das electroenkephalogramm de menschem. *Archiv für Psychiatrie und Nervenkrankheiten, 87,* 527–570.

Berger, H. (1933). Über das Elektrenkephalogramm des Menschen. *Archiv für Psychiatrie und Nervenkrankheiten, 98,* 231–254.

Bernstein, N. (1967). *The coordination and regulation of movements.* London: Pergamon Press.

Binder, J. R., Frost, J. A., Hammeke, T. A., Bellgowan, P. S. F., Rao, S. M., & Cox, R. W. (1999). Conceptual processing during the conscious resting state: A functional MRI study. *Journal of Cognitive Neuroscience, 11*, 80–93.

Binder, P. M. (2008). Frustration in complexity. *Science, 320*, 322–323.

Bitterman, M. E. (1994). The neuroscience of animal intelligence: From the seahare to the seahorse. *Science, 263*, 1635–1637.

Boff, K. R., Kaufman, L., & Thomas, J. P. (Eds.). (1986). *Handbook of perception and human performance.* New York: John Wiley & Sons.

Borg, G., Diamant, H., Strom, L., & Zotterman, Y. (1967). The relation between neural and perceptual intensity: A comparative study of the neural and psychophysical response to taste stimuli. *Journal of Physiology, 192*, 13–20.

Boring, E. G. (1950). *A history of experimental psychology.* New York: Appleton-Century-Crofts.

Bourne, L. E., Jr., Dominowski, R. L., & Loftus, E. F. (1979). *Cognitive processes.* Englewood Cliffs, NJ: Prentice-Hall.

Bowers, J. (2009). On the biological plausibility of grandmother cell: Implications for neural networks in psychology and neuroscience. *Psychological Review, 116*, 220–251.

Boynton, G. M. (2005). Imaging orientation selectivity: Decoding conscious perception in V1. *Nature Neuroscience, 8*, 541–542.

Bradley, C. (1937). The behavior of children receiving Benzedrine. *American Journal of Psychiatry, 94*, 577–585.

Brady, J. V., & Nauta, W. J. (1953). Subcortical mechanisms in emotional behavior: Affective changes following septal forebrain lesions in the albino rat. *Journal of Comparative and Physiological Psychology, 46*, 339–346.

Brambilla, P., Hardan, A., Ucelli di Nemi, S., Perez, J., Soares, J. C., & Barale, F. (2003). Brain anatomy and development in autism: Review of structural MRI studies. *Brain Research Bulletin, 61*, 557–569.

Brandt, T., & Dieterich, M. (2006). The vestibular cortex: Its locations, functions, and disorders. *Annals of the New York Academy of Sciences, 871*, 293–312.

Breiter, H. C., & Rosen, B. R. (1999). Functional magnetic resonance imaging of brain reward circuitry in the human. *Annals of the New York Academy of Sciences, 877*, 523–547.

Bressler, S. L., Tang, W., Sylvester, C. M., Shulman, G. L., & Corbetta, M. (2008). Top-down control of human visual cortex by frontal and parietal cortex in anticipatory visual spatial attention. *Journal of Neuroscience, 28*, 10056–10061.

Brindley, G. S. (1960). *Physiology of the retina and the visual pathway.* London: Edward Arnold.

Britton, J. C., Phan, K. L., Taylor, S. F., Welsh, R. C., Berridge, K. C., & Liberzon, I. (2006). Neural correlates of social and nonsocial emotions: An fMRI study. *NeuroImage, 31*, 397–409.

Broadbent, D. E. (1958). *Perception and communication.* New York: Pergamon Press.

Brodmann, K. (1909). *Vergleichende Lokalisationslehre der Grosshirnrinde in ihren Prinzipien dargestellt auf Grund des Zellenbaues.* Leipzig: Johann Ambrosius Barth Verlag.

Brogden, W. J., & Gantt, W. H. (1937). Cerebellar conditioned reflexes. *American Journal of Physiology, 119,* 277–278.

Brower, M. C., & Price, B. H. (2001). Neuropsychiatry of frontal obe dysfunction in violent and criminal behavior: A critical review. *Journal of Neurology, Neurosurgery, and Psychiatry, 71,* 720–726.

Brown, J. M., & Denney, H. I. (2007). Shifting attention into and out of objects: Evaluating the processes underlying the object advantage. *Perception & Psychophysics, 69,* 606–618.

Buccino, G., Vogt, S., Ritzl, A., Fink, G. R., Zilles, K., Freund, H. J., et al. (2004). Neural circuits underlying imitation of hand actions: An fMRI study. *Neuron, 42,* 323–334.

Bufkin, J. L., & Luttrell, V. R. (2005). Neuroimaging studies of aggressive and violent behavior. *Trauma, Violence & Abuse, 6,* 176–191.

Buller, D. J. (2009). Four fallacies of pop evolutionary psychology. *Scientific American, 300*(1), 74–81.

Burrell, B. (2004). *Postcards from the brain museum.* New York: Broadway Books.

Bush, G., Luu, P., & Posner, M. I. (2000). Cognitive and emotional influences in the anterior cingulate cortex. *Trends in Cognitive Sciences, 4,* 215–222.

Bush, G., Valera, E. M., & Seidman, L. J. (2005). Functional neuroimaging of attention-deficit/hyperactivity disorder: A review and suggested future directions. *Biological Psychiatry, 57,* 1273–1284.

Butter, C. M., Snyder, D. R., & McDonald, J. (1970). Effects of orbital frontal lesions on aversive and aggressive behavior in rhesus monkeys. *Journal of Comparative and Physiological Psychology, 72,* 132–144.

Cabeza, R., & Nyberg, L. (2000). Imaging cognition II: An empirical review of 275 PET and fMRI studies. *Journal of Cognitive Neuroscience, 12,* 1–47.

Callicott, J. H., & Weinberger, D. R. (1999). Neuropsychiatric dynamics: The study of mental illness using functional magnetic resonance imaging. *European Journal of Radiology, 30,* 95–104.

Camerer, C. F. (2008). Neuroeconomics: Opening the gray box. *Neuron, 60,* 416–419.

Campbell, F. W., & Robson, J. G. (1968). An application of Fourier analysis to the visibility of gratings. *Journal of Physiology, 197,* 551–566.

Cariani, P. A. (2004). Temporal codes and computations for sensory representations and scene analysis. *IEEE Transactions on Neural Networks, 15,* 1100–1110.

Carlson, T. A., Schacter, P., & He, S. (2003). Patterns of activity in the categorical representations of objects. *Journal of Cognitive Neuroscience, 15,* 704–717.

Carretie, L., Mercado, F., Hinojosa, J. A. J. A., Martin-Loeches, M., & Sotillo, M. (2004). Vigilance related biases in anxiety through event related potentials. *Journal of Affective Disorders, 78,* 119–130.

Casanova, M. F., Buxhoeveden, D. P., Switala, A. E., & Roy, E. (2002). Minicolumnar pathology in autism. *Neurology, 58,* 428–432.

Castelli, F., Frith, C. D., Happé, F., & Frith, U. (2002). Autism, Asperger syndrome and brain mechanisms for the attribution of mental states to animated shapes. *Brain, 125,* 1839–1849.

Castellucci, V. F., Carew, T. J., & Kandel, E. R. (1978). Cellular analysis of long-term habituation of the gill-withdrawal reflex of *Aplysia californica. Science, 202,* 1306–1308.

Caton, R. (1875). The electric current of the brain. *British Medical Journal, 2,* 278.

Cattell, R. B. (1971). *Abilities: Their structure,growth, and action.* New York: Houghton Mifflin.

Chalke, F., & Ertl, J. P. (1965). Evoked potentials and intelligence. *Life Sciences, 4,* 1319–1322.

Chalmers, D. (1995). Facing up to the problem of consciousness. *Journal of Consciousness Studies, 2,* 200–219.

Charpentier, A. (1891). Analyse experimentale: De quelques elements de la sensation de poids. *Archives de Physiologie Normale and Pathologique, 3,* 122–135.

Chawla, D., Rees, G., & Friston, K. J. (1999). The physiological basis of attentional modulations in extrastriate visual areas. *Nature Neuroscience, 2,* 671–676.

Cheng, D. T., Knight, D. C., Smith, C. N., Stein, S. E., & Helmstetter, F. J. (2003). Function MRI of human amygdala activity during Pavlovian fear conditioning: Stimulus processing versus response expression. *Behavioral Neuroscience, 117,* 3–10.

Cherry, E. C. (1953). Some experiments on the recognition of speech, with one and with two ears. *Journal of the Acoustical Society of America, 25,* 975–979.

Cherry, E. C., & Taylor, W. K. (1954). Some further experiments on the recognition of speech with one and with two ears. *Journal of the Acoustical Society of America, 26,* 554–559.

Chevreul, M. E. (1839). *De la loi du contraste simultane des coleurs et de l'assortiment des object colores.* Paris: Hope and Walsh.

Chiappa, K. H. (1990). Brain stem auditory evoked potential methodology. In K. H. Chiappa (Ed.), *Evoked potentials in clinical medicine* (2nd ed., pp. 173–181). New York: Raven Press.

Chong, T.-J., Cunnington, R., Williams, M. A., Kanwisher, N., & Mattingley, J. B. (2008). fMRI adaptation reveals mirror neurons in human inferior parietal cortex. *Current Biology, 18,* 1576–1580.

Christoff, K., Prabhakaran, V., Dorffman, J., Zhao, Z., Kroger, J. K., Holyoak, J. K., et al. (2001). Rostro-lateral prefrontal cortex involvement in relational integration during reasoning. *NeuroImage, 14,* 1136–1149.

Corbetta, M., Kincade, J. M., & Shulman, G. L. (2002). Neural systems for visual orienting and their relationship to spatial working memory. *Journal of Cognitive Neuroscience, 14,* 508–523.

Corkin, S., Amaral, D. G., Gonzalez, R. G., Johnson, K. A., & Hyman, B. T. (1997). H.M.'s medial temporal lobe lesion: Findings from magnetic resonance imaging. *Journal of Neuroscience, 17,* 3964–3979.

Cosmides, L., & Tooby, J. (2000). Evolutionary psychology and the emotions. In M. Lewis & J. M. Haviland-Jones (Eds.), *Handbook of emotions* (2nd ed., pp. 91–115). New York: Guilford Press.

Costafreda, S. G., Brammer, M. J., David, A. S., & Fu, C. H. Y. (2008). Predictors of amygdala activation during the processing of emotional stimuli: A meta-analysis of 385 PET and fMRI studies. *Brain Research. Brain Research Reviews, 58,* 57–70.

Cowan, N. (1995). *Attention and memory: An integrated framework.* Oxford: Oxford University Press.

Cowey, A., & Irving-Bell, L. (2006). Do parietal cortical lesions impair spatial attention or allocentric spatial perception? *Cortex, 42,* 755–765.

Cox, D. D., & Savoy, R. L. (2003). Functional magnetic resonance imaging (fMRI) "brain reading": Detecting and classifying distributed patterns of fMRI activity in human visual cortex. *NeuroImage, 19,* 261–270.

Craig, J. C., & Rollman, G. B. (1999). Somesthesis. *Annual Review of Psychology, 50,* 305–331.

Craik, F. W., & Lockhart, R. (1972). Levels of processing in human memory: A framework for memory research. *Journal of Verbal Learning and Verbal Behavior, 11,* 671–684.

Crawford, M. B. (2007). The limits of neuro-talk. *New Atlantis (Washington, D.C.),* 19, 65–78.

Crick, F., & Koch, C. (1995). Are we aware of neural activity in primary visual cortex? *Nature, 375,* 121–123.

Crick, F., & Koch, C. (2003). A framework for consciousness. *Nature Neuroscience, 6,* 119–126.

Cross, N. Y. B. (2002). *Electroencephalography (EEG) as a predictor of motor performance.* Unpublished Honors Thesis, Department of Applied Psychology, University of Southern Queensland, Toowoomba, Queensland, Australia.

Culham, J. C., Cavanagh, P., & Kanwisher, N. G. (2001). Attention response functions: Characterizing brain areas using fMRI activation during parametric variations of attentional load. *Neuron, 32,* 737–745.

Culham, J. C., & Kanwisher, N. G. (2001). Neuroimaging of cognitive functions in human parietal cortex. *Current Opinion in Neurobiology, 11,* 157–163.

Culler, E., & Mettler, F. A. (1934). Conditioned behavior in a decorticate dog. *Journal of Comparative Psychology, 18,* 291–303.

Cureton, E. E. (1950). Validity, reliability, and baloney. *Educational and Psychological Measurement, 10,* 94–96.

Damadian, R. (1971). Tumor detection by nuclear magnetic resonance. *Science, 171,* 1151–1153.

Damasio, A. R., & Anderson, S. W. (2003). The frontal lobes. In K. Heilman, M. & E. Valenstein (Eds.), *Clinical Neuropsychology* (4th ed., pp. 404–446). Oxford: Oxford University Press.

Darwin, C. (1872). *The expression of the emotions in man and animals*. London: John Murray.

Davis, F. B. (1971). The measurement of mental capability through evoked potential recording. *Educational Research Bulletin, 1*, 1–171.

Dawson, G. D. (1950). A summation technique for the detection of small evoked potentials. *British Medical Bulletin, 6*, 326–329.

Dehaene, S., Naccache, L., Cohen, L., Le Bihan, D., Mangin, J.-F., Poline, J.-B., et al. (2001). Cerebral mechanisms of word masking and unconscious repetition priming. *Nature Neuroscience, 4*, 752–758.

Delazer, M., Domahs, F., Bartha, L., Brennis, C., Lochy, A., Trieb, T., et al. (2003). Learning complex arithmetic—an fMRI study. *Brain Research. Cognitive Brain Research, 18*, 76–88.

Delgado, J. M. R. (1966). Intracerebral perfusion in awake monkeys. *Archives Internationales de Pharmacodynamie et de Therapie, 161*, 442–462.

Delgado, M. R., Miller, M. M., Inati, S., & Phelps, E. A. (2005). An fMRI study of reward-related probability learning. *NeuroImage, 24*, 862–873.

Del Gratta, C., Penna, S. D., Tartaro, A., Ferretti, A., Torquati, K., Bonomo, L., et al. (2000). Topographic organization of the human primary and secondary somatosensory areas: An fMRI study. *Neuroreport, 11*, 2035–2043.

Dement, W., & Kleitman, N. (1957). Cyclic variations in EEG during sleep and their relation to eye movements, body motility, and dreaming. *EEG and Clinical Neurophysiology, 9*, 673–690.

Demirci, O., Clark, V. P., Magnotta, V. A., Andreasen, N. C., Lauriello, J., Kiehl, K. A., et al. (2008). A review of challenges in the use of fMRI for disease classification: Characterization and a projection pursuit application from a multi-site fMRI schizophrenia study. *Brain Imaging and Behavior, 2*, 207–226.

Dennett, D. C. (1987). Consciousness. In R. L. Gregory (Ed.), *The Oxford companion to the mind* (pp. 160–164). Oxford: Oxford University Press.

Desimone, R., & Duncan, J. (1995). Neural mechanisms of selective attention. *Annual Review of Neuroscience, 18*, 193–222.

Desmedt, J. E., & Cheron, G. (1980). Central somatosensory conduction in man recorded from the neural generators and interpeak latencies in the far-field components recorded from neck and right or left scalp and earlobes. *Electroencephalography and Clinical Neurophysiology, 50*, 382–403.

Desmond, J. E., & Fiez, J. A. (1998). Neuroimaging studies of the cerebellum: Language, learning and memory. *Trends in Cognitive Sciences, 2*, 355–362.

Deutsch, J. A., & Deutsch, D. (1963). Attention: Some theoretical considerations. *Psychological Review, 70*, 80–90.

DeYoe, E. A., Carman, G. J., Bandettini, P., Glickan, S., Wieser, J., Cox, R., et al. (1996). Mapping striate and extrastriate visual areas in human cerebral cortex. *Proceedings of the National Academy of Sciences of the United States of America, 93*, 2382–2386.

Di, H., Boly, M., Wang, X., Ledoux, D., & Laureys, S. (2008). Neuroimaging activation studies in the vegetative state: Predictors of recovery. *Clinical Medicine, 8*, 502–507.

Diamant, H., Oakley, B., Stroem, L., Wells, C., & Zotterman, Y. (1985). A comparison of neural and psychophysical responses to taste stimuli in man. *Acta Physiologica Scandinavica, 64*, 67–74.

Dingman, W., & Sporn, M. B. (1964). Molecular theories of memory. *Science, 144*, 26–29.

Dinstein, I., Thomas, C., Behrmann, M., & Heeger, D. J. (2008). A mirror up to nature. *Current Biology, 18*, R13–R18.

Dinstein, I., Thomas, C., Humphreys, K., Minshew, N., Behrmann, M., & Heeger, D. J. (2010). Normal movement selectivity in autism. *Neuron, 66*, 461–469.

di Pellegrino, G., Fadiga, L., Fogassi, L., Gallese, V., & Rizzolatti, G. (1992). Understanding motor events: A neurophysiological study. *Experimental Brain Research, 91*, 176–180.

Domino, E. F. (2008). Tobacco smoking and MRI/MRS brain abnormalities compared to nonsmokers. *Progress in Neuro-Psychopharmacology & Biological Psychiatry, 32*, 1778–1781.

Donders, F. C. (1868). Die Schnelligkeit psychischer Prozesse [On the speed of mental processes]. *Archiv für Anatomie und Physiologie und wissenschaftliche Medizin*, 657–681.

Doppelmayer, M., Klimesch, W., Stadler, W., Pollhuber, D., & Heine, C. (2002). EEG alpha power and intelligence. *Intelligence, 30*, 289–302.

Doyon, J., & Benali, H. (2005). Reorganization and plasticity in the adult brain during learning of motor skills. *Current Opinion in Neurobiology, 15*, 161–167.

Doyon, J., Penhume, V., & Ungerleider, L. G. (2003). Distinct contribution of the cortico-striatal and cortico-cerebellar systems to motor skill learning. *Neuropsychologia, 41*, 252–262.

Driver, J. (2001). A selective review of selective attention research from the past century. *British Journal of Psychology, 92*, 53–78.

Duncan, J. (1981). Directing attention in the visual field. *Perception & Psychophysics, 33*, 533–547.

Duncan, J. (1984). Selective attention and the organization of visual information. *Journal of Experimental Psychology. General, 113*, 501–517.

Duncan, J. (1995). Attention, intelligence, and the frontal lobes. In M. S. Gazzaniga (Ed.), *The cognitive neurosciences* (pp. 721–733). Cambridge, MA: MIT Press.

Duncan, J., Seitz, R. J., Kolodny, J., Bor, D., Herzog, H., Ahmed, A., et al. (2000). A neural basis for general intelligence. *Science, 289*, 457–460.

Ebbinghaus, H. (1964). *Memory: A contribution to experimental psychology* (Ruger, H. A., & Bussenius, C. E., Trans.). New York: Dover. (Original work published 1885.)

Eckert, M. A., Kamdar, N. V., Chang, C. E., Beckmann, C. F., Greicius, M. D., & Menon, V. (2008). A cross-modal system linking primary auditory and visual cortices: Evidence from intrinsic fMRI connectivity analysis. *Human Brain Mapping, 29*, 848–857.

Edelman, G. M., & Tononi, G. (2000). *A universe of consciousness: How matter becomes imagination.* New York: Basic Books.

Editorial. (2007). Mind games. *Nature, 450,* 457.

Egeth, H., & Yantis, S. (1997). Visual attention: Control, representation, and time course. *Annual Review of Psychology, 48,* 269–297.

Eickhoff, S. B., Weiss, P. H., Amunts, K., Fink, G. R., & Zilles, K. (2006). Identifying human parieto-insular vestibular cortex using fMRI and cytoarchitectonic mapping. *Human Brain Mapping, 27,* 611–621.

Ellingson, R. J. (1965). Brain waves and problems of psychology. *Psychological Bulletin, 53,* 1–34.

Ellingson, R. J. (1966). Relationship between EEG and test intelligence: A commentary. *Psychological Bulletin, 65,* 91–98.

Erickson, R. P. (2008). A study of the science of taste: On the origins and influence of the core ideas. *Behavioral and Brain Sciences, 31,* 59–105.

Erk, S., Spitzer, M., Wunderlich, A. P., Galley, L., & Walter, H. (2002). Cultural objects modulate reward activity. *Neuroreport, 13,* 2499–2503.

Erlanger, J., & Gasser, H. (1937). *Electrical signs of nervous activity.* Philadelphia: University of Pennsylvania Press.

Ertl, J. P., & Shafer, E. W. P. (1969). Brain response correlates of psychometric intelligence. *Nature, 223,* 421–422.

Etkin, A., & Wager, T. D. (2007). Functional neuroimaging of anxiety: A meta-analysis of emotional processing in PTSD, social anxiety disorder, and specific phobia. *American Journal of Psychiatry, 164,* 1476–1488.

Etnier, J. L., Whitwer, S. S., Landers, D. M., Petruzzello, S. J., & Salazar, W. (1996). Changes in electro-encephalographic activity associated with learning a novel motor task. *Research Quarterly for Exercise and Sport, 67,* 272–279.

Falkenstein, M., Hoormann, J., & Hohnsbein, J. (2002). Inhibition related ERP components: Variation with modality, age, and time on task. *Journal of Psychophysiology, 16,* 167–175.

Fan, J., McCandliss, B. D., Fosella, J., Flombaum, J. I., & Posner, M. I. (2005). The activation of attentional networks. *NeuroImage, 26,* 471–479.

Farthing, G. W. (1992). *The psychology of consciousness.* Englewood Cliffs, NJ: Prentice-Hall.

Fecteau, S., Lepage, J. F., & Theoret, H. (2006). Autism spectrum disorder: Seeing is not understanding. *Current Biology, 16,* R131–R133.

Felleman, D. J., & Van Essen, D. C. (1991). Distributed hierarchical processing in the primate cerebral cortex. *Cerebral Cortex, 1,* 1–47.

Fellows, L. K., & Farah, M. J. (2005). Is anterior cingulate cortex necessary for cognitive control? *Brain*, *128*, 788–796.

Feltz, D. L., & Landers, D. M. (1983). The effects of mental practice on motor skill learning and performance: A meta-analysis. *Journal of Sport Psychology*, *5*, 25–57.

Fendrich, R., Wessinger, C. M., & Gazzaniga, M. S. (1992). Residual vision in a scotoma: Implications for blindsight. *Science*, *258*, 1489–1491.

Ferrari, P. F., Gallese, V., Rizzolatti, G., & Fogassi, L. (2003). Mirror neurons responding to the observation of ingestive and communicative mouth actions in the monkey ventral premotor cortex. *European Journal of Neuroscience*, *17*, 1703–1714.

Finan, J. L. (1939). Effects of frontal lobe lesions on temporally organized behavior in monkeys. *Journal of Neurophysiology*, *2*, 208–226.

Finan, J. L. (1942). Delayed response with predelay reinforcement in monkeys after removal of the frontal lobes. *American Journal of Psychology*, *55*, 202–214.

Fink, A., Grabner, R. H., Benedek, M., Reishofer, G., Hauswirth, V., Fally, M., et al. (2009). The creative brain: Investigation of brain activity during creative problem solving by means of EEG and fMRI. *Human Brain Mapping*, *30*, 734–748.

Fink, A., Graif, B., & Neubauer, A. C. (2009). Brain correlates underlying creative thinking: EEG alpha activity in professional vs. novice dancers. *NeuroImage*, *46*, 854–862.

Fink, A., & Neubauer, A. C. (2006). EEG alpha oscillations during the performance of verbal creativity tasks: Differential effects of sex and verbal intelligence. *International Journal of Psychophysiology*, *62*, 46–53.

Fisher, H., Aron, A., & Brown, L. L. (2005). Romantic love: An fMRI study of a neural mechanism for mate choice. *Journal of Comparative Neurology*, *493*, 58–62.

Fitts, P. M. (1954). The information capacity of the human motor system in controlling the amplitude of movement. *Journal of Experimental Psychology*, *47*, 381–391.

Fletcher, P. C., & Henson, R. N. A. (2001). Frontal lobes and human memory: Insights from functional neuroimaging. *Brain*, *124*, 849–881.

Fletcher, P. C., Stephenson, C. M., Carpenter, T. A., & Bullmore, E. T. (2003). Regional brain activations predicting subsequent memory success; an event-related fMRI study of the influence of encoding tasks. *Cortex*, *39*, 1009–1026.

Foote, R. (2007). Mathematics and complex systems. *Science*, *318*, 410–412.

Foxe, J. J., Morocs, I. A., Murray, M. M., Higgins, B. A., Javitt, D. C., & Schroeder, C. E. (2000). Multisensory auditory-somatosensory interactions in early cortical processing revealed by high-density electrical mapping. *Brain Research. Cognitive Brain Research*, *10*, 77–83.

Foxe, J. J., Wylie, G. R., Martinez, A., Schroeder, C. S., Javitt, D. C., Guilfoyle, D., et al. (2002). Auditory-somatosensory multisensory processing in auditory association cortex: An fMRI study. *Journal of Neurophysiology*, *88*, 540–543.

Fransson, P. (2006a). How default is the default mode of brain function? Further evidence from the intrinsic BOLD fluctuations. *Neuropsychologia, 44,* 2836–2845.

Fransson, P. (2006b). How default is the default mode of brain function? *Journal of Cognitive Neuroscience, 18,* 1156–1173.

Franz, S. I. (1912). New phrenology. *Science (N.S.), 35*(896), 321–328.

Freeman, W. J. (2000). *How brains make up their minds.* New York: Columbia University Press.

Freeman, W. J. (2007). 2007 Special Issue: Indirect biological measures of consciousness from field studies of brains as dynamical systems. *Neural Networks (Archive), 20,* 1021–1031.

Fries, P., Womelsdorf, T., Oostenveld, R., & Desimone, R. (2008). The effects of visual stimulation and selective visual attention on rhythmic neuronal synchronization in macaque area V4. *Journal of Neuroscience, 28,* 4823–4835.

Frishman, L. J., Reddy, M. G., & Robson, J. G. (1996). Effects of background light in human dark-adapted electroretinogram and psychophysical threshold. *Journal of the Optical Society of America, 13,* 601–612.

Frost, S. B., Barbay, S., Friel, K. M., Plautz, E. J., & Nudo, R. J. (2003). Reorganization of remote cortical regions after ischemic brain injury: A potential substrate for stroke recover. *Journal of Neurophysiology, 89,* 3205–3214.

Fuster, J. M. (1985). The prefrontal cortex, mediator of cross-temporal contingencies. *Human Neurobiology, 4,* 169–179.

Fuster, J. M. (1989). *The prefrontal cortex: Anatomy, physiology,and the neuropsychology of the frontal lobe* (2nd ed.). New York: Raven Press.

Fuster, J. M. (2000). The module: Crisis of a paradigm (book review). *Neuron, 26,* 51–53.

Fuster, J. M. (2001). The prefrontal cortex—an update: Time is of the essence. *Neuron, 30,* 319–333.

Gabor, D. (1948). A new microscopic principle. *Nature, 161,* 777.

Gabor, D. (1949). Microscopy by reconstructed wave fronts. *Proceedings of the Royal Society of London. Series A, 197,* 454–487.

Galambos, R., & Davis, H. (1943). The response of single auditory nerve fibers to acoustic stimulation. *Journal of Neurophysiology, 6,* 39–57.

Gal, F. J., & Spurzheim, J. C. (1808). *Recherches sur le système nerveux en général, et sur celui du cerveau en particulier.* Paris: Academy de Sciences.

Gallese, V., Fadiga, L., Fogassi, L., & Rizzolatti, G. (1996). Action recognition in the premotor cortex. *Brain, 119,* 593–609.

Gallup, C. G., Jr. (1970). Chimpanzees: Self-recognition. *Science, 167,* 86–87.

Galton, F. (1879). *Hereditary genius: An inquiry into its laws and consequences.* New York: Appleton.

Garner, W. R. (1974). *The processing of information and structure*. Hillsdale, NJ: Erlbaum.

Garrett, A. S., & Maddock, R. J. (2006). Separating subjective emotion from the perception of emotion-inducing stimuli: An fMRI study. *NeuroImage, 33*, 263–274.

Gasser, H. S., & Grundfest, H. (1939). Axon diameter in relation to the spike dimensions and the conduction velocity in mammalian A fibers. *American Journal of Physiology, 127*, 393–414.

Gauthier, I., Hayward, W. G., Tarr, M. J., Anderson, A. W., Skudlarski, P. S., & Gore, J. C. (2002). BOLD activity during mental rotation and viewpoint-dependent object recognition. *Neuron, 34*, 161–171.

Gazzaniga, M. S. (2005). *The ethical brain*. Washington, DC: Dana Press.

Geisler, W. S. (2008). Visual perception and the statistical properties of natural scene. *Annual Review of Psychology, 59*, 167–192.

Gerwig, M., Kolb, F. P., & Timmann, D. (2007). The involvement of the human cerebellum in eyeblink conditioning. *Cerebellum (London), 6*, 38–57.

Ghazanfar, A. A., & Schroeder, C. E. (2006). Is neocortex essentially multisensory. *Trends in Cognitive Sciences, 10*, 278–285.

Gibbs, F. A., Gibbs, E. L., & Lennox, W. G. (1937). Effect on the electroencephalogram of certain drugs which influence nervous activity. *Archives of Internal Medicine, 60*, 154–166.

Gilbert, S. J., Bird, G., Brindley, R., Frith, C. D., & Burgess, P. W. (2008). Atypical recruitment of medial prefrontal cortex in autism spectrum disorder: An fMRI study of two executive function tasks. *Neuropsychologia, 46*, 2281–2291.

Gitelman, D. R., Nobre, A. C., Parrish, T. B., LaBar, K. S., Kim, Y.-H., Meyer, J. R., et al. (1999). A large scale distributed network for covert spatial attention: Further anatomical delineation based on stringent behavioural and cognitive controls. *Brain, 122*, 1093–1106.

Glass, A. (1964). Mental arithmetic and blocking of the occipital alpha rhythm. *Electroencephalography and Clinical Neurophysiology, 16*, 595–603.

Glass, A. L., Holyoak, K. J., & Santa, J. L. (1979). *Cognition*. Reading, MA: Addison-Wesley.

Glees, P., Cole, J., Whitty, C. W. M., & Cairns, H. (1950). The effects of lesions in the cingulate gyrus and adjacent areas in monkeys. *Journal of Neurology, Neurosurgery, and Psychiatry, 13*, 178–190.

Glimcher, P. W., Camerer, C. F., Fehr, E., & Poldrack, R. A. (2009). *Neuroeconomics: Decision making and the brain*. Amsterdam: Elsevier.

Goddard, G. V. (1964). Amygdaloid stimulation and learning in the rat. *Journal of Comparative and Physiological Psychology, 58*, 23–30.

Goff, W. R., Rosner, B. S., & Allison, T. (1962). Distribution of cerebral somatosensory evoked responses in normal man. *Electroencephalography and Clinical Neurophysiology, 14*, 697–713.

Goldberg, E., Colby, C. L., & Duhamel, J.-R. (1990). The representation of visuomotor space in the parietal lobe of the monkey. *Cold Spring Harbor Symposia on Quantitative Biology, 55*, 729–739.

Goldman-Rakic, P. S. (1987). Circuitry of primate prefrontal cortex and regulation of behavior by representational memory. In F. Plum & V. Mountcastle (Eds.), *The Nervous System* (pp. 373–417). Bethesda, MD: American Physiological Society.

Goldman-Rakic, P. S. (1988). Topography of cognition: Parallel distributed networks in primate association cortex. *Annual Review of Neuroscience, 11*, 137–156.

Goltz, F. (1892). Der Hund Ohne Grosshirn. Siebente Abhandlung Uber Die Verrichtungen des Grosshirn. *Pfluegers Archiv, 51*, 570–614.

Goodale, M. A., & Milner, A. D. (1992). Separate visual pathways for perception and action. *Trends in Neurosciences, 15*, 20–25.

Goodale, M. A., & Westwood, D. A. (2004). An evolving view of duplex vision: Separate but interacting cortical pathways for perception and action. *Current Opinion in Neurobiology, 14*, 203–211.

Gopnik, A. (2007). Cells that read minds? What the myth of mirror neurons gets wrong about the human brain. *Slate* http://www.slate.com/id/2165123

Gosselin, N., Samson, S., Adolphs, R., Noulhiane, M., Roy, M., Baulac, M., et al. (2006). Emotional responses to unpleasant music correlates with damage to the parahippocampal cortex. *Brain, 129*, 2585–2592.

Gotch, F., & Burch, C. J. (1899). The electrical response of nerve to two stimuli. *Physiological Reviews, 24*, 421.

Grabner, R. H., Ansari, D., Koschutnig, K., Reishofer, G., Ebner, F., & Neurper, C. (2009). To retrieve or to calculate? Left angular gyrus mediates the retrieval of arithmetic facts during problem solving. *Neuropsychologia, 47*, 604–608.

Grafton, S. T., Hazeltine, E., & Ivry, R. (1995). Functional mapping of sequence learning in normal human. *Journal of Cognitive Neuroscience, 7*, 497–510.

Graham, C., & Hartline, H. K. (1935). The response of single visual sense-cells to lights of different wavelengths. *Journal of General Physiology, 18*, 917.

Granger, C. W. J. (1969). Investigating causal relations by econometric models and cross-spectral methods. *Econometrica, 37*, 424–438.

Gray, J. R., Chabris, C. F., & Braver, T. S. (2003). Neural mechanisms of general fluid intelligence. *Nature Neuroscience, 6*, 316–322.

Green, D. M., & Swets, J. A. (1964). *Signal detection theory and psychophysics*. Huntington, NY: Krieger.

Greene, A. J., Gross, W. L., Elsinger, C. L., & Rao, S. M. (2007). Hippocampal differentiation without recognition: An fMRI analysis of contextual cueing task. *Learning & Memory (Cold Spring Harbor, NY), 14*, 548–553.

Greene, A. J., Gross, W. L., Elsinger, C. L., & Rao, S. M. (2008). Hippocampal differentiation without recognition: An fMRI analysis of the contextual cueing task. *Learning & Memory (Cold Spring Harbor, NY), 14*, 548–553.

Greene, J. D., Sommerville, R. B., Nystrom, L. E., Darley, J. M., & Cohen, J. D. (2001). An fMRI investigation of emotional engagement in moral judgement. *Science, 293,* 2105–2108.

Greenfield, S. A., & Collins, T. F. T. (2005). A neuroscientific approach to consciousness. *Progress in Brain Research, 150,* 11–23.

Grewe, J., Weckstrom, M., Egelhaaf, M., & Warzecha, A.-K. (2007). Information and discriminability as measures of reliability of sensory coding. *PLoS ONE, 12,* 1–7.

Grillner, S., Hellgren, J., Menard, A., Saitoh, K., & Wiksrom, M. A. (2005). Mechanisms for selection of basic motor programs—roles for the striatum and pallidum. *Trends in Neurosciences, 28,* 364–370.

Grill-Spector, K., Kourtzi, Z., & Kanwisher, N. (2001). The lateral occipital complex and its role in object recognition. *Vision Research, 41,* 1409–1422.

Grill-Spector, K., Kushnir, T., Edelman, S., Itzchak, Y., & Malach, R. (1998). Cue-invariant activation in object-related areas of the human occipital lobe. *Neuron, 21,* 191–202.

Grill-Spector, K., & Sayres, R. (2008). Object recognition: Insights from advances in fMRI methods. *Current Directions in Psychological Science, 17,* 73–79.

Grimes, J. (1996). On the failure to detect changes in scenes across saccades. In K. Akins (Ed.), *Perception V 5* (pp. 89–110). New York: Oxford University Press.

Grimm, S., Schmidt, C. F., Bermpohl, F., Heinzel, A., Dahlem, Y., Wyss, M., et al. (2006). Segregated neural representation of distinct emotion dimensions in the prefrontal cortex—an fMRI study. *NeuroImage, 30,* 325–349.

Gross, D. M. (2006). *The secret history of emotion: From Aristotle's "Rhetoric" to modern brain science.* Chicago: University of Chicago Press.

Hadjikhani, N., & de Gelder, B. (2002). Neural basis of prosopagnosia: An fMRI study. *Human Brain Mapping, 16,* 176–182.

Hagen, M. C., Zald, D. H., Thornton, T. A., & Pardo, J. V. (2002). Somatosensory processing in the human inferior prefrontal cortex. *Journal of Neurophysiology, 88,* 1400–1406.

Haider, M., Spong, P., & Lindsley, D. B. (1964). Attention, vigilance, and cortical evoked-potentials in humans. *Science, 145,* 180–182.

Haier, R. J., Jung, R. E., Yeo, R. A., Head, K., & Alkire, M. T. (2004). Structural brain variation and general intelligence. *NeuroImage, 23,* 425–433.

Haier, R. J., Siegel, B. V., Neuchterlein, K. H., Hazlett, E., Wu, J. C., Paek, J., et al. (1988). Cortical glucose metabolic rate correlates of abstract reasoning and attention studied with positron emission tomography. *Intelligence, 12,* 199–217.

Hampton, A. N., & O'Doherty, J. P. (2007). Decoding the neural substrates of reward-related decision making with functional MRI. *Proceedings of the National Academy of Sciences of the United States of America, 104,* 1377–1382.

Hanson, S. J., Matsuka, T., & Haxby, J. V. (2004). Combinatorial codes in ventral temporal lobe for object recognition: Haxby (2001) revisited: Is there a "face" area. *NeuroImage, 23,* 156–166.

Harlow, J. M. (1868). Recovery from the passage of an iron bar through the head. *Publications of the Massachusetts Medical Society, 2,* 327–347.

Harrison, G. W. (2008a). Neuroeconomics: A critical reconsideration. *Economics and Philosophy, 24,* 303–344.

Harrison, G. W. (2008b). Neuroeconomics: A rejoinder. *Economics and Philosophy, 24,* 533–544.

Hartline, H. K. (1938). The response of single optic nerve fibers of the verterbrate eye to illumination of the retina. *American Journal of Physiology, 121,* 400–415.

Hartline, H. K., & Ratliff, F. (1957). Inhibitory interaction of receptor units in the eye of *Limulus. Journal of General Physiology, 40,* 357–376.

Hatfield, B. D., Haufler, A. J., Hung, T.-M., & Spalding, T. W. (2004). Electroencephalographic studies of skilled psychomotor performance. *Journal of Clinical Neurophysiology, 21,* 144–156.

Hauser, M. D., Kralik, J., Botto-Mahan, C., Garrett, M. & Osher, J. (1995). Self-recognition in primates: Phylogeny and the salience of species typical features. *Proceedings of the National Academy of Sciences of the United States of America, 92,* 10811–10814.

Haxby, J. V., Gobbini, M. I., Furey, M. L., Ishai, A., Schouten, J. L., & Pietrini, P. (2001). Distributed and overlapping representations of faces and objects in ventral temporal cortex. *Science, 293,* 2425–2430.

Haynes, J.-D., Deichmann, R., & Rees, G. (2005). Eye-specific effects of binocular rivalry in the human lateral geniculate nucleus. *Nature, 438,* 496–499.

Haynes, J.-D., & Rees, G. (2005). Predicting the orientation of invisible stimuli from activity in primary visual cortex. *Nature Neuroscience, 8,* 686–691.

Hayter, A. L., Langdon, D. W., & Ramnani, N. (2007). Cerebellar contributions to working memory. *NeuroImage, 36,* 943–954.

Hebb, D. O. (1949). *The organization of behavior: A neuropsychological theory.* New York: Wiley.

Hecht, S., Shaler, S., & Pirenne, M. H. (1942). Energy, quanta, and vision. *Journal of General Physiology, 25,* 819–840.

Heilman, K. M., & Valenstein, E. S. (1972). Frontal lobe neglect in man. *Neurology, 22,* 660–664.

Heinzel, A., Hautzel, H., Poeppel, T. D., Boers, F., Beu, M., & Mueller, H.-W. (2008). Neural correlates of subliminal and supraliminal letter processing: An event-related fMRI study. *Consciousness and Cognition, 17,* 699–713.

Helmholtz, H. von. (1850a). Vorlaufige Bericht uber die fortpflanzung-geschwindigkeit der. *Archiv für Anatomie und Physiologie,* 71.

Helmholtz, H. von. (1850b). Über die Theorie der zusammengesetzten Farben. *Archiv für Anatomie, Physiologie und wissenschaftliche Medizin, Berlin,* 461–482.

Helmholtz, H. von. (1867). *Handbuch der physiologischen Optik*. Hamburg: Voss.

Helmholtz, H. von. (1954). *On the sensations of tone as a physiological basis for the theory of music* (Ellis, A. J., Trans.). New York: Dover. (Original work published 1863.)

Hensel, H., & Boman, K. K. A. (1960). Afferent impulses in cutaneous sensory nerves in human subjects. *Journal of Neurophysiology, 23,* 564–578.

Hermann, L. (1870). Eine Erscheinung simultanen Contrastes. *Pflügers Archiv, 3,* 13–15.

Hernandez, L. L., & Lefton, L. A. (1977). Metacontrast as measured under a signal detection method. *Perception, 6,* 695–702.

Hickok, G. (2008). Eight problems for the mirror neuron theory of action understanding in monkeys and humans. *Journal of Cognitive Neuroscience, 21,* 1229–1243.

Hickok, G., Buchsbaum, B., Humphries, C., & Muftuler, T. (2003). Auditory-motor interaction revealed by fMRI: Speech, music, and working memory in Area Spt. *Journal of Cognitive Neuroscience, 15,* 673–682.

Hilgetag, C. C., O'Neil, M. A., & Young, M. P. (1996). Indeterminate organization of the visual system. *Science, 271,* 776–777.

Hirsch, I. J., & Watson, C. S. (1996). Auditory psychophysics and perception. *Annual Review of Psychology, 47,* 461–484.

Hodgkin, A. L. (1937). Evidence for electrical transmission. *Journal of Physiology, 90,* 211.

Hodgkin, A. L. (1948). Repetitive action in nerve. *Journal of Physiology, 107,* 165.

Hofer, A., Siedentopf, C. M., Ischebeck, A., Rettenbacher, M. A., Verius, M., Felber, S., et al. (2006). Gender differences in regional cerebral activity during the perception of emotion: A functional MRI study. *NeuroImage, 32,* 854–862.

Hoffman, J. E., & Subramaniam, B. (1995). The role of visual attention in saccadic eye movements. *Perception & Psychophysics, 57,* 787–795.

Holscher, C. (2003). Time, space and hippocampal functions. *Reviews in the Neurosciences, 14,* 253–284.

Holyoak, K. J., & Morrison, R. G. (2005). Thinking and reasoning: A reader's guide. In K. J. Holyoak & R. G. Morrison (Eds.), *The Cambridge handbook of thinking and reasoning* (pp. 1–12). Cambridge: Cambridge University Press.

Houk, J. C., Buckingham, J. T., & Barto, A. G. (1996). Models of the cerebellum and motor learning. *Behavioral and Brain Sciences, 19,* 368–383.

Hsu, A., Woolley, S. M. N., Fremouw, T. E., & Theunissen, F. E. (2004). Modulation power and phase spectrum of natural sounds enhance neural encoding performed by single auditory neurons. *Journal of Neuroscience, 24,* 9201–9211.

Hubel, D. H., & Wiesel, T. N. (1959). Receptive fields of single neurons in the cat's striate cortex. *Journal of Physiology*, *148*, 574–591.

Hubel, D. H., & Wiesel, T. N. (1965). Receptive fields and functional architecture in two nonstriatal visual areas (18 and 19) of the cat. *Journal of Neurophysiology*, *28*, 229–289.

Huffman, D. A. (1952). A method for the construction of minimum redundancy codes. *Proceedings of the Institute of Radio Engineers*, *40*, 1098–1101.

Hull, C. L. (1943). *Principles of behavior*. New York: Appleton Century.

Hummel, C., Frasnelli, J., Gerber, J., & Hummel, T. (2007). Cerebral processing of gustatory stimuli in patients with taste loss. *Behavioural Brain Research*, *185*, 59–64.

Humphrey, D. G., Kramer, A. F., & Stanny, R. R. (1994). Influence of extended wakefulness on automatic and nonautomatic processing. *Human Factors*, *36*, 652–669.

Hunsley, J., Lee, C. M., & Wood, J. M. (2003). Controversial and questionable assessment techniques. In S. O. Lilienfeld, S. J. Lynn, & J. M. Lohr (Eds.), *Science and pseudoscience in clinical psychology* (pp. 39–76). New York: Guilford Press.

Iacoboni, M. (2009). Imitation, empathy, and mirror neurons. *Annual Review of Psychology*, *60*, 653–670.

Iacoboni, M., Woods, R. P., Brass, M., Bekkering, H., Mazziotta, J. C., & Rizzolatti, G. (1999). Cortical mechanisms of human imitation. *Science*, *286*, 2526–2528.

IAPS. (1999). *International Affective Picture System: Digitized photographs*. Gainesville, FL: The Center for Research in Psychophysiology.

Ihnen, S. K. Z., Church, J. A., Petersen, S. E., & Schlaggar, B. L. (2009). Lack of generalizability of sex differences in the fMRI Bold activity associated with language processes in adults. *NeuroImage*, *45*, 1020–1032.

Ishai, A., Ungerleider, L. G., & Haxby, J. V. (2000a). Distributed neural systems for the generation of visual images. *Neuron*, *28*, 979–990.

Ishai, A., Ungerleider, L. G., Martin, A., Schouten, J. L., & Haxby, J. V. (2000b). Distributed representation of objects in the human ventral visual pathway. *Proceedings of the National Academy of Sciences of the United States of America*, *96*, 9379–9384.

Jacobs, J., Hwang, G., Curran, T., & Kahan, M. J. (2006). EEG oscillations and recognition memory: Theta correlates of memory retrieval and decision making. *NeuroImage*, *32*, 978–987.

Jacobsen, C. F. (1936). Studies of cerebral functions in primates. *Comparative Psychology Monographs*, *13*, 1–60.

Jacobsen, C. F., & Elder, J. H. (1936). Studies of cerebral functions in primates: II The effect of temporal lobe lesions on delayed response on monkeys. *Comparative Psychology Monographs*, *13*, 61–65.

Jacobsohn, P. H. (1995). Horace Wells: Discoverer of anesthesia. *Anesthesia Progress, 42*, 73–75.

Jacoby, L. (1991). A process dissociation framework: Separating automatic from intentional uses of memory. *Journal of Memory and Language, 30*, 513–541.

Jahn, R. G., & Dunne, B. J. (1988). *Margins of reality: The role of consciousness in the physical world*. New York: Harcourt Brace.

James, T. W., Culham, J. C., Humphrey, G. K., Milner, A. D., & Goodale, M. A. (2003). Ventral occipital lesions impair object recognition but not object-directed grasping: An fMRI study. *Brain, 126*, 2463–2475.

James, W. (1890). *The principles of psychology*. New York: Holt.

Jameson, L. C., & Sloan, T. B. (2006). Using EEG to monitor anesthesia drug effects during surgery. *Journal of Clinical Monitoring and Computing, 20*, 445–472.

Jarrard, L. E. (1995). What does the hippocampus really do? *Behavioural Brain Research, 71*, 1–10.

Jastrow, J. (1890). *Time relations of mental phenomena*. New York: Hodges.

Jausovec, N. (2000). Differences in cognitive processes between gifted, intelligent, creative, and average individuals while solving complex problem: An EEG study. *Intelligence, 28*, 213–237.

Jeleazcov, C., & Schwilden, H. (2003). Bispectral analysis does not differentiate between anaesthesia and a linear random process. *Biomedizinische Technik. Biomedical Engineering, 10*, 269–274.

Jenkins, I. H., Brooks, D. J., Nixon, P. D., Frackowiak, R. S. J., & Passingham, R. E. (1994). Motor sequence learning: A study with positron emission tomography. *Journal of Neuroscience, 14*, 3775–3790.

Jewett, D. L., Romano, M. N., & Williston, J. S. (1970). Human auditory evoked potentials: Possible brain stem components detected on the scalp. *Science, 167*, 1517–1518.

Johnson, M. H. (1995). The development of visual attention: A cognitive neuroscience perspective. In M. Gazzaniga (Ed.), The cognitive neurosciences (735–747). Cambridge, MA: MIT Press.

Johnston, W. A., & Heinz, S. P. (1978). Flexibility and capacity demands of attention. *Journal of Experimental Psychology. General, 107*, 420–435.

Johnstone, T., van Reekum, C. M., Oakes, T. R., & Davidson, R. J. (2006). The voice of emotion: An fMRI study of neural responses to angry and happy vocal expressions. *Social Cognitive and Affective Neuroscience, 1*, 242–249.

Jolesz, F. A. (2009). MRI-guided focused ultrasound surgery. *Annual Review of Medicine, 60*, 417–430.

Jones, D. D., & Holding, D. H. (1975). Extremely long-term persistence of the McCollough effect. *Journal of Experimental Psychology. Human Perception and Performance, 1*, 323–327.

Jones, L. M., Fontanini, A., & Katz, D. B. (2006). Gustatory processing: A dynamic systems approach. *Current Opinion in Neurobiology, 16*, 420–428.

Jung, R. E., & Haier, R. J. (2007). The parietal-frontal integration theory (P-FIT) of Intelligence: Converging neuroimaging evidence. *Behavioral and Brain Sciences, 30,* 135–187.

Jurado, M. B., & Rosselli, M. (2007). The elusive nature of executive functions: A review of our current understanding. *Neuropsychology Review, 17,* 213–233.

Just, M. A., Cherkassky, V. L., Keller, T. A., Kana, R. K., & Minshew, N. J. (2007). Functional and anatomical cortical underconnectivity in autism: Evidence from an fMRI study of an executive function task and corpus callosum morphometry. *Cerebral Cortex, 17,* 951–961.

Kaas, J. H. (2004). Neuroanatomy is needed to define the "organs" of the brain. *Cortex, 40,* 207–208.

Kagan, J. (2007). *What is emotion?History, measures, and meanings.* New Haven: Yale University Press.

Kahneman, D. (1973). *Attention and effort.* Englewood Cliffs, NJ: Prentice-Hall.

Kamback, M. C., & Fife, D. D. (1975). Effects of dorsolateral frontal cortical ablations on stimulus equivalence and transpositions in monkeys. *Neuropsychologia, 13,* 307–313.

Kamitani, Y., & Tong, F. (2005). Decoding the visual and subjective contents of the human brain. *Nature Neuroscience, 8,* 679–685.

Kanal, E., & Shellock, F. G. (1992). Patient monitoring during clinical MR imaging. *Radiology, 185,* 623–629.

Kandel, E. R. (1991). Cellular mechanisms of learning and the biological basis of individuality. In E. R. Kandel & J. H. Schwartz (Eds.), *Principles of neural science* (3rd ed., pp. 1009–1032). New York: Elsevier.

Kandel, E., & Freed, D. (1989). Frontal-lobe dysfunction and antisocial behavior: A review. *Journal of Clinical Psychology, 45,* 404–413.

Kandel, E. R., Schwartz, J. H., & Jessell, T. M. (Eds.). (1991). *Principles of neural science* (3rd ed.). New York: Elsevier.

Kaniza, G. (1955). Margini quasi-percettivi in campi con stimolazione omogenea. *Rivista di Psicologia, 49,* 7–30.

Kanwisher, N., McDermott, J., & Chun, M. M. (1997). The fusiform face area: A module in human extrastriate cortex specialized for face perception. *Journal of Neuroscience, 17,* 4302–4311.

Kapogiannis, D., Barbey, A. K., Su, M., Zamboni, G., Krueger, F., & Grafman, J. (2009). Cognitive and neural foundations of religious belief. *Proceedings of the National Academy of Sciences of the United States of America, 106,* 4876–4881.

Karlik, S. J., Heatherley, T., Pavan, F., Stein, J. F., Lebron, F., Rutt, B., et al. (1988). Patient anesthesia and monitoring at a 1.5-T MRI installation. *Magnetic Resonance in Medicine, 7,* 210–211.

Karni, A., Meyer, G., Jezzard, P., Adams, M. M., Turner, R., & Ungerleider, L. G. (1995). Functional MRI evidence for adult motor cortex plasticity during motor skill learning. *Nature, 377,* 155–158.

Kassubek, I., Schmidtke, K., Kimming, H., Lucking, C. H., & Greenlee, M. W. (2001). Changes in cortical activation during mirror reading before and after training: An fMRI study of procedural learning. *Brain Research. Cognitive Brain Research, 10*, 207–217.

Kastner, S., De Weerd, P., Desimone, R., & Ungerleider, L. G. (1998). Mechanisms of directed attention in the human extrastriate cortex as revealed by functional MRI. *Science, 282*, 108–111.

Kastner, S., Pinsk, M., De Weerd, P., Desimone, R., & Ungerleider, L. G. (1999). Increased activity in primary visual cortex during directed attention in the absence of a visual stimulus. *Neuron, 22*, 751–761.

Kastner, S., & Ungerleider, L. G. (2000). Mechanisms of visual attention in the human cortex. *Annual Review of Neuroscience, 23*, 315–341.

Kato, Y., Endo, H., & Kizuka, T. (2009). Mental fatigue and impaired response processes: Event-related brain potentials in a Go-noGo task. *International Journal of Psychophysiology, 72*, 204–211.

Kay, K. N., Naselaris, T., Prenger, R. J., & Gallant, J. L. (2008). Identifying natural images from human brain activity. *Nature, 452*, 353–356.

Kellogg, W. N., Deese, J., Pronko, N. H., & Feinberg, M. (1947). An attempt to condition the spinal dog. *Journal of Experimental Psychology, 37*, 99–117.

Kennard, M. A. (1955). Effect of bilateral ablation of cingulate area on behaviour. *Journal of Neurophysiology, 18*, 159–169.

Killeen, P. R. (2005). An alternative to null hypothesis significance tests. *Psychological Science, 16*, 345–353.

Kim, J. J., & Fanselow, M. S. (1992). Modality-specific retrograde amnesia of fear. *Science, 256*, 675–677.

Kim, J. J., & Thompson, R. F. (1997). Cerebellar circuits and synaptic mechanisms involved in classical eyeblink conditioning. *Transactions in Neural Science, 20*, 177–181.

Kincses, Z. T., Johansen-Berg, H., Tomassini, V., Bosnell, R., Matthews, P. M., & Beckmann, C. F. (2008). Mode-free characterization of brain functional networks for motor sequence learning using fMRI. *NeuroImage, 39*, 1950–1958.

Kirschen, M. P., Chen, S. H. A., Schraedley-Desmond, P., & Desmond, J. E. (2004). Load- and practice-dependent increases in cerebro-cerebellar activation in verbal working memory: An fMRI study. *NeuroImage, 24*, 462–472.

Kirwan, C. B., & Wixted, J. T. (2008). Activity in the medial temporal lobe predicts memory strength, whereas activity in the prefrontal cortex predicts recollection. *Journal of Neuroscience, 28*, 10541–10548.

Kleim, J. A., Barbay, S., & Nudo, R. J. (1998). Functional reorganization of the rat motor cortex following motor skill learning. *Journal of Neurophysiology, 80*, 3321–3325.

Klimesch, W. (1999). EEG alpha and theta oscillations reflect cognitive and memory performance: A review and analysis. *Brain Research. Brain Research Reviews, 29,* 169–195.

Kling, J. W., & Riggs, L. A. (Eds.). (1938). *Woodworth and Schlosberg's experimental psychology.* New York: Holt, Rinehart, and Winston.

Kluver, H. (1937). Certain effects of lesions of the occipital cortex in macaques. *Journal of Psychology, 4,* 383–401.

Kluver, H., & Bucy, P. C. (1937). "Psychic blindness" and other symptoms following bilateral temporal lobectomy in the rhesus monkey. *American Journal of Physiology, 119,* 352–353.

Kluver, H., & Bucy, P. C. (1939). Preliminary analysis of the function of the temporal lobes in monkeys. *Archives of Neurology and Psychiatry, 41,* 979–1000.

Kniermin, J. J., & Van Essen, D. C. (1992). Neuronal responses to static texture patterns in area V1 of the alert macaque monkey. *Journal of Neurophysiology, 67,* 961–980.

Knudsen, E. I. (2007). Fundamental components of attention. *Annual Review of Neuroscience, 30,* 57–78.

Koch, C. (1999). *Biophysics of computation: Information processing in single neurons.* Oxford: Oxford University Press.

Koch, C. (2007). Betting the house on consciousness. *Nature Neuroscience, 10,* 140–141.

Koch, C., & Greenfield, S. (2007). How does consciousness happen? *Scientific American,* (September 16), 76–83.

Koch, C., & Preuschoff, K. (2007). Betting the house on consciousness. *Nature Neuroscience, 10,* 140–141.

Koelsch, S., Fritz, T., von Cramon, D. Y., Muller, K., & Friederici, A. D. (2006). Investigating emotion with music. *Human Brain Mapping, 27,* 239–250.

Konorski, J. (1967). *Integrative activity of the brain.* Chicago: University of Chicago Press.

Kourtzi, Z., & Kanwisher, N. (2000). Activation in human MT/MST by static images with implied motion. *Journal of Cognitive Neuroscience, 12,* 48–55.

Kreezer, G. (1937). The dependence of the electroencephalogram upon intelligence level. *Psychological Bulletin, 34,* 769–770.

Kreezer, G., & Smith, F. W. (1936). Electrical potentials of the brain in certain types of mental deficiency. *Archives of Neurology and Psychiatry, 36,* 1206–1213.

Kriegeskorte, N., Formisano, E., Sorger, B., & Goebel, R. (2007). Individual faces elicit distinct response patterns in human anterior temporal cortex. *Proceedings of the National Academy of Sciences of the United States of America, 104,* 20600–20605.

Kriegeskorte, N., Simmons, W. K., Bellgowan, P. S. F., & Bake, C. I. (2009). Circular analysis in systems neuroscience: The dangers of double dipping. *Nature Neuroscience, 12,* 535–540.

Kroger, J. K., Sabb, F. W., Fales, C. L., Bookheimer, S. Y., Cohen, M. S., & Holyoak, J. K. (2002). Recruitment of anterior dorsolateral prefrontal cortex in human reasoning: A parametric study of relational complexity. *Cerebral Cortex*, *12*, 477–485.

Krueger, F., Spampinato, M. V., Pardin, M., Pajevic, S., Wood, J. N., Weiss, G. H., et al. (2008). Integral calculus problem solving: An fMRI investigation. *Neuroreport*, *19*, 1095–1099.

Kruk, M. R., Westphal, K. G. C., Van Erp, A. M. M., van Asperen, J., Cave, B. J., Slater, E., et al. (1998). The hypothalamus: Cross-roads of endocrine and behavioural regulation in grooming and aggression. *Neuroscience and Biobehavioral Reviews*, *23*, 163–177.

Kuffler, S. W. (1953). Discharge patterns and functional organization of mammalian retina. *Journal of Neurophysiology*, *16*, 37–68.

Laird, A. R., McMillan, K. M., Lancaster, J. L., Kochunov, P., Turkeltaub, P. E., Prado, J. V., et al. (2005). A comparison of label-based review and ALE meta-analysis in the Stroop test. *Human Brain Mapping*, *25*, 6–21.

Lange, L. (1888). Neuue experimente uber den vorgang der einfachen reaction auf sinnesindrucke. *Philosophical Studies*, *4*, 479–510.

Larson, J. A. (1921). Modification of the Marston deception test. *Journal of Criminal Law and Criminology*, *12*, 390–399.

Lashley, K. S. (1950). In search of the engram. *Proceedings of the Society of Experimental Biology*, *4*, 454–482.

Lau, H. C., & Passingham, R. E. (2006). Relative blindsight in normal observers and the neural correlate of consciousness. *Proceedings of the National Academy of Sciences of the United States of America*, *103*, 18763–18768.

Lavie, N. (2000). Selective attention and cognitive control: Dissociating attentional functions through different types of load. In S. Monsell & J. Driver (Eds.), *Attention and performance, vol. 18, Control of cognitive processes* (pp. 175–197). Cambridge, MA: MIT Press.

Lazarus, R. S. (1966). *Psychological stress and the coping process*. New York: McGraw-Hill.

LeDoux, J. E. (1987). Emotion. In F. Plum (Ed.), *Handbook of physiology I: The nervous system* (pp. 419–460). Bethesda, MD: American Physiological Society.

LeDoux, J. E. (1995). Emotion: Clues from the brain. *Annual Review of Psychology*, *46*, 358–372.

LeDoux, J. E. (2000). Emotion circuits in the brain. *Annual Review of Neuroscience*, *23*, 155–184.

LeDoux, J. E. (2002). Cognitive-emotional interactions:Listen to the brain. In R. D. Lane & L. Nadel (Eds.), *Cognitive neuroscience of emotion* (pp. 129–155). New York: Oxford University Press.

Lee, J., Williford, T., & Maunsell, J. H. R. (2007). Spatial attention and the latency of neuronal responses in macaque area V4. *Journal of Neuroscience*, *27*, 9632–9637.

Lettvin, J. Y., Maturana, H. R., McCulloch, W. S., & Pitts, W. H. (1959). What the frog's eye tells the frog's brain. *Proceedings of the Institute of Radio Engineers*, *47*, 1940–1951.

Levy, L. M., Henkin, R. I., Hutter, A., Lin, C. S., Martins, D., & Schellinger, D. (1997). Functional MRI of human olfaction. *Journal of Computer Assisted Tomography, 21*, 849–856.

Lewi, J., Butera, R., & Paninski, L. (2007). Real-time adaptive information-theoretic optimization of neurophysiological experiments. In B. Scholkopf, J. Platt, & T. Hoffman (Eds.), *Advances in neural information processing systems 19* (pp. 857–864). Cambridge, MA: MIT Press.

Lewin, K. (1938). *The conceptual representation and the measurement of psychological forces: Contributions to psychological theory 4.* Durham, NC: Duke University Press.

Lieberman, M. D., Berkman, E. T., & Wager, T. D. (2009). Correlations in social neuroscience aren't voodoo: Commentary on Vul et al. (2009). *Perspectives on Psychological Science, 4*, 299–307.

Likova, L. T., Tyler, C. W., & Wade, R. A. (2003). Brain activation during stereomotion perception: An fMRI study. *Vision, 3*, 802a.

Lindsley, D. B. (1938). Foci of activity of the alpha rhythm in the human electro-encephalogram. *Journal of Experimental Psychology, 23*, 159–171.

Lindsley, D. B. (1944). Electroencephalography. In J. M. Hunt (Ed.), *Personality and the behavior disorders* (pp. 1033–1091). New York: Roland Press.

Ling, G., & Gerard, R. W. (1949). The normal membrane potential of frog sartorius fibers. *Journal of Cellular and Comparative Physiology, 34*, 383–385.

Lingnau, A., Gesierich, B., & Caramazza, A. (2009). Asymmetric fMRI adaptation reveals no evidence for mirror neurons in humans. *Proceedings of the National Academy of Sciences of the United States of America, 106*, 9925–9930.

Liu, T., Shi, J., Zhang, Q., Zhao, D., & Yang, J. (2007). Neural mechanisms of auditory sensory processing in children with high intelligence. *Neuroreport, 18*, 1571–1575.

Livingstone, M., & Hubel, D. H. (1988). Segregation of form, color, movement, and depth: Anatomy, physiology and perception. *Science, 240*, 740–749.

Lloyd, D. (2002). Functional MRI and the study of human consciousness. *Journal of Cognitive Neuroscience, 14*, 818–831.

Locke, J. (1995). *An essay concerning human understanding.* Amherst, NY: Prometheus Books. (Original work published 1690.)

Loftus, E. F.., Coan, J. A., & Pickrell, J. E. (1996). Manufacturing false memories usings bits of reality. In L. M. Reder (Ed.), *Implicit memory and metacognition* (pp. 195–220). Mahwah, NJ: Erlbaum.

Logan, G. D. (1978). Attention in character classification tasks. *Journal of Experimental Psychology. General, 107*, 32–63.

Lombion, S., Comte, A., Tatu, L., Brand, G., Moulin, T., & Millot, J.-L. (2009). Patterns of cerebral activation during olfactory and trigeminal stimulations. *Human Brain Mapping, 30*, 821–828.

Lombroso, C. (1895). *L'homme criminel.* Paris: Alcan.

Loomis, A. L., Harvey, E. N., & Hobart, G. (1935). Potential rhythms of the cerebral cortex during sleep. *Science, 81,* 597–598.

Loomis, A. L., Harvey, E. N., & Hobart, G. A. (1937). Cerebral states during sleep as studied by human brain potentials. *Journal of Experimental Psychology, 21,* 127–144.

Lotto, R. B., & Purves, D. (2000). An empirical explanation of color contrast. *Proceedings of the National Academies of Science of the United States of America, 97,* 12834–12839.

Lotze, M., Braun, C., Birbaumer, N., Anders, S., & Cohen, L. G. (2002). Motor learning elicited by voluntary drive. *Brain, 126,* 866–872.

Luce, R. D. (1986). *Response times: Their role in inferring elementary mental organization.* New York: Oxford University Press.

Lumer, E. D., & Rees, G. (1999). Covariation of activity in visual and prefrontal cortex associated with subjective visual perception. *Proceedings of the National Academy of Sciences of the United States of America, 96,* 1669–1673.

Luna, B., Minshaw, N. J., Garver, K. E., Lazar, N. A., Thulborn, K. R., Eddy, W. F., et al. (2002). Neocortical system abnormalities in autism: An fMRI study of spatial working memory. *Neurology, 59,* 834–840.

Lundberg, L. E., Jorum, E., Holm, E., & Torebjork, E. (1992). Intra-neural electrical stimulation of cutaneous nociceptive fibers in human: Effects of different pulse pattern on the magnitude of pain. *Acta Physiologica Scandinavica, 146,* 41–48.

Lundqvist, D., Flykt, A., & Ohman, A. (1998). *The Karolinska Directed Emotional Faces* [CD-ROM]. Stockholm: Karolinska Institute.

Luria, A. R. (1966). *Higher cortical functions in man.* New York: Basic Books.

Lutzenberger, W., Elbert, T., Birbaumer, N., Ray, W. J., & Schupp, H. (1992). The scalp distribution of the fractal dimension of the EEG and its variation with mental tasks. *Brain Topography, 5,* 27–34.

Lynch, J. C. (1980). The functional organization of posterior parietal association cortex. *Behavioral and Brain Sciences, 3,* 485–534.

Lynch, J. C., & McLaren, J. W. (1989). Deficits of visual attention and saccadic eye movements after lesions of parietooccipital cortex in monkeys. *Journal of Neurophysiology, 61,* 74–90.

Lynch, J. C., Mountcastle, V. B., Talbot, W. H., & Yin, T. C. T. (1977). Parietal lobe mechanisms for directed visual attention. *Journal of Neurophysiology, 40,* 362–389.

MacCorquodale, K., & Meehl, P. E. (1948). On a distinction between hypothetical constructs and intervening variables. *Psychological Review, 55,* 95–107.

Machens, C. K., Gollisch, T., Kolesnikova, O., & Herz, A. V. M. (2005). Testing the efficiency of sensory coding with optimal stimulus ensembles. *Neuron, 47,* 447–456.

MacLean, P. D. (1949). Psychosomatic disease and the "visceral brain": Recent developments bearing on the Papez theory of emotions. *Psychosomatic Medicine, 11,* 338–353.

MacPhail, E. M. (1993). *From the seahare to the seahorse*. New York: Columbia University Press.

Mahon, B. Z., & Caramazza, A. (2008). A critical look at the embodied cognition hypothesis and a new proposal for grounding conceptual content. *Journal of Physiology (Paris), 102,* 59–70.

Maier, A., Wilke, M., Aura, C., Zhu, C., Ye, F. Q., & Leopold, D. A. (2008). Divergence of fMRI and neural signals in V1 during perceptual suppression in the awake monkey. *Nature Neuroscience, 11,* 1193–1200.

Maitra, R. (2009). Assessing certainty of activation or inactivation in test-retest fMRI studies. *NeuroImage, 47,* 88–97.

Mangun, G. R., & Fannon, S. P. (2007). Attention: Control in the visual cortex. *Current Biology, 17,* R170–R172.

Manoach, D. S., Greve, D. N., Lindgren, K. A., & Dale, A. M. (2003). Identifying regional activity associated with temporally separated components of working memory using event related functional MRI. *NeuroImage, 20,* 1670–1684.

Marschner, A., Kalish, R., Vervliet, B., Vansteenwegen, D., & Buchel, C. (2008). Dissociable role for the hippocampus and the amygdala in human cued versus context conditioning. *Journal of Neuroscience, 28,* 9030–9036.

Marsden, C. D., & Obseso, J. A. (1994). The function of the basal ganglia and the paradox of stereotaxic surgery in Parkinson's disease. *Brain, 117,* 877–897.

Marten, K., & Psarakos, S. (1995). Evidence of self-awareness in the bottlenose dolphin (*Tursiops truncatus*). In S. T. Parker, R. W. Mitchell, & M. L. Boccia (Eds.), *Self-awareness in animals and humans* (pp. 361–379). New York: Cambridge University Press.

Martin, S. J., Grimwood, P. D., & Morris, R. G. M. (2000). Synaptic plasticity and memory: An evaluation of the hypothesis. *Annual Review of Neuroscience, 23,* 649–711.

Marx, M. H., & Hillix, W. A. (1963). *Systems and theories in psychology*. New York: McGraw-Hill.

Mashour, G. A. (2006). Monitoring consciousness: EEG-based measures of anesthetic depth. *Seminars in Anesthesia, Perioperative Medicine and Pain, 25,* 205–210.

Masserman, J. H. (1941). Is the hypothalamus a center of emotion? *Psychosomatic Medicine, 3,* 3–25.

Mather, J. A. (2008). Cephalopod consciousness: Behavioral evidence. *Consciousness and Cognition, 17,* 37–48.

Maunsell, J. H. R., & Newsome, W. T. (1987). Visual processing in monkey extrastriate cortex. *Annual Review of Neuroscience, 10,* 363–401.

McCabe, D. P., & Castel, A. D. (2008). Seeing is believing. *Cognition, 107,* 343–362.

McClure, S. M., Li, J., Tomlin, D., Cypert, K. S., Montague, L. M., & Montague, P. R. (2004). Neural correlates of behavioral preferences for culturally familiar drinks. *Neuron, 44,* 379–387.

McCormick, D., & Thompson, R. F. (1984). Cerebellum: Essential involvement in the classically conditioned eyelid response. *Science, 223,* 296–299.

McCulloch, W. S., & Pitts, W. H. (1943). A logical calculus of the ideas immanent in nervous activity. *Bulletin of Mathematical Biophysics, 5,* 115–133.

McCollough, C. (1965). Color adaptiation of edge detectors the human visual system. *Science, 149,* 1115–1116.

McDougall, W. (1926). *An introduction to social psychology.* Boston: Luce.

McGaugh, J. L. (2000). Memory—A century of consolidation. *Science, 287,* 248–251.

McGaugh, J. L. (2004). The amygdala modulates the consolidation of emotionally arousing experiences. *Annual Review of Neuroscience, 27,* 1–28.

McNaughton, N. (1997). Cognitive dysfunction resulting from hippocampal hyperactivity—a possible cause of anxiety disorder. *Pharmacology, Biochemistry, and Behavior, 56,* 603–611.

McRae, K., Ochsner, K. N., Mauss, I. B., Gabrieli, J. J. D., & Gross, J. J. (2008). Gender difference in emotion regulation: An fMRI study of cognitive reappraisal. *Group Processes & Intergroup Relations, 11,* 143–162.

Melcher, D. (2001). Persistence of visual memory for scenes. *Nature, 412,* 401.

Melrose, R. J., Poulin, R. M., & Stern, C. E. (2007). An fMRI investigation of the role of basal ganglia in reasoning. *Brain Research, 1142,* 146–158.

Mesulam, M.-M. (1981). A cortical network for directed attention and unilateral neglect. *Annals of Neurology, 10,* 309–325.

Meunier, M., Cirilli, L., & Bachevalier, J. (2006). Responses to affective stimuli in monkeys with entorhinal or perirhinal cortex lesions. *Journal of Neuroscience, 26,* 7718–7722.

Meyer, D. E., & Kieras, D. E. (1997). A computational theory of executive cognitive processes and multiple task performance: Part 1. Basic mechanisms. *Psychological Review, 104,* 3–65.

Miller, G. (1956). The magical number seven, plus or minus two: Some limits on our capacity for processing information. *Psychological Review, 63,* 81–97.

Miller, G. (2008a). The roots of morality. *Science, 320,* 734–737.

Miller, G. (2008b). Growing pains for fMRI. *Science, 320,* 1412–1414.

Miller, M. B., & Van Horn, J. D. (2007). Individual variability in brain activations associated with episodic retrieval: A role for large scale data bases. *International Journal of Psychophysiology, 63,* 205–213.

Miller, M. B., Van Horn, J. D., Wolford, G. L., Handy, T. C., Valsangkar-Smyth, M., Inati, S., et al. (2002). Extensive individual difference in brain activations associated with episodic retrieval are reliable over time. *Journal of Cognitive Neuroscience, 14,* 1200–1214.

Milner, B. (1963). Effects of different brain lesions on card sorting. *Archives of Neurology, 9,* 100–110.

Mishkin, M. (1954). Visual discrimination performance following partial ablations of the temporal lobe: II. Ventral surface versus the hippocampus. *Journal of Comparative and Physiological Psychology, 47,* 187–193.

Mishkin, M. (1982). A memory system in the monkey. *Philosophical Transactions of the Royal Society of London. Series B, Biological Sciences, 298,* 85–95.

Mishkin, M., & Pribram, K. H. (1954). Visual discrimination performance following partial ablations of the temporal lobe: I. Ventral versus lateral. *Journal of Comparative and Physiological Psychology, 47,* 14–20.

Mittal, S., & Black, P. M. (2006). Intraoperative magnetic resonance imaging in neurosurgery. *Acta Neurochirurgica, 98,* 77–86.

Miyawaki, Y., Uchida, H., Yamashita, O., Sato, M., Morito, Y., Tanabe, H. C., et al. (2008). Visual image reconstruction from human brain activity using a combination of multiscale local image decoders. *Neuron, 60,* 915–929.

Mollaret, P., & Goulon, M. (1959). Le coma depasse: Memoire preliminaire. *Revista de Neurologia, 101,* 3–15.

Monahan, J. S., & Lockhead, G. R. (1977). Identification of integral stimuli. *Journal of Experimental Psychology. General, 106,* 94–110.

Montague, P. R., & Berns, G. S. (2002). Neural economics and the biological substrates of valuation. *Neuron, 36,* 265–284.

Montaser-Kouhsari, L., Landy, M. S., Heeger, D. J., & Larsson, J. (2007). Orientation-selective adaptation to illusory contours in human visual cortex. *Journal of Neuroscience, 27,* 2186–2195.

Monti, M. M., Vanhaudenhuyse, A., Coleman, M. R., Boly, M., Pickard, J. D., Tshibanda, L., et al. (2010). Willful modulation of brain activity in disorders of consciousness. *New England Journal of Medicine, 362,* 579–589.

Moore, E. F. (1956). Gedanken-experiments on sequential machines. In C. E. Shannon & J. McCarthy (Eds.), *Automata studies* (pp. 129–153). Princeton, NJ: Princeton University Press.

Moran, J., & Desimone, R. (1985). Selective attention gates visual process in the extrastriate cortex. *Science, 229,* 782–784.

Moray, N. P. (1959). Attention in dichotic listening: Affective cues and the influence of instructions. *Quarterly Journal of Experimental Psychology, 11,* 56–60.

Morgan, C. L. (1894). *An introduction to comparative psychology.* London: Walter Scott, Limited.

Moruzzi, G., & Magoun, H. W. (1949). Brain stem reticular formation and activation of the EEG. *Electroencephalography and Clinical Neurophysiology, 1,* 455–473.

Muller, J. R., Philiastides, M. G., & Newsome, W. T. (2005). Microstimulation of the superior colliculus focus attention without moving the eyes. *Proceedings of the National Academies of Science of the United States of America, 102,* 524–529.

Mundy-Castle, A. C. (1958). Electrophysiological correlates of intelligence. *Journal of Personality, 26,* 184–199.

Murphy, E. R., Illes, J., & Reiner, P. B. (2008). Neuroethics of neuromarketing. *Journal of Consumer Behaviour, 7,* 293–302.

Murray, S. O., Boyaci, H., & Kersten, D. (2006). The representation of perceived angular size in human primary visual cortex. *Nature Neuroscience, 9,* 429–434.

Nadel, L., & Moscovitch, M. (1997). Memory consolidation, retrograde amnesia and the hippocampal complex. *Current Opinion in Neurobiology, 7,* 217–227.

Nagel, T. (1974). What is it like to be a bat. *Philosophical Review, 83,* 435–450.

Nakao, H. (1958). Emotional behavior produced by hypothalamic stimulation. *American Journal of Physiology, 194,* 411–418.

NAS. (2003). *The polygraph and lie detection: A report by the Committee to Review the Scientific Evidence on the Polygraph, National Research Council of the United States.* Washington, DC: National Academies Press.

Naselaris, T., Prenger, R. J., Kay, K. N., Oliver, M., & Gallant, J. L. (2009). Bayesian reconstruction of natural images from human brain activity. *Neuron, 63,* 902–915.

Neely, J. H. (1977). Semantic priming and retrieval from lexical memory: Role of spreading activation and limited-capacity attention. *Journal of Experimental Psychology. General, 106,* 226–254.

Neisser, U. (1967). *Cognitive psychology.* Englewood Cliffs, NJ: Prentice-Hall.

Neubauer, A. C., & Fink, A. (2009). Intelligence and neural efficiency. *Neuroscience and Biobehavioral Reviews, 33,* 1004–1023.

Neumann, J., Lohmann, G., Derrfuss, J., & von Cramon, D. Y. (2005). The meta-analysis of functional imaging data using replicator dynamics. *Human Brain Mapping, 25,* 165–173.

Newberg, A. B., Pourdehand, M., Alavi, A., & d'Aquili, E. G. (2003). Cortical blood flow during meditative prayer: Preliminary findings and methodological issues. *Perceptual and Motor Skills, 97,* 625–630.

Newman, S. (1999). The medial extended amygdala in male reproductive behavior. *Annals of the New York Academy of Sciences, 877,* 242–257.

Newman, S. D., Carpenter, P. A., Varma, S., & Just, M. A. (2003). Frontal and parietal participation in problem solving in the Tower of London: fMRI and computational modeling of planning and high level perception. *Neuropsychologia, 41,* 1668–1682.

Newman, S. D., Greco, J. A., & Lee, D. (2009). An fMRI study of the Tower of London: A look at problem structure differences. *Brain Research, 1286,* 123–132.

Newman, S. D., Keller, T. A., & Just, M. A. (2007). Volitional control of attention and brain activation in dual task performance. *Human Brain Mapping, 28,* 109–117.

Nickerson, R. S. (2000). Null hypothesis significance testing: A review of an old and continuing controversy. *Psychological Methods, 5,* 241–301.

Nisbett, R. E., & Wilson, T. D. (1977). Telling more than we can know: Verbal reports on mental processes. *Psychological Review, 84,* 231–259.

Norman, D. A. (1968). Toward a theory of memory and attention. *Psychological Review, 75,* 522–536.

NRC. (2009). *Opportunities in neuroscience for future army applications.* Washington, DC: The National Academies Press.

Nunnally, J. C. (1970). *Introduction to psychological measurement.* New York: McGraw Hill.

Oakley, B. (1985). Taste responses of human chorda tympani nerve. *Chemical Senses, 10,* 469–481.

Ochoa, J., & Torebjork, E. (1983). Sensations produced by intraneural microstimulation of single mechanoreceptors units innervating the human hand. *Journal of Physiology, 342,* 633–654.

O'Connor, D. H., Fukui, M. M., Pinsk, M. A., & Kastner, S. (2002). Attention modulates responses in the human lateral geniculate nucleus. *Nature Neuroscience, 5,* 1203–1208.

O'Doherty, J., Dayan, P., Schultz, J., Deichmann, R., Friston, K., & Dolan, R. J. (2004). Dissociable roles of ventral and dorsal striatum in instrumental conditioning. *Science, 304,* 452–454.

Ogawa, H., Wakita, M., Hasegawa, K., Kobayakawa, T., Sakai, N., Hirai, T., et al. (2005). Functional MRI detection of activation in the primary gustatory cortices in humans. *Chemical Senses, 30,* 583–592.

Ogawa, S., Lee, T. M., Kay, A. R., & Tank, D. W. (1990). Brain magnetic resonance imaging with contrast dependent on blood oxygenation. *Proceedings of the National Academies of Science of the United States of America, 87,* 9868–9872.

Ohlendorf, S., Kimmig, H., Glauche, V., & Haller, S. (2007). Gaze pursuit, "attention pursuit" and their effect on cortical activations. *European Journal of Neuroscience, 26,* 2096–2108.

O'Keefe, J., & Dostrovsky, J. (1971). The hippocampus as a spatial map: Preliminary evidence from unit activity in the freely-moving rat. *Brain Research, 34,* 171–175.

O'Keefe, J., & Nadel, L. (1978). *The hippocampus as a cognitive map.* Oxford: Oxford University Press.

Olbrich, S., Mulert, C., Karch, S., Trenner, M., Leicht, G., Pogarell, O., et al. (2009). EEG-vigilance and BOLD effect during simultaneous EEG /fMRI measurement. *NeuroImage, 45,* 319–332.

Olds, J., Disterhoft, J. F., Segal, M., Kornblith, C. L., & Hirsch, R. (1972). Learning centers of rat brain mapped by measuring latencies of conditioned unit responses. *Journal of Neurophysiology, 35,* 202–219.

Olds, J., & Milner, P. (1954). Positive reinforcement produced by electrical stimulation of septal area and other regions of rat brain. *Journal of Comparative and Physiological Psychology, 47,* 419–427.

Olds, M. E., & Olds, J. (1963). Approach-avoidance analysis of rat diencephalon. *Journal of Comparative Neurology, 120,* 259–295.

Olesen, M. D., Westerberg, H., & Klingberg, T. (2004). Increased prefrontal and parietal brain activity after training of working memory. *Nature Neuroscience, 7,* 75–79.

Olshausen, B. A., & Feld, D. J. (2004). Sparse coding of sensory inputs. *Current Opinion in Neurobiology*, *14*, 481–487.

Opitz, B., & Friederici, A. D. (2003). Interactions of the hippocampal system and the prefrontal cortex in learning language-like rules. *NeuroImage*, *19*, 1730–1737.

Orban, P., Peigneux, P., Lungu, O., Albouy, G., Breton, E., Laberenne, F., et al. (2010). The multifaceted nature of the relationship between performance and brain activity in motor sequence learning. *Neuro-Image*, *49*, 694–702.

Ortony, A., & Turner, T. J. (1990). What's basic about basic emotions? *Psychological Review*, *97*, 315–331.

Ostow, M. (1950). Psychic function and the electroencephalogram. *Archives of Neurology and Psychiatry*, *64*, 385–400.

Oswald, W. D., & Roth, E. (1974). Relationships between EEG and intelligence variables. *Psychologische Beiträge*, *16*, 1–47.

O'Toole, A. J., Jiang, F., Abdi, H., Penard, N., Dunlop, J. P., & Parent, M. A. (2007). Theoretical, statistical, and practical perspectives on pattern-based classification approaches to the analysis of functional neuroimaging data. *Journal of Cognitive Neuroscience*, *19*, 1735–1752.

Otten, L. J. (2007). Fragments of a larger whole: Retrieval cues constrain observed neural correlates of memory encoding. *Cerebral Cortex*, *17*, 2030–2038.

Owen, A. M., Coleman, M. R., Boly, M., Davis, M. H., Laureys, S., & Pickard, J. D. (2006). Detecting awareness in the vegetative state. *Science*, *313*, 1402.

Owen, A. M., Downes, J. D., Sahakian, B. J., Polkey, C. E., & Robbins, T. W. (1990). Planning and spatial working memory following frontal lobe lesions in man. *Neuropsychologia*, *28*, 1021–1034.

Panksepp, J. (1982). Toward a general psychobiological theory of emotions. *Behavioral and Brain Sciences*, *5*, 407–467.

Panksepp, J. (1998). *Affective neuroscience: The foundations of human and animal emotions*. Oxford: Oxford University Press.

Papez, J. W. (1937). A proposed mechanism of emotion. *Journal of Neuropsychiatry and Clinical Neurosciences*, *7*, 103–112.

Parker, S. T., Mitchell, R. W., & Boccia, M. L. (1994). *Self-awareness in animals and humans*. New York: Cambridge University Press.

Pashler, H. (1998). *The psychology of attention*. Cambridge, MA: MIT Press.

Patterson, F. (1984). Self-recognition by *Gorilla gorilla gorilla*. *Gorilla*, *7*, 2–3.

Pavlov, I. P. (1960). *Conditioned reflexes: An investigation of the physiological activity of the cerebral cortex* (Anrep, G. V., Trans.). New York: Dover. (Original work published 1927.)

Peachey, N. S., & Seiple, W. H. (1987). Contrast sensitivity of the human pattern electroretinogram. *Investigative Ophthalmology & Visual Science, 28*, 151–157.

Peden, C. J., Menon, D. K., Hall, A. S., Sargentoni, J., & Whitwam, J. G. (1992). Magnetic resonance for the anesthetist. *Anesthesia, 47*, 508–517.

Peirce, C. S., & Jastrow, J. (1884). On small differences of sensation. *Memoirs of the National Academy of Sciences, 3*, 73–81.

Penfield, W. (1933). Wesley M. Carpenter Lecture: Influence of the diencephalon and hypophysis upon general autonomic function. *Bulletin of the New York Academy of Medicine, 9*, 613–637.

Penfield, W., & Rasmussen, T. (1950). *The cerebral cortex of man.* Princeton, NJ: Princeton University Press.

Perenin, M. T., & Jeannerod, M. (1978). Visual function within the hemianopic field following early cerebral hemidecortication in man—I. Spatial localization. *Neuropsychologia, 16*, 1–13.

Peretti, C.-S., Ferreri, F., Blanchard, F., Bakchine, S., Peretti, C. R., Dobrescu, A., et al. (2008). Normal and pathological aging of attention in presymptomatic Huntington's, Huntington's and Alzheimer's disease, and non-demented elderly subjects. *Psychotherapy and Psychosomatics, 77*, 139–146.

Perlstein, W. M., Carter, C. S., Noll, D. C., & Cohen, J. D. (2001). Relation of prefrontal cortex dysfunction to working memory and symptoms in schizophrenia. *American Journal of Psychiatry, 158*, 1105–1113.

Perret, E. (1974). The left frontal lobe of man and the suppression of habitual responses in verbal categorical behavior. *Neuropsychologia, 12*, 323–330.

Persaud, N., McLeod, P., & Cowey, A. (2007). Post-decision wagering objectively measures awareness. *Nature Neuroscience, 10*, 257–261.

Pessoa, L., & Ungerleider, L. G. (2004). Neural correlates of change detection and change blindness in a working memory task. *Cerebral Cortex, 14*, 511–520.

Peterson, L. R., & Peterson, M. J. (1959). Short-term retention of individual verbal items. *Journal of Experimental Psychology, 58*, 193–198.

Pew, R. W. (1974). Human perceptual-motor performance. In B. H. Kantowitz (Ed.), *Human information processing: Tutorial in performance and cognition* (pp. 1–39). Hillsdale, NJ: Erlbaum.

Pfaffmann, C. (1941). Gustatory afferent impulses. *Journal of Cellular and Comparative Physiology, 17*, 243–261.

Pfaffmann, C. (1969). Taste preference and reinforcement. In J. Tapp (Ed.), *Reinforcement and behavior* (pp. 215–241. New York: Academic Press.

Pfingst, B. E. (1988). Comparisons of psychophysical and neurophysiological studies of cochlear implants. *Hearing Research, 34*, 243–251.

Phan, K. L., Wager, T. D., Taylor, S. F., & Liberzon, I. (2002). Functional neuroanatomy of emotion: A meta-analysis of emotion activation studies in PET and fMRI. *NeuroImage, 16,* 331–348.

Phelps, E. A. (2004). Human emotion and memory: Interactions of the amygdala and hippocampal complex. *Current Opinion in Neurobiology, 14,* 198–202.

Phelps, E. A. (2006). Emotion and cognition: Insights from studies of the human amygdala. *Annual Review of Psychology, 57,* 27–53.

Philiastides, M. G., & Sajda, P. (2006). Temporal characteristics of the neural correlates of perceptual decision making in the human brain. *Cerebral Cortex, 16,* 509–518.

Philiastides, M. G., & Sajda, P. (2007). EEG-informed fMRI reveals spatiotemporal characteristics of perceptual decision making. *Journal of Neuroscience, 27,* 13082–13091.

Phillips, R. G., & LeDoux, J. E. (1992). Differential contribution of amygdala and hippocampus to cued and contextual fear conditioning. *Behavioral Neuroscience, 106,* 274–285.

Pinker, S. (1997). *How the mind works.* New York: W. W. Norton & Company.

Pitts, W. H., & McCulloch, W. S. (1947). How we know universals: The perception of auditory and visual forms. *Bulletin of Mathematical Biophysics, 9,* 127–147.

Plaut, D. C., & McClelland, J. L. (2010). Locating object knowledge in the brain: Comment on Bowers' attempt to revive the grandmother cell hypothesis. *Psychological Review, 117,* 284–290.

Plutchik, R. (1991). *The emotions* (rev. ed.). Lanham, MD: University Press of America.

Plutchik, R. (1997). *Circumplex models of personality and emotions.* Washington, DC: American Psychological Association.

Poldrack, R. A. (2006). Can cognitive processes be inferred from neuroimaging data. *Trends in Cognitive Sciences, 10,* 59–63.

Poldrack, R. A., Desmond, J. E., Glover, G. H., & Gabrieli, J. D. E. (1998). The neural basis of visual skill learning: An fMRI study of mirror reading. *Cerebral Cortex, 8,* 1–10.

Poldrack, R. A., Halchenko, Y., & Hanson, S. J. (2009). Decoding the large-scale structure of brain function classifying mental states across individuals. *Psychological Science, 20,* 1364–1372.

Poldrack, R. A., Sabb, F. W., Foerde, K., Tom, S. M., Asarnow, R. F., Bookheimer, S. Y., et al. (2005). The neural correlates of motor skill automaticity. *Journal of Neuroscience, 25,* 5356–5364.

Poppel, E., Held, R., & Frost, D. (1973). Residual visual function in brain wounds involving the central visual pathways in man. *Nature, 243,* 295–296.

Posner, J., Russell, J. A., Gerber, A., Gorman, D., Colibazzi, T., Yu, S., et al. (2009). The neurophysiological basis of emotion: An fMRI study of the affective circumplex using emotion-denoting words. *Human Brain Mapping, 30,* 883–895.

Posner, M. I. (1978). *Chronometric explorations of mind.* Hillsdale, NJ: Erlbaum.

Posner, M. I. (1980). Orienting of attention. *Quarterly Journal of Experimental Psychology, 32*, 3–25.

Posner, M. I. (1988). Structures and functions of selective attention. In T. Boll & B. Bryant (Eds.), *Master lectures in clinical neuropsychology— Brain functions: Research, measurement and practice* (pp. 171–202). Washington, DC: American Psychological Association.

Posner, M. I. (2004a). The achievement of brain imaging: Past and future. In N. G. Kanwisher & J. Duncan (Eds.), *Attention and performance XX* (pp. 505–528). New York: Oxford University Press.

Posner, M. I. (Ed.). (2004b). *Cognitive neuroscience of attention*. New York: Guilford Press.

Posner, M. I. (1995). Attention in cognitive neuroscience: An overview. In M. S. Gazzaniga (Ed.), *The cognitive neurosciences* (pp. 615–624). Cambridge, MA: MIT Press.

Posner, M. I., & Fan, J. (2008). Attention as an organ system. In J. R. Pomerantz (Ed.), *Topics in integrative neuroscience: From cells to cognition* (pp. 31–61). Cambridge: Cambridge University Press.

Posner, M. I., & Petersen, S. E. (1990). The attentional system of the human brain. *Annual Review of Neuroscience, 13*, 25–42.

Posner, M. I., Petersen, S. E., Fox, P. T., & Raichle, M. E. (1988). Localization of cognitive operations in the human brain. *Science, 240*, 1627–1631.

Posner, M. I., & Raichle, M. E. (1994). *Images of the mind*. New York: Scientific American Library.

Posner, M. I., & Raichle, M. E. (1995). Precis of images of mind. *Behavioral and Brain Sciences, 18*, 327–339.

Posner, M. I., & Rothbart, M. K. (2007). Research on attention networks as a model for the integration of psychological science. *Annual Review of Psychology, 58*, 1–23.

Posner, M. I., Snyder, C. R., & Davidson, B. J. (1980). Attention and the detection of signals. *Journal of Experimental Psychology, 109*, 160–174.

Prahakaran, V., Smith, J. A. L., Desmond, J. E., Glover, G. H., & Gabrieli, J. D. E. (1997). Neural substrates of fluid reasoning: An fMRI study of neocortical activation during performance on the Raven's progressive matrices test. *Cognitive Psychology, 33*, 43–63.

Pribram, K. H. (1969). The neurophysiology of remembering. *Scientific American, 220*, 73–86.

Pribram, K. H., Nuwer, M., & Baron, R. J. (1974). The holographic hypothesis of memory structure in brain function and perception. In R. C. Atkinson, D. H. Krantz, R. C. Luce, & P. Suppes (Eds.), *Contemporary developments in mathematical psychology* (pp. 416–467). San Francisco: W. H. Freeman.

Puce, A., Allison, T., Bentin, S., Gore, J. C., & McCarthy, G. (1998). Temporal cortex activation in humans viewing eye and mouth movements. *Journal of Neuroscience, 18*, 2188–2199.

Rachile, M. E. (2006). The brain's (dark energy). *Science, 314*, 1249–1250.

Radio, S. J., Janelle, C. M., Barba, D. A., & Frehlich, S. G. (2001). Perceptual decision making for baseball pitch recognition using P300 latency and amplitude to index attentional processing. *Research Quarterly for Exercise and Sport, 72*, 22–31.

Rampil, I. J. (1998). A primer for EEG signal processing in anesthesia. *Anesthesiology, 89*, 980–1002.

Ranganathan, V. K., Siemionow, V., Liu, J. Z., Sahgal, V., & Yue, G. H. (2004). From mental power to muscle power—gaining strength by using the mind. *Neuropsychologia, 42*, 944–956.

Ranson, S. W. (1934). The hypothalamus: Its significance for visceral innervation and emotional expression. *Transaction of the College of Physicians of Philadelphia, 2*, 222–242.

Raven, J. C. (1936). *Mental tests used in genetic studies: The performance of related individuals on tests mainly educative and mainly reproductive.* Unpublished MSc dissertation. London: University of London.

Raz, A., Lieber, B., Soliman, F., Buhle, J., Posner, J., Peterson, B. S., et al. (2005). Ecological nuances in functional magnetic resonance imaging(fMRI): Psychological stressors, posture, and hydrostatics. *NeuroImage, 25*, 1–7.

Reber, A. S. (1967). Implicit learning of artificial grammars. *Journal of Verbal Learning and Verbal Behavior, 6*, 855–863.

Reber, P. J., Stark, C. E. L., & Squire, L. R. (1998). Cortical areas supporting category learning identified using functional MRI. *Proceedings of the National Academies of Sciences of the United States of America, 95*, 747–750.

Redcay, E., & Courchesne, E. (2005). When is the brain enlarged in autism? A meta-analysis of all brain size reports. *Biological Psychiatry, 58*, 1–9.

Regan, D. (1989). *Human brain electrophysiology: Evoked potentials and evoked magnetic fields in science and medicine.* New York: Elsevier.

Reiss, J. P., Campbell, D. W., Leslie, W. D., Paulus, M. P., Stroman, P. W., Polimeni, J. O., et al. (2005). The role of the striatum in implicit learning: A functional magnetic resonance imaging study. *Neuroreport, 16*, 1291–1295.

Rensink, R. A., O'Regan, J. K., & Clark, J. J. (1997). To see or not to see: The need for attention perceive changes in scenes. *Psychological Science, 8*, 368–373.

Revonsuo, A. (2001). Can functional brain imaging discover consciousness in the brain? *Journal of Consciousness Studies, 8*, 3–23.

Riganello, F., & Sannita, W. G. (2009). Residual brain processing in the vegetative state. *Journal of Psychophysiology, 23*, 18–26.

Rizzolatti, G., Fadiga, L., Fogassi, L., & Gallese, V. (1996). Premotor cortex and the recognition of motor actions. *Brain Research. Cognitive Brain Research, 3*, 131–141.

Robinson, D. L. (1993). The EEG and intelligence: An appraisal of methods and theories. *Personality and Individual Differences, 15*, 695–716.

Robinson, D. N., & Uttal, W. R. (1983). *Foundations of psychobiology.* New York: Macmillan.

Rodriguez, P. F., Aron, A. R., & Poldrack, R. A. (2006). Ventral-striatal/nucleus accumbens sensitivity to prediction errors during classification errors. *Human Brain Mapping, 27*, 306–313.

Rodriguez-Moreno, D., & Hirsch, J. (2009). The dynamics of deductive reasoning: An fMRI investigation. *Neuropsychologia, 47,* 949–961.

Roese, N. J., & Amir, E. (2009). Human-android interaction in the near and distant future. *Perspectives on Psychological Science, 4,* 429–434.

Romanes, G. J. (1883). *Animal intelligence.* New York: D. Appleton and Company.

Rosenthal, R. (1979). The "File Drawer Problem" and tolerance for null results. *Psychological Bulletin, 86,* 638–641.

Roskies, A. (2008). Neuroimaging and inferential distance. *Neuroethics, 1,* 19–30.

Rosner, B. S., & Goff, W. R. (1967). Electrical responses of the nervous system and subjective scales of intensity. In W. D. Neff (Ed.), *Contributions to sensory physiology* (vol. 2, pp. 169–221). New York: Academic Press.

Rossion, B., Caldara, R., Seghier, M., Schuller, A.-M., Lazeyras, F., & Mayer, E. (2003). A network of occipital-temporal face-sensitive areas besides the right middle fusiform gyrus is necessary for normal face processing. *Brain, 126,* 2381–2395.

Roth, B. (1961). The clinical and theoretical importance of EEG rhythms corresponding to lowered vigilance. *Electroencephalography and Clinical Neurophysiology, 13,* 395–399.

Rothstein, H. R., Sutton, A. J., & Borenstein, M. (2005). *Publication bias in meta-analysis.* Chichester: John Wiley & Sons.

Rozell, C. J., Johnson, D. H., Baraniuk, R. G., & Olshausen, B. A. (2008). Sparse coding via threshold and local competition in neural circuits. *Neural Computation, 20,* 2526–2563.

Ruben, J., Krause, T., Taskin, B., Blankenburg, F., Moosmann, M., & Villringer, A. (2006). Subarea-specific suppressive interaction in the BOLD responses to simultaneous finger stimulation in human primary somatosensory cortex: Evidence for increasing rostral-to-caudal convergence. *Cerebral Cortex, 16,* 819–826.

Ruff, C. C., Blankenburg, F., Bjoertomt, O., Bestmann, S., Freeman, E., Haynes, J.-D., et al. (2006). Concurrent TMS-fMRI and psychophysics reveal frontal influences on human retinotopic visual cortex. *Current Biology, 16,* 1479–1488.

Russell, J. A. (1980). A circumplex model of affect. *Journal of Personality and Social Psychology, 39,* 1161–1178.

Sabbagh, M. A., & Taylor, M. (2000). Neural correlates of theory-of-mind reasoning: An event-related potential study. *Psychological Science, 11,* 46–50.

Sakitt, B. (1972). Counting every quantum. *Journal of Physiology, 223,* 131–150.

Sakkalis, V., Zervakis, M., & Micheloyannis, S. (2006). Significant EEG features involved in mathematical reasoning: Evidence from wavelet analysis. *Brain Topography, 19,* 53–60.

Sanes, J. N., & Donoghue, J. P. (2000). Plasticity and primary motor cortex. *Annual Review of Neuroscience, 23,* 395–415.

Sarnrhein, J., von Stein, A., Rappelsberger, P., Petsche, H., Rauscher, F. H., & Shaw, G. L. (1997). Persistent patterns of brain activity: An EEG coherence study of the positive effect of music on spatio-temporal reasoning. *Neurological Research, 19,* 107–116.

SBU. (2008). *EEG-based monitoring of anesthetic depth* (Report Number 2008–02). Stockholm: Swedish Council on Health Technology Assessment.

Schacter, D. L., & Tulving, E. (1994). What are the memory systems of 1994? In D. L. Schacter & E. Tulving (Eds.), *Memory systems* (pp. 1–38). Cambridge, MA: MIT Press.

Schacter, S., & Singer, J. (1962). Cognitive, social, and psychological determinants of emotional states. *Psychological Review, 69,* 379–399.

Schall, U., Johnston, P., Lagopoulos, J., Juptner, M., Jentzen, W., Thienel, R., et al. (2003). Functional maps of Tower of London performance: A positron emission and functional magnetic resonance imaging study. *NeuroImage, 20,* 1154–1161.

Schatpour, P., Molholm, S., Javitt, D. C., & Foxe, J. J. (2006). Spatiotemporal dynamics of human object recognition processing: An integrated high-density electrical mapping and functional imaging study of "closure" processes. *NeuroImage, 29,* 605–618.

Schermer, M. (2008). A new phrenology? *Scientific American* (May 13), 47–48.

Schlinger, H. D. (2005). How the human got its mind: Debunking the last great myth in psychology. *Skeptic, 11,* 48–53.

Schmahmann, J. D. (1997). Rediscovery of an early concept. *International Review of Neurobiology, 41,* 3–27.

Schmahmann, J. D., & Sherman, J. C. (1997). Cerebellar cognitive affective syndrome. *International Review of Neurobiology, 41,* 433–44

Schmidt, E. A., Kineses, W. E., Schrauf, M., Haufe, S., Schubert, R., & Curio, G. (2007). *Assessing drivers' vigilance states during monotonous driving.* Paper presented at the Fourth International Driving Symposium on Human factors in Driver Assessment, Training, and Vehicle Design. Stevenson, WA, July 9–12.

Schmidt, H., Jogia, J., Fast, K., Christodoulou, T., Haldane, M., Kumari, V., et al. (2009). No gender differences in brain activations during the N-back task: An fMRI study in healthy individuals. *Human Brain Mapping, 30,* 3609–3615.

Schmidt, R. A. (1975). A schema theory of discrete motor skill learning. *Psychological Review, 82,* 225–260.

Scoville, W. B., & Milner, B. (1957). Lost of recent memory after bilateral hippocampal lesions. *Journal of Neurology, Neurosurgery, and Psychiatry, 20,* 11–21.

Searle, J. (1980). Minds, brains, and programs. *Behavioral and Brain Sciences, 3,* 415–457.

Sebel, P. S., Bowdle, T. A., Ghoneim, M. M., Rampil, I. J., Padilla, R. E., Gan, T. J., et al. (2004). The incidence of awareness during anesthesia: A multicenter United States study. *Anesthesia and Analgesia, 99,* 833–839.

Seger, C. A., & Cincotta, C. M. (2002). Striatal activity in concept learning. *Cognitive, Affective & Behavioral Neuroscience, 2,* 149–161.

Seghier, M., Dojat, M., Delon-Martyn, C., Rubin, C., Warnking, J., Segebarth, C., et al. (2000). Moving illusory contours activate primary visual cortex. *Cerebral Cortex, 10,* 665–670.

Seghier, M. L., & Vuilleumier, P. (2006). Review: Functional neuroimaging findings on the human perception of illusory contours. *Neuroscience and Biobehavioral Reviews, 30,* 595–612.

Seifritz, E., Di Salle, F., Esposito, F., Herdener, M., Neuhoff, J. G., & Scheffler, K. (2006). Enhancing BOLD response in the auditory system by neurophysiologically tuned fMRI sequence. *NeuroImage, 29,* 1013–1022.

Semon, R. W. (1921). *The mneme.* London: George Allen & Unwin.

Senior, C., Smyth, H., Cooke, R., Shaw, R. L., & Peel, E. (2007). Mapping the mind for the modern market researcher. *Qualitative Market Research: An International Journal, 10,* 153–167.

Seth, A. K., Baars, B. J., & Edelman, D. B. (2005). Criteria for consciousness in humans and other mammals. *Consciousness and Cognition, 14,* 119–139.

Seth, A. K., Dienes, Z., Cleeremans, A., Overgaard, M., & Pessoa, L. (2008). Measuring consciousness: relating behavioral and neurophysiological approaches. *Trends in Cognitive Sciences, 12,* 314–321.

Settlage, P. H. (1939). The effect of occipital lesions on visually-guided behavior in the monkey: I. Influence of the lesions on final capacities in a variety of problem situations. *Journal of Comparative Psychology, 27,* 93–131.

Shaw, G. L., & Bodner, M. (1999). Music enhances spatio-temporal reasoning: Towards a neurophysiological basis using EEG. *EEG and Clinical Neurophysiology, 30,* 151–155.

Sheehan, T. P., Chambers, R. A., & Russell, D. S. (2004). Regulation of affect by the lateral septum: Implications for neuropsychiatry. *Brain Research. Brain Research Reviews, 46,* 71–117.

Shenton, M. E., Dickey, C. C., Frumin, M., & McCarley, R. W. (2001). A review of MRI findings in schizophrenia. *Schizophrenia Research, 49,* 1–52.

Shepard, R. N. (1964a). Attention and the metric structure of the stimulus space. *Journal of Mathematical Psychology, 1,* 54–87.

Shepard, R. N. (1964b). Circularity in judgments of relative pitch. *Journal of the Acoustical Society of America, 36,* 2346–2353.

Sherrington, C. S. (1963). *Man on His Nature.* Cambridge: Cambridge University Press. (Original work published 1940.)

Shiffrin, R. M. (1977). Controlled and automatic human information processing: II. Perceptual learning, automatic attending, and a general theory. *Psychological Review, 84,* 1–66.

Shinkareva, S. V., Mason, R. A., Malave, V. L., Wang, W., Mitchell, T. M., & Just, M. A. (2008). Using fMRI brain activation to identify cognitive states associated with perception of tools and dwellings. *PLoS ONE, 1,* 1–9.

Shurrager, P. S., & Culler, E. (1940). Conditioning in the spinal dog. *Journal of Experimental Psychology*, *26*, 133–159.

Siegel, A., & Flynn, J. P. (1968). Differential effects of electrical stimulation and lesions of the hippocampus and adjacent regions upon attack behavior in cats. *Brain Research*, *7*, 252–267.

Sieving, P. A., & Nino, C. (1988). Scotopic threshold response (STR) of the human electroretinogram. *Investigative Ophthalmology*, *29*, 1608–1614.

Simoncelli, E. P., & Olshausen, B. A. (2001). Natural image statistics and neural representation. *Annual Review of Neuroscience*, *24*, 1193–1216.

Simons, D. J., & Levin, D. T. (1997). Change blindness. *Trends in Cognitive Sciences*, *1*, 261–267.

Simons, J. S., & Spiers, H. J. (2003). Prefrontal and medial temporal lobe interactions in long term memory. *Nature Reviews. Neuroscience*, *4*, 637–648.

Sininger, Y. S., Abadala, C., & Cone-Wesson, B. (1997). Auditory threshold sensitivity of the human neonate as measured by the auditory brainstem response. *Hearing Research*, *104*, 27–38.

Sirotin, Y. B., & Das, A. (2009). Anticipatory haemodynamic signals in sensory cortex not predicted by local neuronal activity. *Nature*, *457*, 475–480.

Skinner, B. F. (1938). *Behavior of organisms*. New York: Appleton-Century.

Smidts, A. (2002). *Kijken in het brein: Over de mogelijkheden van neuromarketing [Brain imaging: Opportunities for neuromarketing]*. Paper presented at the Inaugural Address Rotterdam School of Management, Rotterdam, ERIM-12-MKT.

Smith, C., & Squire, L. R. (2009). Medial temporal lobe activity during the retrieval of semantic memory is related to the age of the memory. *Journal of Neuroscience*, *29*, 930–938.

Smith, E. C. (2006). *Efficient auditory coding* (Unpublished doctoral dissertation), Carnegie Mellon University, Pittsburgh, PA.

Smith, E. C., & Lewicki, M. S. (2006). Efficient auditory coding. *Nature*, *439*, 978–982.

Smith, S. M., Brown, H. O., Toman, J. E. P., & Godman, L. S. (1947). The lack of cerebral effects of D-Tubocurarine. *Anesthesiology*, *8*, 1–14.

Solomon, R. C. (2008). Philosophy of emotions (3rd Edition). In M. Lewis & J. M. Haviland-Jones (Eds.), *Handbook of emotions* (3rd ed., pp. 3–16). New York: Guilford Press.

Somers, D. C., Dale, A. M., Seiffert, A. E., & Tootell, R. B. H. (1999). Functional MRI reveals spatially specific attentional modulation in human primary visual cortex. *Proceedings of the National Academy of Sciences of the United States of America*, *96*, 1663–1668.

Sparks, D. L. (1999). Conceptual issues related to the role of the superior colliculus in the control of gaze. *Current Opinion in Neurobiology*, *9*, 698–707.

Spearman, C. (1904). "General intelligence," objectively determined and measured. *American Journal of Psychology*, *15*, 201–293.

Sperling, G. (1960). The information available in brief visual presentations. *Psychological Monographs, 74*, 1–29.

Spiegel, J. M., Miller, H. R., & Oppenheimer, M. J. (1930). Forebrain and rage reactions. *Journal of Neurophysiology, 3*, 538–548.

Spillmann, L. (1994). The Hermann grid illusion: A tool for studying human perceptive field organization. *Perception, 23*, 691–708.

Spillmann, L. (2009). Phenomenology and neurophysiology correlations: Two approaches to perception research. *Vision Research, 49*, 1507–1521.

Spillmann, L., & Ehrenstein, W. H. (1996). From neuron to gestalt: Mechanisms of visual perception. In R. Greger & U. Windhorst (Eds.), *Comprehensive human physiology* (pp. 861–893). Berlin: Springer-Verlag.

Spydell, J. D., & Sheer, D. E. (1982). Effect of problem solving on right and left hemisphere 40 Hertz EEG activity. *Psychophysiology, 19*, 420–425.

Squire, L. R. (1992). Memory and the hippocampus: A synthesis from findings with rats, monkeys, and humans. *Psychological Review, 99*, 195–231.

Squire, L. R., & Knowlton, B. J. (1995). Memory, hippocampus, and brain systems. In M. S. Gazzaniga (Ed.), *The cognitive neurosciences* (pp. 825–838). Cambridge, MA: MIT Press.

Squire, L. R., Stark, C. E. L., & Clark, R. E. (2004). The medial temporal lobe. *Annual Review of Neuroscience, 27*, 279–306.

Stam, C. J. (2005). Nonlinear dynamical analysis of EEG and MEG: Review of an emerging field. *Clinical Neurophysiology, 116*, 2266–2301.

Stanfield, A. C., McIntosh, A. M., Spencer, M. D., Phillip, R., Faur, S., & Lawrie, S. M. (2008). Towards a neuroanatomy of autism: A systematic review and meat-analysis of structural magnetic resonance imaging studies. *European Psychiatry, 23*, 289–299.

Stark, C. E. L., & Squire, L. R. (2000). Functional magnetic resonance imaging (fMRI) activity in the hippocampal region during recognition memory. *Journal of Neuroscience, 20*, 7776–7781.

Stark, C. E. L., & Squire, L. R. (2001). When zero is not zero: The problem of ambiguous baseline conditions in fMRI. *Proceedings of the National Academy of Sciences of the United States of America, 98*, 12760–12766.

Stearns, P. N. (2000). History of emotions: Issues of change and impact. In M. Lewis & J. M. Haviland-Jones (Eds.), *Handbook of emotions* (pp. 17–29). New York: Guilford Press.

Steffens, B. (2006). *Ibn al-Haytham: First scientist.* Greensboro, NC: Morgan Reynolds Publishing.

Stein, B. E., & Meredith, M. A. (1993). *The merging of the senses.* Cambridge, MA: MIT Press.

Stelmack, R. M., Knott, V., & Beauchamp, C. M. (2003). Intelligence and neural transmission time: A brain stem auditory evoked potential analysis. *Personality and Individual Differences, 34*, 97–107.

Sterman, M. B., & Mann, C. A. (1995). Concepts and applications of EEG analysis in aviation performance evaluation. *Biological Psychology, 40,* 115–130.

Sternberg, R. J. (1985). *Beyond IQ: A triarchic theory of human intelligence.* New York: Cambridge University Press.

Stevens, S. S. (Ed.). (1951a). *Handbook of experimental psychology.* New York: John Wiley & Sons.

Stevens, S. S. (1951b). Mathematics, measurement, and psychophysics. In S. S. Stevens (Ed.), *Handbook of experimental psychology* (pp. 1–49). New York: John Wiley & Sons.

Stewart, D. (2001). *The works of Dugald Stewart* (Vol. III). Charleston, SC: BookSurge Publishing. (Original work published 1829.)

Stiers, P., Peeters, R., Lagae, L., Van Hecker, P., & Sunaert, S. (2006). Mapping multiple visual areas in the human brain with a short fMRI sequence. *NeuroImage, 29,* 74–89.

Stoodley, C. J., Hill, P. R., Stein, J. F., & Bishop, D. V. M. (2006). Auditory event-related potentials differ in dyslexic even when auditory psychophysical performance is normal. *Brain Research, 140,* 190–199.

Strange, B. A., Fletcher, P. C., Henson, R. N. A., Friston, K. J., & Dolan, R. J. (1999). Segregating the functions of human hippocampus. *Proceedings of the National Academies of Sciences of the United States of America, 96,* 4034–4039.

Stroop, J. R. (1935). Studies of interference in serial verbal reactions. *Journal of Experimental Psychology, 18,* 643–662.

Stuss, D. T., & Benson, D. F. (1986). *The frontal lobes.* New York: Raven Press.

Stuss, D. T., & Levine, B. (2002). Adult clinical neuropsychology: Lessons from studies of the frontal lobes. *Annual Review of Psychology, 53,* 401–433.

Suddendorf, T., & Collier-Baker, E. (2009). The evolution of primate visual self-recognition: Evidence of absence in lesser apes. *Proceedings. Biological Sciences, 276,* 1671–1677.

Summerfield, C., Egner, T., Greene, M., Koechlin, E., Mangels, J., & Hirsch, J. (2006). Predictive codes for forthcoming perception in the frontal cortex. *Science, 314,* 1311–1314.

Sutton, B. P., Goh, J., Hebrank, A., Welsh, R. C., Chee, M. W. L., & Park, D. C. (2008). Investigation and validation of intersite fMRI studies using the same imaging hardware. *Journal of Magnetic Resonance Imaging, 28,* 21–28.

Swazy, J. P. (1970). Action prepare and action commune: The localization of cerebral function. *Journal of the History of Biology, 3,* 213–234.

Sylvester, C.-C., Wager, T. D., Lacey, S. C., Hernandez, L. L., Nichols, T. E., Smith, E. E., et al. (2003). Switching attention and resolving interference: fMRI measures of executive functions. *Neuropsychologia, 41,* 357–370.

Talairach, J., & Tournoux, P. (1988). *Co-planar stereotaxic atlas of the human brain: 3-Dimensional proportional system—An approach to cerebral imaging.* New York: Thieme Medical Publishers.

Tateno, A., Jorge, R. E., & Robinson, R. G. (2003). Clinical correlates of aggressive behavior after traumatic brain injury. *Journal of Neuropsychiatry and Clinical Neurosciences, 15*, 155–160.

Teasdale, G., & Jennett, B. (1974). Assessment of coma and impaired consciousness: A practical scale. *Lancet, 2*, 81–84.

Thatcher, R. W., & John, E. R. (1977). *Foundations of cognitive processes.* Hillsdale, NJ: Erlbaum.

Thirion, B., Duchesney, E., Hubard, E., Dubois, J., Poline, J.-B., Lebihan, D., et al. (2006). Inverse retinotopy: Inferring the visual content of images from brain activation patterns. *NeuroImage, 33*, 1104–1116.

Thompson, R. F. (2005). In search of memory traces. *Annual Review of Psychology, 56*, 1–23.

Thompson, R. F., & Kim, J. K. (1996). Memory systems in the brain and localization of a memory. *Proceedings of the National Academies of Sciences of the United States of America, 93*, 13438–13444.

Thompson, T. (2007). *Making sense of autism.* Baltimore: Paul A. Brookes Publishing Co.

Thompson, T. (2008). *Functional analysis of behavior and neuroscience.* Paper presented at the 10th Biannual Symposium on the Silence of Behavior, Guadalajara, Mexico.

Thorndike, E. L. (1898). *Animal intelligence: An experimental study of the associative processes in animals.* New York: Macmillan.

Thorndike, E. L. (1931). *Human learning.* New York: Century.

Thornton, C., & Sharp, R. M. (1998). Evoked responses in anaesthesia. *British Journal of Anaesthesia, 81*, 771–781.

Thurstone, L. L. (1938). *Primary mental abilities.* Chicago: University of Chicago Press.

Toni, I., Krams, M., Turner, R., & Passingham, R. E. (1998). The time course of changes in during motor sequence learning: A whole-brain fMRI study. *NeuroImage, 8*, 50–61.

Tow, P. M., & Whitty, C. W. M. (1953). Personality changes after operations of the cingulate cortex in man. *Journal of Neurology, Neurosurgery, and Psychiatry, 16*, 186–193.

Treisman, A. (1960). Contextual cues in selective listening. *Quarterly Journal of Experimental Psychology, 12*, 242–248.

Treisman, A., & Geffen, G. (1967). Selective attention: Perception or response? *Quarterly Journal of Experimental Psychology, 19*, 1–17.

Treisman, A., & Gelade, G. (1980). A feature integration theory of attention. *Cognitive Psychology, 12*, 97–136.

Trovillo, P. V. (1939a). A history of lie detection. *Journal of Criminal Law and Criminology, 29*, 848–881.

Trovillo, P. V. (1939b). A history of lie detection (Continued from the previous issue). *Journal of Criminal Law and Criminology, 30*, 104–119.

Tufte, E. R. (2001). *The visual display of quantitative information* (2nd ed.). Cheshire, CT: Graphics Press.

Tulving, E. (1972). Episodic and semantic memory. In E. Tulving & W. Donaldson (Eds.), *Organization of memory* (pp. 381–403). New York: Academic Press.

Tunturi, A. R. (1952). A difference in the representation of auditory signals for the left and right ears in the iso-frequency contours of right middle ectosylvian auditory cortex of the dog. *American Journal of Physiology, 168,* 712–727.

Turella, L., Peierno, A. C., Tubaldi, F., & Castiello, U. (2009). Mirror neurons in humans: Consisting or confounding evidence? *Brain and Language, 108,* 10–21.

Turing, A. (1950). Computing machinery and intelligence. *Mind, 59,* 433–460.

Turkeltaub, P. E., Eden, G. F., Jones, K. M., & Zeffiro, T. A. (2002). Meta-analysis of the functional neuroanatomy of single word reading; methodology and validation. *NeuroImage, 16,* 765–780.

Tyndall, J. (1897). *Fragment of science* (Vol. 2, p. 87). New York: Appleton & Company.

Umiltà, M., Kohler, E., Gallese, V., Fogassi, L., Fadiga, L., Keysers, C., et al. (2001). I know what you are doing: A neurophysiological study. *Neuron, 31,* 155–165.

Uncapher, M. R., & Wagner, A. D. (2009). Posterior parietal cortex and episodic encoding: Insights from fMRI subsequent memory effects and dual-attention theory. *Neurobiology of Learning and Memory, 91,* 139–154.

Ungerleider, L. G., Doyon, J., & Karni, A. (2002). Imaging brain plasticity during motor skill learning. *Neurobiology of Learning and Memory, 78,* 553–564.

Urban, B. W. (2002). Current assessment of target and theories of anaesthesia. *British Journal of Anaesthesia, 89,* 167–183.

Uttal, W. R. (1959). A comparison of neural and psychophysical responses in the somesthetic system. *Journal of Comparative and Physiological Psychology, 52,* 485–490.

Uttal, W. R. (1960a). The three stimulus problem: A further comparison of neural and psychophysical responses in the somesthetic system. *Journal of Comparative and Physiological Psychology, 53,* 42–46.

Uttal, W. R. (1960b). Inhibitory interaction of responses to electrical stimuli in the fingers. *Journal of Comparative and Physiological Psychology, 53,* 47–51.

Uttal, W. R. (1967). Evoked brain potentials: Signs or codes? *Perspectives in Biology and Medicine, 10,* 627–639.

Uttal, W. R. (1973). *The psychobiology of sensory coding.* New York: Harper & Row.

Uttal, W. R. (1975). *An autocorrelation theory of form detection.* Hillsdale, NJ: Erlbaum.

Uttal, W. R. (1981). *A taxonomy of visual processes.* Hillsdale, NJ: Erlbaum.

Uttal, W. R. (2000). *The war between mentalism and behaviorism: On the accessibility of mental processes.* Mahwah, NJ: Erlbaum.

Uttal, W. R. (2001). *The new phrenology: The limits of localizing cognitive processes in the brain.* Cambridge, MA: MIT Press.

Uttal, W. R. (2004). *Dualism: The original sin of cognitivism.* Mahwah, NJ: Erlbaum.

Uttal, W. R. (2005). *Neural theories of mind: Why the mind-brain problem may never be solved.* Mahwah, NJ: Erlbaum.

Uttal, W. R. (2007). *The immeasurable mind: The real science of psychology.* Amherst, NY: Prometheus Books.

Uttal, W. R. (2008). *Time, space, and number in physics and psychology.* Cornwall-on-Hudson, NY: Sloan.

Uttal, W. R. (2009a). *Distributed neural systems: Beyond the new phrenology.* Cornwall-on Hudson, NY: Sloan.

Uttal, W. R. (2009b). *Neuroscience in the courtroom: What every lawyer should know about the mind and the brain.* Tucson: Lawyers and Judges.

Uttal, W. R., & Cook, L. (1964). Systematics of the evoked somatosensory cortical potential: A psycho-physical-electrophysiological comparison. *Annals of the New York Academy of Sciences, 112,* 60–80.

Valenstein, E. S. (1986). *Great and desperate cures: The rise and decline of psychosurgery and other radical treatments for mental illness.* New York: Basic Books.

Van Essen, D. C., Anderson, C. H., & Felleman, D. J. (1992). Information processing in the primate visual system: An integrated systems perspective. *Science, 255,* 419–423.

Van Horn, J. D., & Poldrack, R. A. (2009). Functional MRI at the crossroads. *International Journal of Psychophysiology, 73,* 3–9.

Van Norman, G. A. (1999). A matter of life and death: What every anesthesiologist should know about the medical, legal, and ethical aspects of declaring brain death. *Anesthesiology, 91,* 275–287.

Van Orden, G. C., & Paap, K. R. (1997). Functional neuroimages fail to discover pieces of the mind in parts of the brain. *Philosophy of Science, 64,* S85–S94.

Vimal, R. L. P. (2009). Meanings attributed to the term "consciousness." *Journal of Consciousness Studies, 16,* 9–27.

Vogel, W., & Broverman, D. M. (1964). Relationships between EEG and test intelligence: A critical review. *Psychological Bulletin, 62,* 132–144.

Vogel, W., & Broverman, D. M. (1966). A reply to "Relationship between EEG and test intelligence: A commentary." *Psychological Bulletin, 65,* 99–109.

Vogt, B. A., Finch, D. M., & Olson, C. R. (1992). Functional heterogeneity in cingulate cortex: The anterior executive and the posterior evaluative regions. *Cerebral Cortex, 2,* 435–443.

Vuilleumier, P., Armony, J. L., Driver, J., & Dolan, R. J. (2001). Effects of attention and emotion on face processing in the human brain: An event-related fMRI study. *Neuron, 30,* 829–841.

Vul, E., Harris, C., Winkeilman, P., & Pashler, H. (2009). Puzzlingly high correlations in fMRI studies of emotion, personality, and social cognition. *Perspectives on Psychological Science, 4*, 274–290.

Vul, E., & Kanwisher, N. (2010). Begging the question: The nonindependence error in fMRI data analysis. In S. J. Hanson & M. Bunzl (Eds.), *Foundational issues for human brain mapping* (pp. 71–91). Cambridge, MA: MIT Press.

Wager, T. D., & Smith, E. E. (2003). Neuroimaging studies of working memory: A meta-analysis. *Cognitive, Affective & Behavioral Neuroscience, 3*, 255–274.

Wagner, A. D., Maril, A., Bjork, R. A., & Schacter, D. L. (2001). Prefrontal contributions to executive control: fMRI evidence for functional distinctions within lateral prefrontal cortex. *NeuroImage, 14*, 1337–1347.

Waiter, G. D., Deary, I. J., Staff, R. T., Murray, A. D., Fox, H. C., Starr, J. M., et al. (2009). Exploring possible neural mechanisms of intelligence differences using processing seed and working memory tasks: An fMRI study. *Intelligence, 37*, 199–206.

Wandell, B. A., Brewer, A. A., & Dougherty, R. F. (2005). Visual field map clusters in human cortex. *Philosophical Transactions of the Royal Society B, 360*, 693–707.

Ward, J. (1887). Psychological principles III.Attention and the fields of consciousness. *Mind, 12*, 45–67.

Warren, J. F., & Griffiths, T. D. (2003). Distinct mechanisms for processing spatial sequences and pitch sequences in the human auditory brain. *Journal of Neuroscience, 23*, 5799–5804.

Weidner, R., & Fink, G. R. (2007). The neural mechanisms underlying the Muller-Lyer illusion and its interaction with visuospatial judgments. *Cerebral Cortex, 17*, 878–884.

Weisberg, D. S., Keil, F. C., Goodstein, J., Rawsdon, E., & Gray, J. R. (2008). The seductive allure of neuroscience explanations. *Journal of Cognitive Neuroscience, 20*, 470–477.

Weiskrantz, L. (1956). Behavioral changes associated with ablation of the amygdaloid complex in monkeys. *Journal of Comparative and Physiological Psychology, 49*, 381–391.

Weiss, E. M., Siedentopf, C. M., Golaszewski, S., Mottaghy, F. M., Hofer, A., Kremser, C., et al. (2007). Brain activation patterns during a selective attention test—a functional MRI study in healthy volunteers and unmedicated patients during an acute episode of schizophrenia. *Psychiatry Research: Neuroimaging, 154*, 31–40.

Weissman, D. H., Roberts, K. C., Visscher, K. M., & Woldorff, M. G. (2006). The neural basis of momentary lapses in attention. *Nature Neuroscience, 9*, 971–978.

Wendelken, C., Nakhabenko, D., Donohue, S. E., Carter, C. S., & Bunge, S. A. (2008). "Brain is to thought as stomach is to??": Investigating the role of the rosterolateral prefrontal cortex in relational reasoning. *Journal of Cognitive Neuroscience, 20*, 682–693.

Werner, L. A., Folsom, R. C., Manci, L. R., & Syapin, C. L. (2001). Human auditory brainstem response to temporal gaps in noise. *Journal of Speech, Language, and Hearing Research: JSLHR, 44*, 737–750.

Wertheimer, P. M., Jouvet, M., & Descites, J. (1959). Diagnosis of death of the nervous system in comas with respiratory arrest treated by artificial respiration [article in French]. *La Presse Médicale, 67*, 87–88.

Wickelgren, W. A. (1979). *Cognitive psychology*. Englewood Cliffs, NJ: Prentice-Hall.

Wilkinson, F., James, T. W., Wilson, H. R., Gati, J. S., Menon, R. S., & Goodale, M. A. (2000). An fMRI study of the selective activation of human extrastriate form vision areas by radial and concentric gratings. *Current Biology, 10*, 1455–1458.

Williams, R. W., & Herrup, K. (1988). The control of neuron number. *Annual Review of Neuroscience, 11*, 423–453.

Willingham, D. B. (1998). A neuropsychological theory of motor skill learning. *Psychological Review, 105*, 558–584.

Wojciulik, E., & Kanwisher, N. G. (1999). The generality of parietal involvement in visual attention. *Neuron, 23*, 747–764.

Womelsdorf, T., Anton-Erxleben, K., Pieper, F., & Treue, S. (2006). Dynamic shifts of visual receptive fields in cortical area MT by spatial attention. *Nature Neuroscience, 9*, 1156–1160.

Woodworth, R. S., & Sherrington, C. S. (1904). Pseudoaffective reflex and its spinal path. *Journal of Physiology, 31*, 234–243.

Woolsey, C. N. (1961). Organization of the cortical auditory system. In W. A. Rosenblith (Ed.), *Sensory communication* (pp. 235–258). Cambridge, MA: MIT Press.

Wurtz, R. H., & Goldberg, M. E. (1972). The primate superior colliculus and the shift of visual attention. *Investigative Ophthalmology, 11*, 441–450.

Yantis, S., & Johnston, J. C. (1990). On the locus of visual attention: Evidence from focused attention tasks. *Journal of Experimental Psychology. Human Perception and Performance, 16*, 135–149.

Yantis, S., & Serences, J. T. (2003). Cortical mechanisms of space-based and object-based attentional control. *Current Opinion in Neurobiology, 13*, 187–193.

Yarkoni, T. (2009). Big correlations in little studies: Inflated fMRI correlations reflect statistical power—Commentary on Vul et al. (2009). *Perspectives on Psychological Science, 4*, 294–298.

Zedkova, L., Woodward, N. D., Harding, I., Tibbo, P. G., & Purdon, S. D. (2006). Procedural learning in schizophrenia investigated with functional magnetic imaging. *Schizophrenia Research, 88*, 198–207.

Zeineh, M. M., Engel, S. A., Thompson, P. M., & Bookheimer, S. Y. (2003). Dynamics of the hippocampus during encoding and retrieval of face-name pairs. *Science, 299*, 577–580.

Name Index

Subject Index

Accessibility
  arguments for, 15–18
  high-level cognitive skills and, 269, 276
  inaccessibility and, 9, 13–19, 141, 185, 267,
    269–270, 274, 283, 323, 349
  sensation and, 79–82
Acoustic nerve, 53, 64–65, 84–85, 209, 320
Action understanding, 130–136, 391n20
Adenosine monophosphate (AMP), xv
Adrenocorticotropic hormone (ACTH), xv
Affect
  defining, 141–142
  emotion and, 141–142, 160, 167, 169,
    174
  qualia and, 142
Aggression
  emotion studies and, 151–152, 155–156,
    158–159, 171–173, 175, 393n22
  learning and, 203
  regions involved in, 172–173
Agitation, 141, 391n1
Agnosias, 121–122, 390n16, 395n14
Alerting, 231, 256–257
Alertness, 251, 322–328, 361, 399n19, 403n6
Alpha rhythm, 403n6
  high-level cognitive skills and, 290–292,
    305
  skill proficiency and, 331–332
  sleep and, 325–328
Amygdala
  applications and, 342, 345
  centromedial group and, 164

emotion and, 152–155, 158–167, 170, 172,
  392n14
laterobasal group and, 164
learning and, 199–201, 204–205, 209, 213, 215,
  220, 224, 227, 397n26
perception and, 117
superficial group and, 164
Anesthesia
  applications and, 316–323
  biomarkers for, 316–317, 320–321
  cocaine and, 316
  consciousness and, 1, 277, 280, 285, 316–323,
    361, 395n13, 400n4
  electroencephalographs (EEGs) and, 317–320,
    361
  functional magnetic resonance imaging (fMRI)
    and, 321–322
  improved surgical techniques and, 317
  nitrous oxide and, 316
  opium and, 316
  physiological measurements and, 317
Anger, 143, 165, 171, 392n13
*Animal Intelligence: An Experimental Study of the
  Associative Process in Animals* (Thorndike),
  185
Anterior cingulate gyrus, 256
Anterior inferotemporal cortex (AIT), 121–122
Anterior superior insula, 166
Anterior thalamus, 156
Antipsychotic drugs, xiv
Apes, 280
Aplysia californica, 178, 198